EPILEPSY

This book is dedicated to the memory of

Lennart Gram MD

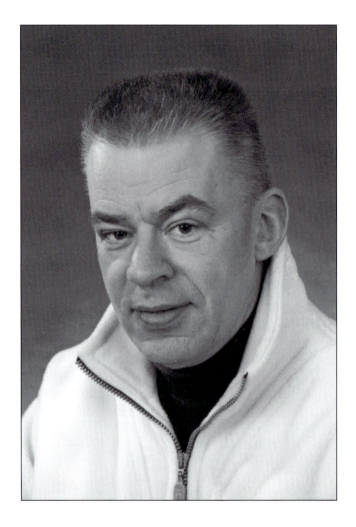

EPILEPSY
Problem Solving in Clinical Practice

Edited by

Dieter Schmidt MD
Emeritus Professor of Neurology
Epilepsy Research Group
Berlin
Germany

Steven C Schachter MD
Medical Director
Office of Clinical Trials and Research
Director of Clinical Research
Comprehensive Epilepsy Center
Beth Israel Deaconess Medical Center, and
Associate Professor of Neurology
Harvard Medical School
Boston, MA
USA

MARTIN DUNITZ

© Martin Dunitz Ltd 2000

First published in the United Kingdom in 2000 by
Martin Dunitz Ltd
The Livery House
7–9 Pratt Street
London NW1 0AE

Tel: +44 (0)207 482 2202
Fax: +44 (0)207 267 0159
E-mail: info@mdunitz.globalnet.co.uk
Website: http://www.dunitz.co.uk

A CIP catalogue record for this book is available
from the British Library

ISBN 1-85317-504-8

Distributed in the United States by:
Blackwell Science Inc.
Commerce Place, 350 Main Street
Malden MA 02148, USA
Tel: 1 800 215 1000

Distributed in Canada by:
Login Brothers Book Company
324 Salteaux Crescent
Winnipeg, Manitoba R3J 3T2
Canada
Tel: 1 204 224 4068

Distributed in Brazil by:
Ernesto Reichmann Distribuidora de Livros, Ltda
Rua Coronel Marques 335
03440-000 São Paulo-SP
Brazil

Composition by Scribe Design, Gillingham, Kent
Printed and bound in Great Britain by Biddles Ltd,
Guildford and King's Lynn

CONTENTS

VIII Childhood epilepsy

IX Prognosis of epilepsy

X Supplemental non-antiepileptic drug therapy

XI The team approach to the treatment of epilepsy

List of contributors

Albert P Aldenkamp MD
Head, Department of Behavioral Science
and Psychological Services, Epilepsiecentrum
Kempenhaeghe, PO Box 61, 5590 AB
Heeze, The Netherlands

Jørgen Alving MD
Department of Neurophysiology, Dianalund
Epilepsy Hospital, DK-4293 Dianalund,
Denmark

Richard E Appleton MD
Consultant Paediatric Neurologist, The
Roald Dahl EEG Unit, Alder Hey
Children's Hospital, West Derby, Liverpool
L12 2AP, UK

Gus A Baker PhD
Senior Lecturer in Clinical
Neuropsychology, University of
Liverpool, Walton Centre, Liverpool L9
1AE, UK

Agostino Baruzzi MD
Professor of Neurology, Istituto Clinica
Neurologica dell'Università di Bologna,
40100 Bologna, Italy

Jürgen Bauer MD
Neurologist, Universitätsklinik für
Epileptologie, Universität Bonn, D-53105
Bonn, Germany

Brian Bell PhD
Research Scientist, Department of
Neurology, University of Wisconsin,
Madison, WI 53792, USA

Anne T Berg PhD
Associate Professor, Department of
Biological Sciences, Northern Illinois
University, DeKalb, IL 60115, USA

Samuel F Berkovic MD, FRACP
Professor of Neurology, The University of
Melbourne, Austin and Repatriation
Medical Centre, Heidelberg, Monash, and
Royal Children's Hospital, Heidelberg,
Melbourne, Victoria, Australia

Warren T Blume MD, FRCP(C)
Professor, Department of Clinical
Neurological Sciences, Epilepsy and Clinical
Neurophysiology, London Health Sciences
Center, University Campus, London,
Ontario, N6A 5A5, Canada

Jane C Casey RN, LCSW
Nurse Clinician, Division of Pediatric
Epilepsy, Johns Hopkins Medical
Institutions, Baltimore, MD 21287, USA

David W Chadwick MD
Professor of Neurology, The Walton Centre
for Neurology and Neurosurgery,
Department of Neurological Science,
Liverpool L9 1AE, UK

Catherine Chiron MD, PhD
Neuropaediatrician, Hôpital Saint Vincent-
de-Paul, Service de Neuropédiatrie et
INSERM Unité 29, Paris, France

Orrin Devinsky MD
Chief, Department of Neurology, Director,
NYU Comprehensive Epilepsy Center, and
Professor of Neurology, NYU School of
Medicine, New York University Hospital
for Joint Diseases, Department of
Neurology, New York, NY 10003, USA

Olivier Dulac MD
Paediatric Neurologist and Professor of
Paediatrics, Hôpital Saint Vincent-de-Paul,
INSERM Unité 29, and Université René
Descartes, Paris, France

Christian E Elger MD, PhD, FRCP
Director, Department of Epileptology,
University of Bonn, D-53105 Bonn,
Germany

John M Freeman MD
Lederer Professor of Pediatric Epilepsy,
Professor of Neurology and Pediatrics,
Director of Pediatric Epilepsy, Johns
Hopkins Medical Institutions, Baltimore,
MD 21287, USA

Elisabeth Gordon BA
Research Associate, NYU–Mount Sinai
Comprehensive Epilepsy Center, New York
University Hospital for Joint Diseases,
Department of Neurology, New York, NY
10003, USA

†Lennart Gram MD
Department of Neurophysiology, Dianalund
Epilepsy Hospital, DK-4293 Dianalund,
Denmark

Thomas Grunwald MD, PhD
Senior Physician (Neurology),
Universitätsklinik für Epileptologie,
Universität Bonn, D-53105 Bonn, Germany

Hajo Hamer MD
Department of Neurology, University of
Marburg, D-35033 Marburg, Germany

Mark Hendriks MD
Clinical Neuropsychologist, Epilepsy
Centre, Dr Hans Berger Clinic, PO Box
90108, 4800 RA Breda, and Lecturer,
Neuro- and Rehabilitation Psychology,
Nijmeegs Institute of Cognition and
Information (NICI), University of
Nijmegen, PO Box 9102, 6500 HC
Nijmegen, The Netherlands

Bruce P Hermann PhD
Professor, Department of Neurology,
University of Wisconsin, Madison, WI
53792, USA

Andrew G Herzog MD, MSc
Associate Professor of Neurology, Harvard
Medical School, and Director,
Neuroendocrine Unit, Beth Israel Deaconess
Medical Center, Boston, MA 02215, USA

Ann Jacoby PhD
Principal Research Associate, Centre for
Health Services Research, University of
Newcastle upon Tyne, Newcastle upon
Tyne NE2 4AA, UK

Anna Kaminska MD
Paediatric Neurologist, Hôpital Saint
Vincent-de-Paul, Service de Neuropédiatrie,
and Université René Descartes, Paris,
France

Pavel Klein MB BChir
Assistant Professor, Director, Epilepsy
Center, and Director, Clinical Neuro-
Endocrinology Unit, Department of
Neurology, Georgetown University Medical
Center, Washington DC 20007, USA

Martin Kurthen MD
Professor of Neurology, Department of
Epileptology, University of Bonn, D-53105
Bonn, Germany

Klaus Lehnertz PhD
Physicist, Universitätsklinik für
Epileptologie, Universität Bonn, D-53105
Bonn, Germany

Thomas Lempert MD
Senior Lecturer, Virchow-Klinikum,
Neurologische Klinik und Poliklinik,
D-13353 Berlin, Germany

† Deceased

Dick Lindhout MD, PhD
Professor of Clinical Genetics and Teratology,
MGC–Department of Clinical Genetics,
Erasmus University Rotterdam, PO Box
1738, 3000 DR Rotterdam, The Netherlands

Jane R McGrogan RD, LD
Dietician, Division of Pediatric Epilepsy,
Johns Hopkins Medical Institutions,
Baltimore, MD 21287, USA

Heinz-Joachim Meencke MD
Professor of Neurology, Chairman of the
Epilepsiezentrum Berlin am Evangelischen
Krankenhaus Königin Elisabeth Herzberge,
D-10362 Berlin, Germany

Lina Nashef MBChB, MRCP, MD
Consultant Neurologist, Kent and
Canterbury Hospital, Canterbury, Kent CT1
3NG, and Honorary Senior Lecturer, King's
Healthcare NHS Trust, King's College
Hospital, London SE5 9RS, UK

Deb K Pal PhD, MRCP
Senior Registrar in Paediatric Neurology,
Neurosciences Unit, Institute of Child
Health, University College Medical School
and Great Ormond Street Hospital for
Children, London WC1N 2AP, UK

A James Rowan MD
Vice-Chairman of Neurology, Mount Sinai
School of Medicine, Neurology Faculty
Associates, New York, NY 10029, USA

Josemir WAS Sander MD
Professor in Clinical Neurology and
Epilepsy, Epilepsy Research Group, Institute
of Neurology, The National Hospital for
Neurology and Neurosurgery, London
WC1N 3BG, UK

Steven C Schachter MD
Medical Director, Office of Clinical Trials
and Research, Director of Clinical
Research, Comprehensive Epilepsy Center,
Beth Israel Deaconess Medical Center, and
Associate Professor of Neurology, Harvard
Medical School, Boston, MA 02215, USA

Ingrid E Scheffer MB BS, PhD, FRACP
Senior Lecturer, Department of Neurology,
The University of Melbourne, Austin and
Repatriation Medical Centre, Monash
Medical Centre, and Royal Children's
Hospital, Heidelberg, Melbourne, Victoria,
Australia

Dieter Schmidt MD
Emeritus Professor of Neurology,
Arbeitsgruppe Epilepsieforschung (Epilepsy
Research Group), D-14163 Berlin, Germany

Bettina Schmitz MD
Senior Lecturer, Virchow-Klinikum,
Neurologische Klinik und Poliklinik,
D-13353 Berlin, Germany

Donald L Schomer MD
Director, Comprehensive Epilepsy Center,
Beth Israel Deaconess Medical Center,
Boston, MA 02215, USA

Michael Seidenberg PhD
Associate Professor, Department of
Psychology, Chicago Medical School,
North Chicago, IL, USA

Hermann Stefan MD
Professor of Neurology, Zentrum Epilepsie
Erlangen, Neurologische Klinik mit
Poliklinik der Universität Erlangen-
Nürnberg, D-91054 Erlangen, Germany

Paolo Tinuper MD
Research Fellow in Neurology, Istituto
Clinica Neurologica dell'Università di
Bologna, 40100 Bologna, Italy

Alan R Towne MD
Associate Professor of Neurology, Chairman
of Adult Neurology, and Director of the
Clinical Neurophysiology Laboratories,
Medical College of Virginia of Virginia
Commonwealth University, PO Box
980577, Richmond, VA 23298, USA

David M Treiman MD
William Dow Lovett Professor and
Chairman, Department of Neurology,
University of Medicine and Dentistry of
New Jersey – Robert Wood Johnson
Medical School, New Brunswick, NJ
08901, USA

Jan Vermeulen MD
Department of Neuropsychology, Epilepsy
Centre 'Meer & Bosch', Heemstede, The
Netherlands

Eileen PG Vining MD
Associate Professor of Neurology and
Pediatrics, Associate Director of Pediatric
Epilepsy, Johns Hopkins Medical
Institutions, Baltimore, MD 21287, USA

Harry van der Vlugt PhD
Neuropsychologist, Department of
Neuropsychology, Tilburg University, 5037
AB Tilburg, The Netherlands

Elizabeth J Waterhouse MD
Assistant Professor of Neurology, Director
of the EEG Laboratory, and Director of the
Adult Seizure Clinic, Medical College of
Virginia of the Virginia Commonwealth
University, PO Box 980577, Richmond, VA
23298, USA

Gary Wendt MD
Assistant Professor, Department of
Radiology, University of Wisconsin,
Madison, WI 53792, USA

Guido Widman MD
Universitätsklinik für Epileptologie,
Universität Bonn, D-53105 Bonn, Germany

Elaine Wyllie MD
Pediatric Epilepsy Program, The Cleveland
Clinic Foundation, Department of
Neurology, Cleveland, OH 44195, USA

Preface

Over the last several years, we have been privileged to witness remarkable achievements in the understanding of clinical epilepsy and the introduction of new options for the treatment of seizures. These developments are superbly detailed in recently published comprehensive textbooks of epilepsy, several of which are longer than classic textbooks of medicine. So why this book?

There remain many clinical problems in the treatment of patients with epilepsy for which there are no easy answers. Indeed, such situations continue to puzzle clinicians and generate heated controversies in the literature and the lecture hall.

The purpose of this book is to identify and tackle these difficult issues. Experts from around the world explain their approach to managing the clinical issues that continue to challenge neurologists and epileptologists.

This book is not meant to be a complete textbook of epilepsy but rather a practical guide to today's vexing problems based on clinical experience. We hope that you will be able to benefit from the collected wisdom of these experts and help to turn today's dilemmas into tomorrow's solutions.

Dieter Schmidt, Berlin
Steven C Schachter, Boston

DIAGNOSTIC ISSUES

I

DIFFERENTIAL DIAGNOSIS OF EPILEPSY

1

Seizures during sleep

Paolo Tinuper and Agostino Baruzzi

On average, one third of the life of a human being is spent sleeping. It is well known that epileptic interictal discharges may be influenced by the state of arousal and that seizures, particularly in some epileptic conditions, may be precipitated by sleep or may occur primarily according to a recognizable circadian rhythm. The relationship between sleep stages and ictal or interictal epileptiform discharges has been exhaustively reviewed.[1,2] The modulation of epileptiform paroxysms during sleep depends on the type of epilepsy and the different electrophysiological status characterizing non-rapid eye movement (NREM) and rapid eye movement (REM) stages. During drowsiness and the first stages of NREM sleep electro-encephalogram (EEG) activity becomes more synchronized, thus facilitating the propagation of epileptiform discharges; muscular tone is diminished but preserved, permitting the clinical manifestation of the seizures. The opposite situation occurs in REM sleep, when EEG activity is desynchronized and postural tone inhibited. The thalamocortical volleys that physiologically evoke the K-complexes and spindles in NREM stages drive burst–pause firing in cortical neurons, facilitating the occurrence of generalized discharges in primary generalized epilepsy. Interictal discharges of localization-related epilepsies tend to propagate during NREM sleep and become topographically restricted in REM stages.

On the other hand, many motor or autonomic phenomena occur during sleep both in physiological and pathological conditions. In clinical practice, this makes it difficult to differentiate epileptic phenomena arising during sleep from other paroxysmal motor phenomena of non-epileptic nature. Video-polysomnographic recordings have much enhanced our knowledge in this field.

This chapter is a brief analysis of the most common epileptic situations related to sleep underlying some particular epileptic syndromes and offers some practical hints for the differential diagnosis between seizures and sleep disorders.

Epilepsy with grand mal seizures on awakening

Epilepsy with grand mal (generalized tonic–clonic) seizures on awakening is a particular form of generalized idiopathic epilepsy (GIE).[3] Onset is in late childhood, adolescence and young adulthood with a frequent genetic trait. Other minor seizures like myoclonic and absence seizures may be associated in the same patients. Generalized tonic–clonic (GTC) seizures appear exclusively or predominantly after awakening or while relaxing.[4–7] Diagnosis is usually straightforward with detailed history-taking, supported by witness description of the seizures. If routine EEG recording is normal in the awake state, EEG after sleep deprivation and during early sleep stages or soon after awakening may be conclusive, disclosing generalized spike-and-wave discharges. In addition, intermittent light stimulation is frequently effective in provoking generalized abnormalities. Some difficulties may arise when patients and witnesses report 'major motor seizures during sleep'. These seizures — characterized by violent motor behaviour mimicking, to inexpert eyes, a GTC — can be observed in nocturnal frontal lobe epilepsy (see later in this chapter). In this condition, however, seizures are very frequent, presenting throughout the night in NREM sleep, and video-polysomnographic recordings promptly disclose focal EEG and semeiological features.

Juvenile myoclonic epilepsy

In juvenile myoclonic epilepsy (JME), another type of GIE, the myoclonic jerks (impulsive petit mal) usually occur after awakening and are often precipitated by sleep deprivation. The seizures consist of sudden short muscle contractions, usually affecting the upper limbs synchronously and symmetrically. If the patient is handling an object it could be thrown away. If the jerks affect the trunk and legs they may provoke a sudden fall, without impairment of consciousness.[8–14] Asymmetric jerks have been described by means of video-polygraphic techniques.[15–17] Absence seizures and GTC seizures may be associated, the latter showing the same circadian distribution with predominance after awakening. Genetic studies suggest a polygenetic mode of inheritance.[18–21] Interictal EEG tracings show generalized bursts of spike and polyspike-and-wave complexes at 3–6 Hz. Rare asymmetric paroxysmal discharges and focal abnormalities are also seen, but with shifting predominance between both hemispheres.[16,22] Photosensitivity is present in 30–42 per cent of the patients and

eye closure can facilitate myoclonias and generalized discharges in ~20 per cent of cases.[23] JME jerks must be differentiated from other paroxysmal non-epileptic motor phenomena during sleep such as physiological hypnic jerks and nocturnal myoclonus (NM), often reported by patients and healthy subjects.[24–27] Physiological hypnic jerks are confined to the moment of falling asleep, whereas JME seizures occur preferably on awakening; hypnic jerks are not accompanied by any epileptiform discharge on EEG. NM consists of a muscle contraction lasting 0.5–4 s affecting flexor muscles of the feet and legs, seldom spreading to the upper limbs. Characteristically, NM appears periodically (each 20–30 s) during light sleep. Differential diagnosis from epileptic phenomena is therefore straightforward. Differentiating JME seizures from jerks in progressive myoclonic epilepsies may be difficult, especially at the onset of the progressive disorders and in some particular forms such as Lafora disease and neuronal ceroid lipofuscinoses that can begin at the same age as JME. However, the progressive course of the disease despite therapy, the appearance of mental deterioration and EEG background worsening as well as the occurrence of myoclonia unrelated to EEG discharges, will establish the correct diagnosis during the follow-up.

Benign epilepsy of childhood with centrotemporal spikes

Sleep is an important activating state of seizures in benign epilepsy of childhood with centrotemporal spikes (BECT).[28–35] This form is the most common partial epilepsy in children (15–24 per cent of all childhood epilepsies).[36] Because of its strong genetic predisposition and appearance in healthy subjects without any

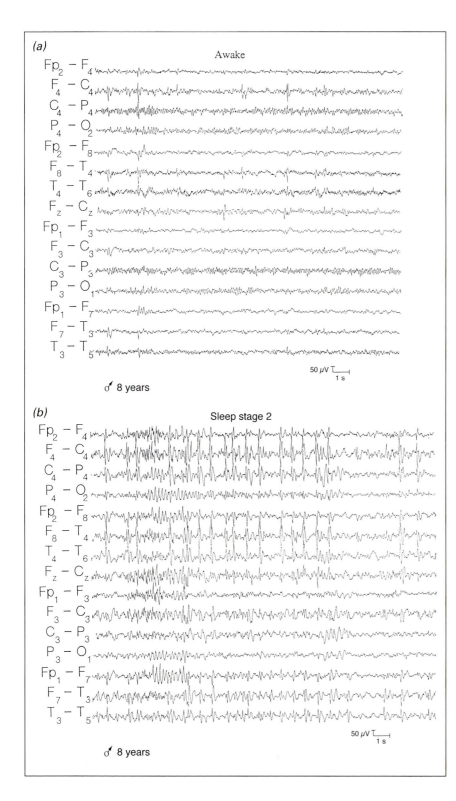

Figure 1.1
(a) During the wake state, isolated spike-and-wave complexes are seen on both centrotemporal regions, predominant on the right. Normal background activity. (b) During sleep stage 2 there is an important activation of abnormalities that maintain the same topography and morphology. Physiological sleep transients are conserved.

evidence of brain lesions, BECT is classified among the idiopathic (with age-related onset) localization-related epilepsies.[3] Onset is around 7 years of age, ranging between 3 and 13 years. Seizures are rare and tend to occur in clusters with prolonged seizure-free intervals. Due to the rarity of the attacks in the majority of patients, the mild aspects of many seizures and their occurrence in sleep in 70–80 per cent of cases, many seizures may remain unnoticed by parents. Typical seizures are characterized by onset with paresthesias in one half of the face, sometimes involving the tongue and lips, followed by clonic jerks involving the same districts, the larynx and pharynx, provoking speech impairment. Clonic movements cause a feeling of suffocation and dysphagia with hypersalivation. Consciousness is retained and patients may be awakened by the seizure. These typical hemifacial seizures may spread to the arm (brachiofacial convulsion) and rarely involve the leg, producing a hemiconvulsive seizure. In this case loss of consciousness may appear. In 7–16 per cent of cases a post-ictal Todd's paresis is observed.[29,37–38] Other rarer seizure types include unilateral tonic–clonic fits and generalized convulsions. In the case of apparent GTC seizures, the observation of a post-ictal focal paresis may suggest the focal onset of the episode. Diagnosis is highly supported by EEG findings. Typical EEG pictures show diphasic high amplitude spikes followed by a slow wave localized on the centrotemporal areas. Activation of EEG abnormalities in drowsiness and sleep is typical and in ~30 per cent of patients spikes appear only during sleep[39] (Figure 1.1). Spikes can remain unilateral, but in ~50 per cent of cases they are bilateral synchronous or asynchronous, often shifting location in subsequent EEG recordings. Other uncommon EEG aspects are the co-existence of occipital spikes or generalized spike-and-wave discharges. In

the presence of a normal child with a normal past medical history, presenting with seizures as classically described in BECT and with the same typical EEG trait, diagnosis is usually clear; further investigations can be avoided and patients and families can be reassured about the good outcome. On the other hand, if these conditions are not fulfilled, magnetic resonance scans should be performed to exclude underlying brain lesions.[40] In children presenting with rare GTC seizures, sleep EEG recording may be useful in detecting typical BECT abnormalities, thus modifying the prognosis and the therapeutic strategy. Another possibility is to disclose EEG aspects typical of BECT in normal children without seizures, while performing EEGs for minor disturbances such as vertigo, trivial head trauma, headache, etc. It must be clear that the diagnosis of BECT, although benign, can only be established in the presence of clinically confirmed seizures.

Rare epileptiform conditions

Other particular rare epileptiform conditions in which sleep plays a fundamental role are the Landau-Kleffner syndrome and continuous spike and waves during sleep.

The Landau-Kleffner syndrome (LKS), first described in 1957,[41] is a functional disorder characterized by an acquired speech disturbance (aphasia and auditory agnosia), occurring in previously age-appropriate children, and accompanied, on EEG, by an almost continuous bitemporal paroxysmal activity. Clinical seizures of various types appear in about two thirds of the patients and have a benign course, responding well to treatment and disappearing in adolescence.[42–48]

In continuous spike and waves during sleep (CSWS)[49–53] EEG paroxysmal activity accounts for at least 85 per cent of sleep and predominates on both frontal areas. Consequently executive and cognitive functions, more than language, are disrupted, leading to severe cognitive and behavioural disturbances. Epileptic seizures are frequent but tend to disappear with treatment and spontaneously in adolescence.

The pathogenetic mechanism of LKS and CSWS is probably the same: the almost continuous paroxysmal EEG activity, interacting with the age-dependent synaptogenesis, produces inappropriate contacts in functional brain areas. The age at onset and the length of time for which this process affects the developing brain will determine the severity and the reversibility of the functional damage. Evaluation of children with suspected LKS or CSWS includes careful neuropsychological testing and repeated EEG recordings during sleep, in addition to a complete neurological and neuroradiological examination. The presence of almost continuous paroxysmal EEG abnormalities during sleep in these conditions help to differentiate them from other disturbances such as autism and developmental dysphasia. The EEG features of LKS and CSWS differ from those recorded in Lennox-Gastaut syndrome, in which sleep EEGs usually show polyspike-and-wave activity and bursts of low amplitude fast activity that may or may not be related to tonic fits.

Nocturnal frontal lobe epilepsy

Localization-related seizures in lesional or cryptogenic partial epilepsy may have a random occurrence. In some patients, irrespective of the clinical form, seizures may acquire a more regular circadian rhythm during the illness and appear preferentially during sleep.

However, there is a peculiar form of partial epilepsy in which seizures appear almost exclusively during sleep. This commonly poses problems of differential diagnosis between epileptic phenomena and other non-epileptic paroxysmal behaviour occurring physiologically or pathologically during sleep. This epileptic condition, described hereafter in more detail, is termed nocturnal frontal lobe epilepsy (NFLE).

The first reports of nocturnal episodes of dyskinetic-dystonic behaviour without any EEG epileptiform ictal pattern were reported in 1981[54] and named first 'hypnogenic' and thereafter 'nocturnal'[55] paroxysmal dystonia (NPD). These reports were then debated by epileptologists, psychiatrists and sleep experts,[56-61] in part because of the term 'dystonia' used to define this condition and because of the difficulties in recording clear-cut interictal and ictal epileptiform abnormalities on EEG in these patients. However, the rarity of EEG correlates in frontal lobe epilepsy is well known and several studies on the semeiological aspects of frontal seizures in drug-resistant epileptic patients undergoing prolonged monitoring for functional neurosurgery described ictal patterns very similar to those observed in NPD.[62-72] Thus it was confirmed once and for all that the so-called NPD is, in fact, a peculiar form of frontal lobe epilepsy.[73]

NFLE seizures are characterized by a sudden arousal from NREM sleep, followed by a complex motor and behavioural activity consisting in cycling or kicking activity of all four limbs, or rocking of the trunk, sometimes with semi-purposeful repetitive movements mimicking sexual or defensive activity. Dystonic or tonic asymmetric postures are frequent. The patients may vocalize, scream or swear and the violence of the behaviour may lead to falling out of bed or physical injury (Figure 1.2). There is no confusional post-ictal

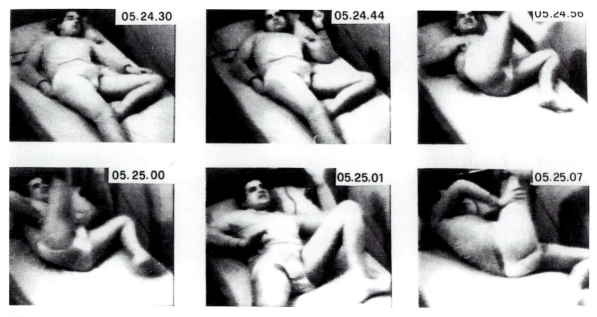

Figure 1.2
Pictures taken from the video-polysomnographic recording of a nocturnal frontal lobe seizure. The patient opens his eyes with a frightened expression; the right arm is rotated inwards and stiff. He seems to be trying to ward off something menacing. He is screaming loudly throughout the episode, lasting 1 min.

state and normally the patient goes back to sleep. Secondary generalization with GTC seizures is extremely uncommon. Some patients may present rare seizures during the wake state, with the same semeiology. Attacks are very frequent and may recur many times every night. Importantly, the seizures conserve the same stereotyped semeiology even over many years in the same patient.[74] Moreover, attacks in the same patient may assume different intensity, but with the same pattern at the onset of the seizures. Brief motor attacks, mimicking a sudden arousal, may represent one fragment of the complete seizure,[75] and they may assume a quasi-periodic occurrence during NREM sleep (Figure 1.3).[76] On the other hand, some patients present prolonged episodes resembling sleepwalking episodes. In

these patients, however, video-polysomnographic recordings disclosed a sustained epileptiform paroxysmal discharge during attacks. These attacks were thus named epileptic nocturnal wandering.[77] It is interesting that some patients may present all the semeiological aspects at the same time or in different stages of the disease, i.e. typical frontal nocturnal seizures, epileptic arousals and epileptic nocturnal wandering episodes (Figure 1.4). Recently, an autosomal dominant form of NFLE (ADNFLE) was identified.[78–81] ADNFLE has been mapped to chromosome 20 in a large Australian family,[82] but heterogeneity has been postulated by other works.[81,83–85] It has become clear that NFLE is a syndrome showing a broad spectrum of paroxysmal epileptiform phenomena.[74,81,86]

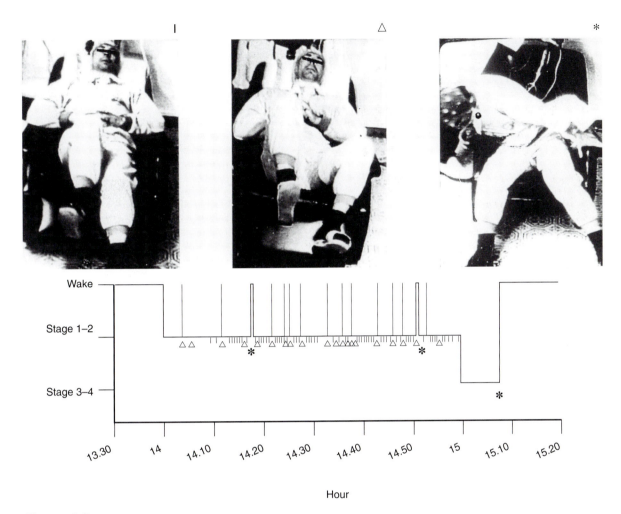

Figure 1.3
Periodism of nocturnal episodes (the following order coincides with the video-polysomnographic recording shown above). (I) brief adduction and flexion of right leg; (Δ) the same movements are followed by opening of the eyes and raising both arms; (*) the same beginning but followed by a complex repetitive motor activity with screaming and vocalization. Sleep histogram shows the periodic occurrence (every 20–40 s) of episodes of different intensity during sleep stages 2–3.

NFLE seizures may pose a serious problem of differential diagnosis vis-à-vis parasomnias like pavor, somnambulism and sleep terrors. It is essential to obtain video-polysomnographic recordings of the attacks in doubtful cases. If more than one attack in the same patient is able to be recorded, the typical stereotypy of the seizures makes the diagnosis clear (Figure 1.5). Some other clinical and polygraphic differential elements are listed in Table 1.1.

Polysomnography is extremely important in differentiating NFLE seizures from psychogenic seizures and other pathological paroxysmal phenomena related to sleep, such as REM sleep

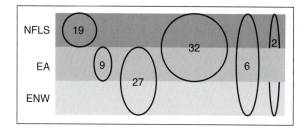

Figure 1.4
Scheme representing the association of different types of seizures in 95 patients with NFLE: 19 had only typical nocturnal frontal lobe seizures (NFLS) and nine only epileptic arousals (EA). In the majority of the patients seizures of different intensity were associated. Six patients showed all three types of seizures. ENW, epileptic nocturnal wandering.

behaviour disorders (RBD) and propriospinal myoclonus. Psychogenic seizures never arise from a true sleep stage, as documented by polygraphic studies.[87] RBD attacks are accompanied by non-stereotyped motor behaviour during REM sleep due to a dysregulation in physiological atonia of this stage,[88] particularly common in degenerative diseases like parkinsonism and multiple system atrophy.[89] Propriospinal myoclonus is a motor phenomenon appearing during drowsiness and characterized, as documented by polygraphic studies,[90–92] by myoclonic activity originating in the axial muscles and propagating rostrally and caudally.

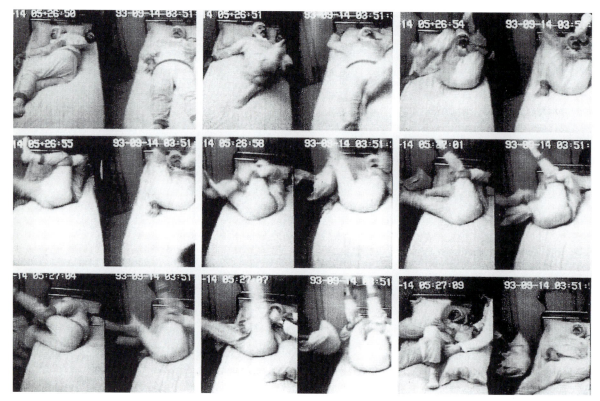

Figure 1.5
Video recording of two different seizures in the same patient on the same night. The onset of the two episodes was synchronized in the split-screen. Note the absolute stereotypy of the motor pattern.

Characteristics	NFLE	Parasomnias (Sleepwalking/sleep terrors)
Positive family history for parasomnias	39%	62–96%
Age at onset (mean)	14 ± 10	Usually <10 years
Age at disappearance	?	7–14 years
Episode frequency/month (mean)	20 ± 11	From <1 to 4
Episode frequency/night (mean)	3 ± 3	One
Sleep stages during which episodes appeared	2 NREM in 65%	3–4 NREM
Episode onset after sleep onset	Any time	First third of the night
Episode duration	From 2 s to 3 min	From 15 s to 30 min
Movements semeiology	Violent, stereotypic	Complex, non-stereotypic
Ictal EEG	Normal in 43%, epileptic in 8%	High amplitude slow waves
Autonomic activation	Present	Present
Triggering factors	None in 79%	Yes

Table 1.1
Elements of differential diagnosis between NFLE and parasomnias (in particular sleepwalking and sleep terrors).

Summary

Sleep may facilitate epileptic seizures, particularly in some forms of epilepsy. Diagnosis may be hampered by the frequent lack of attentive witnesses, the possibility of normal interictal EEG during wakefulness and the presence, during sleep, of other physiological or pathological paroxysmal events. A correct differential diagnosis is based on careful collection of all anamnestic and clinical data and on direct observation of the phenomena by video-polysomnographic techniques.

References

1. Shouse MN, Martins da Silva A. Chronobiology. In: Engel J, Pedley TA, eds. *Epilepsy: a comprehensive textbook*. Philadelphia: Lippincott-Raven, 1997:1917–27.
2. Shouse MN, Martins da Silva A, Sammaritano M. Sleep. In: Engel J, Pedley TA, eds. *Epilepsy: a comprehensive textbook*. Philadelphia: Lippincott-Raven, 1997:1929–42.
3. Commission on Classification and Terminology of the ILAE. Proposal for revised classification of epilepsies and epileptic syndromes. *Epilepsia* 1989;30:389–99.
4. Janz D. The grand mal epilepsies and the sleeping-waking cycle. *Epilepsia* 1962;3:69–109.
5. Janz D. Epilepsy and the sleeping-waking cycle. In: Viken PJ, Bruyn GW, eds. *Handbook of clinical neurology*. Amsterdam: North-Holland, 1974:457–90.
6. Wolf P. Epilepsy with grand mal on awakening. In: Roger J, Dravet C, Bureau M, Dreifuss FE,

Wolf P, eds. *Epileptic syndromes in infancy, childhood and adolescence*, 2nd ed. London: John Libbey, 1992:329–41.

7. Janz D, Wolf P. Epilepsy with Grand Mal on awakening. In: Engel J, Pedley TA, eds. *Epilepsy: a comprehensive textbook*. Philadelphia: Lippincott-Raven, 1997:2347–54.

8. Janz D, Christian W. Impulsiv-petit mal. *Dtsch Z Nervenheilk* 1957;**176**:348.86.

9. Delgado-Escueta AV, Enrile-Bacsal F. Juvenile myoclonic epilepsy of Janz. *Neurology* 1984;**34**:285–94.

10. Janz D. Epilepsy with impulsive petit mal (juvenile myoclonic epilepsy). *Acta Neurol Scand* 1985;**72**:449–59.

11. Dreifuss FE. Juvenile myoclonic epilepsy: characteristics of a primary generalized epilepsy. *Epilepsia* 1989;**30**(Suppl1):51–7.

12. Janz D. Juvenile myoclonic epilepsy. In: Dam M, Gram L, eds. *Comprehensive epileptology*. New York: Raven Press, 1991:171–85.

13. Wolf P. Juvenile myoclonic epilepsy. In: Roger J, Dravet C, Bureau M, Dreifuss FE, Wolf P, eds. *Epileptic syndromes in infancy, childhood and adolescence*, 2nd ed. London: John Libbey, 1992:313–28.

14. Grunewald RA, Panayatopoulos CP. Juvenile myoclonic epilepsy. A review. *Arch Neurol* 1993;**50**:594–8.

15. Canevini MP, Mai R, DiMarco C, et al. Juvenile myoclonic epilepsy of Janz: clinical observations in 60 patients. *Seizures* 1992;**1**:291–98.

16. Lancmann ME, Asconape JJ, Penry JK. Clinical and EEG asymmetries in juvenile myoclonic epilepsy. *Epilepsia* 1994;**35**:302–6.

17. Oguni H, Mukahira K, Oguni M, et al. Video-polygraphic analysis of myoclonic seizures in juvenile myoclonic epilepsy. *Epilepsia* 1994;**35**:307–16.

18. Greenberg DA, Delgado-Escueta AV, Widwlitz H, et al. Juvenile myoclonic epilepsy (JME) may be linked to BF and HLA loci on human chromosome. *Am J Med Genet* 1988;**31**:185–92.

19. Durner M, Sander T, Greenberg DA, Johnson K, Beck-Mannagetta G, Janz D. Localisation of idiopathic generalized epilepsy on chromosome 6p in families of juvenile myoclonic epilepsy patients. *Neurology* 1991;**41**:1651–5.

20. Whitehouse WP, Rees M, Curtis D et al. Linkage analysis of idiopathic generalized epilepsy (IGE) and marker loci on chromosome 6p in families of patients with juvenile myoclonic epilepsy: no evidence for an epilepsy locus in the HLA region. *Am J Hum Genet* 1993;**53**:652–62.

21. Delgado-Escueda AV, Serratosa JM, Liu A, et al. Progress in mapping epilepsy genes. *Epilepsia* 1994;**35**(Suppl1):529–40.

22. Genton P, Salas Puig X, Tunon A, Lahoz C, Del Socorro Gonzales Sanches M. Juvenile myoclonic epilepsy and related syndromes: clinical and neurophysiological aspects. In: Malafosse A, Genton P, Hirsh E, Marescux C, Broglin, Bernasconi R, eds. *Idiopathic generalized epilepsies*. London: John Libbey; 1994:253–65.

23. Wolf P, Goosses R. Relation of photosensitivity to epileptic syndromes. *J Neurol Neurosurg Psychiatr* 1986;**49**:1368–91.

24. Symonds CP. Nocturnal myoclonus. *J Neurol Neurosurg Psychiatr* 1953;**16**:166–71.

25. Lugaresi E, Coccagna G, Mantovani M, et al. The evolution of different types of myoclonus during sleep. *Eur Neurol* 1970;**4**:321–31.

26. Lugaresi E, Coccagna G, Mantovani M, Lebrun R. Some periodic phenomena arising during drowsiness and sleep in man. *Electroencephalogr Clin Neurophysiol* 1972;**32**:701–5.

27. Trenkwalder C, Bucher SF, Oertel WH. Electrophysiological pattern of involuntary limb movements in the restless legs syndrome. *Muscle Nerve* 1996;**19**:155–62.

28. Beaussart M. Benign epilepsy of children with rolandic (centrotemporal) paroxysmal foci: a clinical entity. Study of 221 cases. *Epilepsia* 1972;**13**:795–811.

29. Loiseau P, Beaussart M. The seizures of benign childhood epilepsy with rolandic paroxysmal discharges. *Epilepsia* 1973;**14**:381–9.

30. Lerman P, Kivity S. Benign focal epilepsy of childhood: a follow-up study of 100 recovered patients. *Arch Neurol* 1975;**32**:261–4.

31. Loiseau P, Duche B. Benign childhood epilepsy with centrotemporal spikes. *Clev Clin J Med* 1989;**56**(Supp 1):17–22.

32. Holmes GL. Rolandic epilepsy: clinical and electroencephalographic features. *Epilepsy Res Suppl* 1992;**6**:29–43.

33. Lerman P. Benign partial epilepsy with centrotemporal spikes. In: Roger J, Dravet C,

Bureau M, Dreifuss FE, Wolf P, eds. *Epileptic syndromes in infancy, childhood and adolescence.* 2nd ed. London: John Libbey, 1992: 189–200.

34. Lerman P. Benign childhood epilepsy with centrotemporal spikes (BECT). In: Engel J, Pedley TA, eds. *Epilepsy: a comprehensive textbook.* Philadelphia: Lippincott-Raven, 1997: 2307–14.

35. Wirrel EC. Benign epilepsy of childhood with centrotemporal spikes. *Epilepsia* 1998;**39**(Suppl 4):S32–S41.

36. Cavazzuti GB. Epidemiology of different types of epilepsy in school age children of Modena, Italy. *Epilepsia* 1980;**21**:57–62.

37. Deonna T, Ziegler AL, Desplant PA, van Melle G. Partial epilepsy in neurologically normal children: clinical syndromes and prognosis. *Epilepsia* 1986;**27**:241–7.

38. Wirrel EC, Camfield PR, Gordon KE, Dooley JM, Camfield CS. Benign rolandic epilepsy: atypical features are very common. *J Child Neurol* 1995;**10**:455–8.

39. Blom S, Heijbel J. Benign epilepsy of children with centrotemporal EEG foci. Discharge rate during sleep. *Epilepsia* 1975;**16**:133–40.

40. Santanelli P, Bureau M, Magaudda A, Gobbi G, Roger J. Benign partial epilepsy with centrotemporal (or rolandic) spikes and brain lesion. *Epilepsia* 1989;**30**:182–8.

41. Landau WM, Kleffner FR. Syndrome of acquired aphasia with convulsive disorder in children. *Neurology* 1957;**7**:523–30.

42. Beaumanoir A. The Landau-Kleffner syndrome. In: Roger J, Dravet C, Bureau M, Dreifuss FE, Wolf P, eds. *Epileptic syndromes in infancy, childhood and adolescence.* London: John Libbey, 1985:181–91.

43. Bishop DVM. Age of onset and outcome in 'acquired aphasia with convulsive disorder' (Landau–Kleffner syndrome). *Dev Med Child Neurol* 1985;**27**:705–12.

44. Cole AJ, Andermann F, Taylor L, et al. The Landau–Kleffner syndrome of acquired epileptic aphasia: unusual clinical outcome, surgical experience, and absence of encephalitis. *Neurology* 1988;**38**:31–8.

45. Hirsch E, Marescaux C, Maquet P, et al. Landau–Kleffner syndrome: a clinical and EEG study of five cases. *Epilepsia* 1990;**31**:756–67.

46. Deonna T. Acquired epileptiform aphasia in children (Landau-Kleffner syndrome). *J Clin Neurophysiol* 1991;**8**:288–98.

47. Beaumanoir A. The Landau–Kleffner syndrome. In: Roger J, Dravet C, Bureau M, Dreifuss FE, Wolf P, eds. *Epileptic syndromes in infancy, childhood and adolescence.* 2nd ed. London: John Libbey, 1992:231–43.

48. Deonna T, Roulet E. Acquired epileptic aphasia (AEA): definition of the syndrome and current problems. In: Beaumanoir A, Bureau M, Deonna T, Mira L, Tassinari CA, eds. *Continuous spike and waves during slow sleep: electrical status epilepticus during slow sleep.* London: John Libbey, 1995:37–45.

49. Patry G, Lyagoubi S, Tassinari CA. Subclinical 'electrical status epilepticus' induced by sleep in children. *Arch Neurol* 1971;**24**:242–52:

50. Tassinari CA, Terzano G, Capocchi G, et al. Epileptic seizures during sleep in children: In: Penry JK, ed. *Epilepsy: The 8th International Symposium.* New York: Raven Press, 1977: 345–54.

51. Tassinari CA, Bureau M, Dravet C, Dalla Bernardina B, Roger J. Epilepsy with continuous spikes and waves during slow sleep. In: Roger J, Dravet C, Bureau M, Dreifuss FE, Wolf P, eds. *Epileptic syndromes in infancy, childhood and adolescence.* London: John Libbey, 1985:194–204.

52. Tassinari CA. The problem of 'continuous spikes and waves during slow sleep' or 'electrical status epilepticus during slow sleep' today. In: Beaumanoir A, Bureau M, Deonna T, Mira L, Tassinari CA, eds. *Continuous spike and waves during slow sleep: electrical status epilepticus during slow sleep.* London: John Libbey, 1995:251–5.

53. Smith MC. Landau–Kleffner syndrome and continuous spike and waves during slow sleep. In: Engel J, Pedley TA, eds. *Epilepsy: a comprehensive textbook.* Philadelphia: Lippincott-Raven, 1997:2367–77.

54. Lugaresi E, Cirignotta F. Hypnogenic paroxysmal dystonia: epileptic seizures or a new syndrome? *Sleep* 1981:4:129–38.

55. Lugaresi E, Cirignotta F, Montagna P. Nocturnal paroxysmal dystonia. *J Neurol Neurosurg Psychiatr* 1986;**49**:375–80.

56. Ranja P, Kundra O, Halasz P. Vigilance level-dependent tonic seizures. Epilepsy or sleep disorder? A case report. *Epilepsia* 1983;**24**:725–33.

57. Crowell JA, Anders TF. Hypnogenic paroxysmal dystonia. *J Am Acad Child Psychiatry* 1985;**24**:353–8.

58. Godbout R, Montplaisir J, Roleau I. Hypnogenic paroxysmal dystonia: epilepsy or sleep disorder? A case report. *Clin Electroencephalogr* 1985;**16**:136–42.

59. Lee BI, Lesser RP, Pippenger CE, et al. Familial paroxysmal hypnogenic dystonia. *Neurology* 1985;**35**:1357–60.

60. Berger HJC, Berendse-Versteeg TMC, Joosten EMG. Nocturnal paroxysmal dystonia. *J Neurol Neurosurg Psychiatr* 1987;**50**:647–648.

61. Kovacevic-Ristanovic R, Golbin A, Cartwright R. Nocturnal conversion disorder and nocturnal paroxysmal dystonia. Similarities and treatment. *Sleep Res* 1988;**17**:204.

62. Tharp BR. Orbital frontal seizures. A unique electroencephalographic and clinical syndrome. *Epilepsia* 1972;**13**:627–42.

63. Geier S, Bancaud J, Tailarach J, Bonis A, Szikla G, Enjelvin M. The seizure of frontal lobe epilepsy. *Neurology* 1977;**27**:951–8.

64. Wada JA, Purves SJ. Oral and bimanual-bipedal activity as ictal manifestation of frontal lobe epilepsy. *Epilepsia* 1984;**25**:668.

65. Williamson PD, Spencer DD, Spencer SS, Novelly RS, Mattson RH. Complex partial seizures of frontal lobe origin. *Ann Neurol* 1985;**18**:497–504.

66. Delgado-Escueta AV, Swartz BE, Maldonado HM, Walsh GO, Rand RW, Halgren E. Complex partial seizures of frontal lobe origin. In: Wieser HG, Engel CE, eds. *Presurgical evaluation of epileptics.* New York: Springer-Verlag, 1987:268–99.

67. Waterman K, Purves SJ, Kosaka B, Strauss E, Wada JA. An epileptic syndrome caused by mesial frontal lobe seizure foci. *Neurology* 1987;**37**:577–82.

68. Ajmone Marsan C. Seizures originating from the orbital cortex of the frontal lobe. *Epilepsia* 1988;**29**:208.

69. Morris HH, Dinner DS, Luders H, Wyllie E, Kramer R. Supplementary motor seizures: clinical and electroencephalographic findings. *Neurology* 1988;**38**:1075–82.

70. Wada JA. Nocturnal recurrence of brief, intensely affective vocal and facial expression with powerful bimanual, bipedal, axial, and pelvic activity with rapid recovery as manifestations of mesial frontal lobe seizure. *Epilepsia* 1988;**29**:209.

71. Bancaud J, Talairach J. Clinical semeiology of frontal lobe seizures. In: Chauvel P, Delgado-Escueta AV, Halgren E, Bancaud J, eds. *Frontal lobe seizures and epilepsies.* New York: Raven Press, 1992:3–58. [*Adv Neurol*, Vol. 57.]

72. So NK. Mesial frontal epilepsy. *Epilepsia* 1998;**39**(Suppl 4):49–61.

73. Tinuper P, Cerullo A, Cirignotta F, Cortelli P, Lugaresi E, Montagna P. Nocturnal paroxysmal dystonia with short-lasting attacks: three cases with evidence for an epileptic frontal lobe origin of seizures. *Epilepsia* 1990;**31**:549–56.

74. Tinuper P, Plazzi G, Provini F, Cerullo A, Lugaresi E. The syndrome of nocturnal frontal lobe epilepsy. In: Lugaresi E, Parmeggiani PL, eds. *Somatic and autonomic regulation in sleep.* Milan: Springer, 1997:125–35.

75. Montagna P, Sforza E, Tinuper P, Cirignotta F, Lugaresi E. Paroxysmal arousals during sleep. *Neurology* 1990;**40**:1063–66.

76. Sforza E, Montagna P, Rinaldi R, et al. Paroxysmal periodic motor attacks during sleep: clinical and polygraphic features. *Electroencephalogr Clin Neurophysiol* 1993;**86**:161–6.

77. Plazzi G, Tinuper P, Montagna P, Provini F, Lugaresi E. Epileptic nocturnal wandering. *Sleep* 1995;**18**:749–56.

78. Sheffer IE, Bathia KP, Lopes-Cendes I, et al. Autosomal dominant frontal lobe epilepsy misdiagnosed as sleep disorder. *Lancet* 1994;**343**:515–17.

79. Sheffer IE, Bathia KP, Lopes-Cendes I, et al. Autosomal dominant nocturnal frontal lobe epilepsy: a distinctive clinical disorder. *Brain* 1995;**118**:61–73.

80. Oldani A, Zucconi M, Ferini-Strambi L, Bizozzero D, Smirne S. Autosomal dominant nocturnal frontal lobe epilepsy: electroclinical picture. *Epilepsia* 1996;**37**:964–76.

81. Oldani A, Zucconi M, Asselta A, et al. Autosomal dominant nocturnal frontal lobe epilepsy. A video-polysomnographic and genetic appraisal of 40 patients and delineation of the epileptic syndrome. *Brain* 1998;**121**:205–23.

82. Phillis HA, Sheffer IE, Berkovic SF, Hollway GE, Sutherland GR, Mulley JC. Localisation of gene for autosomal dominant nocturnal frontal lobe epilepsy to chromosome 20q13.2. *Nat Genet* 1995;**10**:117–18.

83. Berkovic SF, Phillis HA, Sheffer IE, et al. Genetic heterogeneity in autosomal dominant nocturnal frontal lobe epilepsy. *Epilepsia* 1995;**36**(Suppl 4):147.

84. Tinuper P, Montagna P, Cerullo A, et al. Autosomal dominant nocturnal epilepsy: a family with brain migration disorder and chromosome 18 duplication. *Epilepsia* 1996;**37**(Suppl 5):37.

85. Mochi M , Provini F, Plazzi G, et al. Genetic heterogeneity in autosomal dominant nocturnal frontal lobe epilepsy. *Ital J Neurol Sci* 1997;**18**:183.

86. Montagna P. Nocturnal paroxysmal dystonia and nocturnal wandering. *Neurology* 1992; **42**(Suppl 6):61–7.

87. Bazil CW, Walczak TS. Effect of sleep and sleep stage on epileptic and non-epileptic seizures. *Epilepsia* 1997;**38**:56–62.

88. Shenck CH, Bundlie SR, Ettinger MG, Mahowald MV. Chronic behavioral disorder of human REM sleep: a new category of parasomnia. *Sleep*1986;**9**:293–308.

89. Plazzi G, Corsini R, Provini F, et al. REM sleep behavior disorders in multiple system atrophy. *Neurology* 1997;**48**:1094–97.

90. Brown P, Thomson PD, Rothwell JC, et al. Axial myoclonus of propriospinal origin. *Brain* 1991;**114**:197–214.

91. Chokroverty S, Walters A, Zimmerman T, Picone A. Propriospinal myoclonus: a neurophysiological analysis. *Neurology* 1992;**42**:1591–95.

92. Montagna P, Provini F, Plazzi G, et al. Propriospinal myoclonus upon relaxation and drowsiness: a cause of severe insomnia. *Mov Disord* 1997;**12**:66–72.

2

Seizures and syncopes

Thomas Lempert

Introduction

Syncope is a transient loss of consciousness and upright posture due to global cerebral ischaemia. The lifetime prevalence of syncope is difficult to assess, but 23 per cent of elderly people remembered previous syncopal attacks.[1] This compares with a lifetime prevalence of unprovoked epileptic seizures of around 5 per cent.[2]

The diagnosis of syncope is made in two steps: first, identifying an attack with loss of consciousness as syncope and secondly, establishing its underlying cause. This article will focus on the recognition of syncope and its differentiation from epileptic seizures, which is a common dilemma in clinical practice. Guidelines for the aetiological work-up of syncope can be found elsewhere.[3,4]

It appears that the most frequent source of diagnostic error is not inaccurate accounts of symptoms from patients or relatives but misconceptions held by doctors.[5] Textbook descriptions of syncope tend to recall the melodramatic faints from Hollywood movies: the actress/patient sighs, sinks to the ground, lies motionless with eyes closed and finally recovers wondering 'Where am I?'. Research into the semeiology of syncope has contested every single element of this stereotype.

To elucidate the phenomenology of syncope we recently videotaped and analysed attacks that were induced by hyperventilation and the Valsalva manoeuvre in healthy volunteers.[6] Previous investigators studied syncope induced by various means such as the Valsalva manoeuvre alone,[7] exposure to acceleration on a centrifuge,[8] venipuncture and blood loss,[9] ocular compression[10-12] and ventricular arrhythmia.[13] The clinical phenomenology, however, proves quite consistent, irrespective of the induction procedure.

We designed our study to observe the motor symptoms of syncope as naturally as possible. Therefore, we did not constrain our subjects but allowed them to fall onto a mat of foam rubber and move freely. Surprisingly, only half of them collapsed flaccidly while the others fell with knees and hips extended (Figure 2.1). Thus, a stiff fall does not necessarily herald a generalized tonic–clonic seizure.

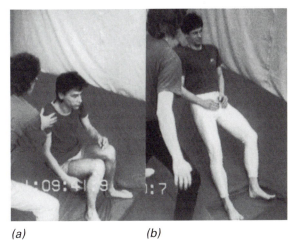

(a)   (b)

Figure 2.1
Variants of syncopal falls: (a) flaccid; (b) stiff.

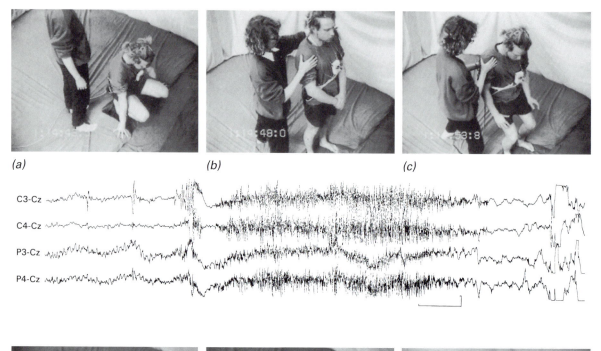

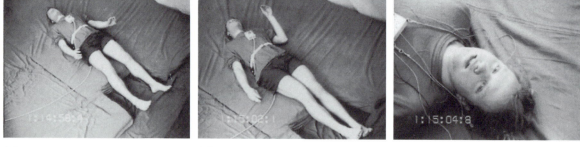

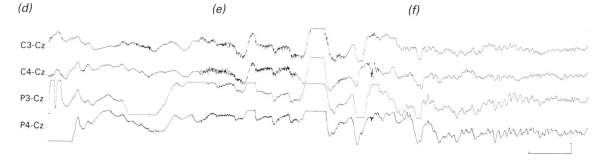

Figure 2.2

Electro-encephalogram during syncope induced by hyperventilation and Valsalva manoeuvre (calibration 1 s, 50 µV). (a) Alpha rhythm while subject hyperventilates in a squatting position. (b) Muscle artifacts during Valsalva manoeuvre. (c) High amplitude slow waves at the onset of syncope. (d) Flattening of the EEG in the presence of bilateral myoclonus. (e) Reappearance of slow wave activity while myoclonus continues. (f) Return of alpha rhythm and consciousness.

Convulsions

The term 'convulsive syncope' implies that there is a peculiar variant of syncope complicated by myoclonic or tonic muscle activity. Moreover, it suggests that an epileptic mechanism may be at work. Both presumptions are erroneous. Convulsions are an integral component of the brain's response to hypoxia and represent the rule rather than the exception. Reported frequencies of seizures associated with syncope vary from 12 per cent[9] to 100 per cent,[14] but most investigators observed them in the order of 70–90 per cent of syncopal episodes.[6–8,10,11,13] High rates were usually obtained from prospective studies and when events were recorded on film or video.[6–8,13]

The fact that convulsions are less often recounted by an ordinary eyewitness reflects their fleeting nature and variable intensity. Syncopal myoclonus may manifest itself as anything from a single twitch of the mouth to a storm of violent jerks affecting the whole body. It is often multifocal with asynchronous muscle jerks in different parts of the body. Alternatively, it may be generalized with bilateral synchronous muscle activation. Both forms of myoclonus may occur during an attack.[6] In contrast to epileptic muscle activity, syncopal myoclonus is not rhythmic and is only rarely sustained for more than half a minute.

Tonic muscle activity during syncope typically consists of head and body extension with either flexion or extension of the arms.[7,9] Usually, it is only mild and does not resemble the forced extensor posturing of a generalized tonic–clonic seizure (GTCS). However, a brief but intense opisthotonic stiffening is a common accompaniment of breath-holding attacks and other forms of childhood syncope.[11]

There is no evidence to suggest that syncopal convulsions reflect epileptic activity of the cerebral cortex. During a syncopal attack, the electro-encephalogram (EEG) shows a quite uniform sequence of generalized slow waves of high amplitude, flattening of the trace, and return of slow waves before normal background activity is restored (Figure 2.2). Epileptic discharges are consistently absent[7,10,13] on both ictal and interictal recordings. Muscle activation during syncope is subcortical and probably originates from abnormal firing of the reticular formation in the lower brainstem.[15] Micro-electrode recordings from experimental animals exposed to total brain ischaemia showed preservation and even increase of neuronal activity in the medullary reticular formation lasting up to 40 s, whereas cerebral cortex potentials ceased after 10 s.[16]

Eye movements

As a rule, eyes are open during syncope, a feature that is shared by epileptic but not by psychogenic seizures.[17] Syncope often starts with a vertical, downbeating nystagmus[11,18] which tends to be missed by observers. The most consistent ocular motor sign is an upward turning of the eyes early in the course of syncope (Figure 2.3).[9,18,19] This may be followed by a lateral deviation[18] which can further complicate the distinction of syncopal and epileptic eye movements. Unlike syncopal eye turns, epileptic eye deviations tend to last longer than just a few seconds.

Automatisms

Automatisms are complex movements performed during impairment of consciousness. They have only rarely been reported in syncope[11] and yet, we observed them in 80 per cent of our subjects.[6] Typical features were lip-licking, chewing, fumbling, reaching for the

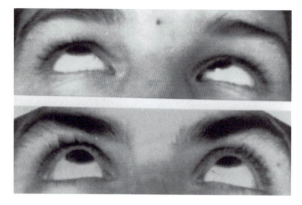

Figure 2.3
Upward eye deviation and slight convergence at the onset of experimentally induced syncope in two subjects.

head, head raising, sitting up, or even standing up while still being unresponsive and amnesic. In contrast to epileptic automatisms these movements were mostly short and solitary rather than repetitive. Occasionally, however, prolonged automatisms during syncope may render the differentiation from complex partial seizures difficult.[11] Similarly misleading may be growling or moaning vocalizations, which we noticed in 40 per cent of subjects.

Hallucinations

Another feature that links the phenomenology of syncope with complex partial seizures is hallucinations. They are usually ignored, because doctors do not ask about them and patients do not volunteer them. However, systematic studies have uncovered them with considerable regularity.[6,7,19,20] In our study, 60 per cent of subjects experienced dream-like hallucinations that were always visual and often also auditory. In some, visual hallucinations were restricted to a perception of grey haze, coloured patches, or glaring lights. Others encountered more complex scenes involving landscapes, familiar situations, or persons. Four subjects had out-of-body experiences. Auditory hallucinations included rushing and roaring sounds, traffic and machine noises, talking and screaming human voices, but never intelligible speech. Unlike epileptic auras, syncopal hallucinations do not precede the attack but rather extend into the reorientation period.[6,19]

Commonly, the emotional experience of syncope was described as detachment, weightlessness, and peace, so that the subjects were reluctant to return to reality. Some compared it with drug or meditation experiences and two were reminded of a previous near-death experience. This similarity led us to speculate that near-death experience may reflect hypoxic disinhibition of the limbic system rather than entry into a transcendental domain.[20]

Incomplete syncope

The two key symptoms of syncope — loss of consciousness and loss of upright posture — may dissociate when cerebral hypoxia is not profound. The more common type of incomplete syncope is falling with at least partial preservation of consciousness, which occurred in 13 out of 56 subjects in our study.[6] These subjects remembered their falls but were not able to count aloud immediately on request. They usually described a state of diminished external awareness, disorientation, and loss of voluntary motor control. These episodes were shorter than complete syncope and only rarely were accompanied by myoclonus or hallucinations. The complementary variant of incomplete syncope — maintenance of upright stance with total loss of awareness and recollection — occurred only once in our series. During the

Precipitant	Pathophysiological mechanism
Standing up	Orthostatic hypotension due to autonomic failure, dehydration, drugs or as an idiopathic disorder in adolescents; anaemia
Carbohydrate meals	Postprandial hypotension of the elderly
Prolonged standing, micturition, pain, invasive medical procedures, glossopharyngeal neuralgia, swallowing, unpleasant sights and smells, psychological shock	Vasovagal (neurally mediated) syncope with reflectory vasodilatation/bradycardia
Heat, alcohol, antihypertensive drugs	Vasodilatation
Coughing, blowing a trumpet, screaming, weight-lifting	Valsalva manoeuvre
Lying supine in advanced pregnancy	Venous obstruction
Hyperventilation ('stuffy air')	Hypocapnic cerebral vasoconstriction
Exertion	Cardiac or pulmonary obstruction, e.g. valve stenosis, myxoma, pulmonary hypertension
Changing body position	Atrial myxoma
Rock concert	Combination of dehydration, prolonged orthostasis, hyperventilation and Valsalva (pressing crowd, screaming)

Table 2.1
Precipitants of syncope: clues for aetiological diagnosis.

attack, the subject staggered around while staring vacantly straight ahead. Although rare, episodes of this kind may be encountered in clinical practice; their differential diagnosis includes complex partial and absence seizures.

Precedents

As a rule of thumb, epileptic seizures occur spontaneously, whereas syncope is provoked by specific actions or circumstances that in about half of the cases can be unearthed by careful history taking. Common precipitants include prolonged standing, violent coughing, micturition, exertion, intake of antihypertensive drugs, nitrates or alcohol, blood loss, venipuncture or other invasive medical procedures, and even attending rock concerts.[21,22] Psychological shock is another frequent precedent of syncope which may render the distinction from hysterical seizures difficult. Identification of precipitating factors provides valuable clues for the pathophysiological mechanisms involved (Table 2.1).

Features	Syncope	GTCS
Duration	Usually <30 s	2–3 min
Precipitating event	~50 per cent	None
Falls	Flaccid or stiff	Stiff
Convulsions	~80 per cent, mostly brief, arrhythmic, multifocal and/or generalized	Always, 2–3 min, rhythmic, generalized
Eyes	Open, transient upward or lateral deviation	Open, often sustained deviation
Hallucinations	Late in the attack	May precede GTCS in focal epilepsy
Colour of the face	Pale	Cyanotic
Hypersalivation, frothing	Absent	Common
Incontinence	Common	Common
Tongue bite	Rare	Common
Post-ictal confusion	<30 s	2–30 min
Creatine kinase	Normal	Often elevated

Table 2.2
Distinctive features of syncope and generalized tonic–clonic seizures (GTCS).

The premonitory symptoms of syncope are manifold;[23] characteristic symptoms are bilateral tinnitus, decreased hearing and 'blackening-out' — a transient amaurosis while consciousness is still preserved — that is caused by the early collapse of retinal perfusion. Light-headedness, confusion, abdominal discomfort, warmth, and faintness are equally common but less specific, as patients may use these terms also to describe an epileptic aura or the sensation that precedes a hysterical seizure. Some well-known epileptic aura phenomena such as tastes, smells, déjà vu experiences, speech disturbances, and unilateral paresthesia do not occur before syncope.[23] Palpitations, although not specific for syncope, are suggestive of an undiagnosed tachycardia that compromises cardiac output.

Post-ictal phenomena

Several post-ictal features are useful to discriminate between syncope and an epileptic seizure. The single most powerful factor is post-ictal confusion as observed by an eyewitness.[24] Reorientation is usually immediate in syncope and does not exceed 30 s even after extended attacks.[13] Thus, any post-ictal disorientation lasting longer than that suggests an epileptic seizure. Likewise, tongue bites point to an epileptic event,[25] but there are exceptions to this rule.[6,11,24] In contrast, urinary incontinence and head injuries appear to be equally common in syncope and GTCS.[24] Exhaustion, sleepiness, vomiting, headaches, and muscle aches may all occur after syncope,[11,24] but tend to be more frequent and severe after GTCS. Table 2.2 summarizes the main features differentiating syncope and GTCS.

Investigations

Although careful history-taking remains indispensable for differentiating seizures and syncope, additional investigations may sometimes help to settle doubtful cases. Creatine kinase plasma concentrations are usually elevated after a GTCS from 2 h onward, but are normal after syncope.[26] Obviously, a negative test on its own is insufficient to diagnose syncope. False negative results and other non-epileptic attacks such as hysterical seizures have to be taken into account. Prolactin levels, which rise within the first hour after a GTCS, may increase[27,28] or remain unchanged[29] after syncope and are therefore not helpful for differential diagnosis.

The diagnostic power of the EEG is often overestimated.[30] Epileptic discharges on an interictal recording certainly support a diagnosis of epilepsy, but do not rule out additional syncopal attacks. A negative EEG does not settle the matter either. Epileptic discharges may be absent in a single interictal EEG even in chronic epilepsy and all the more after seizures related to drug or alcohol withdrawal.[31]

Reproduction of syncope in the laboratory by tilt testing,[32] eyeball pressure,[10,11] or hyperventilation[31] has been advocated to confirm the diagnosis. However, a positive response does not necessarily imply that the patient's habitual attacks are also syncopal in nature.[33,34] Therefore, a relative of the patient should witness the event in the laboratory or review it on video, to confirm its similarity to previous episodes.

Response to anticonvulsants

If a patient with presumed epilepsy continues to have attacks in spite of therapeutic anticonvulsant plasma levels, the diagnosis has to be reconsidered. The literature contains numerous reports of recurrent syncopal episodes due to potentially life-threatening cardiac arrhythmias which were misdiagnosed and treated as epilepsy for several years.[35,36]

Interaction of syncopal and epileptic mechanisms

Many features of syncope may look epileptic but are non-epileptic with regard to their underlying pathophysiology. Exceptionally, however, both syncopal and epileptic mechanisms may be active within one attack. Thus, syncope may provoke an epileptic seizure and vice versa.

Cerebral hypoxia has potent epileptogenic effects, not only after causing structural damage to the cortex,[37] but also at earlier stages. Nevertheless, only about a dozen EEG-documented epileptic seizures evolving from syncope have been reported. Most of them occurred in children in whom syncope was followed by an absence[38–40] or a generalized clonic seizure.[41] In contrast, innumerable other accounts of 'syncope followed by a seizure' have been poorly substantiated and obviously reflect misinterpretation of hypoxic convulsions. A complex partial seizure triggered by syncope has been documented only once.[42]

Practical guidelines for the diagnosis of syncope

- Ask the patient in detail about precipitating events and situations, premonitory and post-ictal symptoms

- Ask an eyewitness about clinical features of the attack

- Remember that tonic and myoclonic convulsions, automatisms, vocalizations, eye deviations and hallucinations may all occur during syncope — it is not their presence or absence but their specific phenomenology that distinguishes syncope from an epileptic seizure

- Arguments for syncope include situational precipitation, blackening-out, brief arrhythmic convulsions and a rapid recovery

- Arguments for a GTCS include specific epileptic aura symptoms such as smells, déjà vu or unilateral paresthesia, a tonic phase followed by sustained, rhythmical and symmetrical myoclonus, salivation, cyanosis, tongue bites and prolonged recovery

- Syncope and epileptic seizures may look similar but their pathophysiology is different — only exceptionally, hypoxic and epileptic mechanisms may interact within a single attack

---

Cardiac arrhythmia is a common accompaniment of epileptic seizures, especially those of temporal lobe origin.[43,44] Only rarely, however, are changes in heart rhythm severe enough to provoke syncope in the course of a complex partial seizure.[45–47] When a patient's history contains elements of both epilepsy and syncope, ictal EEG/electrocardiogram recordings are required to establish the diagnosis and to discriminate atonic drop attacks, another rare complication of temporal lobe epilepsy.[48]

References

1. Lipsitz LA, Wei JY, Rowe JW. Syncope in an elderly institutionalized population. Prevalence, incidence, and associated risk. *Q J Med* 1985; 55:45–55.

2. Hauser WA, Annegers JF, Kurland LT. Incidence of epilepsy and unprovoked seizures in Rochester, Minnesota: 1935–1984. *Epilepsia* 1993;34:453–68.

3. Kapoor WN. Workup and management of patients with syncope. *Med Clin North Am* 1995;79:1153–70.

4. Hopson JR, Kienzle MG. Evaluation of patients with syncope. Separating the 'wheat' from the 'chaff'. *Postgrad Med* 1992;91:321–38.

5. Hoefnagels WA, Padberg GW, Overweg J, Roos RA. Syncope or seizure? A matter of opinion. *Clin Neurol Neurosurg* 1992;94:153–6.

6. Lempert T, Bauer M, Schmidt D. Syncope: a videometric analysis of 56 episodes of transient cerebral hypoxia. *Ann Neurol* 1994;36:233–7.

7. Duvoisin RC. Convulsive syncope induced by the Weber maneuver. *Arch Neurol* 1962; 7:65–72.

8. Whinnery JE, Whinnery AM. Acceleration-induced loss of consciousness. *Arch Neurol* 1990;**47**:764–76.

9. Lin JT, Ziegler DK, Lai CW, Bayer W. Convulsive syncope in blood donors. *Ann Neurol* 1982;**11**:525–8.

10. Gastaut H, Fischer-Williams M. Electroencephalographic study of syncope. Its differentiation from epilepsy. *Lancet* 1957;**2**:1018–25.

11. Stephenson JBP. *Fits and faints*. London: MacKeith Press, 1990.

12. Stephenson JBP. Reflex anoxic seizures and ocular compression. *Dev Med Child Neurol* 1980;**22**:380–6.

13. Aminoff MJ, Scheinmann MM, Griffin JC, Herre JM. Electrocerebral accompaniments of syncope associated with malignant ventricular arrhythmia. *Ann Intern Med* 1988;**108**:791–6.

14. Rossen R, Kabat H, Anderson JP. Acute arrest of cerebral circulation in man. *Arch Neurol Psychiatry* 1943;**50**:510–28.

15. Hallett M, Chadwick D, Adam J, Marsden CD. Reticular reflex myoclonus: a physiologic type of human posthypoxic myoclonus. *J Neurol Neurosurg Psychiatry* 1977;**40**:253–64.

16. Naquet R, Fernandez-Guardiola A. Effects of various types of anoxia on spontaneous and evoked cerebral activity in the cat. In: Gastaut H, Meyer JS, eds. *Cerebral anoxia and the electroencephalogram*. Springfield: Charles C Thomas, 1961:144–63.

17. Schmidt D, Lempert T. Differential diagnosis in adults. In: Dam M, Gram L, eds. *Comprehensive epileptology*. New York: Raven Press, 1990:449–71.

18. Lempert T, von Brevern M. The eye movements of syncope. *Neurology* 1996;**46**:1086–8.

19. Forster EM, Whinnery JE. Recovery from +Gz-induced loss of consciousness: psychophysiologic considerations. *Aviat Space Environ Med* 1988;**59**:517–22.

20. Lempert T, Bauer M, Schmidt D. Syncope and near-death experience. *Lancet* 1994;**344**:829.

21. Ross RT. *Syncope*. London:WB Saunders, 1988.

22. Lempert T, Bauer M. Mass fainting at rock concerts. *N Engl J Med* 1995;**332**:1721.

23. Benke T, Hochleitner M, Bauer G. Aura phenomena during syncope. *Eur Neurol* 1997;**37**:28–32.

24. Hoefnagels WA, Padberg GW, Overweg J, van der Velde EA, Roos RA. Transient loss of consciousness: the value of the history for distinguishing seizure from syncope. *J Neurol* 1991;**238**:39–43.

25. Benbadis SR, Wolgamuth BR, Goren H, Brener S, Fouad-Tarazi F. Value of tongue biting in the diagnosis of seizures. *Arch Intern Med* 1995;**155**:2346–9.

26. Libman MD, Potvin L, Coupal L, Grover SA. Seizure vs. syncope: measuring serum creatine kinase in the emergency department. *J Gen Intern Med* 1991;**6**:408–12.

27. Cordingley G, Brown D, Dane P, Harnish K, Cadmagnani P, O'Hare T. Increases in serum prolactin levels associated with syncopal attacks. *Am J Emerg Med* 1993;**11**:251–2.

28. Oribe E, Amini R, Nissenbaum E, Boal B. Serum prolactin concentrations are elevated after syncope. *Neurology* 1996;**47**:60–2.

29. Anzola GP. Predictivity of plasma prolactin levels in differentiating epilepsy from pseudoseizures: a prospective study. *Epilepsia* 1993;**34**:1044–8.

30. Gibbs J, Appleton RE. False diagnosis of epilepsy in children. *Seizure* 1992;**1**:15–18.

31. Hoefnagels WA, Padberg GW, Overweg J, Roos RA, van Dijk JG, Kamphuisen HA. Syncope or seizure? The diagnostic value of the EEG and hyperventilation test in transient loss of consciousness. *J Neurol Neurosurg Psychiatry* 1991;**54**:953–6.

32. Grubb BP, Gerard G, Roush K, et al. Differentiation of convulsive syncope and epilepsy with head-up tilt testing. *Ann Intern Med* 1991;**115**:871–6.

33. Kapoor WN, Smith MA, Miller NL. Upright tilt testing in evaluation of syncope: a comprehensive review. *Am J Med* 1994;**97**:78–88.

34. Landau WM, Nelson DA. Clinical neuromythology XV. Feinting science: Neurocardiogenic syncope and collateral vasovagal confusion. *Neurology* 1996;**46**:609–18.

35. Schott GD, McLeod AA, Jewitt DE. Cardiac arrhythmias that masquerade as epilepsy. *Br Med J* 1977;**1**:1454–7.

36. Linzer M, Grubb BP, Ho S, Ramakrishnan L, Bromfield E, Estes M. Cardiovascular causes of loss of consciousness in patients with presumed epilepsy: a cause of increased sudden death rate in people with epilepsy? *Am J Med* 1994;**96**:146–54.

37. Madison D, Niedermeyer E. Epileptic seizures resulting from acute cerebral anoxia. *J Neurol Neurosurg Psychiatry* 1970;**33**:381–6.
38. Guerrini R, Battaglia A, Gastaut H. Absence status triggered by pallid syncopal spells. *Neurology* 1991;**41**:1528–9.
39. Battaglia A, Guerrini R, Gastaut H. Epileptic seizures induced by syncopal attacks. *J Epilepsy* 1989;**2**:141–52.
40. Gastaut H, Zifkin B, Rufo M. Compulsive respiratory stereotypies in children with autistic features: polygraphic recording and treatment with fenfluramine. *J Autism Dev Dis* 1995;**17**: 391–406.
41. Aicardi J, Gastaut H, Mises J. Syncopal attacks compulsively self-induced by Valsalva's maneuver associated with typical absence seizures. *Arch Neurol* 1988;**45**:923–5.
42. Bergey GK, Krumholz A, Fleming CP. Complex partial seizure provocation by vasovagal syncope: Video-EEG and intracranial electrode documentation. *Epilepsia* 1997;**38**:118–21.
43. Kothari SS. When epilepsy masquerades as heart disease. Awareness is key to avoiding misdiagnosis. *Postgrad Med* 1990;**88**:167–71.
44. Oppenheimer SM, Cechetto DF, Hachinski VC. Cerebrogenic cardiac arrhythmias. Cerebral electrocardiographic influences and their role in sudden death. *Arch Neurol* 1990;**47**:513–19.
45. Gilchrist JM. Arrhythmogenic seizures: diagnosis by simultaneous EEG/ECG recording. *Neurology* 1985;**35**:1503–6.
46. Constantin L, Martins JB, Fincham RW, Dagli RD. Bradycardia and syncope as manifestations of partial epilepsy. *J Am Coll Cardiol* 1990;**15**:900–5.
47. Reeves AL, Nollet KE, Klass DW, Sharbrough FW, So EL. The ictal bradycardia syndrome. *Epilepsia* 1996;**37**:983–7.
48. Gambardella A, Reutens DC, Andermann F, et al. Late-onset drop attacks in temporal lobe epilepsy: a reevaluation of the concept of temporal lobe syncope. *Neurology* 1994;**44**:1074–8.

3

Rational diagnosis of non-epileptic seizures

Jürgen Bauer

Introduction

Diagnosis of non-epileptic seizures is established by the verification of the suspected non-epileptic seizure type. Excluding the occurrence of epileptic seizures may help to establish the final diagnosis. However, both epileptic and non-epileptic seizures may occur in the same patient.[1]

A non-epileptic seizure is defined as an attack manifesting with the abrupt onset of disturbed cerebral functioning resulting in an impairment of consciousness or focal (excitatory or inhibitory) neurological symptoms.[2,3] Not surprisingly, clinical symptomatology may mimic an epileptic seizure.

The first step in diagnosis is the physician's clinical impression of the reported or observed seizure(s), an impression based on clinical experience. Published videotapes on epileptic and non-epileptic seizures (e.g. Supplements to *Movement Disorders*) enable physicians to improve their knowledge of the phenomenology of different epileptic and non-epileptic seizure types.

The clinical approach to diagnosis of seizure attacks is different in patients with or without an established neurological, psychiatric or internal disease. Most commonly, reported attacks will occur because of a chronic disease pre-existing in a patient, e.g. epilepsy, migraine, cerebrovascular disease, narcolepsia. Only rarely do two different disorders have to be diagnosed in a patient (e.g. the coincidence of epileptic and psychogenic seizures is observed in 5–20 per cent of patients with intractable epileptic seizures).[4]

Exclusion of epileptic seizures

Apart from anamnesis, the diagnosis of epileptic seizures is based on electro-encephalographic (EEG) monitoring during the interictal, and if possible, the ictal phase of the seizure. Results of EEG monitoring depend on seizure type (idiopathic generalized versus symptomatic focal seizures). Principles of EEG investigations have been published and are not reviewed here.[5,6]

It should be borne in mind that sufficient information about a suspected epileptic seizure sometimes can be drawn from post-ictal investigations (Figure 3.1).[7,8] Especially following tonic–clonic seizures, clinical and laboratory findings may indicate the preceding manifestation of an epileptic seizure.[9] The elevation of creatine kinase and post-ictal EEG findings are strong indicators for the previous manifestation of a grand mal.[7] A transient focal neurological deficit coincident with focal slowing in EEG may indicate a focal seizure. However, a rise in serum prolactin can also be demonstrated following syncope, and tongue biting is also seen after psychogenic seizures or, rarely, due to syncope.[7,9]

Time after seizure				
0–30 min	30 min–24 h	24–48 h	48–72 h	72 h–1 week
Prolactin ↑	–	–	–	–
–	Creatine kinase ↑	Creatine kinase ↑	Creatine kinase ↑	–
Todd's paralysis	Todd's paralysis	–	–	–
Petechiae	Petechiae	Petechiae	Petechiae	–
Tongue bite	Tongue bite	Tongue bite	Tongue bite	Tongue bite
Enuresis/encopresis	–	–	–	–
Abnormal EEG	Abnormal EEG	Abnormal EEG	–	–

Figure 3.1
Diagnostic evaluations for the retrospective evaluation of an epileptic seizure.

Seizures with generalized tonic–clonic motor phenomena

Rhythmic generalized tonic–clonic movements in an unconscious patient are typical phenomena of an epileptic grand mal. However, psychogenic seizures, convulsive syncope and hypoglycaemia may mimic this symptomatology.

Psychogenic seizures

With regard to psychogenic seizures, take the opportunity to monitor seizures by video-EEG in various patients in order to become familiar with the corresponding symptomatology, which is helpful in drawing conclusions from seizure descriptions given by other patients.[10] Published videotapes demonstrating such seizures can also be used to enhance clinical experience.

Some clinical criteria that are helpful in distinguishing epileptic from psychogenic seizures are discussed below.

Duration of seizures

Motor movements in grand mal last approximately 62 s.[11] Grand mal-like psychogenic seizures tend to last several minutes or up to an hour.[10]

Phenomenology of seizures

During grand mal, eyes are usually opened; typically during psychogenic seizures they are closed.[12] This finding may, however, vary during the attack. During psychogenic seizures motor phenomena are irregular, arrhythmic and highly frequent.[10] In grand mal, rhythmic powerful cloni are typically observed.[11]

Clinical course of the disease

A seizure-free interval followed by a newly developed seizure type is very likely for the

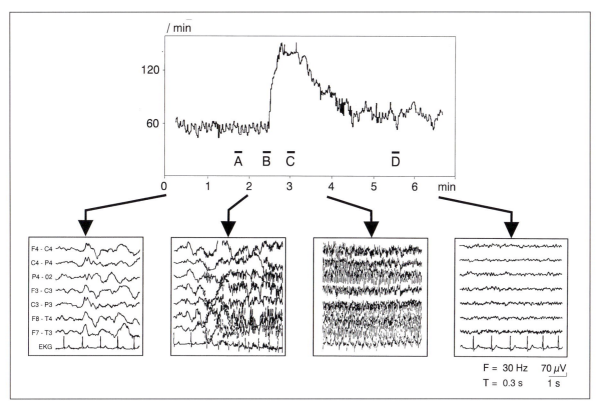

Figure 3.2
Heart rate increase during an epileptic seizure occurring out of sleep (A) documented by ECG and EEG recordings. During the phase of tonic (B)–clonic (C) movements, heart rate increased from 60/min to >120/min. After the seizure, heart rate normalized in the awake patient (D).

diagnosis of psychogenic seizures in a patient who previously suffered from epileptic seizures.[10]

Pitfalls of differential diagnosis
Psychogenic seizures may be observed in patients with abnormal interictal EEG findings (often seen in mentally retarded patients or patients suffering from additional epileptic seizures).[13] Also, cranial magnetic resonance imaging (MRI) may exhibit abnormal findings in such patients (morphology does not necessarily reflect function).[14] Psychogenic seizures

may lead to severe trauma, usually due to an abrupt fall.[10] A seizure manifestation at night does not necessarily mean that the seizure occurred out of sleep (this consequently would exclude psychogenic aetiology of seizures).[10]

Recommended diagnostic procedures
If anamnestic data fail to establish the diagnosis, use the scheme in Figure 3.1. Are there epileptic discharges on post-ictal EEG monitoring?[7] Post-ictal serum prolactin (PRL) can be measured in blood taken 0–30 min after a seizure (increase of serum concentrations is

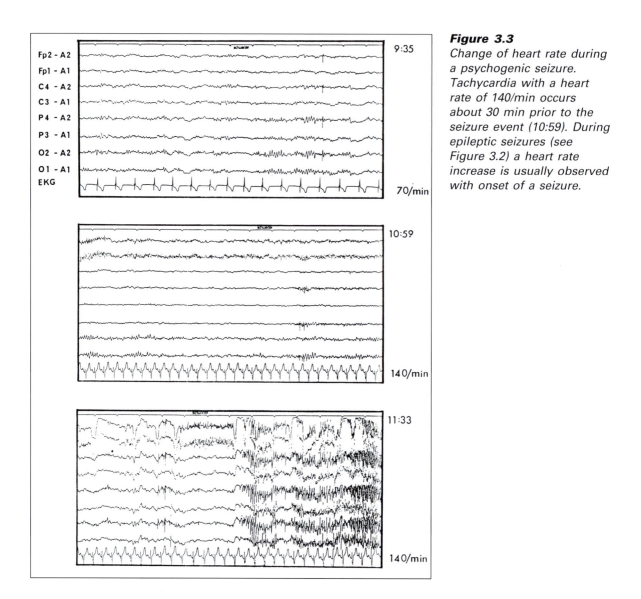

Figure 3.3
Change of heart rate during a psychogenic seizure. Tachycardia with a heart rate of 140/min occurs about 30 min prior to the seizure event (10:59). During epileptic seizures (see Figure 3.2) a heart rate increase is usually observed with onset of a seizure.

observed only in epileptic seizures and syncope).[9]

Post-ictal creatine kinase measurement is typically increased for 12–24 h following a generalized tonic–clonic seizure.[7]

Mobile long-term electroencephalography (MLE) can be carried out. Is there demonstration of epileptic discharges during ictal events?[15] or increase in heart rate during epileptic seizures? (Figures 3.2 and 3.3).[16] Seizure manifestation with onset during sleep excludes psychogenic aetiology.[10]

Suggestive seizure provocation can be performed with simultaneous video-EEG/ECG monitoring. Be sure not to provoke seizures that are untypical for the patient under investigation.[12,17] Demonstration of the recorded seizure to persons who previously observed spontaneous seizures in the patient is recommended. Bazil et al[18] used a saline provocation test in 52 consecutive patients with a tentative diagnosis of epilepsy. In 23 per cent of patients seizures unlike their typical seizures occurred. However, 37 per cent of the patients had typical episodes, reflecting the quantity of patients with psychogenic seizures in an unselected group of patients consulting neurologists about their attacks.

Syncope

Convulsive phenomena during syncope may be mistaken for grand mal (for details see Chapter 2). Usually anamnestic data support the diagnosis.[5,19,20] Aura phenomena are usually (93 per cent in a study by Benke et al[21]) reported in cardiac and vasovagal syncope. Most patients report epigastric, vertiginous, visual or somatosensory experiences. Aura phenomena typically reported in epileptic seizures, such as tastes, smells, déjà vu phenomena, scenic visual perceptions and speech impairments are not observed in syncope.[2]

In epileptic grand mal tonic, posturing is an initial phenomenon of the seizure. In syncope, tonic posturing and mild cloni only occur when asystole lasts longer than 10–15 s, thus, they are observed in the final phase of the attack. However, enuresis and tongue biting have been described, as well as a post-ictal increase of serum prolactin levels.[19]

Interictal EEG monitoring usually does not show abnormal findings in patients with syncope. Gastaut and Fischer-Williams[22] have recorded EEGs during syncope. Following asystole, a stereotyped series of changes occur: after 3–4 s, high-voltage slow activity in the theta range appears. If asystole persists for 8–10 s, slow activity abruptly disappears and the record gets 'flat' unless obscured by tonic electromyographic activity or movement artifact. When cardiac ventricular contractions resume, brain waves reappear in reverse order from their disappearance. In syncope caused by increased intrathoracic pressure the EEG shows generalized slowing, but usually no 'flattening'.[5]

In patients with orthostatic syncope accompanied by dizziness, EEG recordings in erect posture are not helpful in the early stages: subjective dizziness and light-headedness are not associated with significant EEG changes. The same is true for dizziness induced by active or passive head movements. The use of a tilt table is extremely conducive to syncopal manifestations.[23]

Pitfalls of differential diagnosis

In rare cases epileptic seizures may cause asystole induced by spreading epileptic discharges from the temporal lobe to autonomic nuclei (Figure 3.4).[24]

Bergey et al[25] reported on a patient in whom a complex partial seizure was provoked by vasovagal syncope.

Hypoglycaemia

Hypoglycaemia may mimic or induce generalized epileptic seizures, but even complex partial seizures have been reported in a case of insulinoma.[26]

Hypoglycaemia may cause paroxysmal EEG activity that can be confused with seizure activity.[27] The degree of slowing in the EEG combined with epileptic activity may be more or less prominent depending on individual properties.[28] In some patients deep coma and/or major convulsions may occur.[29]

Peri-ictal measurement of blood glucose levels is the most reliable method of establishing this

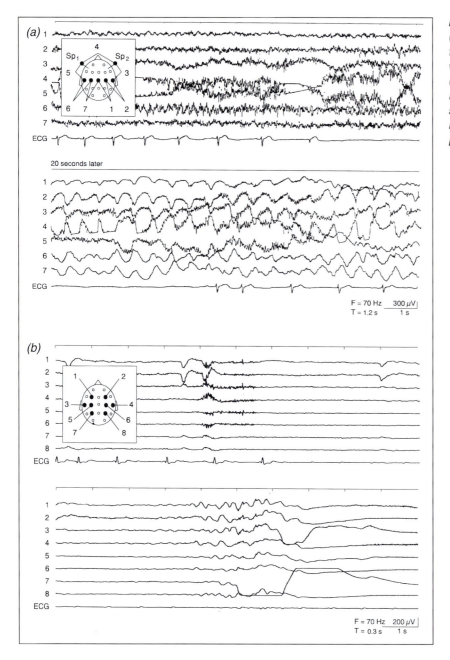

Figure 3.4
(a) Asystole induced by a focal epileptic seizure with left temporal onset. (b) Cardiac asystole resulting in convulsive syncope during which EEG demonstrates paroxysmal slowing.

diagnosis. Phenomena of hypoglycaemia reported by the patients are: sweating, blurred or double vision, confusion, odd behaviour, perioral paresthesia, sensation of cold, tremor, weakness, vertigo, anxiety, hunger, palpitations.[27]

Seizures with focal deficits

Focal epileptic seizures can be mistaken for migraine attacks or transient ischaemic attacks (TIAs) (or vice versa). If EEG fails to establish the diagnosis of a focal epileptic event, differential diagnosis can be difficult in some patients.[5] It is well known that interictal (and even ictal) surface EEG recordings during focal epileptic seizures do not necessarily exhibit focal discharges.[5]

Migraines

A migraine attack is usually characterized by headache, accompanied by focal neurological deficits in the case of migraine accompagnee. Although pain has been described in seizures originating from the parietal lobe this is a rather uncommon phenomenon in epileptic seizures.[30] Studies show that 20–30 per cent of patients with migraine report on auras, developing over 5–20 min, lasting usually <60 min.[31,32] They often occur for periods of an hour, up to several days before the onset of headache.[33,34] Prodromal phenomena include psychological (depression, euphoria, irritability, restlessness, mental slowness, hyperactivity, fatigue and drowsiness), neurological (photophobia, phonophobia and hypersomnia), constitutional and autonomic features.[32,35] Some patients report a poorly characterized feeling that a migraine attack is coming. Although prodromal features vary widely among individuals, they are often consistent within an individual. In migraine, auras usually last longer than 5 min, in epileptic seizures they last <5 min.[36]

EEG performed during migraine aura may show spike activity and may resemble the ictal EEG during an epileptic seizure,[36] apart from the fact that there is no typical propagation or increment in EEG activity as seen in epileptic seizures. In the rare case of recordings made during or shortly after prodromi, EEGs show (a) reduced amplitude or absence of normal rhythms (i.e. alpha or sleep spindles), (b) focal arrhythmic slow activity over the hemisphere appropriate to symptoms, and (c) lateralized or asymmetric rhythmic theta or delta activity.[6] Periodic lateralized epileptiform discharges (PLEDS) may occur in hemiplegic migraine, prolonged migraine aura or incipient migrainous infarction.[37] Patients with common migraine have a normal excess (or, at best, a moderately increased excess) of non-focal theta rhythms in EEG.[38] The EEGs of patients with complex migraine show various abnormalities, determined in part by the severity of symptoms and temporal proximity to prodromi.

Epileptiform discharges are uncommon in migraine, occurring in 8 per cent of cases.[39] Although symptoms in complex migraine may last no longer than 15–45 min, EEG abnormalities resolve slowly over a period of days to a few weeks.[39]

Transient ischaemic attacks

Negative motor phenomena are a possible but rare ictal phenomenon of focal epileptic seizures (more often observed as post-ictal paralysis).[7,40] However, paresis and disturbance of sensory functions usually accompany a transient ischaemic attack (TIA). Common clinical symptoms in carotid TIAs are: sensorimotor phenomena (67–70 per cent), weakness (face, arm or leg; 50–56 per cent), aphasia (45 per cent), sensory phenomena (arm; 44–53 per cent), dysarthria (21–24 per cent), monocular blindness (20–27 per cent).[41] Common symptoms in vertebrobasilar TIAs are: ataxia (60 per cent), vertigo (43 per cent), diplopia (39 per cent), blurred vision (37 per cent), dysarthria (27 per cent).[41] From large series there is evidence that motor symptoms accompany most

TIAs and that typical TIA symptoms are 'negative' (loss of function). Atypical TIA symptoms, possibly mimicking epileptic seizures are: limb-shaking, asterixis, dyskinesia, pure sensory disturbances, speech arrest, visual inversion, auditory hallucinations, anosognosia, akinetic mutism, drop attacks.[42] Most TIAs show rapid onset and brief duration, 24 per cent vanish within 5 min, 39 per cent within 15 min and 50 per cent within 30 min.[43] On average, carotid TIAs last 14 min, while vertebrobasilar TIAs last 8 min.[44]

In a study of 295 patients with TIAs – 270 in carotid territory – EEGs were normal in almost 50 per cent of patients.[45] When abnormal, EEGs showed focal slow wave activity over the appropriate hemisphere. In a patient with apparent TIAs, persistent focal EEG abnormality can signal an infarct. Patients with TIAs in vertebrobasilar territory usually have normal EEGs.[6]

Seizures with drops

Drop attacks may occur with epileptic seizures, syncope, startle reactions and cataplexy. The diagnosis of an epileptic grand mal has been summarized earlier in the chapter. These patients are unconscious, and tonic posturing is an initial phenomenon of the seizure. During syncope, however, tonic posturing is first seen 10–15 s after the loss of consciousness. In startle reactions tonic posturing is related to stimuli, which vary from patient to patient, but are quite constant in a single patient.[30] In some syncopes typical trigger mechanisms (e.g. coughing, micturition) may provoke the attack.[46]

Drops from cataplexy might be mistaken for (myoclonic) astatic seizures in epilepsy. In patients with such epilepsies EEG usually exhibits generalized epileptic discharges, ictally

as well as interictally. Finally, drops in cataplexy are usually triggered by emotion.[47,48]

Cataplexy may occur as the initial or exclusive symptom in patients with the narcolepsia syndrome. All the four typical symptoms (daytime sleepiness, cataplexy, sleep paralysis and hypnagogic hallucinations) occur in only 10 per cent of these patients.[19,49–51] Drops in cataplexy are not as abrupt as in epileptic seizures.

Drop attacks may occur because of vertebrobasilar ischaemia.[52] In a study by Kubala and Millikan[53] this was reported by 29 of 373 patients. Syncope may be related to specific stimuli such as coughing, pressing or micturition. Finally, drop attacks are observed in patients with Parkinson's syndrome or manifest as cryptogenic drop attacks in postmenopausal women.[54,55]

Seizures with transient disturbance of behaviour

Seizures with transient disturbance of behaviour may result from epileptic nonconvulsive status or may reflect parasomnia, psychogenic fugue, narcolepsy, episodic nocturnal wanderings, nocturnal paroxysmal dystonia or transient global amnesia (TGA).

Parasomnias

Parasomnias are undesirable motor, verbal or experiential phenomena that occur during the sleep period. Somnambulism (i.e. clumsy, trance-like behaviour) and night terrors (i.e. intense terror, vocalization, automatic changes) are disorders of arousal, classically occur during the first third of the night, last seconds to minutes and demonstrate a normal waking EEG and paroxysmal slow wave pattern during the event.[51] They might be mistaken for epileptic

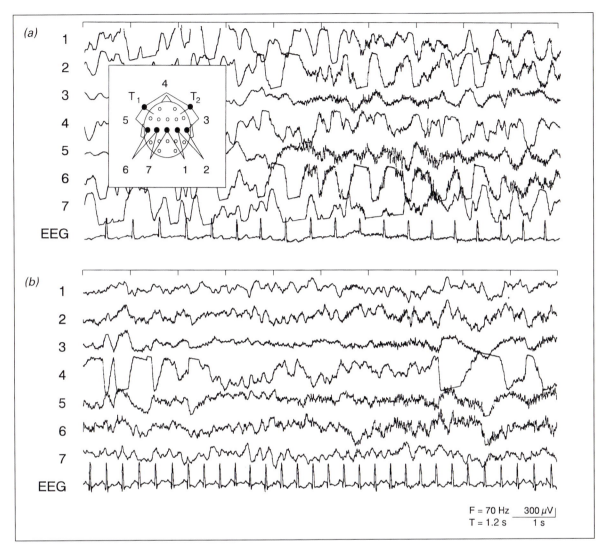

Figure 3.5

(a) EEG taken during sleepwalking. The EEG reveals extremely high amplitude slow waves just preceding the muscular activation and continuing during the first part of the attack. (b) During the attack the sleep stage alters towards stage 2; however, the patient does not wake up during such an attack.

seizures, as about 10 per cent of patients experience epileptic seizures exclusively or predominantly during sleep.[56] If the nocturnal events are ambiguous and occur with a predictable frequency, polysomnography with video-recording will usually permit diagnosis.[57]

Sleepwalking consists of a sequence of complex behaviours that usually occur in the first third of the night during non-REM sleep (sleep stage 3–4). Polysomnography reveals extremely high amplitude EEG slow waves just preceding the muscular activation that ushers in the attack (Figure 3.5).[58] In contrast to nocturnal epileptic seizures, epileptic EEG discharges will not be seen during the episode of sleepwalking. From clinical descriptions it may be difficult to differentiate epileptic seizures from sleepwalking.[59] In some patients this will not be possible without ictal polysomnography.[60]

Narcolepsy

Patients with narcolepsy can show automatic behaviour during which prolonged, complex activities may be performed without conscious awareness or recall.[61–63]

Episodic nocturnal wanderings

Episodic nocturnal wanderings, indistinguishable by history from sleepwalking and sleep terrors, but responding to anticonvulsants, have been described. The patients ambulated, vocalized, and displayed violent behaviour during sleep. Not all exhibited EEG abnormalities in the waking state. There is growing evidence that many of these cases represent epileptic phenomena and are actually ambulatory automatisms.[64–67]

Nocturnal (hypnogenic) paroxysmal dystonia

This is a syndrome characterized by predominantly or exclusively nocturnal episodes of coarse, occasionally violent, movements of limbs associated with tonic spasms, often occurring many times per night. Vocalization or laughter may occur. EEGs between events are normal, and during events they display only movement artifact, without clear evidence of electrical seizure activity.[68,69] Such conditions are thought to be epileptic, possibly of frontal lobe origin.[70,71] Thus, it still remains difficult to establish in all cases of nocturnal paroxysmal dystonia with short-lasting attacks unassociated with epileptic EEG discharges whether they represent a variant of epilepsy or an unrelated paroxysmal disorder.[72,73]

Fugue attacks

During daytime, fugue attacks may reflect psychogenic disturbances of behaviour. Such psychogenic conditions usually last longer than non-convulsive status epilepticus (often days) and patients tend to show spectacular behaviour (e.g. driving a car, having sexual intercourse with strangers).[74] EEG during and after such a fugue is usually normal. Measurement of serum prolactin is not helpful either, as prolactin is not increased even in the course of non-convulsive status epilepticus.[75]

Transient global amnesia

Transient global amnesia may be mistaken for epileptic confusion. However, descriptions of the disorder given by the patients are typical and usually not misleading. There is a more or less sudden onset of severe anterograde amnesia stretching back weeks, months, or longer. The attack lasts several hours. During the attack the patient is fully conscious and has no loss of personal identity. The patient can perform normal everyday activities, but may ask the same question repetitively because of the anterograde amnesia.[76] Finally, ictal EEG will not show epileptiform discharges.

Seizures with generalized myoclonia

There are a variety of types of myoclonus that occur during drowsiness or sleep.[77] Hypnotic jerks might be mixed up with epileptic myoclonia, as occurring in generalized idiopathic seizures. However, the latter seizure type is commonly observed following awakening and has not been described during sleep. Finally, EEG monitoring will exhibit spike–wave patterns in epileptic disorders.[5]

References

1. Ramsay RE, Cohen A, Brown MC. Coexisting epilepsy and non-epileptic seizures. In: Rowan AJ, Gates JR, eds. *Non-epileptic seizures*. Boston: Butterworth-Heinemann, 1993:47–54.

2. Krause KH. Die nichtepileptischen Anfälle. *Nervenarzt* 1984;**55**:507–16.

3. Andermann F. Non-epileptic paroxysmal neurologic events. In: Rowan AJ, Gates JR, eds. *Non-epileptic seizures*. Boston: Butterworth-Heinemann, 1993:111–21.

4. Henry TR, Drury I. Non-epileptic seizures in temporal lobectomy candidates with medically refractory seizures. *Neurology* 1997;**48**:1374–82.

5. Daly DD. Epilepsy and syncope. In: Daly DD, Pedley TA, eds. *Current practice of clinical electroencephalography*. 2nd ed. New York: Raven, 1990:269–334.

6. Daly DD, Markand ON. Focal brain lesions. In: Daly DD, Pedley TA, eds. *Current practice of clinical electroencephalography*. 2nd ed. New York: Raven, 1990:335–70.

7. Bauer J, Elger CE. Objektivierbare Befunde zur retrospektiven Anfallsdiagnostik. *Aktuel Neurol* 1994;**21**:220–3.

8. Bauer J, Güldenberg V, Elger CE. Das 'Forellenphänomen': ein seltenes Symptom epileptischer Anfälle. *Nervenarzt* 1993;**64**:394–5.

9. Bauer J. Epilepsy and prolactin in adults: a clinical review. *Epilepsy Res* 1996;**24**:1–7.

10. Lesser RP. Psychogenic seizures. *Neurology* 1996;**46**:1499–507.

11. Theodore WH, Porter RJ, Albert P, et al. The secondarily generalized tonic-clonic seizure: a videotape analysis. *Neurology* 1994;**44**:1403–7.

12. Flügel D, Bauer J, Käseborn U, Burr W, Elger CE. Closed eyes during a seizure indicate psychogenic etiology: a study with suggestive seizure provocation. *J Epilepsy* 1996;**9**:165–9.

13. Merskey H, Buhrich NA. Hysteria and organic brain disease. *Br J Med Psychol* 1975;**48**: 359–66.

14. Lelliott PT, Fenwick P. Cerebral pathology in pseudoseizures. *Acta Neurol Scand* 1991;**83**: 129–32.

15. Bülau P, Burr W. Die Bedeutung des mobilen Langzeit-EEG und simultanen Doppelbild-Aufzeichnung für die Therapie epileptischer Anfälle. In: Fröscher W, ed. *Aspekte der Epilepsie-Therapie*. Wien Berlin: Ueberreuter Wissenschaft;1989:55–68.

16. Burr W, Bülau P, Elger CE. Does rapid increase in heart rate during sleep support the diagnosis of complex partial seizures? *J Epilepsy* 1994;**7**:321–3.

17. French J. The use of suggestion as a provocative test in the diagnosis of psychogenic non-epileptic seizures. In: Rowan AJ, Gates JR, eds. *Non-epileptic seizures*. Boston: Butterworth-Heinemann, 1993:101–9.

18. Bazil CW, Kothari M, Luciano D, et al. Provocation of non-epileptic seizures by suggestion in a general seizure population. *Epilepsia* 1994;**35**:768–70.

19. Mumenthaler M, ed. *Synkopen und Sturzanfälle*. Stuttgart: Thieme, 1984.

20. Gastaut H. Syncopes: generalized anoxic cerebral seizures. In: Vinken PJ, Bruyn GW, eds. *Handbook of clinical neurology*. Vol 15. Amsterdam: Elsevier, 1974:836–52.

21. Benke TH, Hochleitner M, Bauer G. Aura phenomena during syncope. *Eur Neurol* 1997; **37**:28–32.

22. Gastaut H, Fischer-Williams M. Electroencephalographic study of syncope: its differentiation from epilepsy. *Lancet* 1957;**2**:1018–25.

23. Niedermeyer E. Nonepileptic attacks. In: Niedermeyer E, Lopes Da Silva F, eds. *Electroencephalography*. 3rd ed. Baltimore: Williams & Wilkins, 1993:565–72.

24. Kowalik A, Bauer J, Elger CE. Asystolische Anfälle. *Nervenarzt* 1998;**69**:151–7

25. Bergey GK, Krumholz A, Fleming CP. Complex partial seizure provocation by vasovagal syncope: video-EEG and intracranial electrode documentation. *Epilepsia* 1997;**38**:118–21.

26. Scarpino O, Mauro AM, Del Pesce M. Partial complex seizures and insulinoma: a case report (abstract). *Electroencephalogr Clin Neurophysiol* 1985;**61**:90P.

27. Kaplan PW. Metabolic and endocrine disorders resembling seizures. In: Engel J Jr, Pedley TA, eds. *Epilepsy: a comprehensive textbook*. Philadelphia: Lippincott-Raven, 1997:2661–70.

28. Niedermeyer E. Metabolic central nervous system disorders. In: Niedermeyer E, Lopes Da Silva F, eds. *Electroencephalography*. 3rd ed. Baltimore: Williams & Wilkins, 1993:405–18.

29. Hoefer PFA, Guttmann SA, Sands IJ. Convulsive state and coma in cases of islet cell adenoma of the pancreas. *Am J Psychiatry* 1946;**102**:486–95.

30. Engel J Jr. *Seizures and epilepsy*. Philadelphia: FA Davis, 1989.

31. Silberstein SD, Lipton RB. Migraine. In: Engel J Jr, Pedley TA, eds. *Epilepsy: a comprehensive textbook*. Philadelphia: Lippincott-Raven, 1997:2681–91.

32. Silberstein SD, Young WD. Migraine aura and prodrome. *Semin Neurol* 1995;**15**:175–82.

33. Amery WK, Waelkens J, van den Bergh V. Migraine warnings. *Headache* 1986;**26**:60–6.

34. Blau JN. Migraine prodromes separated from the aura: complete migraine. *BMJ* 1980;**281**: 658–60.

35. Panayiotopoulous CP. Elementary visual hallucinations in migraine and epilepsy. *J Neurol Neurosurg Psychiatry* 1994;**57**:1371–4.

36. Ehrenberg BL. Unusual clinical manifestations of migraine, and 'the borderland of epilepsy' re-explored. *Semin Neurol* 1991;**11**:118–27.

37. Marks DA, Ehrenberg BL. Migraine-related seizures in adults with epilepsy, with EEG correlation. *Neurology* 1993;**43**:2476–83.

38. Slatter KH. Some clinical and EEG findings in patients with migraine. *Brain* 1968;**91**:85–98.

39. Wessely P, Mayr N, Goldenberg G. EEG-Befunde bei komplizierter Migräne. *Z EEG EMG* 1985;**16**:221–6.

40. Guerrini R, Dravet C, Genton P, et al. Epileptic negative myoclonus. *Neurology* 1993;**43**:1078–83.

41. Koudstaal PJ, van Gijn J, Staal P, et al. Diagnosis of TIAs: improvement of interobserver agreement by a checklist in ordinary language. *Stroke* 1986;**17**:723–8.

42. Moroney JT, Sacco RL. Cerebrovascular disorders. In: Engel J Jr, Pedley TA, eds. *Epilepsy: a comprehensive textbook*. Philadelphia: Lippincott-Raven, 1997:2693–704.

43. Levy DE. How transient are transient ischaemic attacks? *Neurology* 1988;**38**:674–7.

44. The Study Group on TIA Criteria and Detection. XI. Transient focal cerebral ischaemia: epidemiological and clinical aspects. *Stroke* 1974;**5**:277–84.

45. Enge S, Lechner H, Logar C, Ladurner G. Clinical value of EEG in transient ischaemic attacks. In: Lechner H, Aranibar A, eds. *EEG and Clinical Neurophysiology*. Amsterdam: Excerpta Medica, 1976:173–80.

46. De Maria AA Jr, Westmoreland BF, Sharbrough FW. EEG in cough syncope. *Neurology* 1984;**34**:371–4.

47. Guillemault C. Narcolepsy syndrome. In: Kryger MH, Roth T, Dement WC, eds. *Principles and practice of sleep medicine*. 2nd ed. Philadelphia: WB Saunders, 1994:549–61.

48. Guillemault C. Idiopathic central nervous system hypersomnia. In: Kryger MH, Roth T, Dement WC, eds. *Principles and practice of sleep medicine*. 2nd ed. Philadelphia: WB Saunders, 1994:562–6.

49. Yoss RE, Daly DD. Criteria for the diagnosis of the narcoleptic syndrome. *Proc Staff Meet Mayo Clin* 1957;**32**:320–8.

50. Daniels LE. Narcolepsy. *Medicine (Baltimore)* 1934;**13**:1–122.

51. Knight F. Syncope in the older patient. Major mechanisms and possible interventions. *Postgrad Med* 1983;**73**:74–80.

52. Kubala M, Millikan C. Diagnosis, pathogenesis and treatment of drop attacks. *Arch Neurol* 1964;**11**:107–13.

53. Mahowald MW, Schenck CH. Sleep disorders. In: Engel J Jr, Pedley TA, eds. *Epilepsy: a comprehensive textbook*. Philadelphia: Lippincott-Raven, 1997:2705–15.

54. Stevens DL, Matthews WB. Cryptogenic drop-attacks: an affliction of women. *BMJ* 1973; I:439–42.

55. Voss R. Klimakterische Blitzsynkopen. Ein Beitrag zur Klinik des Klimakteriums und zur

weiteren Differenzierung der synkopalen Anfälle. *Nervenarzt* 1969;**40**:545–7.

56. Young GB, Blume WT, Wells GA, Mertens WC, Eder S. Differential aspects of sleep epilepsy. *Can J Neurol Sci* 1985;**12**:317–20.

57. Broughton RJ. Polysomnography: principles and applications in sleep and arousal disorders. In: Niedermeyer E, Lopes Da Silva F, eds. *Electroencephalography*. 3rd ed. Baltimore: Williams & Wilkins, 1993:765–802.

58. Keefauver SP, Guillemault C. Sleep terrors and sleepwalking. In: Kryger MH, Roth T, Dement WC, eds. *Principles and practice of sleep medicine*. 2nd ed. Philadelphia: WB Saunders, 1994:567–73.

59. Shouse MN. Epileptic seizure manifestations during sleep. In: Kryger MH, Roth T, Dement WC, eds. *Principles and practice of sleep medicine*. 2nd ed. Philadelphia: WB Saunders, 1994:801–14.

60. Mahowald MW, Schenck CH. Parasomnia purgatory: the epileptic/non-epileptic parasomnia interface. In: Rowan AJ, Gates JR, eds. *Non-epileptic seizures*. Boston: Butterworth-Heinemann, 1993:123–39.

61. Aldrich MS. The neurobiology of narcolepsy. *Prog Neurobiol* 1992;**41**:538–41.

62. Gambardella A, Reutens DC, Andermann F, et al. Late-onset drop attacks in temporal lobe epilepsy: a reevaluation of the concept of temporal syncope. *Neurology* 1994;**44**:1074–8.

63. Lee H, Lerner A. Transient inhibitory seizures mimicking crescendo TIAs. *Neurology* 1990;**40**:165–6.

64. Drake MEJ. Cursive and cursing epilepsy. *Neurology* 1984;**34**:267.

65. Halbreich U, Assael M. Electroencephalogram with sphenoidal needles in sleepwalkers. *Psychiatr Clin* 1979;**11**:213–8.

66. Maselli RA, Rosenberg RS, Spire JS. Episodic nocturnal wanderings in non-epileptic young patients. *Sleep* 1988;**11**:156–61.

67. Pedley TA, Guillemault C. Episodic nocturnal wanderings responsive to anticonvulsant drug therapy. *Ann Neurol* 1977;**2**:30–5.

68. Lugaresi E, Cirignotta F, Montagna P. Nocturnal paroxysmal dystonia. *J Neurol Neurosurg Psychiatry* 1986;**49**:375–80.

69. Montplaisir J, Godbout R, Rouleau I. Hypnogenic paroxysmal dystonia: nocturnal epilepsy or sleep disorder? *Sleep Res* 1985;**14**:193.

70. Meierkord H, Fish DR, Smith SJM, Scott CA, Shorvon SD, Marsden CD. Is nocturnal paroxysmal dystonia a form of frontal lobe epilepsy? *Mov Disord* 1992;**1**:38–42.

71. Tinuper P, Cerullo A, Cirignotta F, Cortelli P, Lugaresi E, Montagna P. Nocturnal paroxysmal dystonia with short-lasting attacks: three cases with evidence for an epileptic frontal lobe origin of seizures. *Epilepsia* 1990;**31**:549–56.

72. Lugaresi E, Montagna P, Cirignotta F. Nocturnal paroxysmal dystonia. In: Kryger MH, Roth T, Dement WC, eds. *Principles and practice of sleep medicine*. 2nd ed. Philadelphia: WB Saunders, 1994:815–7.

73. Fahn S. Movement disorders. In: Engel J Jr, Pedley TA, eds. *Epilepsy: a comprehensive textbook*. Philadelphia: Lippincott-Raven, 1997:2725–38.

74. Flügel D, Bauer J, Elger CE. Kriterien zur Differenzierung epileptischer und psychogener Fugue-Zustände. *Epilepsie-Blätter* 1995;**8**:39–41.

75. Bauer J, Uhlig B, Schrell U, Stefan H. Exhaustion of post-ictal serum prolactin release during status epilepticus. *J Neurol* 1992;**239**:175–6.

76. Warlow C. Disorders of cerebral circulation. In: Walton J. ed. *Brain's diseases of the nervous system*. 10th ed. Oxford: Oxford University Press, 1993:197–268.

77. Hallett M. Myoclonus and myoclonic syndromes. In: Engel J Jr, Pedley TA, eds. *Epilepsy: a comprehensive textbook*. Philadelphia: Lippincott-Raven, 1997:2717–23.

4

Epileptic seizures progressing into non-epileptic conversion seizures

Orrin Devinsky and Elisabeth Gordon

Introduction

Non-epileptic seizures (NES or psychogenic seizures) are common, occurring in approximately 20 per cent of epilepsy monitoring unit admissions and up to 40 per cent of seizure patients in general neurology clinics.[1–3] The clinical appearance of NES can closely resemble epileptic seizures. However, NES result from non-conscious psychological processes that convert psychic conflict into symbolic somatic symptoms for primary or secondary gain while simultaneously preventing conscious awareness of the intent. Common precipitating factors for NES include sexual and physical abuse, other major life stressors, or minor head trauma with claims for disability,[4,5] although frequently neither the provocative factor nor the mechanisms underlying the conversion symptoms are readily identified.

In this chapter, we will review the diagnosis of NES and the historical basis for the association of epilepsy and hysteria. We will then discuss the clinical entity of NES occurring during or immediately after epileptic seizures in the context of the pathophysiology of conversion symptoms.

Diagnosis of NES

The diagnosis of NES can present a challenge to the physician because the clinical features can mimic diverse forms of epileptic seizures. No single feature is pathognomonic of NES. Generalized convulsive or focal motor movements and subjective symptoms (e.g. episodic sensory and experiential phenomena) are all part of the wide clinical spectrum of NES. The clinical diagnosis of NES is difficult and has traditionally relied on identifying bizarre or atypical paroxysmal behavioral changes, especially in patients with known psychological or psychiatric disorders. The understanding of the behavioral spectrum of epileptic and non-epileptic seizures has been radically transformed by information obtained from video-electro-encephalogram (EEG) monitoring. Consequently, video-EEG recording of spontaneous or suggestion-induced NES events is a valuable and reliable diagnostic procedure.[6,7]

The historical features traditionally associated with NES are a histrionic (hysterical) personality style, la belle indifference (unconcern for deficits or problems), depression, anxiety disorder, and a history of physical or sexual abuse. However, these features are neither exclusive to nor always found in NES patients. While identification of these historical features can help elucidate the etiology of the conversion symptoms and may impact treatment, these features alone cannot reliably distinguish NES from epileptic seizures. Furthermore, although the presence of one or more historical features may raise the suspicion of NES, their diagnostic value is reduced by the co-occurrence in many patients of NES and epilepsy or of epileptic seizures and psycho-pathology.

Issues of primary or secondary gain are often identified in NES patients, but may be absent in patients with NES and present in those with epileptic seizures. Primary gain occurs when the elaboration of the NES allows the patient to express an internal need or conflict that has been suppressed from becoming conscious. For example, after being raped, the patient's anger and fear may be symbolically expressed as a seizure. Secondary gain occurs when the NES are a means of gaining support from people or social services that the patient might otherwise not obtain. Alternatively, the NES may allow the patient to avoid an unpleasant situation. In many cases, the psychic mechanism underlying psychogenic seizures is never identified, because patients may be extremely resistant to psychological or psychiatric intervention. In those cases where the underlying mechanism contributing to conversion symptoms remains undefined, psychiatric intervention can be helpful.

The common belief that a history of seizures triggered by emotional factors supports the diagnosis of NES is not substantiated by clinical data.[8] More patients with epileptic than non-epileptic seizures report that emotional stress provokes seizures. Uncontrolled seizures despite high dosages of an antiepileptic drug (AED) or multiple AEDs, or frequent emergency room visits or hospitalizations should suggest the possible diagnosis of NES; but these factors are also quite consistent with medically refractory epileptic seizures. An atypical emotional reaction to a seizure (i.e. unconcern after a 'convulsive episode' or excessive crying) can suggest NES, but is also non-specific. For example, some patients with tonic–clonic seizures have little awareness of the seizures, especially if they occur during sleep and are not associated with tongue biting or other physical trauma. Conversely, NES can be associated with self-inflicted or accidental injuries. A history of physical or emotional abuse or psychiatric disorders is more common among patients with NES than epileptic seizures, but may also occur in patients with epileptic seizures. In the past, attacks which occurred during sleep were often considered to be epileptic or a sleep disorder; however, it is now clear that NES can occur during apparent sleep.[9]

Psychiatric disorders other than conversion can cause NES.[10] Among these, anxiety disorders are most common, followed by all forms of psychotic disorders and impulse control problems associated with attention deficit disorder. This non-conversion NES group of patients does not show a female predominance (as in the conversion group) and is significantly less likely to be characterized by physical or sexual abuse in childhood or adolescence compared with conversion NES patients. Malingering is difficult to distinguish from a conversion disorder, especially in cases with secondary gains involving employment, disability or litigation. Intentional (malingering) and unconscious (conversion) mechanisms probably co-exist in many patients. For instance, patients with risk factors for NES may sustain head trauma or other stressors for which they seek legal compensation. In such cases, both the susceptibility to post-traumatic stress disorder as well as the possibility of legal compensation may be important.

Epilepsy and hysteria

Throughout history, seizures have been closely linked to hysteria. Hippocrates distinguished hysterical from epileptic convulsions by apply-ing digital pressure to the patient's abdomen. If the patient perceived the pressure, the disorder was classified as hysteria, if not, the diagnosis was epilepsy. The modern history of hysteria and epilepsy began with Willis. In 1684, he was the first to suggest that hysteria was a disorder of brain function and he emphasized the association between epilepsy and hysteria, speculating that both disorders shared a similar mechanism.[11] The co-existence of hysteria (conversion disorder) and epilepsy within the same patient was first recognized in 1836 by Beau.[12] Shortly afterwards, Esquirol[13] observed 'hysteric patients who are at the same time epileptics. . . With a little practice one could recognize very well, when the attacks are separate, to which of the two diseases the convulsions belong to which the patient is actually prey.' Around the same time, Landouzy[14] postulated 'the coexistence of two neuroses, with distinct attacks', to which he gave the name 'hystero-epilepsy with separate crises.' Subsequently, the co-existence of the two disorders was discussed by Trousseau,[15] Dostoyevsky,[16] D'Olier[17] and Gowers,[18] with attention focused on differentiating the two types of seizures. Perhaps the greatest contri-bution was made by Charcot, who described four patterns of co-existent hysteria and epilepsy: (1) hysteria supervening in a patient already epileptic, (2) epilepsy supervening in a patient already hysteric, (3) convulsive hysteria co-existing with epileptic vertigo, and (4) epilepsy developing upon the results of hyste-ria, non-convulsive (e.g. contracture, anesthe-sia) (quoted by D'Olier).[17] The most common pattern of the dual diagnosis is a patient with epilepsy who subsequently develops NES.[3]

Studies show that 10–45 per cent of patients with NES have a history of current or past epileptic seizures.[3,19–21] Much of the variance in the reported range of the NES patients who also have a history of epileptic seizures reflects inclusion criteria — e.g. evidence of active epilepsy versus past history of epileptic seizures, evidence to support epilepsy (e.g. spikes versus well-documented epileptic seizures). In a patient with co-existing epilepsy and NES, the features of the NES usually differ from those of the patient's typical epileptic seizure[3] and often occur as multiple types of different events. However, the overall character of the NES may be similar to a patient's epilep-tic seizures. For example, if the patient experi-ences tonic–clonic seizures, the NES may mimic a tonic–clonic seizure.

An epileptic seizure that is functionally elaborated into a conversion seizure was first suggested by Gowers,[18] who presented a case in which a minor seizure was elaborated into a conversion seizure. Recently, Kapur and colleagues[22] reported three patients studied with depth electrodes in whom hippocampal electrographic discharges were followed by psychogenic unresponsiveness (Table 4.1). We studied three patients with video-EEG record-ings in whom non-epileptic seizures developed during or immediately after an epileptic seizure. In contrast to those reported by Kapur et al, these NES included motor features and mimicked complex partial seizures with automatisms (Table 4.2).

Case reports

Case 1

A 12-year-old girl who had had medically refractory partial seizures since the age of eight was referred for presurgical evaluation. She had video-EEG-documented epileptic and non-epileptic seizures with numerous admissions to multiple epilepsy centers, and >50 emergency room visits. High doses of four AED drugs given as monotherapy or polytherapy, with high serum concentrations, had been used over

Patient no.	Age and sex	Type of epilepsy	Psychiatric diagnosis	EEG or invasive electrodes	Features of epileptic seizures	Features of NES
1	22F	Partial epilepsy	Non-psychotic depression and conversion disorder with NES	• Right hippocampal seizures with spread to multiple bilateral sites during the behavioral epileptic seizure • Right hippocampal subclinical electrographic discharges	• 6 CPS: (60–100 s) epigastric sensation and auditory and visual illusions, impaired consciousness and oral and hand movements • Amnestic for the events • 37 electrographic hippocampal seizures that were subclinical or auras	• Onset after hippocampal seizure (5 min, 26 s), • Flaccid and unresponsive to noxious stimuli • Amnestic for events
2	21F	Partial epilepsy	Mild depression and conversion disorder with NES	• Left hippocampal onset with bilateral spread on frontotemporal depth and subdural electrodes in epileptic seizure • Left hippocampal activity during subclinical seizures	• 5 CPS: (<50 s) characterized by dizziness, impaired consciousness and non-stereotyped automatisms involving all limbs • Amnestic for the events • 34 electrographic hippocampal seizures were subclinical or auras	• Onset after hippocampal seizure (60 s) • Motionless and unresponsive • Amnestic for the events
3	34F	Partial epilepsy	Chronic anxiety, irritability, conversion disorder with NES	• CPS right hippocampal onset with aura, spreading to bilateral frontotemporal electrodes • Left hippocampal and temporal pole activity in one seizure preceding psychogenic unresponsiveness • Unilateral hippocampal activity during subclinical seizures (depth electrodes)	• 8 CPS: (1 min duration) aura of déjà vu and micropsia, nonsense speech and later oral automatisms • 145 unilateral hippocampal electrographic seizures that were subclinical or auras	• Onset after hippocampal seizure (40 s) • Motionless and unresponsive • Amnestic for the event

Abbreviations: EEG, electro-encephalogram; M, male; F, female; R, right; L, left; NES, non-epileptic seizure; CPS, complex partial seizure.

Table 4.1
Clinical features of Kapur's[22] patients with partial seizures temporally associated with non-epileptic seizures.

Patient no.	Age and sex	Type of epilepsy	Psychiatric diagnosis	EEG or invasive electrodes	Imaging studies	Features of epileptic seizures	Features of NES
1	12F	Partial epilepsy	Conversion disorder with NES	Right frontotemporal and parietal rhythmic 5.5 Hz ictal (surface EEG) theta discharge	MRI-right frontoparietal cortical dysplasia	• Simple partial seizures of 90 s duration • Continuous automatisms: repeatedly struck bed with left fist and writhed from side to side	• 10.5 min • Motor activity would stop and start again • Punching and hitting move-ments (see text)
2	62M	Partial epilepsy	Conversion disorder with NES	Right frontotemporal rhythmic ictal 2–3 Hz delta activity persisted through NES (surface EEG)	MRI-enhancing tumor without mass effect in right fronto-temporal region	• Simple partial seizures of fear that occasionally generalized	• 20 s • Bizarre, complex, purposeful motor activity (e.g. held bed-rails and shook wildly while verbally responsive)
3	36M	Partial epilepsy	Conversion disorder with NES	Right frontopolar, orbitofrontal and anterior temporal basal rhythmic theta activity (subdural EEG)	Initial MRI — increased signal in both mesial temporal regions and right orbitofrontal region suggesting encephalitis	• 30–45 s • Axial movements, clonic lower extremity movements, right hand automatisms and moaning, verbally unresponsive	• 7 events characterized by 5–25 min unresponsiveness, rapid breathing, turning to either side, repetitive flexion of both arms, stiffening, fetal position and moaning

Abbreviations: EEG, electro-encephalogram; M, male; F, female; NES, non-epileptic seizure; MRI, magnetic resonance imaging.

Table 4.2
Clinical features of case reports described in text of partial seizures temporally associated with non-epileptic seizures.

the preceding 4 years. Current seizure frequency averaged three per week. Attacks were characterized by auditory hallucinations of a male voice, vertigo, hand automatisms, screaming and impairment of consciousness. Episodes usually lasted 2–3 min, but occasionally lasted longer than 10 min.

The patient had been subjected to repeated sexual abuse by a cousin two summers before presentation. MRI revealed right frontoparietal cortical dysplasia, with thickened cortex around the sensorimotor and posterior parietal cortices.

Several complex partial seizures and two NES were recorded with video-EEG monitoring.

During one partial seizure, she said, 'oh, no, here it comes.' She then repeatedly struck the bed with her left hand, which was held in a fisted position and called, 'no, no, no.' Subsequently she began to writhe from side to side screaming 'stop it, stop it' and to bang even more forcibly. During the event, she 'appeared to be fighting off an assailant' according to the nurse who witnessed the event and by independent analysis of the videotape. At the time when she was unresponsive and saying 'here it comes,' there was a rhythmic 5.5 Hz theta discharge over the right frontotemporal and parietal regions. Subsequently, a normal background returned (between intermixed muscle and movement artifact) and for 10.5 min she displayed punching and hitting movements that differed from those associated with the ictal EEG discharge. These 'fighting off' movements and her saying 'stop it, stop it' (which were similar to her isolated NES), would stop and then restart, and could be both provoked and terminated by suggestive techniques.

During another video-EEG-documented spell, a simple partial seizure of her stereotypic auditory aura progressed to a complex partial seizure which further evolved into a NES. This interpretation was supported by the following observations: (1) presence of the definite rhythmic theta (overlying her dysplastic cortex) during the simple and complex partial seizure portions, (2) absence of EEG changes during the non-epileptic portion, (3) stopping and starting again of motor activity during the non-epileptic portion in contrast to the continuous automatisms during the many stereotypic epileptic events, (4) the 90-s duration of the partial seizure activity and the non-epileptic component that continued for 10.5 min, and (5) the ability of suggestive techniques to reproduce and stop behaviors that were identical to her non-epileptic events.

Case 2

A 62-year-old man with a right frontotemporal glioma, treated with chemotherapy and radiation therapy, had both partial seizures and atypical seizures strongly suggestive of NES. Neurological examination revealed behavioral disinhibition with loud and excessive speech discourse. There was impaired dexterity in the left hand and increased left-sided deep tendon reflexes. MRI revealed an enhancing tumor in the right frontotemporal region, without mass effect.

During the video-EEG monitoring three types of seizures were recorded: epileptic, simple partial and secondarily generalized tonic–clonic; spontaneous conversion non-epileptic (CNES); and non-epileptic induced and terminated by suggestion and by normal saline injection, and characterized by complex, purposeful motor activities. One ictal event was notable: a simple partial seizure with electrographic changes during which the patient concurrently experienced a conversion seizure. At the onset the patient complained to the nurse of fear and the EEG registered rhythmic 2–3 Hz delta activity over the right frontotemporal region, which was not present on his baseline EEG. The EEG activity persisted throughout the simple partial seizure with no additional abnormal EEG changes during the conversion event. As the patient continued to speak to the nurse, he experienced a conversion event in which he held both bed-rails, shook wildly from side to side for 20 s, then asked the nurse, 'Did you see that?'. Subsequently, the ictal discharge waxed and waned for six min, and then the prolonged simple partial seizure progressed to a secondarily generalized tonic–clonic seizure. The conversion seizure that occurred during the simple partial seizure was similar to other, isolated CNES.

Case 3

A 36-year-old right-handed man was referred for presurgical evaluation. He had been well until 18 months earlier, when he developed subacute onset of lethargy, agitation, tonic–clonic seizures and confusion followed by unresponsiveness. A lymphocytic pleocytoisis in his spinal fluid and bilateral increased signal in both mesial temporal regions and the right orbitofrontal region strongly suggested encephalitis. Extensive serological and spinal fluid tests for viral pathogens were negative. He was treated with acyclovir. He developed refractory partial epilepsy, with approximately three complex partial seizures per day despite treatment with multiple AEDs, used alone and in combination.

Video-EEG monitoring studies at another epilepsy centre revealed partial seizures with bilateral EEG changes occurring more than 30 s after the onset of prominent axial movements and right arm automatisms. In addition, numerous atypical episodes (e.g. curling into a fetal position and moaning for 30 min) occurred that were not associated with EEG changes. These events were diagnosed as NES. Repeat scalp/sphenoidal video-EEG monitoring at our center supported the diagnosis of co-existing epileptic and non-epileptic seizures.

After initiation of psychotherapy and psychopharmacotherapy, the patient underwent evaluation with bilateral subdural strip electrodes, with extensive coverage over both temporal and frontal regions. Six typical partial seizures were recorded. Electrographic onset was characterized by rhythmic theta activity over right frontopolar, orbitofrontal and anterior temporal basal regions. Clinically, the seizures consisted of axial movements, clonic lower extremity movements, right hand automatisms and moaning. The patient was unresponsive during the seizures, which lasted 30–45 s. He also had five prolonged events (>5 min) which were not associated with EEG changes and had atypical features. These NES consisted of prolonged unresponsiveness, rapid breathing, turning to either side, repetitive flexion of both arms, assuming a fetal position and moaning.

Two events documented on the subdural strip recordings revealed rhythmic theta discharges arising from the right anteromesial temporal and orbitofrontal regions lasting 10–20 s, during which time the patient pressed the event button to indicate a 'feeling.' Following the offset of the EEG discharge he became unresponsive, stiffened, developed rapid and labored breathing, right or left arm tremors, and made intermittent choking sounds for 8–12 min. These were clinically and electrographically consistent with NES.

Partial seizures: elaboration into non-epileptic seizures

As these three cases illustrate, conversion NES can occur almost immediately after or during epileptic seizures, suggesting that the experience of having a seizure can, in susceptible individuals, provoke a NES. However, in most patients with co-existing epileptic and non-epileptic seizures, the two different types of attack are clinically and temporally distinct.[3] In all three of the cases described above the conversion symptoms developed during the epileptic seizure or within seconds of seizure offset. Each patient had partial epilepsy with right temporal or right hemispheric foci. We found no personal or literature cases in which conversion symptoms were followed by epileptic seizures, other than the possible cases reported by Gowers[18] and D'Olier,[17] and Kapur's recent cases.[22]

Gowers[18] first reported hysteria developing as an elaboration of a simple partial seizure or during the post-ictal period. He described patients passing 'into a condition of hysteroid convulsion' during the 'dazed' state after complex partial ('petit mal') and, less often, after tonic–clonic seizures. His cases probably include post-ictal confusional states with agitation and disinhibited behavior, as well as post-ictal NES. Gowers also described patients with attacks intermediate between epilepsy and hysteria, 'in which the characters of the two forms are combined at the same time, and are not merely associated in consecutive development.'

Kapur and colleagues[22] reported three patients with documented partial seizures originating in the hippocampus in whom depth electrode recordings documented an electrographic discharge limited to the hippocampus and temporal pole followed by unresponsiveness that was presumed to be a psychogenic elaboration of a simple partial seizure. Two of the patients reported a typical aura during the EEG discharge that preceded the unresponsiveness. These events of impaired responsiveness were clinically atypical and were not associated with automatisms or depth EEG changes. Each patient had one event; the events lasted 20 s, 60 s, and 326 s respectively. The authors suggest individual predisposition to conversion symptoms, the stressful hospital setting and the ictal discharge as contributing factors to the psychogenic episodes.

In our cases, the temporal proximity of epileptic and non-epileptic seizures may be either coincidental or pathogenically related. However, the infrequent occurrence of partial seizures in these three patients and the occurrence of NES during or immediately after the epileptic event strongly suggest a pathogenic relationship. In case 1, the patient's complex partial seizures often involved screaming. Ictal activation of limbic vocalization and emotional areas may have triggered memories of prior rape, leading to the conversion symptoms of vocally and physically 'fighting off an assailant.' In case 2, ictal fear superimposed on the right hemisphere dysfunction with prominent interictal behavioral disinhibition may have facilitated the elaboration of conversion symptoms. The event in which patient 2 held the bed-rails and shook wildly was not consistent with a frontal lobe complex seizure. The atypical features of well-preserved responsiveness and memory, lack of EEG changes, attention-seeking statements, and marked difference compared with his stereotypic partial seizures support the diagnosis of NES.

Pathophysiology of conversion symptoms

What non-conscious process mediates conversion symptoms and which anatomic structures and networks are activated and inhibited? The pathophysiology of conversion disorder may best be approached simultaneously from dynamic and neurological perspectives, as Charcot attempted.

The understanding of the pathogenesis of conversion disorder has advanced little since Janet postulated dissociation and Freud conceived conversion as the relevant mechanisms. Extensive discussion of psychodynamic factors and of issues related to primary and secondary gain has not provided a scientific framework to refute or prove these hypotheses. Risk factors for conversion disorder, including female sex, physical or sexual abuse, other emotional traumas and mild head injury are well defined.[23–27] However, the cognitive and cerebral processes that transform a stressful life event to physical symptoms produced outside of conscious awareness remain mysterious.

Conversion disorder reflects an impairment of emotional regulation, manifesting as a simultaneous restriction in the conscious fields of attention, memory, and emotions, and excessive involvement of non-conscious processes in behavioral expression. Conversion or somatic symptoms are manifestations of previously suppressed emotional memories and are produced 'intentionally' by non-conscious networks. These networks may actively prevent conscious awareness of the intent, or the failure to recognize non-consciously generated behavior may reflect neurological impairment. Patients typically perceive their symptoms as spontaneous and 'organic', often rejecting the 'psychological' explanation.

The mechanisms by which a partial seizure triggers or contributes to a psychogenic NES remain uncertain, but may involve factors associated with the development of conversion disorder (e.g. prior psychiatric disorders, emotional traumas, or current stressors) as well as organic factors (e.g. underlying brain dysfunction or ictal discharge). Bennett, in 1878,[28] recognized that patients with neurological disorders have an increased frequency of conversion disorder.[29–31] Conversion symptoms can develop in patients with neurological disorders such as epilepsy, traumatic brain injury, and multiple sclerosis.[29–32] Neurological disorders may predispose to conversion symptoms by illness-induced stress. However, the lack of a similar association between serious non-neurological medical disorders (e.g. heart failure or cancer) and conversion symptoms suggests that physical illness is not the principal factor. Alternatively, impaired cerebral regulation of emotion, impulse control and self-monitoring may contribute to the elaboration of conversion symptoms. Therefore, neurological disorders that impair emotional or self-monitoring functions, such as seizures, may contribute to the manifestation of conversion symptoms.

The right hemisphere is dominant in emotional perception and expression.[33,34] While both frontal lobes are critical in self-monitoring and mediating behavioral inhibition,[35–37] the right frontal lobe may dominate in controlling impulses.[35,37] The right hemisphere may often express emotional behaviors without conscious awareness. For example, in our daily behavior, we say and do things that are self-generated, but the psychological motivation (which may be readily apparent to a family member) is not recognized, or is recognized only in hindsight. Lack of awareness for motivations and mechanisms underlying emotional feelings and actions may result from processes occurring outside conscious awareness or from active suppression of conscious awareness.

The emotional network centered in the right hemisphere may repress or positively redirect traumatic experiences and memories. Further, right hemisphere dysfunction can impair conscious awareness of (1) body parts, (2) neurological deficits (e.g. anosognosia), (3) sensory input, and (4) emotional and (5) social cues.[38] This would suggest that pathological involvement of the right hemisphere might be critical in conversion disorder.[38] Notably, all of our cases had right hemisphere onset seizures.

In a personal observation of a consecutive series of conversion NES patients, right hemisphere lesions outnumbered left hemisphere lesions 32 to 9 (78 per cent; $p<0.05$). Right hemisphere lesions may simultaneously impair the capacity to 'process' negative emotions and maintain awareness of the disordered somatic (e.g. anosognosia) and self-generated (e.g. conversion) disorders. The failure to recognize non-consciously produced conversion symptoms may reflect both active inhibition and impairment of perceptual modules.

In 1859, Briquet[39] observed that 'there are three left-sided hysterical anesthetics existing for every right-sided one.' Further research has shown that there is a preponderance of left body symptoms in conversion disorder, hypochondriasis and somatiform rheumatic pain.[40,41] Similar findings were reported in large clinical experiences[42–45] and in recent reviews and clinical studies.[46–48] The left-sided symptom preference is not explained by the least functional deficit — the 'most convenient symptom' (non-dominant) theory — as both right- and left-handed patients show the same preponderance of left-sided conversion symptoms.[49]

Modern imaging techniques can also help to define the functional anatomy of conversion. A positron emission tomography study of script-driven imagery in patients with post-traumatic stress disorder[50] revealed that during traumatic script recall, blood flow increased in right hemisphere limbic, paralimbic and visual areas. When a woman with left-sided conversion paralysis attempted to move her weak left leg, she failed to activate the right primary motor cortex, but activated right orbitofrontal and anterior cingulate cortex.[51] This suggests that these two areas inhibit prefrontal (willed) effects on the right primary motor cortex when the patient tries to move her left leg.

The observation that right hemisphere disorders can facilitate the development of conversion symptoms does not imply that the conversion symptoms arise exclusively from the right hemisphere. Conversion symptoms can occur in patients with unilateral dominant hemisphere or bihemispheric lesions,[52] suggesting that dysfunction outside the non-dominant hemisphere can also contribute to the development of conversion symptoms. A purely organic pathogenesis is unlikely in most conversion patients, as the disorder often develops in young women exposed to adverse environmental influences or personality development without the co-occurrence of neurological disease. However, in many of these patients, excessive effects of, or impaired capacities to process, negative emotional stimuli by the right hemisphere may contribute to conversion symptom development.

Summary

Simple partial seizures may trigger or be temporally linked with subsequent non-epileptic seizures. The three patients described in the case reports had video-EEG-documented partial seizures that were temporally related to non-epileptic seizures which started either during or immediately following the epileptic seizure. These cases support Gowers' (1885)[18] assertion that minor seizures can elaborate into hysterical seizures. In each patient, the partial seizures arose from right frontotemporal regions. In these patients, epileptic seizures were infrequent and the temporally associated conversion attack was probably triggered or caused, in part, by the preceding seizure. Ictal activation of emotions or disruption of impulse control and self-monitoring may have contributed to these non-epileptic events.

References

1. Rowan AJ, Gates JR. *Non-epileptic seizures.* Boston: Butterworth-Heinemann, 1993.

2. Bazil CW, Kothari M, Luciano D, et al. Provocation of non-epileptic seizures by suggestion in a general seizure population. *Epilepsia* 1994;**35**:768–70.

3. Devinsky O, Sanchez-Villasenor F, Vasquez B, Kothari M, Alper K, Luciano D. Clinical profile of patients with epileptic and non-epileptic seizures. *Neurology* 1996;**46**:1530–3.

4. Alper K, Devinsky O, Perrine K, Vazquez B, Luciano D. Nonepileptic seizures and childhood sexual and physical abuse. *Neurology* 1993;**43**:1950–3.

5. Barre E, Krumholz A, Bergey GK, et al. Nonepileptic seizures following head injury. *Epilepsia* 1998;**39**:427–31.

6. Luther JS, McNamara JO, Carwile S, Miller P, Hope V. Pseudoepileptic seizures: methods and video analysis to aid diagnosis. *Ann Neurol* 1982;**12**:458–62.

7. Walczak TS, Williams DT, Berten W. Utility and reliability of placebo infusion in the evaluation of patients with seizures. *Neurology* 1994;**44**:394–9.

8. Luciano D, Perrine K, Clayton B, Devinsky O. Stress as a seizure precipitant and its relationship to ictal focus. *Epilepsia* 1992;**33**(Suppl 3):130.

9. Thacker K, Devinsky O, Perrine K, Alper K, Luciano D. Nonepileptic seizures during apparent sleep. *Ann Neurol* 1993;**33**:414–8.

10. Alper K, Devinsky O, Perrine K, Luciano D. Psychiatric classification of nonconversion nonepileptic seizures. *Arch Neurol* 1995;**52**:199–201.

11. Veith I. *Hysteria: the history of the disease.* Chicago, IL: University of Chicago Press, 1965.

12. Beau B. Recherches statistiques pour servir a l'histoire de l'epilepsie et de l'hysterie. *Arch Generales Medecine* (2e serie) 1836;**11**:328–52.

13. Esquirol E. *Des maladies mentales.* Vol I. Paris: J S Chaude, 1838: 284.

14. Landouzy H. *Trait de l'hysterie.* Paris: J B & G Balliere, 1846.

15. Trousseau A. *Clinique medicale de l'Hotel-Dieu de Paris.* 3rd ed. Vol II. Paris, 1868. Cited by D'Olier.

16. Dostoyevsky F. *The brothers Karamzov.* (Translated by D. Magarshack). Harmondsworth: Penguin Books, 1881:712.

17. D'Olier M. On the coexistence of hysteria and epilepsy, with distinct manifestations of two neuroses. *Alienist Neurologist* 1882;**3**:178–93.

18. Gowers WR. Attacks intermediate between hysteria and epilepsy. In: *Epilepsy: borderland of epilepsy.* London: William Wood and Co., 1885: 190–2.

19. Lesser RP, Luders H, Dinner DS. Evidence for epilepsy is rare in patients with psychogenic seizures. *Neurology* 1983;**33**:502–4.

20. Krumholz A, Neidermeyer E. Psychogenic seizures: a clinical study with follow-up data. *Neurology* 1983;**33**:498–502.

21. Meierkord H, Will B, Fish D, Shorvan S. The clinical features and prognosis of pseudoseizures diagnosed using video-EEG telemetry. *Neurology* 1991;**41**:1643–6.

22. Kapur J, Pillai A, Henry TR. Psychogenic elaboration of simple partial seizures. *Epilepsia* 1995;**36**:1126–30.

23. Reed JL. The diagnosis of hysteria. *Psychol Med* 1975;**5**:13–17.

24. Alper K, Devinsky O, Perrine K, Vazquez B, Luciano D. Nonepileptic seizures and childhood sexual and physical abuse. *Neurology* 1993;**43**:1950–3.

25. Harris MB, Dreary IJ, Wilson JA. Life events and difficulties in relation to the onset of globus pharyngis. *J Psychosom Res* 1996;**40**:603–15.

26. Barry E, Krumholz A, Bergey GK, Chatha H, Alemayehu S, Grattan L. Nonepileptic posttraumatic seizures. *Epilepsia* 1998;**39**:427–31.

27. Westbrook LE, Devinsky O, Geocadin R. Nonepileptic seizures after head injury. *Epilepsia* 1998;**39**:978–82.

28. Bennett AH. Case of cerebral tumour-symptoms simulating hysteria. *Brain* 1878;**1**:114–20.

29. Slater E. Diagnosis of hysteria. *BMJ* 1965;**1**:1395–9.

30. Mersky H, Buhrich NA. Hysteria and organic brain disease. *Br J Med Psychol* 1975;**48**:359–66.

31. Caplan LR, Nadelson T. Multiple sclerosis and hysteria. *JAMA* 1980;**243**:2418–21.

32. Lesser RP. Psychogenic seizures. In: Pedley TA, Meldrum BS, eds. *Recent advances in epilepsy.* Vol 12. Edinburgh: Churchill Livingstone, 1985:273–96.

33. Cancilliere AEB, Kertesz A. Lesion localization in acquired deficits of emotional expression and comprehension. *Brain Cogn* 1990;**13**:133–47.

34. Heilman KM, Bowers D. Emotional disorders associated with hemispheric dysfunction. In: Fogel BS, Schiffer RB, eds. *Neuropsychiatry.* Baltimore: Williams & Wilkins, 1995:401–6.

35. Cummings JL, Mendez MF. Secondary mania with focal cerebro-vascular lesions. *Am J Psychiatry* 1984;**141**:1084–7.

36. Robinson RG, Kubos KL, Starr LB, Rao K, Price TR. Mood disorders in stroke patients: importance of location of lesion. *Brain* 1984;**107**:81–93.

37. Starkstein SE, Pearlson GD, Boston J, Robinson RJ. Mania after brain injury. *Arch Neurol* 1987;**17**:445–7.

38. Devinsky O. Neurological aspects of the conscious and unconscious mind. *Ann NY Acad Sci* 1997;**835**:321–9.

39. Briquet P. *Traite clinique et therapeutique de l'hysterie.* Paris: Baillière, 1859.

40. Halliday J. Psychological factors in rheumatism. *BMJ* 1937;**1**:264–9.

41. Kenyon FE. Hypochondriasis: a clinical study. *Br J Psychiatry* 1964;**110**:478–88.

42. Richer P. *Etudes cliniques sur la grande hysterie ou hystero-epilepsie.* 2nd ed. Paris: Delahaye and Lacrosnier, 1885.

43. Purves-Stewart J. *The diagnosis of nervous diseases.* London: Butler and Tamner, 1924.

44. Ferenczi S. *Further contributions to the theory and technique of psychoanalysis.* London: Hogarth Press, 1926:110–17.

45. Engel G. Conversion symptoms. In: MacBryde CM, Blacklow RS, eds. *Signs and symptoms: applied pathologic physiology and clinical interpretation.* 5th ed. Lippincott: Philadelphia, 1970:650–8.

46. Galin D, Diamond R, Braff D. Lateralization of conversion symptoms: more frequent on the left. *Am J Psychiatry* 1977;**134**:578–80.

47. Axelrod S, Noonan M, Atanacio B. On the laterality of psychogenic somatic symptoms. *J Nerv Ment Dis* 1980;**168**:517–25.

48. Ley RG. An archival examination of an asymmetry of hysterical conversion symptoms. *J Clin Neuropsychol* 1980;**2**:1–9.

49. Stern DB. Handedness and the lateral distribution of conversion reactions. *J Nerv Ment Dis* 1977;**164**:122–8.

50. Rauch SL, VanderKolk BA, Fisher RE, et al. A symptom provocative study of posttraumatic stress disorder using positron tomography and script-driven imagery. *Arch Gen Psychiatry* 1996;**53**:380–7.

51. Marshall JC, Halligan PW, Fink GR, Wade DT, Frackowiak RS. The functional anatomy of a hysterical paralysis. *Cognition* 1997;**64**:B1–B8.

52. Krahn LE, Rummans TA, Sharbrough FW, Jowsey SG, Cascino GD. Pseudoseizures after epilepsy surgery. *Psychosomatics* 1995;**36**:487–93.

II

AGE-RELATED DIAGNOSTIC ISSUES

5

Partial seizures in children and adults: are they different?

Hajo Hamer and Elaine Wyllie

Introduction

Epilepsy is a common medical condition, affecting 0.5–1 per cent of all children in industrialized countries.[1] The age-specific incidence is very high during the first few months of life and falls significantly after the first year of life.[2,3] It stays relatively stable through the first decade of life and falls again during adolescence. Among all incidence cases, partial seizures contribute > 50 per cent of the classified seizure types.[3,4] While generalized seizures may be more frequent in the first year of life, the incidence of partial seizures increases with age up to the age of 10 years.[5]

The International Classification of Epileptic Seizures (ICES)[6] defines partial seizures as 'those in which, in general, the first clinical and electro-encephalographic changes indicate initial activation of a system of neurons limited to part of one cerebral hemisphere.' Based on this definition, several previous reports have characterized the semeiology of partial seizures in children[7–13] and a limited number of video-electro-encephalogram (EEG) studies focused on partial seizure semeiology in infants.[14–19] The data available suggest that semeiology in young children and infants with partial seizures may be significantly different from that in adolescents and adults.[9,12,14]

In contrast to partial seizures, the concept of localization-related or focal epilepsies is broader, sometimes moving beyond focal features in clinical seizures or ictal EEG. The classification from the International League Against Epilepsy (ILAE)[20] defines partial epilepsies as 'epileptic disorders in which seizure semeiology or findings at investigation disclose a localized origin of the seizures.' This wider concept allows for the inclusion of seizures involving bilateral motor movements that occur with focal EEG seizures[14,15,17] or epileptic spasms with generalized electrodecrement on EEG that may be due to focal epileptogenic lesions seen on neuroimaging.[21–23] Focal epilepsies can be further subdivided into idiopathic and symptomatic subgroups. In symptomatic focal epilepsies, the epileptogenic lesion is usually localized in one cerebral hemisphere, while idiopathic syndromes may involve homologous epileptogenic regions in both hemispheres.[24] At the present time, very few data are available from video-EEG studies of children with idiopathic focal epilepsy.

This review will address the seizure semeiology in symptomatic focal epilepsies of infancy and childhood and focus on semeiological differences between children and adults in relation to identification of potential candidates for epilepsy surgery.

Complex partial seizures

According to the ICES definition,[6] complex partial seizures are focal seizures associated with an alteration in consciousness at onset or with simple partial onset followed by impairment of consciousness. Automatisms may or may not be present. Using this definition, Duchowny[16] studied 14 infants under 2 years of age with complex partial seizures and lateralized ictal EEG. Seizure semeiology most frequently included behavioral arrest and tonic extension of the arms, and sometimes chewing, sucking, mouthing or blinking. Yamamoto and colleagues[12] compared complex partial seizures in 15 infants younger than 2 years of age with those of 23 children aged 3–13 years. They found that seizures in infants were longer in duration and had simpler, predominantly oral automatisms. In addition, children aged 4 years and younger were more likely to have tonic or myoclonic movements during partial seizures. In a study of temporal lobe epilepsy, Brockhaus and Elger[9] compared the seizure semeiology of young children (18 months–6 years) with older children and adolescents (8–16 years). Young children lacked auras and complex automatisms, but often had symmetric motor phenomena. The authors concluded that some young children may be appropriate candidates for epilepsy surgery despite 'atypical' seizure semeiology. In contrast, older children had seizures with semeiological features resembling those of adults, including auras, complex fine motor automatisms and dystonic posturing. Similarly, in a study of older children and adolescents aged 5–18 years, Holmes[7] concluded that complex partial seizures in this age group were similar to those seen in adult patient populations.

Most of the video-EEG studies of infants and young children[14,15,17,19] noted difficulties in assessing the level of consciousness during seizures. Reactivity to an examiner was variable during the seizures, and amnesia for ictal events could not be assessed in these preverbal patients. Even if a child seems unresponsive, this does not necessarily mean that consciousness is impaired, as behavioral responses may be prevented by motor phenomena or the child may be preoccupied with the ictal sensory or motor phenomena he or she is experiencing. Therefore, it frequently is not feasible to use the seizure classification proposed by the ILAE[20] with its initial focus on impairment or preservation of consciousness in the differentiation of simple and complex partial seizures. Dravet et al[15] proposed the term 'undetermined partial seizures' while Nordli et al[17] suggested the term 'behavioral seizures' for seizures with undetermined level of consciousness associated with an abrupt change of behavior (typically quiet) without other overt features. In contrast, Duchowny[16] accepted the term 'complex partial seizures' based on failure to attract the attention of the child during the seizure. In two studies from our institution, Acharya et al[14] and Hamer et al[19] used the term 'hypomotor seizure' to describe seizures characterized by arrest or significant decrease of behavioral motor activity with undetermined level of consciousness. Hypomotor seizures comprised 20 per cent of the recorded seizure types in a series of 76 children under 3 years of age and were compatible with either a focal, multifocal or a generalized epileptogenic process.[19] Nordli et al[17] similarly reported 'behavioral seizures' in seven of 20 infants with focal or generalized epilepsy. In a study of 23 patients aged 2–24 months with partial epilepsy defined by localized ictal EEG and neuroimaging, Acharya et al[14] found hypomotor seizures in seven patients with EEG seizures arising from temporal or temporo-parietal regions.

Several authors[9,10,13,14,17,19] have noted that seizures with prominent complex automatisms are rare in infants and young children. In this age group, automatisms, if present, tend to be subtle and predominantly oral. Occasionally patients have simple gross motor movements of the proximal extremities during seizures.[11] Karbowski et al[25] proposed the term 'temporal pseudoabsence' to emphasize that decreased behavioral activity was more prominent than automatisms in their study of infants with temporal lobe epilepsy. The notable lack of automatisms in infants and young children may reflect the extreme end of an age-related spectrum in which subtle oral and manual automatisms first appear in the second and third year of life with gradual evolution to more complex and vigorous automatisms throughout childhood.[11] This is not surprising, because ictal automatisms may be considered release phenomena[26] and infants do not command the repertoire of fine motor movements that are typically seen later in life. In contrast, older children and adolescents can exhibit the full range of automatisms as expressed in adults.[27]

Motor seizures

Focal motor seizures with localized clonic, tonic or atonic features are seen throughout infancy, childhood and adolescence, and can reliably be assumed to be due to a focal or multifocal epilepsy in children as well as in adults.[9,14,17,19,28] Clonic seizures indicate ictal activation of the contralateral rolandic motor areas, while atonic phenomena may be caused by involvement of prefrontal negative motor areas.[29] The clinical features are consistently contralateral to the side of EEG seizure onset.[14,19]

Versive seizures are characterized by forced, involuntary, sustained and extreme movements of the head and/or eyes to one side and may indicate seizure onset in the contralateral hemisphere, including ictal activation of the frontal eye field.[28] In infants and young children,

however, versive seizures provide challenges for interpretation. In a study of 76 patients younger than 3 years of age, Hamer and colleagues[19] found that most of the unnatural ictal head and eye turning movements could not be confidently classified as versive seizures because they were not sufficiently extreme, pronounced and sustained for this characterization. Even among five patients with seizures classified as versive seizures, the movement was contralateral to the side of seizure onset in four patients and ipsilateral in one case.[19] We agree with Jayakar and Duchowny[11] that head and eye turning during seizures in infants and young children must be interpreted cautiously with respect to the side of seizure origin.

Many studies have noted bilateral motor phenomena, including clonic, myoclonic, tonic and atonic features, during partial seizures in infants and young children.[12–14,16,17,27] Dravet et al[15] described several children with clinically generalized motor seizures with localized EEG ictal patterns. Similarly, Hamer et al[19] reported that almost half of all seizures with generalized motor symptomatology at seizure onset in their patients under 3 years of age were associated with focal or lateralized EEG ictal findings. The mechanism of clinically generalized seizure manifestations in infantile focal epilepsies is not clear. Acharya et al[14] hypothesized that early ictal activation of mesial frontal structures in this age group may lead to generalized motor features in focal epilepsies. On the other hand, Chugani et al[30] reported activation of subcortical structures on positron emission tomography (PET) studies during generalized epileptic spasms in infants with focal epilepsy. Epilepsy syndromes cannot be assumed to be generalized in infants and young children on the basis of clinically generalized seizure semeiology alone. More detailed testing may be necessary including video-EEG monitoring, magnetic resonance imaging (MRI) and PET scans. These studies may reveal the patients with generalized motor seizures who may be appropriate candidates for epilepsy surgery.

Bilateral eye blinking has been observed infrequently during partial seizures in children.[14,16,19] It has been interpreted as an automatism[16] or as involuntary clonic activity.[14,19] In the setting of focal epilepsy, bilateral blinking may possibly be more common in infants than in adults, but the underlying mechanism is unclear. In older patients, unilateral blinking has been noted with partial epilepsy[31] and bilateral blinking is most often observed with generalized absence seizures.[32]

Although generalized tonic seizures and generalized clonic seizures are each frequent seizure types in infants and children, seizures with the typical generalized tonic–clonic evolution appear to be infrequent in this age group.[17,19] Brockhaus and Elger[9] reported typical tonic–clonic seizures only in children older than 6 years of age, while children under 6 years old did not show this seizure type. The reason for this is unknown but it may represent the immature dendritic development and myelin formation and imperfect synchronization of both hemispheres in the first years of life.[33] However, the lack of generalized tonic–clonic seizures in these video-EEG studies contrasts with reports of a high frequency of generalized tonic–clonic seizures in the setting of simple or complex febrile convulsions in infants and young children.[34,35] This discrepancy may be due to the fact that seizure semeiology of febrile convulsions is typically derived from the description of parents or other witnesses, while the above-mentioned observations[9,17,19] came from expert review of videotaped seizures. In studies based on witnesses' reports, it may be possible that some generalized tonic seizures and generalized clonic seizures were combined into a single description of generalized tonic–clonic seizures.

Infantile spasms

In infants and young children, epileptic spasms usually occur in generalized epilepsies due to a variety of diffuse brain insults.[36,37] However, spasms may also be seen occasionally in the setting of focal epilepsies.[14,15,17,19,21,22,38,39] In focal as well as in generalized processes, epileptic spasms usually occur in clusters. Typically, they consist of an abrupt initial movement followed by a longer tonic-like muscle contraction,[19] involving prominent axial features with truncal and neck flexion and proximal arm extension and abduction. Within a cluster, there tends to be a build-up of shorter spasms at the beginning to longer and harder spasms as the cluster progresses, followed by gradually shortened and milder spasms towards the end of the cluster.

Several authors have reported patients who presented with epileptic spasms and hypsarrhythmia but became seizure free after resection of a focal lesion identified by neuroimaging.[14,21,23,38,39] The most commonly reported epileptogenic lesion in surgical series of children with infantile spasms has been focal cortical dysplasia,[21] especially in the temporo-parieto-occipital region. However, frontal or temporal tumors have also been noted.[9,23,40] An important sign of an underlying focal epileptogenic process may be a past or current history of partial seizures in addition to epileptic spasms.[12,14,40,41]

Age-related seizure semeiology in the presurgical evaluation of localization-related epilepsy

Several seizure manifestations are clearly age-dependent. West syndrome with epileptic spasms, for example, has a peak of age of onset at 5–6 months and rarely begins after 1 year of age.[33,42] In addition, several seizure types may occur sequentially at different ages in the same patient with unchanged pathology. Partial seizures may precede generalized infantile spasms followed by the development of Lennox-Gastaut syndrome with tonic and atonic seizures.[43] In children older than 5 or 6 years of age, the adult spectrum of seizure symptomatology becomes more prominent.[9]

Seizure manifestations can substantially contribute to the epilepsy diagnosis and help define therapeutic options with respect to the choice of antiepileptic drugs or candidacy for epilepsy surgery. However, the interpretation of seizure manifestations may be more difficult in infants and young children than in older patients. Seizure characteristics signalling localized onset in older patients may be absent or unidentifiable in infants. An aura, for example, is an important clue for focal seizure onset in older children and adults, but sensory phenomena are difficult to detect and rarely observed during video-EEG monitoring in preverbal infants and young children.[14,17,19,44] In the setting of bilateral motor seizure semeiology in infants and children, a significant asymmetry of epileptic spasms or tonic seizures may be a clue to an underlying focal epilepsy.[19] As mentioned above, a history of focal seizures may also be an important hint. When well-localized EEG ictal patterns are absent, other helpful interictal EEG signs include focal attenuation of beta activity or sleep spindles, focal slowing or predominance of interictal epileptiform discharges over one brain region. Neurological examination may show evidence for unilateral hemispheric dysfunction with decreased movement of one arm or gaze preference to one side. Focal hyperperfusion may be evident in ictal single photo emission computed tomography (SPECT) scans.[45,46] Sharp waves may be seen over the zone of cortical abnormality during intraoperative electrocorticography.[47] MRI and PET scans are of critical importance in identifying focal cortical lesions in the presurgical evaluation of epileptic infants and children with suspected focal epilepsy.[21,44,45] In infants, as in children and adults, however, the location of a focal epileptogenic lesion must be defined by convergence of results from video-EEG monitoring, anatomical and functional neuroimaging, clinical examination and other testing.[44]

Summary

Epilepsies with onset in infancy and early childhood, although a heterogenous group, share some special characteristics which may be due to the immaturity of the brain. The repertoire of clinical seizure manifestations in infants and young children is limited. The main seizure types include clonic seizures, tonic seizures, epileptic spasms and hypomotor seizures characterized by arrest or significant decrease of behavioral motor activity with indeterminate level of consciousness.[19] Focal motor seizures are reliably associated with contralateral focal EEG ictal patterns and focal epilepsy syndromes, while hypomotor and generalized motor seizures may occur with either focal or generalized EEG ictal patterns in focal, multifocal, or generalized epilepsy syndromes. Therefore, generalized motor semeiology does not reliably predict a generalized epileptic process in this age group. More extensive evaluation, including video-EEG monitoring and neuroimaging, may be appropriate in selected infants with these seizure types to clarify possibilities for epilepsy surgery. Greater maturity during late childhood, usually older than 5 or 6 years of age, and adolescence are associated with increasing frequency of generalized tonic–clonic seizures, 'absence seizures' and seizures with complex ictal automatisms, while seizure types characteristic of infancy, such as epileptic spasms, decrease in frequency.

References

1. Hauser WA. Epidemiology of epilepsy in children. *Neurosurg Clin North Am* 1995;6:419–29.

2. Camfield C, Camfield P. Epidemiology of epilepsy in children less than age 16 based on a regional population. *Epilepsia* 1994;35(Suppl 8):149.

3. Hauser WA, Annegers JF, Rocca WA. Descriptive epidemiology of epilepsy: contributions of population-based studies from Rochester, Minnesota. *Mayo Clin Proc* 1996;71:576–86.

4. Joensen P. Prevalence, incidence and classification of epilepsy in the Faroes. *Acta Neurol Scand* 1986;74:150–5.

5. Sidenvall R, Forsgren I, Blomquist HK, et al. A community-based prospective incidence study of epileptic seizures in children. *Acta Paediatr* 1993;82:60–5.

6. Commission on Classification and Terminology of the International League Against Epilepsy. Proposal for revised clinical and electroencephalographic classification of epileptic seizures. *Epilepsia* 1981;22:489–501.

7. Holmes GL. Partial complex seizures in children: an analysis of 69 seizures in 24 patients using EEG FM radiotelemetry and videotape recording. *Electroencephalogr Clin Neurophysiol* 1984;57:13–20.

8. Bye AME, Foo S. Complex partial seizures in young children. *Epilepsia* 1994;35:482–8.

9. Brockhaus A, Elger CE. Complex partial seizures of temporal lobe origin in children of different age groups. *Epilepsia* 1995;36:1173–81.

10. Blume WT. Clinical profile of partial seizures beginning at less than four years of age. *Epilepsia* 1989;30:813–19.

11. Jayakar P, Duchowny MS. Complex partial seizures of temporal lobe origin in early childhood. *J Epilepsy* 1990;3:41–5.

12. Yamamoto N, Watanabe K, Negoro T, et al. Complex partial seizures in children: ictal manifestations and their relation to clinical course. *Neurology* 1987;37:1379–82.

13. Wyllie E, Chee M, Granström ML, et al. Temporal lobe epilepsy in early childhood. *Epilepsia* 1993;34:859–68.

14. Acharya JN, Wyllie E, Lüders HO, et al. Seizure symptomatology in infants with localization-related epilepsy. *Neurology* 1997;48: 189–96.

15. Dravet C, Catani C, Bureau M, Roger J. Partial epilepsies in infancy: a study of 40 cases. *Epilepsia* 1989;30:807–12.

16. Duchowny MS. Complex partial seizures of infancy. *Arch Neurol* 1987;44:911–14.

17. Nordli DR, Bazil CW, Scheuer ML, Pedley TA. Recognition and classification of seizures in infants. *Epilepsia* 1997;38:553–60.

18. Oller-Daurella L, Oller LFV. Partial epilepsy with seizures appearing in the first three years of life. *Epilepsia* 1989;30:820–6.

19. Hamer HM, Wyllie E, Lüders HO, et al. Symptomatology of epileptic seizures in the first three years of life. *Epilepsia* 1999; in press.

20. Commission on Classification and Terminology of the International League Against Epilepsy. Proposal for revised classification of epilepsies and epileptic syndromes. *Epilepsia* 1989;30: 389–99.

21. Chugani HT, Shewmon DA, Shields WD, et al. Surgery for intractable infantile spasms: neuroimaging perspectives. *Epilepsia* 1993;34:764–71.

22. Koo B, Hwang P. Localization in focal cortical lesions influences age of onset of infantile spasms. *Epilepsia* 1996;37:1068–71.

23. Wyllie E, Comair YG, Kotagal P, et al. Epilepsy surgery in infants. *Epilepsia* 1996;37:625–37.

24. Zupanc ML. Update on epilepsy in pediatric patients. *Mayo Clin Proc* 1996;71:899–916.

25. Karbowski K, Vassella F, Pavlincova E, Nielsen J. Psychomotorische Anfälle bei Säuglingen und Kleinkindern. *Z EEG-EMG* 1988;19:30–4.

26. Penry JK. Perspectives in complex partial seizures. *Adv Neurol* 1975;11:1–14.

27. Aicardi J. Epilepsies with affective-psychic manifestations and complex partial seizures. In: Aicardi J, ed. *Epilepsy in children*. 2nd ed. New York: Raven Press, 1994:165–206.

28. Wyllie E, Lüders H, Morris HH, et al. The lateralizing significance of versive head and eye movements during epileptic seizures. *Neurology* 1986;36:606–11.

29. Lüders HO, Lesser RP, Dinner DS, et al. A negative motor response elicited by electrical

stimulation of the human frontal cortex. *Adv Neurol* 1992;**57**:149–57.

30. Chugani HT, Shewmon DA, Sankar R, et al. Infantile spasms. II. Lenticular nuclei and brain stem activation on positron emission tomography. *Neurology* 1992;**31**:212–19.

31. Benbadis SR, Kotagal P, Klem GH. Unilateral blinking — a lateralizing sign in partial seizures. *Neurology* 1996;**46**:45–8.

32. Penry JK, Porter RJ, Dreifuss FE. Simultaneous recording of absence seizures with videotape and electroencephalography. A study of 374 seizures in 48 patients. *Brain* 1975;**98**:427–40.

33. Aicardi J. Overview: syndromes of infancy and early childhood. In: Engel J Jr, Pedley TA, eds. *Epilepsy: a comprehensive textbook*. Philadelphia: Lippincott-Raven, 1998:2263–5.

34. Hirtz DG, Camfield CS, Camfield PR. Febrile Convulsions. In: Engel J Jr, Pedley TA, eds. *Epilepsy: a comprehensive textbook*. Philadelphia: Lippincott-Raven, 1998:2483–88.

35. Nelson KB, Ellenberg JH. Prognosis in children with febrile seizures. *Pediatrics* 1978; **61**:720–7.

36. Chevrie JJ, Aicardi J. Convulsive disorders in the first year of life. Neurologic and mental outcome and mortality. *Epilepsia* 1978;**19**: 67–74.

37. Cavazutti GB, Ferrari P, Lalla M. Follow-up of 482 cases with convulsive disorders in the first year of life. *Dev Med Child Neurol* 1984; **26**:425–37.

38. Kotagal P, Cohen BH, Hahn JF. Infantile spasms in a child with brain tumor: seizure-free outcome after resection. *J Epilepsy* 1995;**8**: 57–60.

39. Wyllie E, Comair YG, Kotagal P, et al. Seizure outcome after epilepsy surgery in children and adolescents. *Ann Neurol* 1998;**44**:740–48.

40. Asanuma H, Wakai S, Tanaka T, Chiba S. Brain tumors associated with infantile spasms. *Pediatr Neurol* 1995;**12**:361–4.

41. Chugani HT, Shields WD, Shewmon DA, et al. Infantile spasms: I. PET identifies focal cortical dysplasia in cryptogenic cases for surgical treatment. *Ann Neurol* 1990;**27**:406–13.

42. Meencke HJ, Gerhard C. Morphological aspects of aetiology and the course of infantile spasms (West-Syndrome). *Neuropediatrics* 1985;**16**:59–66.

43. Yamamoto N, Watanabe K, Negoro T, et al. Partial seizures evolving to infantile spasms. *Epilepsia* 1988;**29**:34–40.

44. Wyllie E. Epilepsy surgery in infants. In: Wyllie E, ed. *The treatment of epilepsy: principles and practice*. 2nd ed. Baltimore: Williams & Wilkins, 1997:1087–96.

45. Kuzniecki RI. Neuroimaging in pediatric epilepsy. *Epilepsia* 1996;**37**(Suppl 1):S10–S21.

46. Harvey AS, Berkovic SF. Functional neuroimaging with SPECT in children with partial epilepsy. *J Child Neurol* 1994;**9**(Suppl 1): S71–S81.

47. Peacock WF, Comair Y, Chugani HT, et al. Epilepsy surgery in childhood. In: Lüders HO, ed. *Epilepsy Surgery*. New York: Raven Press, 1991:589–98.

6

Diagnosis and treatment of seizures in the elderly: current recommendations

A James Rowan

Introduction

Seizures are relatively common in the elderly as reported in the careful epidemiological studies by Hauser et al.[1] Despite their high incidence, approaching 140/100,000 at age 80,[1] seizures in the elderly are almost certainly underdiagnosed. Several factors may account for this apparent discrepancy. In the first place there is limited awareness of the scope of the problem in the elderly. Thus, caregivers and professional personnel are less likely to think of seizures in this age group when confronted with episodic changes in behavior. Moreover, the seizure manifestations themselves, with the exception of generalized tonic–clonic seizures, are not well understood. Both these factors constitute an educational challenge. This chapter will outline the special features of seizure diagnosis in the elderly along with treatment considerations for this age group.

Diagnosis

Hauser[2] reports that the incidence of complex partial seizures, the most common seizure type in adults, rise sharply after the age of 60. This is in contrast to children, in whom generalized tonic convulsions are most frequently encountered. Partial seizures, with or without secondary generalization, account for the majority if not all seizures encountered in the elderly. Primary generalized seizures that persist into late life are thought to be rare, although their incidence is unknown. The clinical characteristics of seizure types in the elderly have been considered to be similar to those of younger individuals; however, this concept is based on incomplete data. Older patients with seizures appear to have a lower frequency than younger individuals and usually do not undergo video-EEG monitoring: therefore, details of seizure phenomenology are not well documented in this age group. There is some preliminary evidence that partial seizures in the elderly may be less elaborate than in younger adults.[3] Not only may the seizures themselves differ between older and younger age groups, but there is evidence that the post-ictal state differs in the two groups. The post-ictal state in the elderly may be quite prolonged— sometimes extending to days, even weeks.[4] The disability may take the form of memory loss, general cognitive decline, or an increase in the extent of focal neurological disabilities such as hemiparesis or aphasia. These sequelae are likely to affect quality of life more profoundly than the seizure itself.

Seizures themselves may have serious consequences for the aged. For example, there is increased risk of fracture due to osteoporosis along with an increased risk of intracranial hemorrhage. The latter may take the form of a subdural hematoma or an intracerebral hemorrhage. Vulnerability to the former is increased by the presence of cerebral atrophy, common in older individuals.

Elderly individuals, particulary those with cognitive decline, display intermittent behaviors that mimic those of complex partial seizures (CPS). Repetitive motor activity such as rubbing, rocking and orofacial movements are common and in themselves may not distinguish the two conditions. Yet in the long-stay setting, where dementias are common, it is likely that complex partial seizures are underdiagnosed. This is due not only to lack of familiarity with overt symptoms suggestive of CPS, but also the limited presence of personnel in such facilities. Moreover, there is a deficiency in the education of caregivers regarding seizure types other than overt convulsions. Furthermore, evidence is available indicating that EEG studies are infrequently performed in the majority of long-stay patients.[5] This is in sharp contrast to imaging studies that are performed in the majority of younger patients. It is likely that sensitivity to the possibility of seizures in patients with fluctuating mental status would not only increase the likelihood of diagnosing seizures on clinical grounds, but also lead to ordering EEG studies that might support the diagnosis. The solution to the problem of maximizing the diagnosis of seizures in the elderly rests on an educational program, both for personnel in chronic care facilities and for physicians who care for the elderly.

A major diagnostic pitfall with the elderly is the differentiation of neurogenic syncope from an epileptic seizure. In general, syncope poses little diagnostic difficulty. A careful history, eliciting typical premonitory symptoms, a brief loss of consciousness and rapid recovery are characteristic. With an elderly person, however, such details may not be recalled. Indeed, a common history is that the patient simply was found on the floor, suffering from an unwitnessed fall. Such cases deserve a thorough evaluation, including the cerebrovascular and cardiovascular systems, and also appropriate EEG studies. Neurogenic syncope may also be complicated by convulsive activity.[6] In particular, if the patient is unable to fall to a horizontal position (e.g. while sitting), cerebral ischemia is likely to continue with resultant clonic or tonic motor activity. Under these circumstances, returning the patient to a recumbant position leads to rapid recovery. It should be noted that EEG recording during a convulsive syncopal attack reveals diffuse slowing, which may progress to marked depression of amplitude resembling an isopotential record. There is no epileptiform activity, and treatment with antiepileptic drugs (AEDs) is not indicated.

Intermittent cardiac arrhythmias such as atrial fibrillation, supraventricular tachycardias and Stokes-Adams attacks are associated with syncope. The attack may resemble neurogenic syncope and may also be followed by convulsive movements or tonic posturing. Resolution of the arrhythmia and restoration of adequate cerebral blood flow will lead quickly to recovery.

In general, differentiating a transient ischemic attack (TIA) from an epileptic seizure is not difficult. The typical TIA is characterized by transient neurological dysfunction such as hemiparesis or hemiplegia, or hemisensory symptoms such as paresthesiae. Attacks may last from minutes to hours, followed by complete recovery. In as much as negative motor symptoms are unusual in epileptic seizures—although they have been described[7]—such attacks are diagnosed correctly. If a TIA results in brief sensory events, the differentiation may be more difficult. A rapid march of symptoms in an anatomically understandable sequence may suggest an epileptic etiology, but cannot be considered definitive. Unfortunately, the EEG may not be helpful because of the difficulty of recording a localized epileptiform discharge in the Rolandic area. In patients with simple partial seizures, the yield on EEG is as low as 10 per cent.[8] In doubtful cases, it is probably most reasonable to treat the patient with antiplatelet therapy and monitor the clinical response. AEDs should be used only if there is a strong suspicion of epilepsy.

So-called drop attacks fall within the differential diagnosis of epilepsy in older persons. These episodes are characterized by a sudden fall to the ground, sometimes with serious injury. The patient recovers rapidly and may deny loss of consciousness. The etiology of these attacks is often unclear, although in many cases vertebrobasilar ischemia is suspected. The EEG is devoid of epileptiform activity.

A more difficult problem in differentiating TIAs from epilepsy is that of episodic dysphasia or aphasia, especially in patients who have a previous history of a left hemispheric stroke. Epileptic aphasia is well described,[9] and even simple partial epilepticus characterized by aphasia may occur. Again, the pattern of development of the aphasia may provide the correct diagnosis. We have observed a patient during continuous video-EEG monitoring who developed an expressive aphasia during neuropsychological testing. The aphasia began with mild word-naming difficulty, progressing to paraphasic errors, unintelligible speech and muteness. The developing aphasia was accompanied by left frontal ictal activity. With cessation of the electrographic ictus, gradual and complete recovery ensued. There was no associated motor activity or apparent alteration of awareness. It should be emphasized that such aphasic episodes would go unnoticed unless the patient was speaking. This is pointed up by the fact that other episodes of similar electrographic ictal activity were recorded in this patient, during which he was reading (or appeared to be reading) a newspaper without any evidence of apparent clinical dysfunction. Although uncommon, epileptic aphasia should be considered in patients with episodic language disturbance.

Metabolic and toxic disorders may lead to seizures in the elderly as in other age groups. In new onset seizures, consideration should always be given to such conditions as hypoglycemia, hyponatremia and renal or hepatic disease. Thorough laboratory testing will usually confirm the diagnosis. It should be noted that in certain toxic and metabolic states including hypocalcemia, hyponatremia, and lithium intoxication, the EEG may show epileptiform discharges, often multifocal in location.

Special mention is made of transient global amnesia (TGA). TGA is a condition most frequently seen in the elderly and is characterized by the acute onset of memory loss with a defect in short-term storage. Registration and remote memory remain intact. Patients are able to carry out various activities and to converse, although they are bewildered and ask questions repeatedly. The average duration of an episode is 7–9 h.[10] The EEG during an attack is normal and displays no epileptiform activity.[11] In many cases the cause appears to be ischemia in the deep temporal structures. Although originally described as a once-in-a-lifetime event, multiple attacks may occur. Because a post-ictal confusional state following a complex partial seizure may be prolonged in the elderly, an episode of TGA should be differentiated from a complex partial seizure with appropriate EEG studies.

The elderly appear to be particularly prone to the development of non-convulsive status epilepticus (NCSE). The clinical presentation is a change in mental status, ranging from mild confusion or forgetfulness to unresponsiveness.[12] There may be waxing and waning of cognitive function, or an enduring state suggestive of dementia. Attacks of NCSE may last for hours, days, or even months. Unless the appropriate diagnosis is entertained, such patients may wrongly be considered for nursing home placement. The most common cause of NCSE in the elderly is drug withdrawal, particularly the benzodiazepines. Other psychotropic drugs have been implicated. Thus, in such cases, a careful inquiry into the patient's medication history is critical.

Case report

A 67-year-old former registered nurse was evaluated for cognitive decline of 3 months duration. She had a history of complex partial seizures for many years and currently was receiving carbamazepine and gabapentin. The patient was hospitalized in December 1995 for hypertension. During her hospital stay she became agitated and reported hallucinations. There was no overt seizure activity and her carbamazepine levels were therapeutic. She was treated with haloperidol up to a dose of 30 mg/day. Thereafter she was described as being confused and functioning poorly. After discharge she continued to experience impaired cognitive function with mental slowing and forgetfulness. She could no longer perform activities of daily living. Haloperidol was discontinued with no improvement. The patient had a history of post-ictal psychosis in the past, and during one episode she displayed hyper-religiosity.

One month after discharge she was described as withdrawn and non-communicative much of the time. In February 1996 she had an EEG which was described as diffusely slow with background disorganization. On examination the patient was confused and quiet, dressed in her nightclothes with an overcoat. There was severe impairment of recall and prolonged response latency. She could follow simple commands. The formal neurological examination was normal although the gait was slowed. Review of the February 1996 EEG revealed synchronous epileptiform discharges with runs of sharp–slow complexes. She was sent to the EEG laboratory where the EEG revealed a similar picture. Administration of 0.5 mg intravenous (i.v.) lorazepam abolished the ictal patterns, and the patient was started on low dose valproate. Her family and physicians noted a remarkable improvement in her cognition within days. An EEG 2 weeks later was mildly abnormal owing to mildly excessive diffuse theta activity. On a subsequent visit she was impeccably dressed and coifed, articulate, conversational, and full of personality. She reported that during her ictal confusion she felt as if she were in a daze. She was amnestic for much of the previous 3 months. Plans for her placement in a skilled nursing facility were canceled.

Treatment considerations

In the past, little attention has been paid to the unique problems of treating the elderly person with seizures. Indeed, the general tendency has been to follow the same guidelines for both older and younger adults when choosing an appropriate AED and its dose. This approach is fraught with pitfalls. It does not take into consideration the metabolic changes that occur with age, the increased incidence of intercurrent illnesses, changes in the brain leading to increased vulnerability to the effects of drugs, and the long list of other medications taken by many elderly patients. Moreover, the response to and tolerability of antiepileptic drugs in the elderly differs from that of younger persons.

Consider the physiological changes in various organ systems. With age, there is increasing atrophy of the gastric mucosa along with a decline in gastric motility. These factors potentially affect the absorption of pharmacological agents including AEDs although, in general, absorption of drugs is generally adequate.[13] Erratic absorption can lead to fluctuating serum levels of AEDs with the potential for intermittent drug toxicity.

Renal function is another important consideration in the treatment of the elderly patient. Creatinine clearance declines linearly after the age of 20, reaching values 50 per cent lower at age 80.[14] Clearly this decline has implications for the choice of an AED for the elderly. Some AEDs are extensively metabolized by the liver, whereas others are excreted essentially unchanged by the kidney.

Changes in hepatic function are also characteristic of the aging process. Hepatic blood flow declines with age as does liver size itself.[15] There may also be changes in oxidative metabolism, but none in hepatic conjugation.[13]

Another consideration is the change in the ratio of lean to fat body mass.[16] With age, lean body mass declines, whereas there is an increase in the percentage of fat. This feature of aging affects the distribution of drugs, in particular those (such as diazepam), that are highly lipophilic.

Serum albumin plays an important role when considering use of highly bound protein drugs such as phenytoin and valproate. There tends to be a decline in albumin with age, but the most important factor is the often precipitous decrease in the face of acute illness. With very low albumin, toxic side effects of highly bound drugs quickly appear.

The elimination half-lives of AEDs determine dosing schedules and are well documented for all AEDs, however, these data may not apply to the elderly. There is some evidence that the half-life of some drugs may be considerably prolonged in the elderly (Cloyd J; personal communication). In addition, the zero-order or exponential kinetics of phenytoin have been demonstrated to be much steeper in the elderly than in young patients. This kinetic change may give rise to toxicity in older patients if the drug is administered at dosing schedules appropriate for younger subjects.

An additional factor of importance is the probability of altered pharmacodynamics in the elderly. The presence of cerebral atrophy and chronic cerebral lesions such as infarcts would appear to place the patient at increased risk for adverse effects of AEDs, even in the face of no significant pharmacokinetic change. Evidence for this concept is limited. However, there are data to suggest that older patients are more prone to the sedative side effects of benzodiazepines than younger patients when the drugs are given at similar unbound serum concentrations.[17,18] This potential factor may underlie side effects such as sedation and should be a consideration, even in the face of so-called therapeutic levels.

Selection of an appropriate AED for the elderly

At this point in time, those concerned with the treatment of epilepsy are enjoying a surfeit of riches. We now have double the number of useful AEDs in the armamentarium thanks to the intensive AED development program of the NIH and the pharmaceutical industry. Previously it was necessary to juggle a few drugs, principally carbamazepine, and valproate, in combinations or as monotherapy, or sometimes to resort to more toxic drugs in cases of refractory epilepsy. The advent of new drugs including gabapentin, lamotrigine, topiramate, and tiagabine has markedly broadened the treatment possibilities. These new drugs have come along since 1993, and their possibilities are just beginning to be realized. Wide experience is now available with gabapentin and lamotrigine, and the use of topiramate and tiagabine is accelerating. These developments are particularly intriguing for the elderly, for the older agents all have intrinsic disadvantages for this population.

The 'old' AEDs

Phenytoin, which has now been on the market for ~60 years, is widely used, especially in North America, and has a track record of efficacy and safety. Despite some inherent disadvantages it remains a standard to which other compounds are compared. As with many drugs that have been available for a long time, there is a certain comfort level with phenytoin, and many prescribed it because of the lack of familiarity with newer compounds. Phenytoin is the only AED with an exponential kinetic profile. If phentyoin's kinetics are well understood, including age-related differences, this does not necessarily confer a disadvantage. On the other hand, many cases of phenytoin toxicity and even increased seizures are directly due to unexpected rapid rises and falls in phenytoin concentration. This danger is increased in the elderly because rise in concentration with comparable dose increase is steeper than that seen in younger patients. Another problem with phenytoin is its high degree of protein binding. Phenytoin competes with other protein-bound drugs, resulting in changes in phenytoin concentration or decreased effectiveness of co-medications. The list of drugs that interact with phenytoin is lengthy. Therefore, this is a major consideration in the elderly who take an average of four to six drugs for various medical conditions, and in some cases many more. One major advantage of phenytoin is its availability as an intravenous preparation. This allows for continuing treatment if oral medications cannot be taken, and for loading with the drug in emergency situations such as repeated seizures. Another advantage is the cost of the drug; phenytoin is one of the least expensive AEDs on the market.

Carbamazepine has been available in North America for nearly 25 years. This AED has gained the status of first-line therapy for partial seizures, although it required many years for the compound to gain this status. It appears that clinicians, a generally conservative group, are slow to accept newer therapies. Carbamazepine has many advantages including linear kinetics, twice-daily dosing for the extended release preparation and proven efficacy. Protein binding is lower than for phenytoin, but drug interactions do occur. Hyponatremia, a well-known effect of carbamazepine, is usually mild and without clinical implications. Hyponatremia of mild to moderate degree appears to be more common than in younger subjects, but the clinical relevance of this factor is unknown as yet. Carbamazepine has dose-related side effects, the most common of which are visual disturbances, dizziness and unsteadiness. Diarrhoea may be a problem in some patients. The central nervous system (CNS) side effects are readily reversible by lowering the dose.

Valproate has been available for over 20 years and has become one of the top standard drugs for treatment of epilepsy. It has a broader spectrum than phenytoin or carbamazepine and is effective in primary generalized seizures. Valproate is also effective in many patients with partial onset seizures, especially those that are secondarily generalized.[19] The drug has a relatively short half-life and requires divided dosing. A new extended release preparation will offer twice-daily dosing with more stable serum levels. Valproate is highly protein bound and is prone to drug interactions. When used with enzyme-inducing AEDs, it is difficult to achieve high valproate levels. The most common side effects are tremor, weight gain, and in some cases hair loss. Thrombocytopenia with risk of hemorrhage occurs infrequently.

The new AEDs

Gabapentin is related to the neurotransmitter γ-aminobutyric acid (GABA) and was designed to cross the blood–brain barrier. Although the drug does not appear to act at postsynaptic GABA receptors in the brain, it does raise whole brain GABA levels, and gabapentin binding sites exist throughout the brain. Gabapentin is effective in the treatment of partial onset seizures. The drug is not metabolized and is excreted unchanged by the kidney. There are no drug interactions. Because of an elimination half-life of 7–9 h, three times daily dosing is recommended. Side effects are few with the exception of CNS-related symptoms at the beginning of therapy. These symptoms may include mild drowsiness or unsteadiness and usually disappear after 1 or 2 weeks.

Lamotrigine is a phenyltriazine that demonstrates a weak antifolate property. The drug is active at sodium-dependent channels, appears to inhibit glutamate release and blocks rapid neuronal firing. Lamotrigine is well absorbed and demonstrates linear kinetics. It is ~55 per cent protein bound. The drug is extensively metabolized by the liver, and only ~10 per cent of the drug is excreted unchanged by the kidney. The elimination half-life is 24 h, which allows twice-daily dosing. However, when lamotrigine is given concomitantly with enzyme-inducing drugs its half-life is reduced by 50 per cent. Conversely, when given with valproate, an enzyme inhibitor, its half-life is doubled. There are no other clinically relevant drug interactions. Lamotrigine is effective in partial onset seizures and may have a broader spectrum of action. There is evidence from comparative trials that lamotrigine's efficacy is similar to carbamazepine and phenytoin. The drug has a favorable side-effect profile. Mild CNS effects may occur at the onset of treatment. Rash has been reported in ~10 per cent of patients receiving lamotrigine, and severe rash with exfoliation has been reported. There is some evidence that slow titration of the drug may decrease the incidence of rash.

Topiramate was recently approved for use as add-on therapy in partial seizures, although there is some evidence that it may have a much broader spectrum of action. It is active at sodium-dependent sodium channels and may modulate GABA-A receptors. The drug is a weak carbonic anhydrase inhibitor, but this activity is not thought to be important in its mechanism of action. The drug is well absorbed, is weakly protein bound, and demonstrates linear kinetics. It is not extensively metabolized, and excretion is mainly via the kidneys. Topiramate's elimination half-life of 20–24 h permits twice-daily dosing. Both phenytoin and carbamazepine decrease topiramate concentration by 40 per cent, and topiramate increases phenytoin concentration by ~25 per cent. There are no other important drug interactions. Mild neurotoxicity may be seen at the beginning of treatment. Weight loss has been reported, and changes in mental status have been observed at high doses in patients on polytherapy.

Tiagabine is the most recently approved AED in the USA and has a unique mode of action. It selectively blocks the uptake of GABA into presynaptic neurons, thus increasing the concentration of GABA in the extracellular space. The drug is approved as add-on therapy for partial-onset seizures. Incomplete data are available for efficacy in other seizure types. Tiagabine is highly protein bound and extensively metabolized in the liver. Its elimination half-life is about 9 h, and divided dosing is recommended. Pharmacokinetics in the elderly are the same as in younger patients. A sustained release version of the drug is under development. When given with enzyme-inducing AEDs, the dose of tiagabine must be increased to achieve concentrations comparable to those obtained during tiagabine monotherapy. Otherwise, the drug has no important drug interactions. Tiagabine has a favorable side-effect profile, mainly comprising transient CNS effects at the onset of therapy. Changes in mental status have been observed at high doses.

Veterans' administration (VA) cooperative study No. 428, treatment of seizures in the elderly population

VA Cooperative Study No. 428 is the first large-scale study of the treatment of seizures in the elderly. The trial began in January 1998 and is expected to continue for 5 years. It is planned to enroll > 700 patients at 18 sites across the USA. The study is a double-blind, parallel group trial to determine the comparative efficacy and tolerability of three AEDs: carbamazepine, gabapentin and lamotrigine. Target doses for the three drugs are lower than those usually recommended for adults. Dosage adjustment is permitted throughout the trial depending on the patient's clinical course. The primary outcome measure is retention in the trial for 12 months, a measure of a drug's efficacy and tolerability. Extensive information regarding the clinical aspect of seizures in the elderly, seizure types and frequency, and specific side effects will be obtained along with measures of cognitive function, mood and quality of life. It is

expected that the comparative data obtained during the trial will lead to an improvement both in seizure management and quality of life for the elderly patient with seizures.

The ideal AED

The ideal AED, of course, does not exist. None the less, there is a continuing effort to approach the ideal as evidenced by the remarkable research efforts of the past 20 years. When evaluating the characteristics of existing AEDs, the following attributes of an ideal AED should be borne in mind:

1. Highly effective
2. Broad spectrum
3. A number of identified cellular actions
4. Linear pharmacokinetics
5. No dose-related adverse effects
6. No organ toxicity
7. Fast titration
8. An available intravenous preparation
9. Inexpensive

In particular clinical situations, some of the above characteristics will be more important than others. For example, rapid titration is a key advantage when seizure frequency is relatively high. In emergency situations, linear pharmacokinetics would be less important than availability of an intravenous preparation. When treating a specific type of seizure, a drug's broad spectrum may not be particularly relevant. These and other related issues form the basis for the following discussion of AED selection.

A rational approach to AED selection for the elderly

Because the aging process influences the features of epilepsy as well as the pharmacokinetic and pharmacodynamic characteristics

Features	Younger patients	Older patients
Seizure frequency	Often high	Low
Post-ictal state	Relatively brief	Relatively prolonged
Potential for injury	Relatively low	Relatively high
Etiology	Many	Few
Response to AEDs	Variable (poor to excellent)	Usually good (incomplete data available)
Tolerance to AEDs	Variable (usually good)	Often poor (incomplete data available)
Required doses of AEDs	Higher	Lower
Speed of AED titration	Higher	Lower

Table 6.1
Epilepsy in younger versus older patients.

of antiepileptic drugs, there is a need for a unique approach to treatment of the elderly. Table 6.1 summarizes the comparative characteristics of epilepsy in the young and the old. The differences between these broad age groups underlie the treatment considerations outlined below.

As suggested above, few data are available concerning treatment of the elderly. Most clinical trials of AEDs exclude the elderly, partly because this age group tends to take a variety of medications and to suffer from one or more concomitant medical diseases. Of course, these factors reflect the reality of caring for elderly patients and must be considered when choosing an appropriate AED. Until more definitive data are available, such as may derive from the VA Cooperative Study, the rational selection of an AED for the elderly patient must depend on available information concerning efficacy and side-effect profiles as well as the patient's individual circumstances.

An early decision confronting the physician is whether to use one of the standard AEDs or one of the newer compounds. The standard AEDs have the advantage of familiarity based on extensive track records. As noted above,

prescribing patterns change slowly; thus comfort when prescribing the newer AEDs will come gradually. None the less, the new drugs should be considered seriously in appropriate cases. As the following discussion will make clear, no one treatment is suitable for all patients.

The primary consideration is whether acute treatment, i.e. loading with an AED, is indicated. Such a case might involve a patient with the new onset of two consecutive seizures, with or without complete interictal recovery. The choices are limited, but most would agree that i.v. phenytoin or fosphenytoin, or oral phenytoin would be indicated. Phenobarbital may also be used, but its sedation constitutes a major disadvantage in the elderly. Valproate is available in an i.v. preparation and might be considered in secondarily generalized seizures, although its efficacy in an acute situation is less well documented than in the case of phenytoin.

With respect to chronic AED therapy after i.v. loading, phenytoin may be continued as an oral preparation, an advantage not shared by the benzodiazepines. At a later time, consideration may be given to crossing over to another agent, e.g. one of the new AEDs.

When there is lack of urgency—e.g. a patient who developed his/her first complex partial seizure 1 or 2 weeks ago—treatment with oral medication without a loading dose is usually indicated. Here, speed of titration, side-effect profile and extent of drug interactions of the AED become prime considerations. For many patients, gabapentin would appear to be an excellent choice. Its safety profile and lack of drug interactions approach the ideal AED for the elderly patient. In addition, titration can be fairly rapid, e.g. a reasonable program might be titration to a dose of 1500 mg/day over 2 weeks. One disadvantage of gabapentin is its recommended three times daily dosing schedule. Because of the lack of drug interactions, gabapentin may be added safely to an existing AED regimen. In fact, adding gabapentin to a patient's AED program after he/she has been treated acutely with phenytoin and is on maintenance therapy is suggested as a rational therapeutic choice for many patients.

Lamotrigine is also a good choice for the elderly because of its favorable side-effect profile, twice-daily dosing, and lack of drug interactions when used as monotherapy. The problem of rash is potentially limiting, but slow titration apparently reduces this complication. For the elderly, titration to a dose of 150 mg/day can be achieved within 6 weeks. Slow titration, however, is a disadvantage when more rapid attainment of a therapeutic dose is required. If a patient is already being treated with standard AEDs, monotherapy with lamotrigine can be achieved readily by crossing over systematically.[20]

At the time of writing, carbamazepine is considered the treatment of choice for partial onset seizures and, among the older drugs, it is probably the first for the elderly. The worldwide acceptance of carbamazepine has come about because of its efficacy, relatively good tolerability and predictable pharmacokinetics. Does carbamazepine approach the ideal AED?

No, but as already indicated, clinicians feel comfortable with this compound and know it well enough to deal with the dose-related side effects. Titration in the elderly should be relatively slow, aiming for a dose between 400 and 600 mg/day, achieved over about 4 weeks. As with other AEDs, serum levels in the low therapeutic range should be sufficient to achieve seizure control and minimize side effects. Based on available data, carbamazepine is a reasonable, if not the first, choice for treatment of seizures in the elderly.

Valproate is a consideration when the patient has secondarily generalized tonic–clonic convulsions, with or without isolated complex partial seizures. As with other highly protein-bound AEDs, care must be taken when the patient is taking multiple co-medications. The side effects of tremor and weight gain may be limiting factors.

Tiagabine and topiramate await further experience before any recommendation can be made for the elderly. None the less, should other agents fail or be inappropriate, these AEDs should be considered. At the time of writing, tiagabine may be the better choice of the two because of its favorable side-effect profile, specific mechanism of action and lack of drug interactions.

Summary

In summary, choice of the most appropriate AED for the elderly patient must be customized and appropriate to the clinical problem. Of the new AEDs, at the time of writing, gabapentin and lamotrigine appear to offer distinct advantages in the elderly. These agents may not be suitable for all, and carbamazepine may be preferable in some circumstances. Regardless of the agent chosen it is imperative that the AED be introduced slowly and titrated to a daily dose that is on average lower than that used in younger adults. No specific guidelines are available, but the suggestions for carbamazepine, gabapentin and lamotrigine derive from the protocol for the VA Cooperative Study. Bear in mind that the so-called therapeutic ranges of the older AEDs do not apply to the elderly, mainly due to an overall decreased tolerability for drugs in this age group. A useful guide would be to aim for a 'low therapeutic' serum level, increasing the dose if necessary. Finally, successful treatment of the elderly rests on detailed knowledge of the characteristics of both the old and new AEDs, a clear understanding of the unique features of the elderly patient, and the careful application of this knowledge to the specific clinical picture.

References

1. Hauser WA, Annegers JF, Kurland LT. The incidence of epilepsy and unprovoked seizures in Rochester, Minnesota, 1935–1984. *Epilepsia* 1993;**34**:453–68.
2. Hauser WA. Epidemiology of seizures and epilepsy in the elderly. In: Rowan AJ, Ramsay RE, eds. *Seizures and epilepsy in the elderly*. Boston: Butterworth-Heinemann, 1997:7–18.
3. Tuniper P. The altered presentation of seizures in the elderly. In: Rowan AJ, Ramsay RE, eds. *Seizures and epilepsy in the elderly*. Boston: Butterworth-Heinemann, 1997:123–30.
4. Tallis R. Antiepileptic drug trials in the elderly: rationale, problems and solutions. In: Rowan AJ, Ramsay RE, eds. *Seizures and epilepsy in the elderly*. Boston: Butterworth-Heinemann, 1997:311–20.
5. Rowan AJ, Ramsay RE. Unpublished data.
6. Lempert T, Bauer M, Schmidt D. Syncope: a videometric analysis of 56 episodes of transient cerebral hypoxia. *Ann Neurol* 1994;**36**:233–7.
7. Penfield W, Jasper H. *Epilepsy and the functional anatomy of the brain*. Boston: Little Brown, 1954:269–70.
8. Devinsky O, Kelley K, Porter RJ, Theodore WH. Clinical and electroencephalographic features of simple partial seizures. *Neurology* 1988;**38**:1347–52.
9. Rosenbaum DH, Siegel M, Barr WB, Rowan AJ. Epileptic aphasia. *Neurology* 1986;**36**: 281–4.
10. Caplan LR. Transient global amnesia. In: Vinken PJ, Bruyn GW, Klawans H, eds. *Handbook of clinical neurology*. Amsterdam: Elsevier Science Publishing, 1985:205–18.
11. Gloor P. The EEG during transient global amnesia. *Electroencephalogr Clin Neurophysiol*; in press.
12. Guberman A, Cantu-Reyna G, Stuss D, Broughton R. Nonconvulsive generalized status epilepticus: clinical features, neuropsychological testing, and long-term follow-up. *Neurology* 1994;**36**:1284–91.
13. Vestal RE, Cusack BJ. Pharmacology and aging. In: Schneider EL, Rowe JW, eds. *Handbook of the biology of aging*. 3rd ed. San Diego: Academic Press, 1990:349–83.
14. Rowe JW, Andres RA, Tobin JD, et al. The effect of age in creatinine clearance in man: a cross sectional and longitudinal study. *J Gerontol* 1976;**31**:155–63.
15. Woodhouse KW, Wynne HA. Age-related changes in liver size and hepatic blood flow. The influence on drug metabolism in the elderly. *Clin Pharmacokinet* 1988;**15**:287–94.
16. Novak LP. Aging, total body potassium, fat free mass and cell mass in males and females between the ages 18 and 85 years. *J Gerontol* 1972;**27**:438–43.
17. Feely J, Coakley D. Altered pharmacodynamics in the elderly. *Clin Geriatr Med* 1990;**6**: 269–83.
18. Greenblatt DJ, Harmatz JS, Shapiro L, et al. Sensitivity to triazolam in the elderly. *N Engl J Med* 1991;**324**:1691–8.
19. Mattson RH, Cramer JA, Collins JF and the VA Epilepsy Cooperative Study No. 264 Group. A comparison of valproate with carbamazepine for the treatment of partial seizures and secon-

darily generalized tonic-clonic seizures in adults. *N Engl J Med* 1992;**327**:765–71.

20. De Toledo J, Rowan AJ, Uthman BM, et al. Conversion to lamotrigine monotherapy: an open label study on the efficacy in primary and partial epilepsies and influence of inducing and non-inducing antiepileptic drugs on the rate of initiation. (Submitted to *Epilepsia*).

III
ROLE OF DIAGNOSTIC TESTS IN CLINICAL EPILEPSY PRACTICE

7

Rational diagnosis of subtle and non-convulsive status epilepticus

Alan R Towne and Elizabeth J Waterhouse

Introduction

Status epilepticus (SE) is a major neurological and medical emergency, requiring acute medical management to avoid significant morbidity and mortality. Recent articles have indicated that the mortality of SE in the general population remains high, approaching 22 per cent, and is higher still in the elderly, ~30 per cent.[1,2] Non-convulsive status epilepticus (NCSE) is becoming increasingly recognized as a relatively common, and certainly underdiagnosed, form of SE.

Classification

The definition of NCSE has been controversial. Gastaut,[3] Treiman,[4] Krumholz et al[5] and others have used the term to refer only to absence or complex partial SE (CPSE). Gastaut[3] suggested that the term 'absence SE' be applied to all cases of generalized NCSE that lack focal electrographic findings. However, Tomson et al[6] and others have pointed out that CPSE may rapidly generalize, making later-stage CPSE electrographically indistinguishable from absence SE. As more clinical and electrographic cases of absence SE and CPSE have been described in the literature, the need for a widely accepted and unambiguous NCSE classification scheme has become increasingly clear.

The confusion surrounding the definition of absence SE led to the initial belief that absence SE comprised the majority of cases of NCSE, while CPSE was relatively rare.[7–10] With prolonged electro-encephalogram (EEG) monitoring, examples of generalized electrographic SE have demonstrated initial focal onset, or waxing and waning focal features. These cases, which might previously have been considered absence SE, have been appropriately recognized as CPSE with secondary generalization.[6,11–15]

In the last decade, the term 'subtle SE' has been added to the lexicon. While Treiman[4] considers it a form of generalized convulsive SE, others consider it a form of NCSE. There is still no widespread consensus in the classification of SE or NCSE.

A significant number of NCSE cases occur in intensive care unit (ICU) patients. These patients, of course, may have severe metabolic, neurologic or systemic problems that may predispose them to NCSE. NCSE should be suspected in any ICU patient who is comatose, without other clear etiology, or in any patient who had convulsive SE which stopped, without subsequent improvement in the level of consciousness.

Epidemiology

Recent studies have indicated that the total incidence of SE (overt and non-convulsive) is much higher than previously thought. A retrospective study of SE found the incidence of SE as 18.3 per 100,000, but this is probably an underestimate.[16] A prospective population-based epidemiologic study of SE in Richmond, Virginia, indicated that the minimum incidence of SE in the Richmond area was 41 per 100,000 people per year.[2] SE episodes occurred with a frequency of 50 episodes per 100,000 people per year. Based on the 1990 census US population of 249,924,000, the Richmond epidemiologic data were projected to determine the national incidence of SE. Based on this estimate, 102,000–152,000 patients experiencing 126,000–195,000 SE events would be predicted in the US per year. Data from this study also suggest that ~10 per cent of patients with SE have a non-convulsive presentation.

Absence status epilepticus

Clinical description

Absence SE is also known as spike–wave stupor, petit mal status, prolonged petit mal automatism, epilepsia minoris continua, and status pyknolepticus.[17-20] While some researchers have reported that absence SE is the most common form of NCSE,[17,18] more recent studies have suggested that CPSE and other types of NCSE occur more commonly.[6,21] Some of these discrepancies are attributable to the controversies surrounding the classification of absence SE, described above. For the purposes of this chapter, absence SE is considered as lasting at least 30 min and is associated with any of the following changes from baseline EEG: (1) typical 3 Hz generalized spike–wave discharges on EEG, usually occurring in people with a history of absence epilepsy; (2) atypical generalized spike–wave or polyspike-and-wave discharges at frequencies other than 3 Hz,

usually occurring in patients with a history of epilepsy (such as Lennox–Gastaut syndrome, juvenile myoclonic epilepsy or other myoclonic epilepsies); (3) de novo occurrence of typical generalized 3 Hz rhythmic spike–wave discharges in adults not previously known to have epilepsy, usually with an identifiable precipitating factor (such as drug administration or withdrawal).

Absence SE presents clinically with a prolonged episode of confusion, or 'epileptic twilight state'. Clinically, these patients demonstrate consistently clouded consciousness or confusion that may range from subtle to obvious to the observer. Complete unresponsiveness is rare. Some patients in absence SE are still able to function, but may appear slightly less alert than usual or demonstrate a relative paucity of speech. These behaviors may be interpreted as psychiatric illness.[20,22] There may be occasional associated blinking or myoclonic twitches. Absence SE tends to occur as a prolonged single attack rather than as a series of repetitive events, and there is usually retained partial responsiveness rather than total unresponsiveness.

Patient population

While absence SE can occur in patients of any age, 75 per cent of cases occur before the age of 20, usually in patients who have already been diagnosed with epilepsy.[18] Absence SE occurs in 3 per cent of all patients with absence seizures and 10 per cent of adults with persistent absence seizures that began in childhood.[17,20,23] In population-based studies, absence SE has accounted for 1.2–3.5 per cent of all SE.[16,28]

Absence SE may be precipitated de novo in older adults by benzodiazepine withdrawal.[11] Other precipitating factors include the administration of carbamazepine with primary generalized epileptiform EEG patterns, amitriptyline toxicity, thyroxine, metrizamide neurotoxicity, hypocalcemia, hyponatremia and alcoholism.[18-20,25-34]

Differential diagnosis

The differential diagnosis of absence SE includes CPSE, post-ictal confusional state, psychiatric states, or encephalopathy due to toxic, metabolic, ischemic, inflammatory or post-traumatic causes.

Diagnostic evaluation

EEG is of paramount importance in making the diagnosis of absence SE, or any kind of NCSE. The EEG characteristically shows generalized 2–4 Hz spike and slow-wave complexes, or polyspike-and-wave complexes, often maximal at the bifrontal head regions. The spike–wave pattern may be continuous, or almost continuous, with intervals of arrhythmic spike and wave, polyspike activity or semi-rhythmic slow wave activity. The interictal EEG may demonstrate brief bursts of generalized 2–3 Hz spike-and-wave activity. In one electrographic study of NCSE, a typical spike–wave pattern was seen in 4 cases (7 per cent).[35] Electrographically, absence SE is differentiated from CPSE by the absence of focal electrographic ictal activity, and by the presence of monomorphic generalized rhythmic 3 Hz spike–wave discharges.

A careful family history should be obtained to see if there are relatives with epilepsy. Metabolic evaluation should be performed and, if clinically indicated, a drug screen should be sent.

Treatment

If at all possible, an EEG should be performed prior to treatment, in order to confirm the diagnosis. While other types of NCSE require emergent treatment, absence SE is not a life threatening disorder and has a very low associated morbidity and mortality.[1] Therefore, the patient may be treated with oral or parenteral antiepileptic medication. In a hospitalized patient, IV diazepam (0.2–0.3 mg/kg), or lorazepam (0.07 mg/kg) are preferred, although either of these drugs may precipitate respiratory depression and the need for endotracheal intubation. Other available parenteral agents include IV acetazolamide,[36] which is considered safer, but less effective, than benzodiazepines, and IV valproate, which may prove advantageous in the urgent treatment of absence SE. While benzodiazepines are very effective at restoring normal clinical responsiveness and EEG activity, they exert only a transient effect, and a long-acting antiepileptic drug is usually needed in the long term. First-line oral antiepileptic drugs that are effective for absence SE are ethosuximide and valproate. Other drugs that may also be effective include lamotrigine, clonazepam and topiramate.

Aggressive treatment of absence SE with general anesthesia or barbiturates is not indicated because of the low morbidity and mortality associated with this condition. However, absence SE must be differentiated from other types of NCSE, which may also cause a decreased level of responsiveness and require urgent treatment.[19] In patients with *de novo* absence SE, benzodiazepine therapy alone may terminate the SE and, if the precipitating agent is removed, long-term antiepileptic drug therapy may not be needed.

Prognosis

The prognosis of typical absence SE is favorable.[2,18] While a patient may experience recurrent episodes of absence SE, no deaths or long-term morbidity have been reported.

However, in patients with Lennox–Gastaut syndrome and atypical absence SE the prognosis is poor, with persistent, often intractable, seizures and developmental delay. The unfavorable outcomes in this group of patients are most likely due to the underlying encephalopathy rather than the SE itself.[3,37]

Complex partial status epilepticus (CPSE)

Clinical description

CPSE was first described by Gastaut et al in 1956.[38] This entity is also known as psychomotor status, status psychomotricus, and temporal lobe status epilepticus. CPSE is defined as 30 min or more of discrete or continuous partial seizures without full recovery of consciousness in between. The characteristic clinical manifestation is impairment of consciousness, which can vary from mild alteration in mentation to complete unresponsiveness. CPSE also may be characterized by a cyclic pattern in which phases of unresponsiveness alternate with partially responsive phases. During the periods of partial responsiveness, automatisms and abnormal speech patterns may be present. During the unresponsive phase, complete speech arrest usually occurs, occasionally accompanied by stereotyped automatisms.[9] The clinical manifestations of CPSE are varied and may be difficult to differentiate from generalized NCSE. The accompanying behavior can range from confusion to bizarre or psychotic-type behavior. Lateralizing or localizing neurological deficits can also be seen, such as aphasia or ictal paresis. While the duration of CPSE is usually 30 min to several hours, recent reports have described examples of CPSE lasting for months, indicating that prolonged fugue states can be caused by CPSE.

Patient population

Thirty to fifty per cent of patients have a history of seizures prior to developing CPSE. In those patients who develop CPSE without an antecedent history, CPSE occurs most

Alcohol withdrawal
Anoxia
Antiepileptic drug withdrawal
Cerebrovascular
    arteriovenous malformation
    intracerebral hemorrhage
    ischemic stroke
    subarachnoid hemorrhage
    subdural hemorrhage
    venous sinus thrombosis
CNS infection
Congenital brain abnormalities
Dementia
Drug overdose
Electroconvulsive therapy
Epilepsy
Fever
Generalized convulsive seizures
Hyperventilation
Hypoxia
Inborn errors of metabolism
Leptomeningeal carcinomatosis
Menstruation
Metabolic
Mitochondrial disorder
Photic stimulation
Postcerebral angiography
Postmyelography
Postoperative
Sepsis
Sleep deprivation
Thrombotic thrombocytopenic purpura
Trauma
Tumor

Table 7.1
Etiologies and precipitants of non-convulsive status epilepticus (NCSE).

commonly in adult patients with symptomatic neurological disease such as herpes simplex encephalitis and cerebral infarction. In patients with a history of epilepsy, precipitating factors include recent infection and inadequate anticonvulsant levels. CPSE has also been reported after cerebral angiography and can be associated with thrombotic thrombocytopenic purpura (Tables 7.1 and 7.2).[39]

The incidence of CPSE is difficult to assess because the paucity of clinical symptoms may not raise the suspicion of possible SE, and because there are few population-based studies. A population-based study done in Richmond, Virginia, revealed that CPSE represented ~ 5 per cent of the total number of convulsive and non-convulsive SE episodes and 35 per cent of non-convulsive episodes. Other studies have demonstrated that CPSE comprises 10–40 per cent of all cases of NCSE.

Baclofen
Carbamazepine
Cephalosporins
Ciprofloxacin
Cyclosporin
Haloperidol
Ifosfamide
Lidocaine
Lithium
Metrizamide
Metronidazole
OKT3
Penicillins
Phenothiazines
Theophylline
Thyroxine
Trimethoprim-sulfa

Table 7.2
Drugs implicated as precipitants of non-convulsive status epilepticus (NCSE).

Differential diagnosis

CPSE should be suspected in any patient being evaluated for confusion or unresponsiveness. Other conditions that may be confused with CPSE include absence status epilepticus, prolonged post-ictal states, psychiatric syndromes (such as somatoform disorder and psychosis) and cerebral circulation disorders, including transient ischemic attacks and stroke with delirium. Other conditions, such as encephalopathies, migraine and transient global amnesia, also need to be considered in the differential diagnosis.

Diagnostic evaluation

To prevent serious morbidity and mortality, CPSE must be promptly diagnosed and treated. Among patients with convulsive SE, mortality ranges from 10–40 per cent, depending on the etiology, duration of SE and the response to treatment. Recent studies have indicated that CPSE is also associated with increased morbidity and mortality. Identification of CPSE may be delayed in those patients who are comatose and do not present with clinical manifestations which suggest ongoing seizure activity. Thus, EEG confirmation is mandatory to make the diagnosis of this condition. Recent studies of SE in comatose patients reveal that ~ 10 per cent of the patients are in electrographic SE, despite the fact that the patient may not demonstrate obvious clinical activity, or only subtle clinical manifestations.[40] Thus, patients who have persistent alterations of mental status should be evaluated immediately by EEG.

EEG findings in CPSE are varied, with some patients demonstrating intermittent partial seizures and post-ictal alterations between seizures, and other patients demonstrating continuous EEG abnormalities. The EEG may

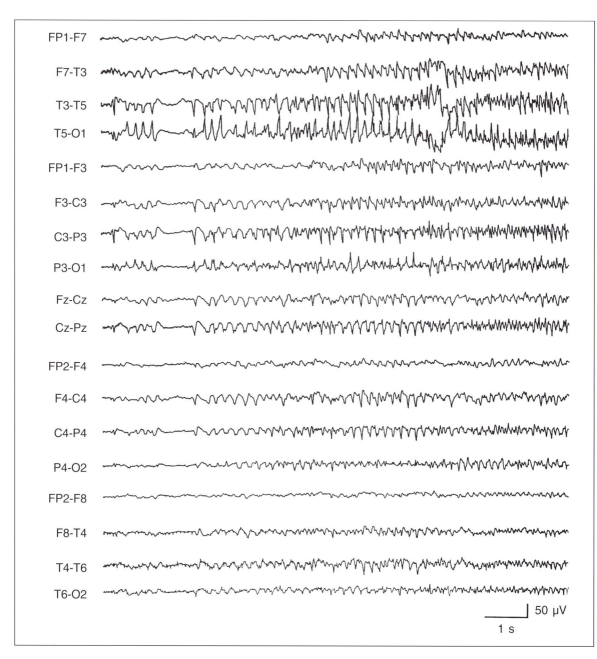

Figure 7.1
Complex partial status epilepticus (CPSE). Rhythmic left posterior temporal sharp waves with secondary generalization.

demonstrate polyspike discharges, regular sharp or slow waves, spike and slow-wave discharges and rhythmic slowing (Figure 7.1). The focal onset of the seizure may not be apparent in a patient with a generalized EEG pattern. As the seizure progresses, the EEG may reveal a diffuse, regular high-amplitude, slow-wave abnormality without definite focal features.[19] Williamson et al[41] performed depth electrodes in patients with intractable partial epilepsy during episodes of NCSE. They concluded that CPSE may be more likely in patients with extratemporal epileptogenic zones, and scalp EEG monitoring alone may result in an underestimate of patients who develop CPSE.[41–43]

The diagnostic evaluation of patients with CPSE should also include studies to identify the etiology of the event. These studies include laboratory tests to investigate the possibility of metabolic disorders, infections, toxic exposure and withdrawal conditions. Neuroimaging studies, such as computed tomography (CT) or MRI, can reveal abnormalities which may have a diagnostic value. Although not usually performed, ictal SPECT can also provide information concerning the localization of the seizure, especially in atypical cases.

Treatment

The treatment of CPSE is similar to that of subtle NCSE. Benzodiazepines, such as diazepam, lorazepam or midazolam, are usually used as first-line choices. A benzodiazepine is generally followed by IV fosphenytoin. In those patients with a prior history of intractable complex partial seizures, surgical intervention may be considered.

Prognosis

The prognosis of CPSE is variable and depends upon multiple factors, including the age of the patient, seizure duration and etiology.[1] This condition can be associated with increased neurological deficits in some patients and is associated with increased mortality. Some of this increased mortality is secondary to the underlying cause. There is evidence that persistent memory and behavioral sequelae can appear as a result of CPSE.[44] There are also reports of patients who have recovered from prolonged CPSE without any permanent neurologic deficits.[45]

Simple partial status epilepticus (SPSE)

Clinical description

SPSE is a relatively rare seizure type in comparison with the other NCSE types. Shorvon[46] divides SPSE into two types—with and without motor phenomena. There exist multiple SPSE types with varied symptomatology, which are defined as seizure activity lasting 30 min or more, without loss or severe alteration of consciousness. Following Gastaut, non-convulsive SPSE can be classified within the following categories: (1) sensory SPSE; (2) visual SPSE; (3) acoustic SPSE; (4) olfactory SPSE; (5) gustatory SPSE; (6) autonomic SPSE; (7) dysphasic or aphasic SPSE.[3] This last type can be further subdivided into expressive versus receptive aphasic SPSE. Some authors include Landau–Kleffner syndrome (LKS) and continuous spike-and-wave during slow sleep (CSWS), two childhood epileptic syndromes, under the entity of aphasic SPSE.[47]

A literature review may suggest that these types of SE are extremely rare. However, detection may be difficult because they may not be recognized easily by clinical or EEG criteria. The most well documented of these types of seizures is aphasic SPSE. Aphasic SPSE is characterized by aphasia, sometimes associated with agraphia and alexia. It can be divided into intermittent versus continuous. During the intermittent type, language is disturbed only during the seizures, with normal oral expression between them. In the other type, the language disturbance persists during the inter-ictal period.

Patient population

Due to the rarity of published reports, it is difficult to establish the prevalence of SPSE. Its clinical symptoms vary widely and may be difficult to identify. Some cases of SPSE have been misdiagnosed as CPSE. In addition, the EEG is not always diagnostic. The onset of SPSE varies, with entities such as LKS beginning most commonly between the ages of 3–8 years, and SPSE with sensory, visual, acoustic, olfactory, autonomic or gustatory symptoms being reported most commonly in adults.

Differential diagnosis

SPSE may be confused with CPSE. The difference between these two types is determined by the presence or absence of altered consciousness, which may be difficult to assess, especially if the patient is uncooperative or aphasic. Psychiatric disturbances must also be considered. Behavioral changes, such as fear, panic and irritability, can be seen in some types of SPSE with autonomic symptoms. Cases of dysphasic, aphasic and sensory SPSE need to be differentiated from cerebrovascular ischemic events.

Diagnostic evaluation

The EEG is essential in establishing the diagnosis of SPSE, although frequently the scalp EEG is non-diagnostic and may even demonstrate no abnormalities. Frequently, the diagnosis can only be made by depth electrodes. Wieser,[47] who has recorded combined surface and depth EEG during SPSE, has demonstrated that there may be localized high frequency 'tonic' discharges, but more frequently the discharges consist of rhythmic clonic patterns with sharp slow-wave complexes at a frequency of ~0.3–3 per s. Other EEG findings include a waxing and waning pattern, and continuously repetitive rhythmic spike discharges.

Brain imaging studies, preferably MRI with gadolinium, should be performed to investigate the possibility of underlying focal structural abnormality causing SPSE.

Treatment

SPSE is usually well controlled by benzodiazepines such as diazepam, lorazepam or midazolam.

Prognosis

In non-convulsive SPSE there appears to be no mortality and little or no risk of secondary brain damage. However, in the childhood epileptic syndromes—LKS and CSWS—the neuropsychological outcomes are poor.

Subtle SE and generalized electrographic SE

Clinical description

The term 'subtle SE' denotes a form of generalized SE with minimal clinical signs.[49] Generalized electrographic SE may have no associated clinical signs. Uncertainty in the classification of NCSE is common because impaired consciousness may result from the initial or precipitating illness, making application of current terminology (absence SE, SPSE, CPSE) difficult.

Many NCSE patients are critically ill.[50,51] Clinical manifestations range from coma without other manifestations of seizures, to subtle convulsive movements, including rhythmic twitching of the limbs, trunk or face, or jerking conjugate eye movements. Less commonly, patients may be awake, with confusion, slowed responses and catatonia.[52] NCSE may present as prolonged confusion following convulsions, with clinical manifestations of eye blinking and rolling, automatisms, neglect, psychotic symptoms or agitated behavior.[53,54] Underlying etiologies of post-convulsive NCSE include hypoxia, infection, CVA, metabolic abnormalities, tumor, subdural hemorrhage, or withdrawal from ethanol or antiepileptic drugs.[21,50]

It is becoming increasingly recognized that subtle NCSE may persist, even after the clinical manifestations of convulsive SE resolve.[14,55] Treiman[56] has described the clinical manifestations of inadequately treated generalized convulsive SE (GCSE) as an evolution from overt to increasingly subtle activity, until ultimately the patient appears comatose and motionless, with persistent ictal activity on the EEG.[56] He postulated that inadequately treated GCSE causes an ictal encephalopathy which results, eventually, in clinical/electrographic dissociation and the evolution from overt to subtle seizure activity. *De novo* subtle or electrographic generalized SE may occur without ever being associated with overt clinical seizure activity.

Patient population

Subtle SE and electrographic SE are more common than was previously thought.[40,50,57,58] The incidence of electrographic SE after control of clinical SE was 14 per cent in the Richmond, Virginia, population-based study of SE.[21] Studies of patients with altered consciousness or coma have documented subtle or electrographic SE in over one third of those in whom the diagnosis was considered.[57,58] Another study looked at patients who had generalized electrographic SE, identified by EEG. Most were comatose, and 38 per cent had never had clinical seizures. Clinical SE had occurred in 40 per cent of this group, but most of these patients were thought to have stopped seizing and ongoing electrographic SE was unsuspected in 81 per cent of these patients.[50] In the ICU, NCSE is common, occurring in 8 per cent of ICU patients with altered consciousness or coma.[40]

NCSE, or subtle SE, commonly occurs after convulsive SE has stopped. In a study of generalized electrographic SE found on EEG, 40 per cent of patients demonstrated clinical SE, but these patients were thought to have stopped seizing.[50] In the Richmond study, 14 per cent of patients who clinically stopped seizing continued to demonstrate electrographic SE and 34 per cent had seizures, of which two thirds had non-convulsive seizures.[21]

Differential diagnosis

The differential diagnosis of subtle SE and generalized electrographic SE includes other causes of coma, such as metabolic encephalopathy, infection, tumor, stroke, prolonged post-ictal state, systemic or central nervous system infection, hypoxia/anoxia, sedative drugs and the other etiologies included in Tables 7.1 and 7.2.[14,27–34,50,59–64] CPSE may have minor clinical manifestations and bilateral EEG changes, making differentiation from subtle SE and generalized electrographic SE a clinical challenge.

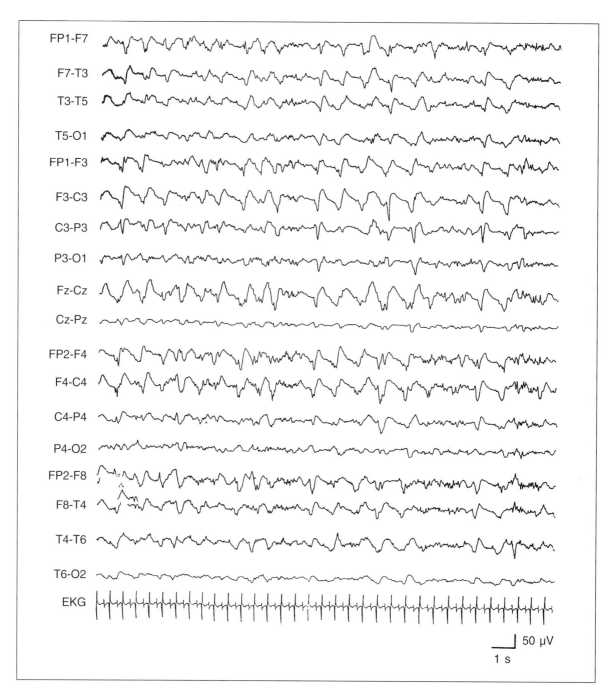

Figure 7.2
Generalized non-convulsive status epilepticus (NCSE). Bifrontally predominant 1 Hz rhythmic sharp and slow-wave complexes.

Diagnostic evaluation

As with all cases of NCSE, the EEG is of paramount importance in diagnosis. Treiman[46] has described a sequence of EEG changes that are frequently observed during GCSE. Initially, there are discrete electrographic seizures beginning with low-voltage fast activity, often focal, that evolves with increasing amplitude and decreasing frequency. There is usually a great deal of muscle artifact that obscures the cerebral activity on the EEG. When clonic activity stops, low-voltage activity occurs. Seizures continue to occur, and ictal discharges wax and wane, without a clear-cut beginning or end. Rhythmic activity is almost continuous, speeding up and slowing down. Finally, intervals of relative voltage suppression occur between bursts of epileptiform discharges and the suppressed intervals progressively lengthen. Eventually, periodic discharges occur on a suppressed background.[65–67]

Varying EEG presentations of NCSE have been described.[21,51,52,54, 58,68] The EEG typically shows either sharp waves, spikes or rhythmic slow-wave activity that is generalized, but may have a focal predominance. The frequency is most often 2–4 Hz, but may initially be faster or slower (Figure 7.2).

Evaluation of the underlying cause of NCSE should include metabolic laboratory studies and cerebrospinal fluid analysis to rule out systemic infection, and obtaining a brain imaging study, preferably MRI.

Treatment

Treatment should be initiated with intravenous administration of a benzodiazepine, which may also aid in diagnosis by causing rapid, although usually transient, attenuation of electrographic ictal activity. Comatose patients with NCSE should be treated with long-term anticonvulsant drugs. Since they are often critically ill, drug treatment may be limited by hypotension, organ failure or other factors. However, since these patients are usually intubated and artificially ventilated, drug-induced respiratory depression is usually not an issue. If the NCSE is suspected to be due to withdrawal from an antiepileptic agent, this drug should be replaced to a high therapeutic serum concentration. A loading dose of intravenous phenytoin or fosphenytoin is usually given, unless there are specific contraindications. If electrographic ictal activity persists, a burst–suppression pattern can be obtained on the EEG using anesthetic doses of pentobarbital, diazepam, midazolam or propofol. Intravenous benzodiazepines have the advantage of a short half-life, however, they may prove ineffective if prolonged treatment (more than several days) is required. Propofol is also clinically short acting, conferring the ability to decrease the infusion rate and quickly assess the patient's baseline level of consciousness.

It is generally considered that treatment with anticonvulsant agents, even to anesthetic levels, is warranted, given the evidence that suggests that the seizure activity associated with SE injures the nervous system, with an increase in morbidity and mortality associated with prolonged SE.[69–73] The approach to patients who are awake, but confused, is less clear-cut. In these patients, efforts may be made to treat with a benzodiazepine and phenytoin or fosphenytoin, while trying to avoid intubation and further deterioration in the level of consciousness. Patients may be given phenytoin, carbamazepine or valproic acid orally, or via NG tube in an effort to boost drug levels to the therapeutic range. Antiepileptic drugs should be titrated upward to clinical response or side effects.

Prognosis

There is a significant morbidity and mortality associated with subtle SE, electrographic SE and postconvulsive NCSE. Mortality rates range from 57 to 87 per cent.[50,74] Predictors of poor outcome include anoxic etiology and coma at the time of presentation.[50] Multivariate logistic regression analysis of nonconvulsive seizures in the ICU using continuous EEG monitoring demonstrated that only seizure duration and delay in diagnosis were significantly associated with increased mortality.[74] There was no significant difference in mortality between patients who had clinical seizures initially and those who did not.[50]

Patients with generalized NCSE who are not comatose generally have a better prognosis.[52,54,74] In a series of patients whose NCSE manifested as confusion following convulsions, all recovered, despite a delayed response to treatment. Many of these patients had a prior history of epilepsy.[54] Even when there is no prior history of epilepsy, NCSE presenting with confusion often responds well to medication, although recurrences are common.[75]

References

1. Towne AR, Pellock JM, Ko D, DeLorenzo RJ. Determinants of mortality in status epilepticus. *Epilepsia* 1994;35:27–34.
2. DeLorenzo RJ, Hauser WA, Towne AR, et al. A prospective, population-based epidemiologic study of status epilepticus in Richmond, Virginia. *Neurology* 1996;46:1029–35.
3. Gastaut H. Classification of status epilepticus. In: Delgado-Escueta AV, Wasterlain CG, Treiman DM, Porter RJ, eds. *Status epilepticus*. New York: Raven Press, 1983:15–35.
4. Treiman DM, Status epilepticus. *Clin Neurology* 1996;5:821–39.
5. Krumholz A, Sung GY, Fisher RS, et al. Complex partial status epilepticus accompanied by serious morbidity and mortality. *Neurology* 1995;45:1499–504.
6. Tomson T, Svanborg E, Wedlund JE. Nonconvulsive status epilepticus: High incidence of complex partial status. *Epilepsia* 1986;27: 276–85.
7. Jagoda A, Riggio S. Nonconvulsive status epilepticus in adults. *Amer J Emerg Med* 1988;6:250–4.
8. Celesia G. Modern concepts of status epilepticus. *JAMA* 1976;235:1571–4.
9. Treiman D, Delgado-Escueta A. Complex partial status epilepticus. In: Delgado-Escueta AV, Wasterlain CG, Treiman DM, Porter RJ, eds. *Status epilepticus*. New York: Raven Press, 1983:69–81.
10. Gastaut H, Tassinari C. Status epilepticus. In: Gastaut H, ed. *Handbook of Electroencephalography and Clinical Neurophysiology*. Vol. 13A. Amsterdam: Elsevier, 1975:39–45.
11. Tomson T, Lindborn U, Nilsson BY. Nonconvulsive status epilepticus in adults: Thirty-two consecutive patients from a general hospital population. *Epilepsia* 1992;33:829–35.
12. Roger J, Lob H, Tassinari CA. Status epilepticus. In: Vinken PJ, Bruyn GW, eds. *Handbook of clinical neurology*. Vol. 15, *The epilepsies*. Amsterdam: Elsevier, 1974:145–99.
13. Markand ON, Wheeler GL, Pollack SL. Complex partial status epilepticus (psychomotor status). *Neurology* 1978;28:189–95.
14. DeLorenzo RJ, Garnett LK, Towne AR, et al. Comparison of status epilepticus with prolonged seizure episodes lasting from 10–29 minutes. *Epilepsia* 1999:submitted.
15. Jaitly RK, Sgro JA, Towne AR, et al. Prognostic

value of EEG monitoring after status epilepticus, a prospective adult study. *J Clin Neurophysiol* 1997;**14**:326–34.

16. Hesdoffer DC, Logroscino G, Cascino G, et al. Incidence of status epilepticus in Rochester, Minnesota, 1965–1984. *Neurology* 1998;**50**:735–41.

17. Andermann F, Robb JP. Absence status: a reappraisal following review of thirty-eight patients. *Epilepsia* 1972;**13**:177–87.

18. Porter RJ, Penry JK. Petit mal status. In: Delgado-Escueta AV, Wasterlain CG, Treiman DM, Porter RJ, eds. *Status epilepticus*. New York: Raven Press, 1983:61–7.

19. Engel JE Jr. Status epilepticus. In: Engel JE Jr, ed. *Seizures and epilepsy*. Philadelphia: FA Davis, 1989:A:256–80.

20. Cascino G.D. Nonconvulsive status epilepticus in adults and children. *Epilepsia* 1993;**34**(Suppl 1):S21–8.

21. DeLorenzo RJ, Waterhouse EJ, Towne AR, et al. Persistent nonconvulsive status epilepticus after the control of convulsive status epilepticus. *Epilepsia* 1998;**39**:833–40.

22. Berkovic SF, Bladin PF. Absence status in adults. *Clin Exp Neurol* 1983;**19**:198–207.

23. Hauser WA. Status epilepticus: frequency, etiology, and neurological sequelae. In: Delgado-Escueta AV, Wasterlain CG, Treiman DM, Porter RJ, eds. *Status epilepticus*. New York: Raven Press, 1983:3–14.

24. DeLorenzo RJ, Pellock JM, Towne AR, Boggs JG. Epidemiology of status epilepticus. *J Clin Neurol* 1995;**12**:316–25.

25. Thomas P, Beaumanoir A, Genton P, et al. 'De novo' absence status of late onset: report of 11 cases. *Neurology* 1992;**42**:104–10.

26. Vignaendra V, Frank AO, Lim CL. Clinical note: absence status in a patient with hypocalcemia. *Electroencephalogr Clin Neurophysiol* 1977;**43**:429–33.

27. Obeid T, Yaqub B, Panayiotopoulos C, et al. Absence status epilepticus with computed tomographic brain changes following metrizamide myelography. *Ann Neurol* 1988;**24**:582–4.

28. Pritchard PB, O'Neal DB. Nonconvulsive status epilepticus following metrizamide myelography. *Ann Neurol* 1984;**16**:252–4.

29. Callahan DJ, Noetzel MJ. Prolonged absence status epilepticus association with carbamazepine therapy, increased intracranial pressure, and transient MRI abnormalities. *Neurology* 1992;**42**:2198–201.

30. Snead OC, Hosey LC. Exacerbation of seizures in children by carbamazepine. *N Engl J Med* 1985;**313**:916–21.

31. Vollmer NE, Weiss H, Beanland C, Krumholz A. Prolonged confusion due to absence status following metrizamide myelography. *Arch Neurol* 1985;**42**:1005–8.

32. Ahmed I, Pepple R, Jones RP. Absence status epilepticus resulting from metrizamide and omnipaque myelography. *Clin Electroencephalogr* 1988;**19**:37–42.

33. Sundaram MB, Hill A, Lowry N. Thyroxine-induced petit mal status epilepticus. *Neurology* 1985;**35**:1792–3.

34. Wagner JH. Another report of nonconvulsive status epilepticus after metrizamide myelography. *Ann Neurol* 1995;**18**:369–70.

35. Granner MA, Lee IK. Nonconvulsive status epilepticus: EEG analysis in a large series. *Epilepsia* 1994;**35**:42–7.

36. Browne TR, Mikati M. Status epilepticus. In: Ropper AH, Kennedy SF, eds. *Neurological and neurosurgical intensive care*. Rockville: Aspen, 1988:269–88.

37. Dulac O, N'Guyen T. The Lennox–Gastaut syndrome. *Epilepsia* 1993;**34**(Suppl 7):S7–17.

38. Gastaut H, Roger J, Roger A. Sur la signification de certaines fugues epileptiques: etat de mal temporal *Revue Neurologique* 1956;**94**:298–301.

39. Garrett WT, Chang CW, Bleck TP. Altered mental status in thrombotic thrombocytopenic purpura is secondary to nonconvulsive status epilepticus. *Ann Neurol* 1996;**40**:245–6.

40. Towne AR, Boggs JG, Smith JR, DeLorenzo RJ. Status epilepticus in patients in whom EEGs were obtained for the evaluation of coma. *Neurology* 1995;**45**(Suppl 4):A424.

41. Williamson PD, Spencer DD, Spencer SS, et al. Complex partial status epilepticus: A depth-electrode study. *Ann Neurol* 1985;**18**:647–54.

42. Williamson PD, Spencer DD, Spencer SS, et al. Complex partial seizures of frontal lobe origin. *Ann Neurol* 1985;**18**:497–504.

43. Williamson PD. Complex partial status epilepticus. In: Engel J Jr, Pedley TA, eds. *Epilepsy:*

a comprehensive textbook. Philadelphia: Lippincott-Raven, 1997:618–723.

44. Young GB, Jordan GJ. Do nonconvulsive seizures damage the brain?—Yes. *Arch Neurol* 1998;**55**:117–19.

45. Aminoff MJ. Do nonconvulsive seizures damage the brain?—No. *Arch Neurol* 1988;**55**:119–20.

46. Shorvon S. *Status epilepticus*. New York: Cambridge University Press, 1994.

47. Wieser HG. Simple partial status epilepticus. In: Engel J Jr, Pedley TA, eds. *Epilepsy: a comprehensive textbook*. Philadelphia: Lippincott-Raven, 1997:709–21.

48. Wieser HG, Williamson PD. Ictal semeiology. In: Engel J Jr, ed. *Surgical treatment of the epilepsies*, 2nd ed. New York: Raven Press, 1993:161–71.

49. Treiman DM, DeGiorgio CMA, Salisbury SM, Wickboldt CL. Subtle generalized convulsive status epilepticus. *Epilepsia* 1984;**25**:653.

50. Drislane FW, Schomer DL. Clinical implications of generalized electrographic status epilepticus. *Epilepsy Res* 1994;**19**:111–21.

51. Jordan KG. Status epilepticus: A perspective from the neuroscience intensive care unit. *Neuro Surg Clin North Am* 1994;**5**:671–86.

52. Guberman A, Cantu-Reyna G, Stuss D, Broughton R. Nonconvulsive generalized status epilepticus: clinical features, neurophysiological testing, and long-term follow-up. *Neurology* 1986;**36**:1284–91.

53. Lee SI. Nonconvulsive status epilepticus: ictal confusion in later life. *Arch Neurol* 1985;**42**:778–781.

54. Fagan KJ, Lee SI. Prolonged confusion following convulsions due to generalized nonconvulsive status epilepticus. *Neurology* 1990;**40**: 1689–94.

55. Bauer G, Aichner F, Mayr U. Nonconvulsive status epilepticus: postictal confusional state: EEG. *Eur Neurol* 1982;**21**:411–19.

56. Treiman DM. Generalized convulsive status epilepticus in the adult. *Epilepsia* 1993;**34** (Suppl 1):S2–11.

57. Privitera M, Hoffman M, Moore JL, Jester D. EEG detection of nontonic-clonic status epilepticus in patients with altered consciousness. *Epilepsy Res* 1994;**18**:155–66.

58. Lowenstein DH, Aminoff MJ. Clinical and EEG features of status epilepticus in comatose patients. *Neurology* 1992;**42**:100–4.

59. Bhardwaj A, Badesha PS. Ifosfamide-induced nonconvulsive status epilepticus. *Ann Pharmacother* 1995;**29**:1237–9.

60. Varma NK, Lee SI. Nonconvulsive status epilepticus following electroconvulsive therapy. *Neurology* 1992;**42**:263–4.

61. Vickrey BG, Bahls FH. Nonconvulsive status epilepticus following cerebral angiography. *Ann Neurol* 1989;**25**:199–201.

62. Wengs WJ, Talwar DT, Bernard J. Ifosfamide-induced nonconvulsive status epilepticus. *Arch Neurol* 1993;**50**:1104–5.

63. Zak R, Solomon G, Petito F, Labar D. Baclofen-induced generalized nonconvulsive status epilepticus. *Ann Neurol* 1994;**36**:113–14.

64. Klion AD, Kallsen J, Cowl CT, Nauseef WM. Ceftazidime-related nonconvulsive status epilepticus. *Arch Intern Med* 1994;**154**:586–9.

65. Treiman DM, Walton NY, Kendrick C. A progressive sequence of electroencephalographic changes during generalized convulsive status epilepticus. *Epilepsy Res* 1990;**5**:49–60.

66. Treiman DM. Generalized convulsive, nonconvulsive, and focal status epilepticus. In: Feldman E, ed. *Current diagnosis in neurology*. St Louis: Yearbook, Inc, 1994:11–18.

67. Treiman DM. Electroclinical features of status epilepticus. *J Clin Neurophysiol* 1995;**12**: 343–62.

68. Towne AR, Waterhouse EJ, Boggs JG. Prevalence of non-convulsive status epilepticus in comatose patients. *Neurology* 1999:submitted.

69. Meldrum BS, Vigouroux RA, Brierley JB. Systemic factors and epileptic brain damage. *Arch Neurol* 1973;**29**:82–7.

70. Sloviter RS. 'Epileptic' brain damage in rats induced by sustained electrical stimulation of the perforant path. I Acute electrophysiological and light microscopic studies. *Brain Res Bull* 1983;**10**:675–97.

71. Rowan AJ, Scott DF. Major status epilepticus: a series of 42 patients. *Acta Neurol Scand* 1970;**46**:573–84.

72. Oxbury JM, Whitty CWM. Causes and consequences of status epilepticus in adults: a study of 86 cases. *Brain* 1971;**94**:733–44.

73. Aminoff MJ, Simon RP. Status epilepticus: causes, clinical features and consequences in 98 patients. *Am J Med* 1980;**69**:657–66.

74. Young GB, Jordan GJ, Doig GD. An assessment of nonconvulsive seizures in the intensive care unit using continuous EEG monitoring: an investigation of variables associated with mortality. *Neurology* 1996;**47**:83–9.

75. Dunne JW, Summers QA, Stewart-Wynne EG. Nonconvulsive status epilepticus: a prospective study in an adult general hospital. *Q Medical* 1987;**62**:117–26.

8

Diagnosis of cortical and subcortical dysplasias in epilepsy

Heinz-Joachim Meencke

Introduction

Developmental disturbances are the most frequent findings in epilepsies, with a rate of 63 per cent.[1] Besides severe malformations, slight developmental disturbances are gaining increasing clinical interest. These slight developmental disturbances are summarized under the term 'cortical dysplasia' from the clinical point of view. This increased clinical interest is related to the development of surgery for seizures resistant to pharmacotherapy and to the improvement of neuroimaging methods.

The developmental disturbances described in this chapter occur during the second and third periods of fetal brain development. Specific brain malformations are related to different stages of fetal brain development. Current neurobiological knowledge makes it possible to establish six fundamental steps in the development of the nervous tissue:

1. Cellular proliferation of the periventricular matrix zone.
2. Neuronal migration within the glial fiber tracks with the inside/outside mode.
3. Neuronal cell death with apoptosis.
4. Further differentiation of neuronal and glial cell elements.
5. Axonal and dendritic outgrowth.
6. Synaptogenesis.

At present, it is impossible to present a classification of brain malformations on the basis of these neurobiologically defined steps of brain development. Moreover, the detailed aetiopathogenesis of a distinct malformation is speculative, because several steps of the developmental process are involved in any one distinct type of malformation. In some malformations the genetic background is known, on the other hand many malformations are the result of epigenetic factors. In particular, the relationship between the genetic background of a distinct epilepsy syndrome and its association with a distinct malformation is not known. Because of the uncertainty of the neurobiological background of the aetiopathogenesis of many malformations there is continuing controversy about the classification of brain malformations.

Bresler[2] was the first to use the term 'dysplasias of the cerebral cortex' strictly for developmental disturbances and to separate them from the residual lesions of the cortex related to ischemia. Today the entire spectrum of developmental malformations is summarized under the term dysplasias of the cerebral cortex (Table 8.1). Figure 8.2 shows the macroscopically visible disturbances such as pachygyria, polymicrogyria, heterotopia, and also slight developmental disturbances such as dystopic Cajal cells, protusions, clusters and abnormal laminar architecture, which Meencke and Veith described, together with other slight architec-

Agyria (lissencephaly)	Leptomeningeal glioneuronal heterotopias
Pachygyria	Persistence of Cajal cells
Heterotopia	Columnar arrangement
Nodular	Abnormal laminar architecture
Laminar	Focal dysplasia of the cerebral cortex
Polymicrogyria	
Nodular cortical dysplasia	

(Modified from Bresler, 1899)[2]

Table 8.1
Dysplasias of the cerebral cortex.

tural disturbances, under the term microdysgenesis[3] (Figure 8.1). The term 'focal dysplasia of the cerebral cortex' is also included in this group. This term was introduced by Taylor et al[4] and describes a distinct type of cortical dysplasia which is not macroscopically visible with a normal thickness of the cortex. This is ignored in many current publications which use the term in respect to this paper, but illustrate macroscopically visible enlarged regional developmental disturbances not comparable with the primary description. Also, Vinters and co-workers[5] proposed a limited definition of neocortical dysplasia which included predominantly morphological criteria of the microdysgenesis described by Meencke and Veith,[3] adding the polymicrogyria and some elements of changes of the neuronal body (Table 8.2). On a pathological basis, Kuzniecky and co-workers produced a classification of focal

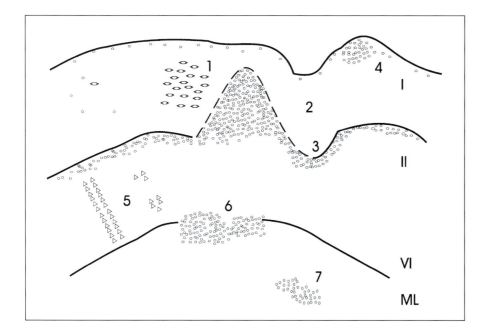

Figure 8.1
Heteromorphism of microdysgenesis. (1) Diffuse and localized increase of dystopic neurons; (2) nerve cell protrusions; (3) pits and hollows; (4) subpial nerve cell nests; (5) architectural disturbances of deeper cortical zone; (6) indistinct border zone; (7) dystopic neurons in the white matter.

1. Cortical laminar disorganization
2. Single heterotopia white manner neurons
3. Neurons in the cortical molecular layer
4. Persistent remains of the subpial granular cell layer (SGL)
5. Marginal glioneural heterotopia
6. Polymicrogyria
7. White matter neuronal heterotopia
8. Neuronal cytomegaly with associated cytoskeletal abnormalities
9. Balloon cell change

(Modified from Vinters et al, 1993)[5]

Table 8.2
Cortical dysplasia.

cortical dysplasias comprised of two types:[6] type I with only changes of cortical architecture and type II with additional abnormal cell proliferation and differentiation, all with macroscopically visible cortical changes. It should be kept in mind that the term cortical dysplasia is a diagnostic hotchpotch encompassing a large variety of morphological changes; in the main the neuropathologist is able to give the final diagnosis. From a practical point of view, especially for clinical and imaging aspects, a phenomenological classification which differentiates between microscopically and macroscopically visible dysplasias is preferable (Figure 8.2). At present it is usually only possible to demonstrate the macroscopically visible changes with imaging methods, but the close correlation of imaging results and neuropathological analysis will improve the capacity to demonstrate slight developmental disturbances by imaging methods.

Epilepsy surgery has made an important contribution to the understanding of dysplasias

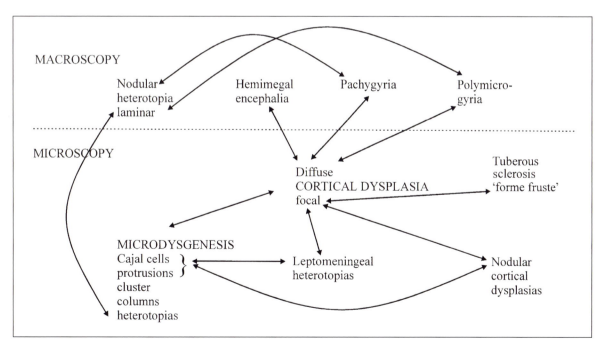

Figure 8.2
Phenomenological transition between different dysplasias.

and at the same time has improved the capabilities of presurgical monitoring to define the epileptogenic lesion. The neuropathological diagnosis of cortical dysplasia in resected specimens is affected by fundamental methodological problems. The demonstration of very slight developmental disturbances depends on adequate neuroanatomical topographic orientation. Neuronal density, lamination and gyration of the cortex are defined by the direction and level of the cut through the cortical specimen. This definition is usually possible in autopsy material, but is difficult and sometimes impossible in biopsy studies. Slight architectural disturbances of the cortex without abnormal cell elements therefore require quantitative morphometric studies. Clearly defined histological criteria are needed for these studies; if these are missing, the validity of the results is limited.

In vivo diagnosis by imaging methods

Magnetic resonance imaging (MRI)

The use of imaging methods considerably improves the syndrome diagnosis. The specification of the syndrome diagnosis is very important for an individual patient's therapy and prognosis. Although genetic studies and genetic counselling need a precise syndrome separation, epilepsy surgery primarily requires a clear morphological diagnosis by imaging methods to separate the epileptogenic lesion and to give a clear definition of the relationship between the lesion and the irritative and ictogenic zone.[7] MRI is the best method for in vivo imaging.

Positron emission tomography (PET) and single photon emission computed tomography (SPECT), both functional imaging methods, are additional techniques that can clarify functional aspects of anatomical deviations. In pediatric epileptology ultrasound is sometimes also used. MRI is the structural imaging modality of choice for the investigation of patients with epilepsy and suspected developmental malformations. Although computerized tomography (CT) can detect some of these malformations, it cannot be used as a definite diagnostic technique in the classification of these disorders. MRI should include T1-weighted and T2-weighted sequences to cover the entire brain in at least two planes. It should be borne in mind that MRI covers two aspects: imaging of the macroscopic anatomy and of the tissue quality.

Normal MRI procedures are carried out in spin–echo sequences (SE). Imaging of the anatomy is predominantly done by T1-weighted images with additional inversion recovery mode. The inversion recovery mode allows a clear definition of the anatomy. The new technology with gradient echo (GE) imaging with three-dimensional (3-D) data aquisition improves the analysis of detailed anatomical changes. The technique allows the analysis of very thin slices (1 mm thick), which avoids projection-related artifacts. The imaging of tissue quality, on the other hand, reveals a number of pathological deviations. These aspects are best analysed with T2-weighted images and the fluid attenuated inversion recovery (FLAIR) technique. Sometimes it is not possible to define the pathological architecture of the cortex by the macroscopical structure in the T1 inversion recovery mode alone. In these cases the FLAIR technique helps to focus on the pathological region (Figure 8.3), because this technique increases the signal that results from pathological tissue composition. MRI 3-D–FT data aquisition techniques should be performed, if available. Reformatting of multiple planes should be carried out in the analysis of these

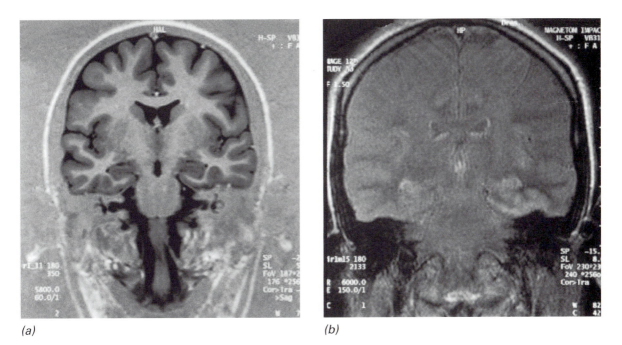

(a)   *(b)*

Figure 8.3
(a) MRI, T1–IR mode. Suspicious architecture of the parahippocampal gyrus on the left side. (b) MRI, FLAIR technique. Signal increase of the parahippocampal gyrus on the left side.

images. This helps to separate normal cortical migration from clearly dysplastic changes. Figure 8.4 shows a schematic proposal for the step by step approach to diagnostic evaluation using MRI. MRI is first performed in three planes in SE with T1-weighted imaging, including inversion recovery mode, T2-weighted images and the FLAIR technique. If the MRI is negative, video-EEG monitoring should be used to generate a localization hypothesis. With this localization hypothesis a special MRI should be performed in this region with very thin slices (if possible in GE mode), including T1 inversion recovery and FLAIR mode and reconstruction of 3-D multiple planes. Indirect signs of pathological changes can be indicated by changes in relaxation times, differences in the cortical

thickness and the transition between cortex and subcortical white matter.

PET/SPECT

Functional isotope brain studies, including PET and SPECT, have a limited role in the investigation of patients with cortical developmental malformations and epilepsy unless surgery is contemplated. Interictal PET and ictal SPECT studies may be useful in the delineation of the main areas of epileptogenesis in some individuals with these malformations.

However, these studies can contribute information about functional aspects of morphological disturbances. In particular, PET studies

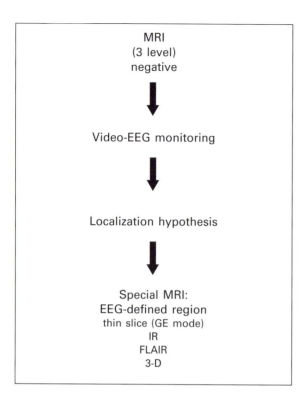

Figure 8.4
Diagnostic stages in MRI investigation.

can demonstrate abnormal receptor functions that are associated with the MRI findings, often far outside the restricted morphological lesions. This is shown even in patients with focal cortical dysplasias.[8] These widespread functional disturbances probably reflect the poor outcome after epilepsy surgery in some cases with focal cortical dysplasias. However, at present there are no predictors available that would allow the association of different functional disturbances with specific anatomical lesions.

Ultrasound (US) studies

Ultrasound studies are used in pediatric epileptology, but they are not adequate for the investigation of slight (microscopic) changes. Subcortical gray matter heterotopias are not demonstrable with this method. Two aspects can be demonstrated:

1. Changes associated with cortical dysplasias, e.g. clefts (schizencephaly) or pathological gyration (lissencephaly).
2. Severe macroscopic changes such as nodules and giant cell astrocytomas in some cases of tuberosclerosis.

These studies are limited and the results should be verified by MRI studies, related to the clinical situation and required therapeutic decisions.

Neuropathological and imaging aspects of cortical dysplasia

Table 8.3 shows the proportional rates of migrational disturbances which reflect the pathological findings summarized under the term cortical dysplasias.

	Controls (n=7374)	Epilepsies (n=591)
Microdysgenesis	6*	37.7
Heterotopia	0.6	5.3
Microgyria	1	4.7
Pachygyria	0.25	1.9

*n = 150 (Meencke and Veith, 1992)

Table 8.3
Proportional rates of migrational disturbances (%).

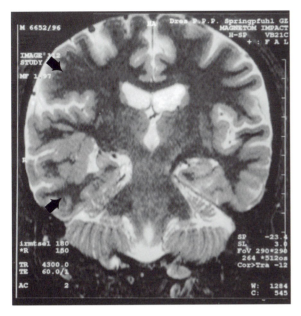

Figure 8.5
*MRI, T1–IR mode. Polymicrogyria in the
perisylvian region of the right side.*

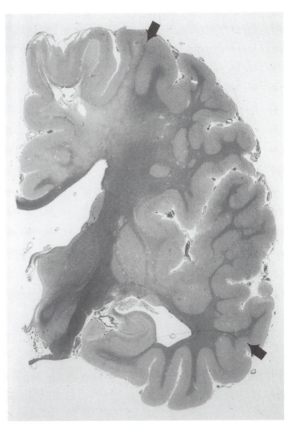

Figure 8.6
*Neuropathological specimen of the left
hemisphere. Polymicrogyria with subcortical
nodular heterotopias is shown between the
arrows.*

One feature that is definitely demonstrable
by MRI is the frequent finding of **polymicrogyria** as shown in Figure 8.5. The cortical
changes are clearly related to the vascular territory of the mid-cerebral artery. The pathological specimen (Figure 8.6) indicates that this
kind of cortical deviation is predominantly
associated with subcortical nodular heterotopias. Meencke and Veith provided evidence
that this type of disturbance is related to
metabolic disturbances in the fetal period
restricted to distinct vascular territories.[9] The
polygyric cortex is normally made up of four
layers: the molecular layer, a dense cell layer, a
low density cell layer (containing a horizontal
plexus of myelinated fibers) and a deep cell
layer with the transition zone to the subcortical white matter. On occasion some patients
have macroscopically normal configuration of
the gyrus or even a less folded configuration,
which supports the diagnosis of a pachygyric
cortex. In some of these cases, pathological
studies clearly demonstrate the polygyric type
of cortex, as shown in Figure 8.7. Therefore a
radiological appearance of pachygyria is not
necessarily confirmed pathologically. The
polygyric changes can be very discrete and
circumscribed (Figure 8.8), with only a discol-
ored thicker cortex and an indistinct transition
to the subcortical white matter.

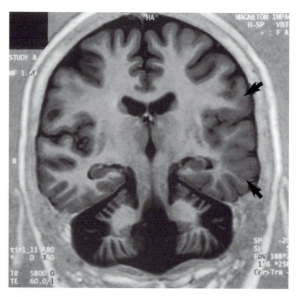

Figure 8.8
MRI, T1–IR mode. Restricted polygyric cortex shown between the arrows of the left perisylvian region.

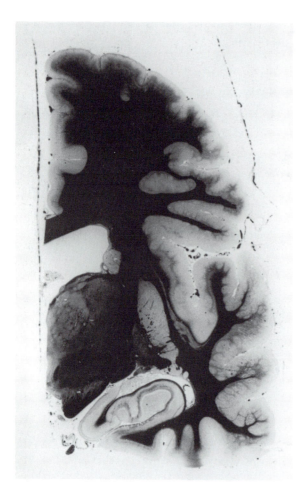

Figure 8.7
Neuropathological specimen of the left hemisphere. The pachygyric aspect of the cortex shows a clear polymicrogyric pathology.

However, this MRI finding is not only related to polygyric pathology. Figure 8.9 shows comparable circumscribed changes of the cortical configuration in the basal lateral left temporal lobe. The cortex is thicker, the internal border of the white matter is folded and the gyration of the surface also seems to be changed. The pathological study shows a feature which is predominantly described as

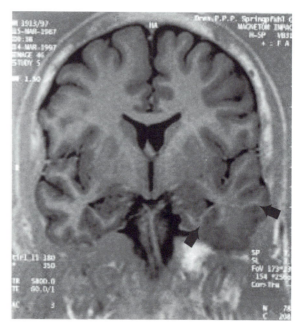

Figure 8.9
MRI, T1–IR mode. Disturbances of the architecture of the basal temporal cortex (see Figure 8.10).

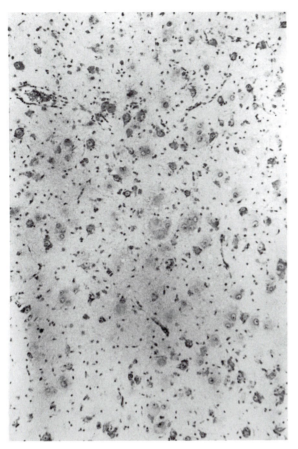

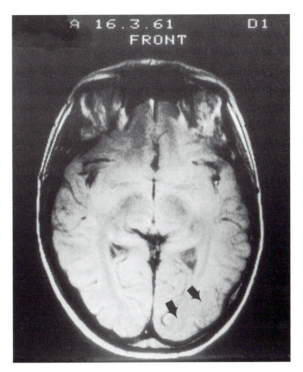

Figure 8.11
MRI, T1 mode. Circumscribed left occipital pachygyria.

Figure 8.10
Neuropathology of the lesion from Figure 8.9. This shows unlayered change of intracortical architecture with bizarre cells and clustering.

cortical dysplasia (Figure 8.10). There is an unlayered change in intracortical architecture with bizarre cells and clustering.

In cases with these types of pathology sometimes even the inversion recovery mode is not able to delineate the pathological cortical area clearly (see Figure 8.3). Then, as mentioned above, the FLAIR technique is helpful for focusing on the pathological area.

Pachygyrias are less frequent in epilepsies than other abnormalities, but nevertheless these changes are also demonstrable by imaging methods. Figure 8.11 shows a circumscribed area of pachygyria in the occipital lobe and Figure 8.12 shows bilateral pachygyria in the parieto-temporal areas, but it is very difficult to differentiate these changes clearly from polymicrogyria by imaging methods, as mentioned above. The diagnosis can be made, if, as usually shown, the cortical changes are correlated with the subcortical laminar heterotopias (Figure 8.13). This provides evidence that the pachygyria and subcortical laminar heterotopias represent different aspects and stages of the same pathological event.

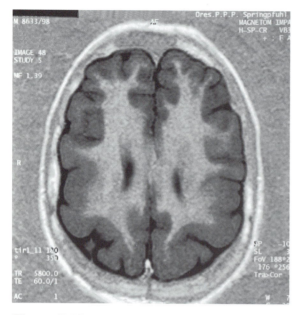

Figure 8.12
MRI, T1–IR mode. Widespread bilateral pachygyric cortex.

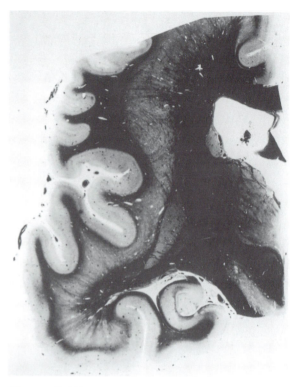

Figure 8.13
Neuropathological specimen of the right hemisphere with pachygyric cortex of the temporal lobe and subcortical laminar heterotopias.

Subcortical heterotopias are the most frequent findings of migration disturbances in epilepsy. The nodular heterotopias are predominant, occurring in >70 per cent of cases. Heterotopic gray matter does not represent dysplasias of the cerebral cortex in a strict sense. Yet it is appropriate to consider them in this chapter as they are formed from the same pool of cells as the cortex. Recent studies demonstrated that almost all cases with heterotopias also had disturbances of the overlying cortex (Table 8.4).[9,10]

	MD	MD Pachygyria	MD Microgyria	MD Microgyria + pachygyria
Nodular	8	2	9	2
Nodular/laminar			3	4
Laminar		1	1	

MD, microdysgenesis; (Meencke et al, 1998)[10]

Table 8.4
Combination of heterotopias and cortical disturbances.

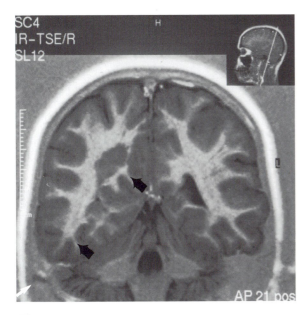

Figure 8.14
MRI, T1–IR mode. Nodular heterotopias in the right occipital lobe.

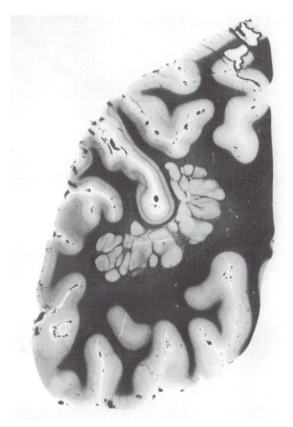

Figure 8.15
Neuropathological specimen of an occipital lobe with macroscopically normal overlying cortex.

Nodular heterotopias can be separated clearly, as shown in Figure 8.14. The pathological specimen shown in Figure 8.15 demonstrates that the overlying cortex can be macroscopically unsuspicious. Also, laminar heterotopias (Figure 8.16) can be demonstrated clearly with the macroscopically normal cortex, but histology shows widespread microdysgenesis.

The periventricular heterotopias make up a separate entity with a clear genetic background (Figure 8.17). Also, in these cases histologically there is a widespread cortical pathology (Table 8.5).

The cortical changes overlying heterotopic masses point to the fact that the slight intracortical changes of development, especially of migration and cell differentiation, cannot be demonstrated by current imaging methods.

Localized intracortical changes have been verified in secondary generalized symptomatic/ cryptogenic epilepsies (West syndrome, Lennox-

Pathology	Number
Microdysgenesis	3
Microdysgenesis + micropolygyria	1
Microdysgenesis + localized dysplasia	2
Total	6

(Meencke et al 1998)[10]

Table 8.5
Periventricular heterotopias and associated disturbances.

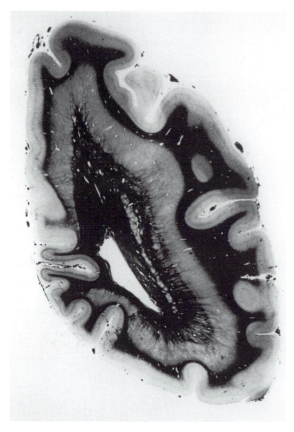

Figure 8.16
Neuropathological specimen of an occipital lobe with laminar heterotopias and a pachygyric cortex.

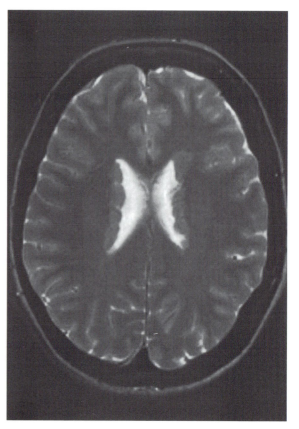

Figure 8.17
MRI, T2 mode. Periventricular bilateral heterotropias.

Gastaut syndrome).[11] Figure 8.18 shows a large localized protrusion of neurons up to the pia. Most cases show intracortical clustering, as can be seen in Figure 8.19. Even this clearly localized protrusion, which is demonstrable histologically, is not demonstrable by current imaging methods.

MRI does not add anything to the diagnosis of the slight developmental disturbances shown in generalized idiopathic epilepsies. Single cell heterotopias in the molecular layer and in the subcortical white matter cannot be shown by MRI (Figure 8.20).

It seems unlikely that these slight developmental disturbances can be visualized in the near future, given current restrictions on image resolution. The question arises whether other indirect parameters — that are related to these minimal developmental disturbances — could be demonstrated more easily. Four aspects seem to be important:

1. Thickness of the cortex.
2. Density of the cortex.
3. Pattern of gyration.
4. Larger dystopic masses: (a) within the cortex, (b) outside the cortex.

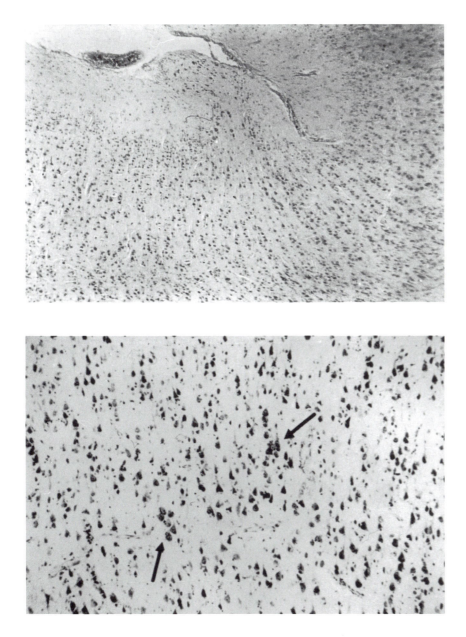

Figure 8.18
Localized protrusions of the cortex (paraffin and Nissl's stain).

Figure 8.19
Intracortical clustering of neurons (paraffin and Nissl's stain).

Even for these aspects the image resolution is critical. Extremely thin slices (<1 mm) are required (GE mode) to allow high resolution analysis of cortical areas and of the cortex at the white matter junction.

Pathological specimens have shown that the thickness of the cortex can be changed in cases with more prominent microdysgenesis with secondary generalized or focal epilepsies.[12,13] In contrast, pathological examinations of

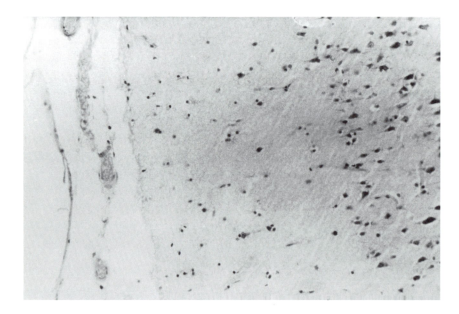

Figure 8.20
Single cell heterotopias in the molecular layer of the cortex (paraffin and Nissl's stain).

patients with primary generalized epilepsies show no alteration of cortical thickness, compared with non-epileptic controls.[14] High resolution scanning will also allow better delineation of gray and white matter, and the gray and white matter transition, changes that have been demonstrated in pathological specimens.[14]

Changes in gyration pattern are easily visible in patients with the more severe changes of pachygyria and polymicrogyria. Even more localized changes could be demonstrated if imaging was carried out with ultra-thin sections. Slight changes in the gyration pattern might be identified by fractal analysis.

Larger dystopic neuronal masses outside the cortex are easily visible by MRI imaging. Dystopic masses within the cortex, like the focal protrusions of the whole cortical lamina, are likely to be demonstrated by the use of thin sections. So far the demonstration of single dystopic neurons or swarms of single dystopic neurons (cortical and subcortical) has been limited.[15]

In summary, MRI can demonstrate a large variety of migration disturbances, however, the minimal developmental disturbances remain a significant challenge for this method.

References

1. Meencke H-J, Veith G. Migration disturbances in epilepsy. *Epilepsy Res* 1992; **9**(Suppl 9): 31–40.
2. Bresler J. Clinical and pathological–anatomical aspects of microgyria. *Arch Psychiat* 1899;**31**: 566–73.
3. Meencke H-J, Veith G. Neuropathological aspects of myoclonic–astatic *petit mal* (Lennox-syndrome). In: Kruse R, ed. *Epilepsie 84*. Reinbeck: Eichhorn Presse, 1985.
4. Taylor DC, Falconer MA, Bruton CJ, Corsellis JAN. Focal dysplasia of the cerebral cortex in

epilepsy. *J Neurol Neurosurg Psychiatry* 1971; **34**:369–87.

5. Vinters HV, De Rosa MJ, Farrell MA. Neuropathologic study of resected cerebral tissue from patients with infantile spasms. *Epilepsia* 1993;**34**:772–9.

6. Kuzniecky R, Garcia JH, Faught E, Morawetz RB. Cortical dysplasia in temporal lobe epilepsy: magnetic resonance imaging correlations. *Ann Neurol* 1991;**29**:293–8.

7. Lüders HO, Awad I. Conceptual considerations. In: Lüders HD, ed. *Epilepsy surgery*. New York: Raven Press, 1992.

8. Chugani HT. Functional imaging in cortical dysplasia: positron emission tomography. In: Guerrini R, et al, eds. *Dysplasias of cerebral cortex and epilepsy*. New York: Lippincott-Raven, 1996:169–74.

9. Meencke H-J, Vieth G. Perisylvian malformation-vascular aetiology? In: Tuxham I, Holthausen H, Boenigk H, eds. *Paediatric epilepsy syndromes and their surgical treatment*. London: John Libbey, 1997:190–9.

10. Meencke H-J, Veith G. Disturbances of cortical architecture associated with different types of heterotopias. *Epilepsia* 1998; **39**(Suppl 6): 231.

11. Meencke H-J, Gerhard C. Morphological aspects of aetiology and the course of infantile spasms (West syndrome). *Neuropediatrics* 1985;**16**:59–66.

12. Meencke H-J, Janz D. Neuropathological findings in primary generalized epilepsies: a study of eight cases. *Epilepsia* 1984;**25**:8–21.

13. Meencke H-J. Neuron density in the molecular layer of the frontal cortex in primary generalized epilepsy. *Epilepsia* 1985;**26**:450–4.

14. Meencke H-J. The density of dystrophic neurons in the white matter of the gyrus frontalis inferior in epilepsies. *J Neurol* 1983; **230**:171–81.

15. Chiron C, Dulac O, Nultin C, Depas G. Functional imaging in cortical dysplasia: SPECT. In: Guerrini R, et al. *Dysplasias of cerebral cortex and epilepsy*. New York: Lippincott-Raven, 1996:175–9.

9

Rational diagnosis of genetic epilepsies

Ingrid E Scheffer and Samuel F Berkovic

Introduction

In the 4th century BC, Hippocrates of Cos, the Greek physician many regard as the father of medicine, is attributed as saying of epilepsy 'And they who first referred this disease to the gods ... have given out that the disease is sacred ... Its origin is hereditary, like that of other diseases'.[1] The hereditary nature of epilepsy has long plagued people with the disorder. For example, the old Hebrew text, the Talmud, advised against taking a wife from an epileptic family. The ancient Scots 'instantly gelded' any man with the falling sickness, any such woman was 'kept from all company of men; and if by chance, ... found to be with child, she and her brood were buried alive: and this was done for the common good, lest the whole nation should be injured or corrupted'.[2] Until as recently as the middle of the 20th century, restrictive laws on marriage were placed on persons with epilepsy in at least 19 North American states.[3] Thus, the social stigma pervading epilepsy today arises not from the unpredictable nature of the attacks alone, but also from recognition of its genetic implications.

Despite widespread acknowledgement of the role of genetic factors in epilepsy, understanding the genetics of the epilepsies had been relatively limited until the latter part of the 20th century. It took a long time to establish that epilepsy was not one disorder, but rather a group of disorders, more appropriately regarded as 'the epilepsies'. Progress was made with the evolution of the International League Against Epilepsy's (ILAE) classification, which differentiated types of epileptic seizures,[4] followed by the revised classification incorporating epileptic syndromes in 1989.[5] The classification makes the important division of the epilepsies into generalized and partial epilepsies which are then broken down into idiopathic and symptomatic categories, providing a framework for research into the genetics of the epilepsies.

Clinical approach

Clinical clues to a genetic aetiology

The routine evaluation of a patient with epilepsy involves a comprehensive account of the patient's attacks and past medical history, as well as a full general and neurological examination. Although a family history is usually taken, it may be cursory if the clinician feels it is not relevant, or if he or she is not skilled in constructing a pedigree. In fact, a detailed family history is often the most important pointer to a genetic aetiology. A formal pedigree can be taken relatively quickly but should denote both sides of the patient's family and clearly indicate the relationship of the patient to other affected individuals (Table 9.1). A history

Name and date of birth of individuals
Maiden names of partners
Countries of origin of ancestors
Consanguinity
Obstetric history (miscarriages, stillbirths, neonatal deaths)
Ask about any seizures (not just epilepsy), including febrile convulsions, nocturnal or paroxysmal attacks
Ask patient to obtain data from other family members
Ask older family members, particularly women
Recheck data on follow-up visits
Update pedigree when new individuals become affected or new children are born

Table 9.1
Check-list for routine pedigree construction.

of epilepsy is not sufficient. The clinician should enquire whether family members have had any type of paroxysmal attack including febrile convulsions or isolated seizures. The patient often may not know much about their family history but should be encouraged to talk to the mothers in the family and any elderly matriarchs who may know of early childhood attacks in other family members, long since forgotten. Thus, it is common that the family history is 'fleshed out' by the patient who provides more significant detail at subsequent visits.

Attention to detail is important in constructing a pedigree. It is worth recording the date of birth (if known) of family members, maiden names of partners and the country of origin of a person's ancestors. Often, first names recur in a family tree and the date of birth is essential to prevent confusion among family members with the same name.

When taking the family history it is also important to ask about the patient's mother's obstetric history. If the patient's mother had an undue number of miscarriages or stillbirths, this may point to a genetic aetiology following sex-linked dominant inheritance with lethality in males. Some rare developmental malformations which may cause epilepsy have recently been recognized with this inheritance pattern which is easily missed if the salient questions are not asked.[6–12]

The familial nature of the patient's epilepsy may only become apparent with time, as further extended family history comes to light or new members of the family develop epilepsy. The older generations may initially be reticent to discuss a family history of seizures as they feel guilty about 'passing on' a disorder. With gentle education regarding genetic issues, as well as time, they may volunteer carefully guarded family secrets of major relevance.

Many individuals presenting with their first seizure have a distant relative with a history of seizures. It is unusual to obtain a family history suggestive of single-gene inheritance, such as an autosomal dominant or recessive or sex-linked pattern. Where there are a large number (e.g. 5 or 6) of affected family members over multiple generations (multiplex family), single-gene inheritance should not be dismissed if a few key individuals are not affected as they may be non-penetrant carriers of epilepsy genes. Epilepsy in multiplex families may also be following polygenic inheritance which, in some instances, can be impossible to differentiate from monogenic inheritance.

Family studies: research

There are a number of research strategies available to the clinical geneticist of the epilepsies. The first is genetic epidemiology, which uses a population-based approach. Theoretically, genetic epidemiology would be the ideal way to study the aetiological factors underlying the epilepsies; however, the search for epilepsy genes is dependent upon accurate diagnosis of epilepsy syndromes. There is no straightforward biological marker for affected status for epilepsy, which may be evanescent, unrecognized or misdiagnosed, making population-based studies very difficult to interpret. Population-based studies are further complicated by phenotypic and genotypic heterogeneity, already shown in a number of epilepsy syndromes (see below).

A second method is to focus on small families with multiple (~3–5) affected individuals. This method is valuable for recessive conditions, particularly if studying families from a geographic isolate, and led to identifying the genetic basis of Unverricht–Lundborg disease.[13] Such studies have been used extensively for juvenile myoclonic epilepsy (JME) and led to controversial results, partly because of the likelihood of underlying genetic heterogeneity (see below). In earlier studies of children with benign childhood epilepsy with centro-temporal spikes (BCECTS), a high rate of seizure disorders and epileptiform abnormalities in their families led the authors to postulate autosomal dominant inheritance, probably due to skewed ascertainment as they chose families where siblings had BCECTS, an uncommon clinical scenario.[14]

The third approach, and the one favoured here, is the study of large multi-generational, or multiplex, families which are an invaluable resource in studying disorders with complex inheritance such as epilepsy. Families with a large number of individuals with seizures are rare, but are more likely to have seizure disorders following single-gene inheritance. Studies of multiplex families with seizures have been fruitful in identifying new inherited epilepsy syndromes and in isolating genes for idiopathic epilepsies (see below).[15]

Multiplex families are ideal for clarifying the interrelationships of epilepsy syndromes, as they allow analysis of the phenotypic variation deriving from a relatively homogeneous genetic pool. The ILAE classification does not presently incorporate all phenotypes commonly observed, one common example being febrile seizures occurring in mid-childhood.[5] By studying the variety of epilepsy phenotypes within a multiplex family, an understanding of the seizure disorders arising from a single mutation can be developed and the classification improved; for instance, the relationship between febrile seizures and the generalized epilepsies can be examined (see below). Further, as opposed to the undoubted value of the classification in diagnosing individuals, when families are evaluated, heterogeneous phenotypes are observed. Understanding the familial interrelationships of phenotypes is a critical prerequisite for molecular genetic studies.

Detailed family studies are not realistically possible within the day-to-day practice of the clinician, as a single large family with 30 affected individuals takes a year to undergo a comprehensive assessment. Large multiplex families are virtually never referred to the clinical researcher as a *fait accompli* in terms of numbers of affected individuals or clinical detail. The usual situation is that the researcher begins with a kindred of 4 or 5 affected family members. The researcher then contacts all branches of the family, over as many generations as can be ascertained, looking for a history of seizures in any individual. Affected branches of a family often do not know of the existence of more distantly related individuals with epilepsy. This process may involve contacting hundreds of family members and isolating those branches of the family with a history of seizures for a more detailed study (Figure 9.1).

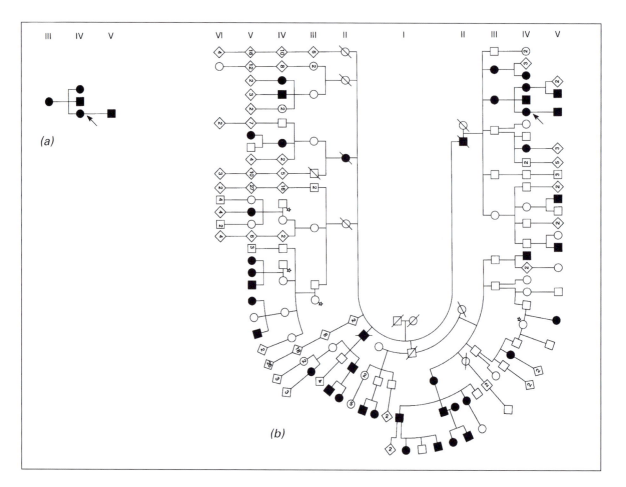

Figure 9.1

How a pedigree grows. (a) The number of affected individuals in the family when first ascertained at routine clinical assessment. (b) The 42 affected individuals when the family were studied in detail, of whom 26 had epilepsy consistent with the GEFS+ spectrum[19] and 21 had the SCN1B mutation.[20]

Individuals in these branches are then interviewed in detail for a history of seizures, obtaining both personal and eyewitness accounts, particularly from the mothers of affected family members. It is important to interview both affected and unaffected family members as it is not unusual to find that individuals have previously had undiagnosed or misdiagnosed seizures.[16–18] A neurological examination is performed on all family members as well as a careful inspection for dysmorphic features and neurocutaneous stigmata.

Partners who have married into the family must also be questioned regarding the presence of seizures both in themselves and in their extended family of origin. Bilineal inheritance of seizures is common, which is not surprising given the frequency of the epilepsies and febrile convulsions in the general population.[19] The finding of bilineal inheritance naturally alters the interpretation of the inheritance pattern of seizure disorders in a family, making polygenic inheritance considerably more likely in a family previously presumed to have autosomal dominant inheritance.[20]

Investigations centre around the electro-encephalogram (EEG). All family members should have routine EEG studies, or sleep EEG studies if possible, to look for the presence of epileptiform abnormalities. EEG studies are of variable value depending on the epilepsy syndrome in question. In some inherited epilepsies [e.g. autosomal dominant nocturnal frontal lobe epilepsy (ADNFLE)], interictal studies are normal in affected individuals,[17] while in others epileptiform discharges may be found in clinically unaffected family members.[21,22] In the latter situation, the epileptiform activity may represent a marker of carrier state in an inherited epilepsy syndrome with incomplete penetrance. Interpretation of the findings of EEG studies should take into account the age-dependent nature of some epileptiform abnormalities, such as centro-temporal spikes in BCECTS and 3 Hz generalized spike-and-wave in the idiopathic generalized epilepsies. Thus, EEG studies in later life may not give any information regarding an adult's affected status. Epileptiform discharges may also be state dependent so that they are only apparent if a sleep recording is obtained. In summary, the EEG has a role in family studies but is by no means the definitive marker of affected status.

Other investigations depend on the clinical setting. For example, in partial epilepsies, magnetic resonance imaging (MRI) studies of the brain allow analysis of the structure of the brain in the search for either inherited malformations or alternative aetiologies of an individual's seizures. Functional investigations, such as inter-ictal positron emission tomography (PET) and single photon emission computed tomography (SPECT), and ictal SPECT often help in localization of seizure origin. Definitive ictal studies require video-EEG monitoring which may be performed on key affected individuals in a family. In some families, more sophisticated clinical evaluation may be indicated, such as formal neuropsychological or speech pathology assessments depending on the clinical context.[22,23]

Molecular genetic studies

The epileptologist with an interest in clinical genetics has a unique opportunity to collaborate with molecular geneticists in discovering genes for epilepsy. As multiplex families are relatively genetically homogeneous, they provide the best approach for molecular genetic studies, as shown by successful molecular genetic studies in a variety of other complex disorders.[24] Large families allow an 'affected only' molecular analysis to be used. In a disorder such as epilepsy, unaffected status can be difficult to prove: subtle seizures may remain undiagnosed or misdiagnosed despite detailed interviewing; reliance on an abnormal EEG trait has a number of inherent problems (see above); in autosomal dominant disorders, penetrance is not usually full. Misdiagnosis of affected status confounds the molecular genetic analysis making linkage studies much less likely to succeed.

A blood sample for molecular genetic studies should therefore be taken from all family members when they undergo detailed assessment. Molecular studies involve two principal stages. The first is mapping the disorder to a specific part of the genome, which then allows the molecular biologist to pursue the second stage, identification of the mutation in the gene associated with the disorder.

Once the entire family has been studied, their blood samples can be used in linkage studies. In order for the molecular biologist to begin molecular studies, the affected status of family members must be determined by the clinical researcher. The research team must be scrupulous about this data which should not be manipulated to fit the linkage data, as this practice is fraught with danger. When the molecular geneticist asks the clinician whether they are certain if a specific individual who appears as a recombinant on the linkage data is definitely affected, the clinician must be precise about that person's affected status whether it be affected, unaffected or, rarely, uncertain.

It should be stressed that family studies are a dynamic evolving story often incomplete in the first few months or even years of the project. Over many years, new branches of affected individuals in a family crop up which may change the clinical picture and make molecular studies viable. Linkage studies require accurate information on a large number of individuals. As a rule of thumb, a minimum of 10 individuals affected with a specific epilepsy syndrome is required to produce a significant log of the odds (LOD) score. A LOD score of 3 is considered consistent with linkage in a kindred. Such a LOD score may be difficult to discern from the linkage data resulting from a routine screen of around 200 markers spanning the entire human genome. Indeed, only a hint of linkage may be initially ascertained on a screen of a family with more than 20 affected individuals. These hints of linkage are then pursued with vigour and critical analysis of any potential recombinants. More specific markers are identified to precisely map the disorder.

Candidate gene approach

Once a disorder is mapped to a specific part of the genome, the locations of known genes in that region of the chromosome are scrutinized as likely candidate genes. Positional candidate genes are known genes localized to a linked chromosomal region which could conceivably be related to the trait under study because of their function and/or pattern of expression.[25] Such candidate genes are targeted first for further analysis. For example, in epilepsy, attention has focused on genes associated with excitatory neurotransmitters, such as glutamate, and inhibitory neurotransmitters, such as gamma-aminobutyric acid (GABA). Techniques such as single strand conformational polymorphisms and DNA sequencing are employed to identify a mutation in a gene in affected individuals.

Physical mapping and isolation of new genes

When no positional candidate genes are identified, or a mutation is not found by direct analysis of promising candidate genes, the more arduous approach when dealing with a sufficiently narrow genomic region is to search for new genes. This is achieved through the use of integrated physical genetic maps of the human genome using contigs of a range of artificial chromosomes, such as yeast artificial chromosomes, anchored to polymorphic markers for linkage analysis. Such work is facilitated by the increasing availability of expressed sequence tags which are sequences from transcribed genes available in the public domain. These are mapped to chromosomal regions where their respective genes are localized and they provide sequence information.[25]

Evaluation of candidate genes

Once a specific mutation in a gene is identified in affected family members and obligate carriers, and is not present in unaffected family members or controls, it is unlikely to be an innocent polymorphism. Nevertheless, the onus is on the investigator to show that the mutation is responsible for the clinical disorder. In the case of epilepsy, evidence that the mutation is pathogenic can either be obtained from electrophysiological studies demonstrating that the mutation alters the normal function of the gene, transgenic animal models expressing a related phenotype, or therapeutic interventions based on modification of the underlying genetic defect. The aim of such functional studies is to strengthen the association between a genetic mutation and a specific disorder.

An alternative approach to functional studies is to find a family with the same epilepsy syndrome with a mutation in the same gene, again implicating the gene in a causative role. Another angle is to show a mutation in a related gene for individuals with the same phenotype, such as the second potassium-channel mutation in benign familial neonatal convulsions on chromosome 8 (see below). Whichever strategy is used, identification of epilepsy genes is the first step to improving understanding of the mechanisms of epilepsy and potential therapeutic manoeuvres.

Genetics of epilepsy syndromes: current understanding

Generalized epilepsies

When a clinician considers the question of genetic epilepsies, the idiopathic generalized epilepsies (IGE), such as childhood absence epilepsy (CAE), juvenile absence epilepsy (JAE) and JME, spring to mind.[5] In contrast, the symptomatic generalized epilepsies are usually thought of as acquired disorders where genetic factors are discounted as being of little relevance. Our understanding of the interrela-

tionship of the idiopathic and symptomatic epilepsies is changing and genetic factors may be of significant importance in both settings.

IGE with simple inheritance

Only rare generalized epilepsy syndromes follow monogenic inheritance, e.g. benign familial neonatal convulsions (BFNC), a true idiopathic epilepsy with a good prognosis, and a few progressive conditions with symptomatic generalized epilepsy.

BFNC

BFNC typically begins on days 2–3 of life in an otherwise well neonate who develops bilateral clonic or tonic seizures with or without apnoea.[26] The attacks generally cease after about a week and the interictal EEG is normal. Although classified as a generalized epilepsy, ictal EEG studies showed both generalized and focal onset.[27] Approximately 5 per cent of these infants develop later febrile seizures and 11 per cent later afebrile seizures. Cognitive and neurological development is normal.[28]

BFNC follows autosomal-dominant inheritance with high penetrance, and linkage was first demonstrated in a US family to chromosome 20q13.2 in 1989.[29] Confirmation of linkage has been reported in other US, French, Canadian and Australian families, and this locus was deemed EBN1.[30–33] Locus heterogeneity exists with a second locus (EBN2) on 8q, described in 1993,[34,35] and there is evidence for a third locus with some families not linking to either 20q or 8q.[36]

Only in 1998 was a gene for BFNC cloned, a newly identified voltage-gated potassium-channel gene KCNQ2.[37,38] KCNQ2 bears some similarity to a gene on chromosome 11 associated with the prolonged QT syndrome, a disorder of cardiac conduction. BFNC families showed a variety of mutations affecting the ion channel, the 6th transmembrane domain and the C-terminal. In a family with a C-terminal mutation, the phenotype did not follow the archetypal BFNC picture, with some infants having seizures in the first few months of life rather than in the neonatal period. A similar gene, *KCNQ3*, was found on chromosome 8q at *EBN2*.[39] Other potassium channels in the brain are likely candidate genes for the BFNC families not yet linked.

IGE with complex inheritance

Family studies of the common syndromes of the IGE suggest that their inheritance is complex rather than monogenic.[40] Complex inheritance is implied not only by genetic analyses but also by the observations that specific syndromes described in the classification have considerable nosological overlap, and different syndromes are frequently found within one family.[41–43]

Recent twin studies incorporating the concept of epilepsy syndromes found that concordant monozygotic twin pairs had the same specific IGE syndrome, implying that each syndrome is genetically derived.[44] In contrast, dizygotic twin pairs, where both are affected, show a mixed picture of epilepsy syndromes, akin to siblings and families of probands with IGE.[41–43] Models of complex inheritance applied to IGE family studies are consistent with a multiplicative effect of multiple contributing loci.[45,46]

JME

JME, originally coined 'impulsive *petit mal*' by Janz, is characterized by adolescent onset of generalized tonic–clonic seizures (GTCS) and myoclonic seizures, and accounts for ~8 per cent of patients with epilepsy.[43] Recognition of the genetic aetiology of JME grew from the finding that 30 per cent of patients had relatives with seizures compared with 7 per

cent of patients with symptomatic or focal epilepsies.[43,47–50] Twin studies added further evidence, as dizygotic twins were concordant for any IGE whereas monozygotic twins were concordant for the specific IGE syndrome, such as JME.[51] A variety of models of inheritance of JME have been postulated, including autosomal dominant, autosomal recessive,[52] two-locus[21] and polygenic models.[47,49,50,53,54]

Genetic studies have largely focused on multiple small kindreds with JME and produced controversial results. In 1988, Greenberg et al[21] reported that a JME locus lay on chromosome 6p close to the human leucocyte antigens (HLA) complex. A significant LOD score was obtained only if asymptomatic relatives with abnormal EEG were classified as affected, although many of the EEG abnormalities were not 'epileptiform' in nature. Further studies using different models, both replicated[55–57] and disputed the findings.[58–60] In some instances the findings may have been based on clinically different subsets, such as those incorporating individuals with absence epilepsies,[58,59] but others employed pure JME kindreds and were unable to confirm the mapping data.[60] However, confirmation of a 6p locus came with data from a single large family mapping to 6p21.2-p11, which implied that this JME locus lay more than 30 centimorgans centromeric to the HLA region, expanding the putative region for the locus for JME.[61] This locus *EJM1* was considered to map only 'classical JME', which included myoclonus and GTCS alone, and excluded individuals with typical absence seizures or 3 Hz spike–wave discharges.[61] Further work on the relationship of other IGE syndromes in families of JME patients and the 6p locus looked at families ascertained through probands with pure adolescent onset of grand mal seizures (GTCS) alone without myoclonic seizures. Greenberg et al[62] found that families of individuals with generalized tonic–clonic seizures on awakening (GTCA) showed suggestive evidence of linkage to the 6p locus; whereas families of adolescents with grand mal occurring at any time of day did not link to this region. The current status is that the chromosome 6p locus, designated '*EJM1*', is thought to predispose to a trait expressed either as clinical JME, its associated EEG abnormality or, according to some workers, IGE, and lies between the HLA region and the centromere.

There is no doubt that locus heterogeneity exists for JME, as for all the common generalized epilepsy syndromes, which partially explains the linkage inconsistencies.[59] The controversial findings in JME may, however, relate to problems inherent in mapping complex diseases which require higher thresholds to suggest significant linkage.[63] With the exception of the single large family reported, the studies suggesting linkage to chromosome 6p may be intrinsically flawed by failing to reach significant linkage for a complex disorder.[59,60] Even if this is the case, the 6p locus cannot be excluded categorically as a subset of families may link to this region and, in complex diseases, it is impossible to exclude any region of the genome until all cases are accounted for by known genes.[64]

Following the isolation of a gene for an idiopathic epilepsy in the neuronal nicotinic acetylcholine receptor (nAChR) α4 subunit (see below), genes encoding nAChR subunits were considered candidate-susceptibility loci for other idiopathic epilepsies.[65] Parametric and non-parametric linkage analyses of 34 JME families recently mapped the majority of these families to chromosome 15q14, a region harbouring the gene for the α7 subunit of the nAChR, now a candidate gene for JME.[53]

Other IGE

The Italian study of families with at least three cases of IGE in one or more generations found that phenotypic heterogeneity was common, with only 25 per cent of families having concordance of phenotypes such as GTCS or febrile convulsions among all affected individuals. A higher concordance was noted with first-degree relatives in every form of IGE, whereas different phenotypes were more likely with more distant relatives.[41]

Zara et al[46] performed non-parametric analysis on these families and found evidence for linkage to chromosome 8q24, in the same region previously linked for BFNC[34] and subsequently linked in a family with persisting absence and GTCS.[66] Interestingly, they did not find evidence of linkage to the JME locus on chromosome 6p.[46] The same group has also mapped an unusual generalized epileptiform EEG trait in an Italian family with IGE to chromosome 3p.[67]

Sander and colleagues studied families ascertained through probands with absence epilepsies, either CAE or JAE, looking for evidence of linkage to *EJM1*. They found significant evidence against linkage, concluding that *EJM1* confers genetic susceptibility to CAE and JAE only in families where one member has JME.[58] Recently, two reports of linkage of absence epilepsies have been made, however, neither are for classical CAE. In one family with linkage to chromosome 1p, absence seizures persisted and evolved into a JME phenotype.[68] The second linkage involved an Indian pedigree, with persisting absence seizures and GTCS, which was mapped to chromosome 8q24, the same region as IGE family studies.[66]

A large European group has also looked at a cluster of GABA subunit genes on chromosome 15 for linkage in families with IGE. They found a hint of linkage in families with JME, but clearly this finding needs to be replicated.[69]

Symptomatic generalized epilepsies with simple inheritance

There are over 200 rare Mendelian disorders for which seizures are a symptom of a more widespread disorder of the central nervous system, such as tuberous sclerosis or neurofibromatosis. Although a number of the disorders with symptomatic generalized epilepsy have been mapped, and the genes cloned, information on the genes underlying these symptomatic epilepsies is unlikely to contribute to our understanding of the neurobiology of the epilepsies *per se*. Similarly, an array of chromosomal anomalies may be associated with seizures such as trisomies 13, 18 and 21, but these large stretches of DNA do not lend themselves to the discovery of epilepsy genes and are not dealt with further here.[70]

Progressive myoclonus epilepsies (PME)

PME form an enlarging group of rare monogenic symptomatic epilepsies characterized by myoclonic seizures, generalized epilepsy and progressive neurological deterioration with ataxia and dementia. A full analysis of the current clinical and molecular understanding of PME can be found elsewhere.[71-73]

Symptomatic generalized epilepsies (SGE) with complex inheritance

SGE, such as West syndrome and the Lennox-Gastaut syndrome (LGS), have generally been attributed to acquired causes such as birth asphyxia and not regarded as having a significant genetic aetiology. There is increasing evidence, however, that some of the SGE, such as myoclonic-astatic epilepsy and certain cerebral malformations have a genetic basis.[6,7,11,12]

Myoclonic-astatic epilepsy (MAE)

MAE falls under the rubric of LGS, but Doose differentiates it by normal early development, the almost total absence of tonic seizures, irregular generalized fast spike-and-wave on EEG and a variable prognosis.[5,74] MAE is thought to have a genetic aetiology, a factor helpful in differentiating it from LGS. Doose regards inheritance of MAE as polygenic with little non-genetic variability.[74,75] Doose's family studies found that about one third of MAE probands had a family history of seizures which typically consisted of febrile and afebrile GTCS in early childhood.[74,76] The inheritance pattern of MAE has become clearer with delineation of generalized epilepsy with febrile seizures plus (GEFS+). There is now strong evidence that some cases of MAE are due, in part, to a single gene disorder (see below).

Febrile convulsions

Febrile convulsions affect 2–5 per cent of children.[77,78] A family history of seizures occurs in over half of children with febrile seizures.[79] Various genetic models for the inheritance of febrile seizures have been proposed, including autosomal dominant,[80,81] autosomal recessive[82] and polygenic or multi-factorial models.[40,83,84] There is no doubt that febrile seizures are genetically heterogeneous, as evidenced by a complex segregation analysis of 467 families performed by Rich et al.[85] They proposed that single febrile seizures were associated with polygenic inheritance while three or more febrile seizures followed a single-major-locus model with nearly dominant seizure susceptibility. Further support for this hypothesis comes from the finding that the recurrence risk of seizures in children with febrile seizures is increased with a family history of febrile seizures[86,87] or generalized epilepsy.[88-90]

Autosomal dominant febrile seizures

A number of studies have reported large multigenerational families where febrile seizures appear to follow autosomal dominant inheritance or polygenic inheritance with a single-major-locus predominating.[91-94] In these families, ~50 per cent of first-degree relatives of probands were affected, and there tended to be unilateral inheritance of febrile seizures from either the maternal or paternal line.[94] Rare individuals in these families developed later temporal lobe epilepsy associated with hippocampal sclerosis, particularly if they were subject to prolonged febrile seizures in childhood.[91,92] Pure autosomal dominant febrile seizures are genetically heterogeneous with two loci identified to date, on chromosomes 8q13-21[92] and 19p13.3,[93,95] but some kindreds do not link to these loci.[96]

GEFS⁺

GEFS⁺ is a common, recently described autosomal dominant syndrome that crosses the human-made boundaries of idiopathic and symptomatic generalized epilepsies, and the artificial separation of the epilepsies from febrile convulsions.[97] GEFS⁺ is characterized by a spectrum of epilepsy phenotypes ranging from febrile seizures to febrile seizures plus (FS⁺) (where febrile seizures continue past 6 years of age or are associated with afebrile GTCS), to FS⁺ sometimes associated with myoclonic, absence or atonic seizures to MAE (see below).

GEFS⁺ is genetically heterogeneous with mapping of two large multiplex families to chromosome 2q and 19q.[20,98] In the 19q family, the genetic mutation has very recently been isolated in the β1 subunit of the sodium channel, which will focus attention on other sodium-channel genes as likely candidates for febrile seizures and generalized epilepsies.[20]

Partial epilepsies

Even as recently as the mid-1980s, genetically determined epilepsies were thought to manifest as generalized rather than focal epilepsies, with the recognized exception of the benign partial epilepsies of childhood.[70,99] The concept of an idiopathic partial epilepsy has been less readily accepted, perhaps because it is intuitively more appealing to imagine that a genetically-based enhancement of neuronal excitability would affect all neurons and result in a generalized seizure, rather than have a localized effect.[25,70] In contrast, partial epilepsies have generally been regarded as essentially acquired disorders associated with structural lesions.

The main exception has been the idiopathic localization-related epilepsies (or benign partial epilepsies of childhood), which include BCECTS, and childhood epilepsy with occipital paroxysms. The idiopathic partial epilepsies have been thought to have a genetic aetiology,[14,100,101] but the precise mode of inheritance of the common forms remains elusive and may well be multi-factorial.[102] The new group of monogenic partial epilepsy syndromes has greatly expanded in recent years.

Idiopathic partial epilepsies with simple inheritance

Benign familial infantile convulsions (BFIC)

The concept of benign infantile convulsions was first introduced by Fukuyama in 1963, referring to a single seizure occurring in infancy often associated with a family history of seizures.[103] Later, further Japanese workers reported the same condition[104] and, more recently, the autosomal dominant inheritance of BFIC was brought to the fore by Vigevano et al (Table 9.3).[105]

BFIC typically begins at 6 months (range 4–8 months) with a cluster of partial seizures. Clusters of 4–10 seizures per day occur over 2–4 days. Partial seizures with secondary generalization are characterized by psychomotor arrest, head and eye deviation with varying laterality, and tonic–clonic manifestations.

Epilepsy syndrome	Linkage	Gene
Generalized epilepsies		
Benign familial neonatal convulsions	20q	KCNQ2‡
	8q	KCNQ3‡
Idiopathic generalized epilepsy, unspecified	8q*	?
	3p*	?
Juvenile myoclonic epilepsy	6p†	?
	15q*	?
Persisting absence with later myoclonic epilepsy	1p*	?
Persisting absence with tonic–clonic seizures	8q*	?
Generalized epilepsy with febrile seizures plus	2q*	?
	19q	SCN1B§
Partial epilepsies		
Benign familial infantile convulsions	19q	?
	16	?
Autosomal dominant nocturnal frontal lobe epilepsy	20q	CHRNA4¶
	15q24	
Partial epilepsy with auditory features	10q	?
Familial partial epilepsy with variable foci	2q*	?
Special syndromes		
Febrile seizures	8q*	?
	19p*	?

*Single report to date in epilepsies with complex inheritance, so linkage should be regarded as tentative.
†See text for discussion.
‡KCNQ2 and KCNQ3 are novel neuronal potassium-channel genes.
§SCN1B is the gene for the β1 subunit of the sodium channel
¶CHRNA4 is the gene for the α4 subunit of the neuronal nicotinic acetylcholine receptor.

Table 9.2
Molecular genetics of idiopathic epilepsies.

Interictal EEG is normal and ictal recordings show central-occipital onset.[105,106] Development, examination and imaging are normal. Seizures are easily controlled with antiepileptic therapy and later seizures are rare. In family studies, seizures do not begin in the neonatal period nor after the 8th month.[106–108]

Molecular genetic studies in BFIC have excluded the locus for BFNC on chromosome 20q.[109] Italian families have been mapped to a locus on chromosome 19q.[110] BFIC is a genetically heterogeneous disorder, as not all families map to the 19q region (unpublished data). A cluster of families from Northern France with BFIC and paroxysmal choreo-athetosis has recently been linked to the pericentromeric region of chromosome 16 (Table 9.2).[111]

Autosomal dominant nocturnal frontal lobe epilepsy (ADNFLE)

ADNFLE is characterized by childhood onset of clusters of violent nocturnal motor seizures (Table 9.3). Onset typically occurs at ~8 years and the individual is woken within 2 h of falling asleep with either thrashing or tonic attacks, often with clonic components. Attacks often begin with a non-specific aura and awareness may be retained throughout the brief seizure. Individuals have an average of 7 attacks over a few hours. Seizures are often undiagnosed or misdiagnosed as sleep disorders, such as night-mares or night terrors, psychiatric diagnoses, such as hysteria, or movement disorders. Since the original report of families studied in Australia, Britain and Canada,[16,17] families have been recognized around the world.[112-114]

In the largest Australian family studied, with 27 affected individuals, the gene was mapped to chromosome 20q13.2.[115] Using a candidate gene approach, a mutation was identified in the α4 subunit of the neuronal nAChR in this family.[65] Subsequently, a Norwegian family has been reported with a different mutation of the same gene.[116] ADNFLE is genetically heterogeneous with the majority of families not having mutations of the α4 subunit and a further locus has recently been identified on chromosome 15q.[117]

Familial temporal lobe epilepsy

FTLE was first recognized through twin studies where concordant monozygotic twin pairs with mild, easily treatable temporal lobe epilepsy were identified (Table 9.3). Typically, simple partial seizures, characterized by psychic or autonomic phenomena, begin in adolescence or early adult life. Infrequent complex partial and secondarily generalized seizures occur. EEG studies show sparse interictal temporal epilepti-form abnormalities in around one quarter of patients and structural neuroimaging is normal. Multiplex families show inheritance suggestive

of an autosomal dominant pattern with penetrance of 60 per cent. The subtle nature of symptoms means that a significant number of individuals have escaped diagnosis until under-going detailed clinical study.[18]

While the seizures of FTLE are suggestive of mesial temporal (limbic) origin, a family with autosomal dominant partial epilepsy, charac-terized by seizures of probable lateral temporal origin, was described by Ottman et al.[118] Individuals in this family have simple partial seizures with auditory hallucinations such as ringing or humming. Molecular genetic studies linked this family to chromosome 10q but no gene has been identified. FTLE is genetically heterogeneous as the families with mesial FTLE do not link to the 10q region.[18]

Autosomal dominant rolandic epilepsy with speech dyspraxia (ADRESD)

ADRESD was described in a single Australian family (Table 9.3).[23] In this disorder, the typical seizures of BCECTS occurred in mid-childhood accompanied by centro-temporal spikes on EEG. In this family, epilepsy followed autoso-mal dominant inheritance and was associated with speech dyspraxia and cognitive impair-ment. Clinical anticipation was found, suggest-ing the possibility of a triplet repeat expansion as the genetic basis of this disorder. The family is too small for linkage studies to map the disease locus to define a region of the genome which might contain a repeat expansion responsible for this disorder. Interestingly, a family with severe orofacial dyspraxia, studied intensively in the UK,[119-121] has recently been linked to chromosome 7q31,[122,123] but this locus has been excluded in ADRESD.[124]

Familial partial epilepsy with variable foci (FPEVF)

FPEVF has also been described in a single Australian family with 10 affected individuals

	Familial partial epilepsy with variable foci (FPEVF)	Autosomal dominant nocturnal frontal lobe epilepsy (ADNFLE)	Familial temporal lobe epilepsy (FTLE)	Autosomal dominant rolandic epilepsy with speech dyspraxia (ADRESD)	Benign familial infantile convulsions (BFIC)
Age of onset					
Mean (years)	13	11.7	24	5	0.5
Median (years)	10	8	19	6	0.5
Range (years)	0.75–43	0.17–52	10–63	1–10	0.3–0.7
Partial seizure					
Semiology	Heterogeneous	Frontal	Temporal	Rolandic	Partial
Timing	Any time	Clusters in sleep	Usually diurnal	Sleep	Cluster over few days
EEG studies					
Interictal epileptiform	Variable foci, often active	Normal	Normal or infrequent temporal spikes	Active centro-temporal discharges especially in sleep, age dependent	Normal
Ictal	Congruent with interictal focus	Artefact or frontal activity	Temporal	Centro-temporal phase reversal	Occipitoparietal
Epileptiform in clinically unaffected individuals	Yes	No	No	No	?
Penetrance	62 per cent	69 per cent	60 per cent	~100 per cent	?
Linkage	?2q	20q (2 families) 15q non-20q	10q (1 family) non-10q	No	19q 16 (choreo-athetosis)

Table 9.3
Autosomal dominant partial epilepsies.

over 4 generations.[22] This disorder is intriguing, as partial seizures originate in different parts of the cerebral cortex in different family members. The seizure origin varied between individuals with seizures arising from the frontal, temporal, occipital and centro-parietal regions. In each individual, seizure semiology correlated with the epileptiform focus on EEG studies, which were often active, particularly in sleep. Two individuals without seizures had epileptiform abnormalities in EEG studies. There is suggestive evidence of linkage in this family to chromosome 2. The inherited nature of FPEVP may be overlooked because of relatively low penetrance and because of the variability in age of onset and electroclinical features between affected family members (Table 9.3).

Idiopathic partial epilepsies with complex inheritance

BCECTS

The syndrome of BCECTS accounts for one sixth of all childhood epilepsies.[125,126] BCECTS is a benign syndrome with a genetic aetiology, although the inheritance pattern remains unclear. It has been suggested that the EEG abnormality, rather than the seizure disorder, follows autosomal dominant inheritance.[101] Genetic studies of BCECTS showed an increase in epileptiform abnormalities in the EEGs of relatives of probands.[100] Clinical studies alone are not suggestive of a monogenic inheritance pattern but, when the EEG trait is analysed, an autosomal dominant pattern with variable age-dependent penetrance has been hypothesized,[14,101] although it is generally thought that BCECTS follows complex inheritance.

Attempts to map BCECTS have been unsuccessful to date. Exclusion of linkage of BCECTS to the *EJM1* locus on chromosome 6p,[127] and to the BFNC loci *EBN1* and *EBN2*, have been reported.[128]

Symptomatic partial epilepsies with simple inheritance

There are many Mendelian symptomatic epilepsies where partial seizures may occur in addition to generalized convulsions, such as the neurocutaneous syndromes of tuberous sclerosis and neurofibromatosis, reflecting the coexistence of both focal and diffuse cerebral abnormalities. As stated above, with regard to the symptomatic generalized epilepsies with simple inheritance, progress in mapping and cloning genes responsible for these disorders is unlikely to lend specific understanding to the mechanisms underlying the epilepsies.

Northern epilepsy syndrome

The northern epilepsy syndrome is an autosomal recessive syndrome described in north Finland.[129] It is characterized by progressive cerebral, cerebellar and brainstem atrophy beginning in normal children at ~5–10 years with seizures which may be febrile, generalized or partial. A slowly progressive dementia occurs with ataxia and eventual visual failure; seizures become rare by middle age. This rare condition maps to chromosome 8p but the gene is unknown.[130]

Symptomatic partial epilepsies with complex inheritance

Despite early contentions that temporal lobe epilepsy occurring in siblings could be attributed solely to their passage from the same uterus through the same birth canal,[131] there has been emerging evidence of a role for genetic factors in the partial epilepsies. Temporal lobe epilepsy, the most common partial epilepsy, may be mild and easily treated, thereby escaping diagnosis or not drawing attention to the significance of a family history (see above). In contrast, patients with refractory partial epilepsy make up a large proportion of a neurologist's practice and lesional aetiologies, particularly hippocampal sclerosis, are increasingly evident with more sophisticated structural and functional imaging techniques. Nevertheless, formalized study of these populations has suggested that genetic factors here also play a part. Andermann and

colleagues found that relatives of patients with partial epilepsy were more likely to have EEG abnormalities than relatives of controls and concluded that these findings supported the unitary concept of the epilepsies where partial epilepsies resulted from acquired lesions in individuals with an underlying epileptic predisposition.[40,132,133]

References

1. Hippocrates. *The genuine works of Hippocrates — Vol. I & II*. London: The Sydenham Society, 1849:847.
2. Burton, R. *The anatomy of melancholy. Volume 1*. London: Everyman's Library, 1932:216.
3. Kimball OP. On the inheritance of epilepsy. *Wisconsin Med J* 1954;**53**:271–6.
4. Commission of Classification and Terminology of the International League Against Epilepsy. Proposal for revised clinical and electroencephalographic classification of epileptic seizures. *Epilepsia* 1981;**22**:489–501.
5. Commission on Classification and Terminology of the International League Against Epilepsy. Proposal for revised classification of epilepsies and epileptic syndromes. *Epilepsia* 1989;**30**:389–99.
6. Huttenlocher PR, Taravath S, Mojtahedi S. Familial periventricular heterotopias and seizures in four generations. *Ann Neurol* 1991;**30**:461.
7. Eksioglu YZ, Scheffer IE, Cardenas P, et al. Periventricular heterotopia: an X-linked dominant epilepsy locus causing aberrant cerebral cortical development. *Neuron* 1996;**16**:77–87.
8. Palmini A, Andermann F, Aicardi J, et al. Diffuse cortical dysplasia, or the 'double cortex' syndrome: the clinical and epileptic spectrum in 10 patients. *Neurology* 1991;**41**:1656–62.
9. Pinard JM, Motte J, Chiron C, et al. Subcortical laminar heterotopia and lissencephaly in two families: a single X linked dominant gene. *J Neurol Neurosurg Psychiatry* 1994;**57**:914–20.
10. Des Portes V, Pinard JM, Smadja D, et al. Dominant X linked subcortical laminar heterotopia and lissencephaly syndrome (XSCLH/LIS): evidence for the occurrence of mutation in males and mapping of a potential locus in Xq22. *J Med Genet* 1997;**34**:177–83.
11. Ross ME, Allen KM, Srivastava AK, et al. Linkage and physical mapping of X-linked lissencephaly/SBH (XLIS): a gene causing neuronal migration defects in human brain. *Hum Mol Genet* 1997;**6**:555–63.
12. Gleeson JG, Allen KM, Fox JW, et al. *Doublecortin*, a brain-specific gene mutated in human X-linked lissencephaly and double cortex syndrome, encodes a putative signaling protein. *Cell* 1998;**92**:63–72.
13. Lehesjoki A-E, Koskiniemi M, Sistonen P, et al. Localization of a gene for progressive myoclonus epilepsy to chromosome 21q22. *Proc Natl Acad Sci USA* 1991;**88**:3696–9.
14. Heijbel J, Blom S, Rasmuson M. Benign epilepsy of childhood with centrotemporal EEG foci: a genetic study. *Epilepsia* 1975;**16**:285–93.
15. Berkovic SF, Scheffer IE. Epilepsies with single gene inheritance. *Brain Dev* 1997;**19**:13–18.
16. Scheffer IE, Bhatia KP, Lopes-Cendes I, et al. Autosomal dominant frontal epilepsy misdiagnosed as sleep disorder. *Lancet* 1994;**343**:515–17.

17. Scheffer IE, Bhatia KP, Lopes-Cendes I, et al. Autosomal dominant nocturnal frontal lobe epilepsy. A distinctive clinical disorder. *Brain* 1995;**118**:61–73.

18. Berkovic SF, McIntosh A, Howell RA, et al. Familial temporal lobe epilepsy: a common disorder identified in twins. *Ann Neurol* 1996;**40**:227–35.

19. Singh R, Scheffer IE, Crossland K, Berkovic SF. Generalized epilepsy with febrile seizures plus: a common, childhood-onset genetic epilepsy syndrome. *Ann Neurol* 1999;**45**:75–81.

20. Wallace RH, Singh R, Scheffer IE, et al. A sodium channel subunit SCN1B mutation is responsible for febrile seizures and generalised epilepsy. *Nat Genet* 1998;**19**:366–70.

21. Greenberg DA, Delgado-Escueta AV, Widelitz H, et al. Juvenile myoclonic epilepsy (JME) may be linked to the BF and HLA loci on human chromosome 6. *Am J Med Genet* 1988;**31**:185–92.

22. Scheffer IE, Phillips HA, O'Brien CE, et al. Familial partial epilepsy with variable foci: a new partial epilepsy syndrome with suggestion of linkage to chromosome 2. *Ann Neurol* 1998;**44**:890–9.

23. Scheffer IE, Jones L, Pozzebon M, et al. Autosomal dominant rolandic epilepsy and speech dyspraxia: a new syndrome with anticipation. *Ann Neurol* 1995;**38**:633–42.

24. Lander ES, Schork NJ. Genetic dissection of complex traits. *Science* 1994;**265**:2037–48.

25. Pandolfo M. Clinical genetic and molecular genetic approaches to the familial partial epilepsies. In: Berkovic SF, Genton P, Hirsch E, Picard F, eds. *Genetics of focal epilepsies: Clinical aspects and molecular biology.* London: John Libbey & Co. Ltd, 1999:15–32.

26. Rett A, Teubel R. Neugeborenenekrampfe im rahmen einer epileptisch belasteten familie. *Wien Klin Wochenschr* 1964;**76**:609–13.

27. Bye AME. Neonate with benign familial neonatal convulsions: recorded generalized and focal seizures. *Pediatr Neurol* 1994;**10**: 164–5.

28. Plouin P. Benign familial neonatal convulsions. In: Malafosse A, Genton P, Hirsch E, Marescaux C, Broglin D, Bernasconi R, eds. *Idiopathic Generalized Epilepsies: clinical, experimental and genetic aspects.* London: John Libbey & Co. Ltd, 1994:39–44.

29. Leppert M, Anderson VE, Quattlebaum T, et al. Benign familial neonatal convulsions linked to genetic markers on chromosome 20. *Nature* 1989;**337**:647–8.

30. Malafosse A, Leboyer M, Dulac O, et al. Confirmation of linkage of benign familial neonatal convulsions to D20S19 and D20S20. *Hum Genet* 1992;**89**:54–8.

31. Leppert M, McMahon WM, Quattlebaum TG, et al. Searching for human epilepsy genes: a progress report. *Brain Pathology* 1993; **3**:357–69.

32. Ronen GM, Rosales TO, Connolly Y, et al. Seizure characteristics in chromosome 20 benign familial neonatal convulsions. *Neurology* 1993;**43**:1355–60.

33. Berkovic SF, Kennerson ML, Howell RA, et al. Phenotypic expression of benign familial neonatal convulsions linked to chromosome 20. *Arch Neurol* 1994;**51**:1125–8.

34. Lewis TB, Leach RJ, Ward K, et al. Genetic heterogeneity in benign familial neonatal convulsions: identification of a new locus on chromosome 8q. *Am J Hum Genet* 1993;**53**: 670–5.

35. Steinlein O, Schuster V, Fischer C, Haussler M. Benign familial neonatal convulsions: confirmation of genetic heterogeneity and further evidence for a second locus on chromosome 8q. *Hum Genet* 1995;**95**:411–15.

36. Lewis TB, Shevell MI, Andermann E, et al. Evidence of a third locus for benign familial convulsions. *J Child Neurol* 1996; **11**:211–14.

37. Singh NA, Charlier C, Stauffer D, et al. A novel potassium channel gene, KCNQ2, is mutated in an inherited epilepsy of newborns. *Nat Genet* 1998;**18**:25–9.

38. Biervert C, Schroeder BC, Kubisch C, et al. A potassium channel mutation in neonatal human epilepsy. *Science* 1998;**279**:403–6.

39. Charlier C, Singh NA, Ryan SG, et al. A pore mutation in a novel KQT-like potassium channel gene in an idiopathic epilepsy family. *Nat Genet* 1998;**18**:53–5.

40. Andermann E. Genetic studies of epilepsy in Montreal. In: Anderson VE, Hauser WA, Leppik IE, Noebels JL, Rich SS, eds. *Genetic strategies in epilepsy research.* Amsterdam: Elsevier, 1991:129–37.

41. Italian League Against Epilepsy Genetic Collaborative Group. Concordance of clinical forms of epilepsy in families with several affected members. *Epilepsia* 1993;**34**:819–26.

42. Reutens DC, Berkovic SF. Idiopathic generalized epilepsy of adolescence: are the syndromes clinically distinct? *Neurology* 1995;**45**:1469–76.

43. Janz D, Durner M, Beck-Mannagetta G, Pantazis G. Family studies on the genetics of juvenile myoclonic epilepsy (epilepsy with impulsive petit mal). In: Beck-Mannagetta G, Anderson VE, Doose H, Janz D, eds. *Genetics of the epilepsies*. Berlin: Springer-Verlag, 1989:43–52.

44. Berkovic SF, Howell RA, Hay DA, Hopper JL. Epilepsies in twins: genetics of the major epilepsy syndromes. *Ann Neurol* 1998;**43**: 435–45.

45. Risch N. Linkage strategies for genetically complex traits. 1) Multilocus models. *Am J Hum Genet* 1990;**54**:222–8.

46. Zara F, Bianchi A, Avanzini G, et al. Mapping of genes predisposing to idiopathic generalized epilepsy. *Hum Mol Genet* 1995;**4**:1201–7.

47. Delgado-Escueta AV, Enrile-Bacsal F. Juvenile myoclonic epilepsy of Janz. *Neurology* 1984; **34**:285–94.

48. Janz D, Christian W. Impulsiv-petit mal. *J Neurol* 1957;**176**:346–86.

49. Tsuboi T, Christian W. On the genetics of the primary generalized epilepsy with sporadic myoclonias of impulsive petit mal type. *Humangenetik* 1973;**19**:155–82.

50. Delgado-Escueta AV, Greenberg D, Weissbecker K, et al. Gene mapping in the idiopathic generalized epilepsies: juvenile myoclonic epilepsy, childhood absence epilepsy, epilepsy with grand mal seizures, and early childhood myoclonic epilepsy. *Epilepsia* 1990;**31**:S19–29.

51. Berkovic SF, Howell RA, Hay DA, Hopper JL. Epilepsies in twins. In: Wolf P, ed. *Epileptic seizures and syndromes*. London: John Libbey, 1994:157–64.

52. Panayiotopoulos CP, Obeid T. Juvenile myoclonic epilepsy: an autosomal recessive disease. *Ann Neurol* 1989;**25**:440–3.

53. Elmslie FV, Rees M, Williamson MP, et al. Genetic mapping of a major susceptibility locus for juvenile myoclonic epilepsy on chromosome 15q. *Hum Mol Genet* 1997; **6**:1329–34.

54. Greenberg DA, Delgado-Escueta AV, Maldonado HM, Widelitz H. Segregation analysis of juvenile myoclonic epilepsy. In: Beck-Mannagetta G, Anderson VE, Doose H, Janz D, eds. *Genetics of the epilepsies*. Berlin: Springer-Verlag, 1989:53–61.

55. Weissbecker KA, Durner M, Janz D, et al. Confirmation of linkage between juvenile myoclonic epilepsy locus and the HLA region of chromosome 6. *Am J Med Genet* 1991; **38**:32–6.

56. Durner M, Sander T, Greenberg DA, et al. Localization of idiopathic generalized epilepsy on chromosome 6p in families of juvenile myoclonic epilepsy patients. *Neurology* 1991; **41**:1651–5.

57. Greenberg DA, Delgado-Escueta AV. The chromosome 6p epilepsy locus: exploring mode of inheritance and heterogeneity through linkage analysis. *Epilepsia* 1993; **34**:S12–S18.

58. Sander T, Hildmann T, Janz D, et al. The phenotypic spectrum related to the human epilepsy susceptibility gene 'EJM1'. *Ann Neurol* 1995;**38**:210–17.

59. Whitehouse WP, Rees M, Curtis D, et al. Linkage analysis of idiopathic generalized epilepsy (IGE) and marker loci on chromosome 6p in families of patients with juvenile myoclonic epilepsy: no evidence for an epilepsy locus in the HLA region. *Am J Hum Genet* 1993;**53**:652–62.

60. Elmslie FV, Williamson MP, Rees M, et al. Linkage analysis of juvenile myoclonic epilepsy and microsatellite loci spanning 61cM of human chromosome 6p in 19 nuclear pedigrees provides no evidence for a susceptibility locus in this region. *Am J Hum Genet* 1996;**59**:653–63.

61. Liu AW, Delgado-Escueta AV, Serratosa JM, et al. Juvenile myoclonic epilepsy locus in chromosome 6p21.2-p11: linkage to convulsions and electroencephalography trait. *Am J Hum Genet* 1995;**57**:368–81.

62. Greenberg DA, Durner M, Resor S, et al. The genetics of idiopathic generalized epilepsies of adolescent onset: differences between juvenile

myoclonic epilepsy and epilepsy with random grand mal and with awakening grand mal. *Neurology* 1995;**45**:942–6.

63. Lander E, Kruglyak L. Genetic dissection of complex traits: guidelines for interpreting and reporting linkage results. *Nat Genet* 1995;**11**:241–7.

64. Thomson G. Identifying complex disease genes: progress and paradigms. *Nat Genet* 1994;**8**:108–10.

65. Steinlein OK, Mulley JC, Propping P, et al. A missense mutation in the neuronal nicotonic acetylcholine receptor α4 subunit is associated with autosomal dominant nocturnal frontal lobe epilepsy. *Nat Genet* 1995;**11**:201–3.

66. Fong CG, Shah PU, Huang Y, et al. Childhood absence epilepsy in an Indian (Bombay) family maps to chromosome 8q24. *Neurology* 1998;**50**:357 (abst).

67. Zara F, Labuda M, Bianchi A, et al. Evidence for a locus predisposing to idiopathic generalized epilepsy and spike-wave EEG on chromosome 3p14.2-p12.1. *Am J Hum Genet* 1997;**61**:41 (abst).

68. Westling B, Weissbecker K, Serratosa JM, et al. Evidence for linkage of juvenile myoclonic epilepsy with absence to chromosome 1p. *Am J Hum Genet* 1996;**59**:241 (abst).

69. Sander T, Kretz R, Williamson MP, et al. Linkage analysis between idiopathic generalized epilepsies and the GABA(A) receptor alpha5, beta3 and gamma3 subunit gene cluster on chromosome 15. *Acta Neurol Scand* 1997;**96**:1–7.

70. Andermann E. Genetic aspects of the epilepsies. In: Sakai T, Tsuboi J, eds. *Genetic aspects of human behaviour*. Tokyo: Igaku-Shoin, 1985:129–45.

71. Berkovic SF, Andermann F, Carpenter S, Wolfe LS. Progressive myoclonus epilepsies: specific causes and diagnosis. *N Engl J Med* 1986;**315**:296–305.

72. Marseille Consensus Group. Classification of progressive myoclonus epilepsies and related disorders. *Ann Neurol* 1990;**28**:113–16.

73. Berkovic SF. Progressive myoclonus epilepsies. In: Engel J Jr, Pedley TA, eds. *Epilepsy: a comprehensive textbook*. Philadelphia: Lippincott-Raven, 1998:2455–68.

74. Doose H. Myoclonic astatic epilepsy of early childhood. In: Roger J, Bureau M, Dravet Ch, Dreifuss FE, Perret A, Wolf P, eds. *Epileptic syndromes in infancy, childhood and adolescence*, 2nd edn. London: John Libbey, 1992:103–14.

75. Doose H, Baier WK. Epilepsy with primarily generalized myoclonic-astatic seizures: a genetically determined disease. *Eur J Pediatr* 1987;**146**:550–4.

76. Doose H, Ritter K, Volzke E. EEG longitudinal studies in febrile convulsions. Genetic aspects. *Neuropediatrics* 1983;**14**:81–7.

77. Verity CM, Butler NR, Golding J. Febrile convulsions in a national cohort followed up from birth. I-Prevalence and recurrence in the first five years of life. *BMJ* 1985;**290**: 1307–10.

78. Duchowny M. Febrile seizures in childhood. In: Wyllie E, ed. *The treatment of epilepsy*. Philadelphia: Williams & Wilkins, 1993:647–53.

79. Lennox WG, Lennox MA. *Epilepsy and related disorders*. Boston: Little, Brown & Co, 1960.

80. Frantzen E, Lennox-Buchthal M, Nygaard A, Stene J. A genetic study of febrile convulsions. *Neurology* 1970;**20**:909–17.

81. Lennox-Buchthal MA. Febrile convulsions. A reappraisal. *Electroencephalogr Clin Neurophysiol* 1973;**S32**:1–132.

82. Schuman SH, Miller LJ. Febrile convulsions in families: findings in an epidemiologic survey. *Clin Pediatr* 1966;**5**:604–8.

83. Fukuyama Y, Kagawa K, Tanaka K. A genetic study of febrile convulsions. *Eur Neurol* 1979; **18**:166–82.

84. Gardiner RM. Genes and epilepsy. *J Med Genet* 1990;**27**:537–44.

85. Rich SS, Annegers JF, Hauser WA, Anderson VE. Complex segregation analysis of febrile convulsions. *Am J Hum Genet* 1987;**41**: 249–57.

86. Berg AT, Shinnar S, Hauser WA, Leventhal JM. Predictors of recurrent febrile seizures: a metaanalytic review. *J Pediatr* 1990;**116**: 329–37.

87. Van Esch A, Steyerberg EW, Berger MY, et al. Family history and recurrence of febrile seizures. *Arch Dis Childhood* 1994;**70**: 395–9.

88. Nelson KB, Ellenberg JH. Prognosis in children with febrile seizures. *Pediatrics* 1978; **61**:720–7.

89. Verity CM, Golding J. Risk of epilepsy after febrile convulsions: a national cohort study. *BMJ* 1991;**303**:1373–6.

90. Annegers JF, Hauser WA, Shirts SB, Kurland LT. Factors prognostic of unprovoked seizures after febrile convulsions. *N Engl J Med* 1987;**316**:493–8.

91. Maher J, McLachlan RS. Febrile convulsions. Is seizure duration the most important predictor of temporal lobe epilepsy? *Brain* 1995;**118**:1521–8.

92. Wallace RH, Berkovic SF, Howell RA, et al. Suggestion of a major gene for familial febrile convulsions mapping to 8q13-21. *J Med Genet* 1996;**33**:308–12.

93. Dubovsky J, Weber JL, Orr HT, et al. A second gene for familial febrile convulsions maps on chromosome 19p. *Am J Hum Genet* 1996;**59**:A223 (abst).

94. Maher J, McLachlan RS. Febrile convulsions in selected large families: a single-major-locus mode of inheritance? *Dev Med Child Neurol* 1997;**39**:79–84.

95. Johnson EW, Dubovsky J, Rich SS, et al. Evidence for a novel gene for familial febrile convulsions, FEB2, linked to chromosome 19p in an extended family from the midwest. *Hum Mol Genet* 1998;**7**:63–7.

96. McLachlan RS, Racacho LJ, Maher J, et al. Exclusion of the familial febrile convulsions locus at 8q13–21 for linkage in two large kindreds segregating febrile seizures: evidence for genetic heterogeneity. *Epilepsia* 1996;**37**:114 (abst).

97. Scheffer IE, Berkovic SF. Generalized epilepsy with febrile seizures plus. A genetic disorder with heterogeneous clinical phenotypes. *Brain* 1997;**120**:479–90.

98. Lopes-Cendes I, Scheffer IE, Berkovic SF, et al. Mapping a locus for idiopathic generalized epilepsy in a large multiplex family. *Epilepsia* 1996;**35**:127 (abst).

99. Delgado-Escueta AV, Treiman DM, Walsh GO. The treatable epilepsies. *N Engl J Med* 1983;**308**:1508–14.

100. Bray PF and Wiser WC. Evidence for a genetic etiology of temporal-central abnormalities in focal epilepsy. *N Engl J Med* 1964;**271**:926–33.

101. Bray PF, Wiser WC. Hereditary characteristics of familial temporal-central focal epilepsy. *Pediatrics* 19965;**36**:207–11.

102. Doose H, Baier WK. Benign partial epilepsy and related conditions: multifactorial pathogenesis with hereditary impairment of brain maturation. *Eur J Pediatr* 1989;**149**:152–8.

103. Fukuyama Y. Borderland of childhood epilepsy, with special references to febrile convulsions and so-called infantile convulsions. *Seishin Igaku* 1963;**5**:211–23.

104. Fukuyama Y. A short reflection on Japanese contributions to pediatric epileptology — Thanks in return. *Brain Dev* 1995;**17**:1–16.

105. Vigevano F, Di Capua M, Fusco L, et al. Sixth-month benign familial convulsions. *Epilepsia* 1990;**31**:613.

106. Vigevano F, Fusco L, Di Capua M, et al. Benign infantile familial convulsions. *Eur J Pediatr* 1992;**151**:608–12.

107. Dordi B, De Marco P, Biamino P, Tabiadon G. Benign infantile familial convulsions. *Neurology* 1993;**43**:A245 (abst).

108. Hauser E, Seidl R, Tenner W, et al. Benign infantile familial convulsions. *Eur J Pediatr* 1995;**154**:499–500.

109. Malafosse A, Beck C, Bellet H, et al. Benign infantile familial convulsions are not an allelic form of the benign familial neonatal convulsions gene. *Ann Neurol* 1994;**35**:479–82.

110. Guipponi M, Rivier F, Vigevano F, et al. Linkage mapping of benign familial infantile convulsions (BFIC) to chromosome 19q. *Hum Mol Genet* 1997;**6**:473–7.

111. Szeptowski P, Rochette J, Berquin P, et al. Familial infantile convulsions and paroxysmal choreoathetosis: a new neurological syndrome linked to the pericentromeric region of human chromosome 16. *Am J Hum Genet* 1997;**61**:889–98.

112. Oldani A, Zucconi M, Ferini-Strambi L, et al. Autosomal dominant nocturnal frontal lobe epilepsy: electroclinical picture. *Epilepsia* 1996;**37**:964–76.

113. Magnusson A, Nakken KO, Brubakk E. Autosomal dominant frontal epilepsy. *Lancet* 1996;**347**:1191–2.

114. Khatami R, Neumann M, Kolmel HW. A family with frontal lobe epilepsy and mental retardation. *Epilepsia* 1997;**38**:200 (abst).

115. Phillips HA, Scheffer IE, Berkovic SF, et al. Localization of a gene for autosomal dominant nocturnal frontal lobe epilepsy to chromosome 20q13.2. *Nat Genet* 1995;**10**: 117–18.

116. Steinlein OK, Magnusson A, Stoodt J, et al. An insertion mutation of the *CHRNA4* gene in a family with autosomal dominant nocturnal frontal lobe epilepsy. *Hum Mol Genet* 1997;**6**:943–8.

117. Phillips HA, Scheffer IE, Crossland KM, et al. Autosomal dominant nocturnal frontal-lobe epilepsy: genetic heterogeneity and evidence for a second locus at 15q24. *Am J Hum Genet* 1998;**63**:1108–16.

118. Ottman R, Risch N, Hauser WA, et al. Localization of a gene for partial epilepsy to - chromosome 10q. *Nat Genet* 1995;**10**:56–60.

119. Hurst JA, Baraitser M, Auger E, et al. An extended family with a dominantly inherited speech disorder. *Dev Med Child Neurol* 1990;**32**:352–5.

120. Gopnik M. Feature-blind grammar and dysphasia. *Nature* 1990;**344**:715.

121. Vargha-Khadem F, Watkins K, Alcock K, et al. Praxic and nonverbal cognitive deficits in a large family with a genetically transmitted speech and language disorder. *Proc Natl Acad Sci USA* 1995;**92**:930–3.

122. Fisher SE, Vargha-Khadem F, Watkins K, et al. Localisation of a gene implicated in a severe speech and language disorder. *Am J Hum Genet* 1997;**61**:A28 (abst),

123. Fisher SE, Vargha-Khadem F, Watkins KE, et al. Localisation of a gene implicated in a severe speech and language disorder. *Nat Genet* 1998;**18**:168–70.

124. Scheffer IE. Autosomal dominant rolandic epilepsy with speech dyspraxia. In: Berkovic SF, Genton P, Hirsch E, Picard F, eds. *Genetics of focal epilepsies: Clinical aspects and molecular biology*. London: John Libbey & Co. Ltd, 1999:109–14.

125. Lerman P. Benign partial epilepsy with centro-temporal spikes. In: Roger J, Bureau M, Dravet Ch, Dreifuss FE, Perret A, Wolf P, eds. *Epileptic syndromes in infancy, childhood and adolescence*, 2nd edn. London: John Libbey, 1992:189–200.

126. Lerman P. Benign childhood epilepsy with centrotemporal spikes (BECT). In: Engel J Jr, Pedley TA, eds. *Epilepsy: a comprehensive textbook. Volume 3*. Philadelphia: Lippincott-Raven, 1998:2307–14.

127. Whitehouse W, Diebold U, Rees M, et al. Exclusion of linkage of genetic focal sharp waves to the HLA region on chromosome 6p in families with benign partial epilepsy with centrotemporal sharp waves. *Neuropediatrics* 1993;**24**:208–10.

128. Neubauer BA, Moises HW, Lassker U, et al. Benign childhood epilepsy with centrotemporal spikes and electroencephalography trait are not linked to EBN1 and EBN2 of benign neonatal familial convulsions. *Epilepsia* 1997;**38**:782–7.

129. Hirvasniemi A, Lang H, Lehesjoki A-E, Leisti J. Northern epilepsy syndrome: an inherited childhood onset epilepsy with associated mental deterioration. *J Med Genet* 1994;**31**:177–82.

130. Tahvanainen E, Ranta S, Hirvasniemi A, et al. The gene for a recessively inherited human childhood progressive epilepsy with mental retardation maps to the distal short arm of chromosome 8. *Proc Natl Acad Sci USA* 1994;**91**:7267–70.

131. Penfield W, Paine K. Results of surgical therapy for focal epileptic seizures. *Can Med Assoc J* 1955;**73**:515–31.

132. Andermann E. Multifactorial inheritance in the epilepsies. In: Canger R, Angeleri F, Penry JK, eds. *Advances in epileptology: XIth epilepsy international symposium*. New York: Raven Press, 1980:297–309.

133. Andermann E, Straszak M. Family studies of epileptiform EEG abnormalities and photosensitivity in focal epilepsy. In: Akimoto H, Kazamatsuri H, Seino M, Ward A, eds. *Advances in epileptology: XIIIth epilepsy international symposium*. New York: Raven Press, 1982:105–12.

IV

IDENTIFYING CANDIDATES FOR EPILEPSY SURGERY

10

Early recognition of surgically amenable epilepsy syndromes

Hermann Stefan

Introduction

Surgical treatment of pharmacoresistant epilepsies has increased considerably over the past few years. This is due to several factors: the gain in experience concerning epilepsy surgery of different epilepsy syndromes, development of new diagnostic techniques and application of new surgical techniques. Since there are many patients with pharmacoresistant epilepsies, the question arises: How can patients be selected for surgical treatment?

After several months of unsuccessful drug treatment, a practitioner should refer the patient to a specialist for further treatment. In general, medical intractability can be assessed within 2 years. In infants with catastrophic epilepsies, i.e. daily seizures, a quick decision is necessary. For the assessment of medical intractability in adult patients, usually antiepileptic drugs in mono- and polytherapy are required. Monotherapy should be increased in dosages up to the occurrence of side effects if seizures cannot be controlled and/or intolerable side effects are occurring. In the case of a surgically amenable epilepsy syndrome, intensive presurgical evaluation is indicated.[1]

Spectrum of methods for surgery

In addition to the classical temporal lobe 'en bloc' or 'standard' resection, several modifica-

tions, e.g. selective amygdalohippocampectomy or tailored resections, have been developed for epilepsy surgery in temporal lobe epilepsies. In extratemporal lobe epilepsies, individual tailoring of partial lobectomies, or even lesionectomies, can be performed. As well as the resection of epileptogenic brain tissue, the inhibition of propagation of epileptic activity by means of transection (callosotomy or multiple subpial transection) is also a possibility. If the epileptogenic lesion is partially overlapping the functionally important area, a combination of resection with an extention to functional epilepsy surgery, i.e. transection in the eloquent area, can be carried out. Alternative surgical procedures—if resection or transection is not considered—are vagus stimulation and, still in the experimental phase, radiosurgery (performed by the γ-knife technique). Alternatively, radiotherapy can also be carried out by fractionated low-dose stereotactic radiation using a linear accelerometer. Whereas different types of resections have been performed in thousands of patients, the results of transection and other techniques are, up to now, reported in smaller numbers of patients. In an overview, in 8,234 patients who underwent epilepsy surgery, a resection in the temporal lobe was performed in 66 per cent, a resection in extratemporal lobe epilepsies in 13 per cent, lesionectomy in 5 per cent, hemispherectomy in 5 per cent and corpus callosotomies in 10 per cent of the cases.[2] From

Mesial temporal lobe epilepsy (MTLE)	Extratemporal epilepsies	Possible catastrophic epilepsy in infancy and childhood	Other lesional syndromes
Febrile seizures first year of life Spontaneous complex partial second half of first decade Epigastric aura (fear, déjà vu, etc.) Secondary generalized seizure and isolated aura Silent periods several years Loss of aura (bilateralization?)	**Frontal** 1. SP*, CP†, frequent, cluster, sudden onset and end, little post-ictal confusion, hypermotor, bizarre 2. Silent areas (polar) 3. M2E-seizure (from first frontal gyrus) supplementary motor area (SMA), mesial parietal 4. Frontal except lateralized clonic seizures rarely lateralization or localization by seizure signs **Parietal** Somatosensory aura in 50 per cent, sometimes vertigo or movement sensation **Occipital** Ictal amaurosis Elementary visual hallucinations	Diffuse hemispheric syndromes Hemimegencephaly Extensive cortical malformation Tuberous sclerosis Sturge–Weber syndrome Rasmussen encephalitis Multifocal Lennox–Gastaut syndrome Frequent seizures and/or status epilepticus Generalized motor seizures Tonic seizures Atypical absences Drop attacks Slow spike–wave 30–50 per cent etiology detectable	Low-grade glial neoplasia Highest potential for epileptogenesis Different lesions in different lobes, e.g. cortical dysplasia Cavernous hemangioma Trauma Focal encephalitis Cysticercosis, etc.
Special diagnostic techniques EEG temporal mesial spikes MR hippocampal atrophy MR-spectroscopy: NAA‡ decrease	**Special diagnostic technique** MRI (1 mm), fast ictal SPECT		**Special diagnostic technique** For detection of cortical malformation, high resolution MRI and inversion recovery

*Simple partial.
†Complex partial.
‡N-acetyl-aspartate.

Table 10.1
Recognition criteria for surgically amenable epilepsy syndromes and special diagnostic techniques that may be helpful for early recognition.

the analyses of the outcome of surgically treated patients (seizure control, side effects and psychosocial development), several outlines can be obtained for the early recognition of surgically amenable epilepsy syndromes.

Epilepsy syndromes

Syndromes amenable for epilepsy surgery

Focal lesional epilepsies can be recognized early as surgically amenable epilepsy syndromes (Table 10.1).[3] This most often concerns temporal lobe epilepsies but also extratemporal lobe epilepsies. Epilepsy surgery is often indicated early in life in diffuse hemispheric syndromes if there is a regional accentuation, for instance, in hemimegencephalia, Sturge–Weber syndrome, cortical malformation, Rasmussen's syndrome, HHE syndrome and infantile spasms. In catastrophic epilepsy syndromes in infants a surgical intervention has to be carried out early in the disorder. In focal cryptogenic epilepsies, patients with mesial temporal lobe epilepsy syndrome are also possible candidates for epilepsy surgery, especially if it coincides with an indication for unilateral epileptic activity. Cryptogenic extratemporal lobe epilepsies are difficult to localize and do not therefore belong to the early surgically amenable epilepsy syndromes. Resection can be performed only in a limited number of those patients who have undergone major invasive diagnostic explorations. Multifocal drug-resistant epilepsies can be treated by multi-lobar resections or, for instance, in the case of Lennox–Gastaut syndrome, by means of callosotomy. Generalized motor seizures (tonic), atypical absence seizures and drop attacks frequently occur in patients with Lennox–Gastaut syndrome. In 30–50 per cent of cases no etiology can be detected. In the other half of patients, birth injuries, encephalitis or tuberous sclerosis, etc., can be detected. In multifocal epilepsies, callosotomy may be used for the treatment if the patient has a drug refractory epileptic syndrome, no resectable focus, generalized seizures, or partial seizures with secondary generalization causing falling and no profound mental retardation.[2,4]

Syndromes not amenable for epilepsy surgery

The following are not surgically amenable: idiopathic generalized epilepsies or syndromes in childhood with spontaneous remission, like benign rolandic epilepsy syndrome; childhood epilepsy with occipital spikes; benign psychomotor epilepsy; benign seizures in the temporal lobe in adolescence. In addition, syndromes with fatal metabolic or degenerative disorders, as well as electrolytic or hypoglycemically-induced seizures, are not suited for epilepsy surgery because of the rapid fatal progression of the underlying disease (e.g. ceroid lipofuscinosis, Alpers disease). Besides these exclusional syndromatic criteria, any severe medical systemic illness or metabolic disease affecting the central nervous system may present a contraindication for epilepsy surgery. Other criteria which have to be considered are the neurological function of the patient: age; IQ (IQ <70 often argues against resective surgery); psychic condition (e.g. missing motivation, missing cooperation or ability to cooperate, or a fixed psychosis). Concerning seizure type, the individual disability, as a consequence of the seizure, has to be taken into account. Most often, simple partial seizures (except epilepsia partialis continua) do not disable a patient enough to indicate epilepsy surgery. Frequency and duration of the seizures also depend on the individual impact of the daily life and professional work of a patient. The number of antiepileptic drugs which should have been applied to the patient depend on the seizure syndrome and presumed operability of the patient's type of epilepsy.

Recognition criteria

Before a decision on surgical treatment can be taken, the following criteria have to be considered individually. Did the medically non-responsive patient receive adequate medical therapy? Using a clinical history, neurological examination, magnetic resonance imaging (MRI), electroencephalogram (EEG), and neuropsychology testing the following should be answered:

- seizure classification, additional psychogenic attacks

- definition of the epileptic syndrome
- hints for possible overlap of epileptogenic area with functional area
- prediction of etiology by means of MRI (static lesion, tumor, malformation, non-lesional)
- uni- or bilateral EEG changes
- IQ, memory, psychosis, coping feasibility, cooperation.

Considering this check-list, patients with amenable epilepsy syndromes have to be analyzed individually, for instance, using a rating scale (Figure 10.1) for probable clinical localization, hypothesis and operability. After having estimated the localization and operation probability, the decision for further drug treatment or surgical therapy can finally be taken (Figure 10.2).

Epileptic syndrome	**1** Mesial temporal cryptogenetic, cavernoma or atrophy	**0** Pachygyria	**–1** Cryptogenic generalized
Probability of localization and surgery	**1** Electrophys. unifocal congruent with imaging	**0** Temporal + extratemporal unilateral	**–1** Multifocal bitemporal + extratemporal and functional zone
Drug intractability	**1** > Three-drug side effects	**0** Three	**–1** < Three
Psychosocial plasticity	**1** Coping capability	**0**	**–1** Low IQ and cooperation

Figure 10.1
Exemplary proposal for rating scales used individually as an additional guide for decision-making as an indication for preoperative monitoring in epilepsy surgery.

Removable epileptogenic lesion	Resection Uni–multilobar
Epileptogenic area in eloquent area	Multiple subpial transection (MST)
Large non-removable lesion	Partial resection or transection, MST, callosotomy
Multifocal generalized (LGS, bilateral poly-microgyry, double cortex)	Callosotomy
Large epileptogenic area (diffuse hemispheric)	Hemispherectomy, hemispherotomy
Inoperability by resection or transection	Vagus stimulation, radiotherapy?

Figure 10.2
Potential operative strategies in different conditions of patients with pharmacoresistant epilepsies.

Final decision strategies

From clinical experience, it is very important to mention that for further decisions to be made the physician and patient must have similar expectations concerning the benefit and risk of further diagnostic and surgical procedures. For further steps to be taken the patient's subjective opinion is a necessary additional guide. This also concerns the extent of the clinical localization hypothesis, i.e. the electrophysiological invasive or non-invasive confirmation of the epileptogenic tissue and, if necessary, the functionally eloquent brain area. Depending on the results of this more or less invasive presurgical exploration, a decision has to be taken on the individual selection of one of the available surgical methods, like resection, transection, vagus stimulation or radiotherapy (Figures 10.3 and 10.4). In cases of overlapping of epileptogenic and functionally important areas, e.g. in the central region or a language area, more patients can be treated

TLE	TLE	IDIOPATH. GENERALIZED
(Tumor, angioma)	Cryptogenic (a) right → preoperative diagnostics (b) left → more extensive drug treatment before preoperative diagnostics?	New AED
right or left → preoperative diagnostics		
EXTRATEMPORAL (a) non-lesional → more extensive drug treatment? (b) cortical malformation → more extensive drug treatment? Multiple subpial transection?	FLE (a) right lesional → preoperative diagnostics (b) left lesional → multiple subpial transection?	MULTIFOCAL GENERALIZED e.g. LGS n. vagus stimulation Callosotomy

Figure 10.3
Estimated chances for localization probability and successful surgery. It is assumed that the left hemisphere is dominant. FLE, frontal lobe epilepsy; LGS, Lennox–Gastaut syndrome; TLE, temporal lobe epilepsy.

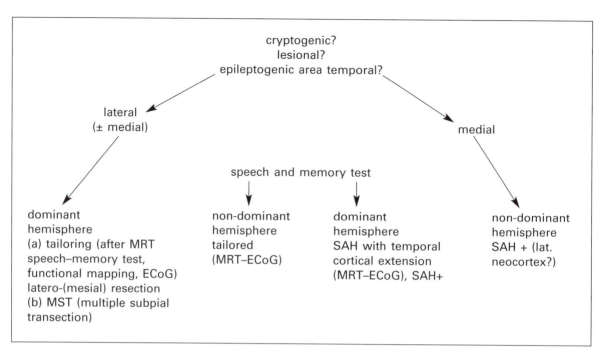

Figure 10.4

Different surgical approaches depending on localization in the dominant or non-dominant hemispheres and functional individual reserve capacity of the brain. SAH, selective amygdalohippocampectomy; +, additional temporobasal and neocortical extension.

surgically than in former times. This is due to the combination of partial resection and transection. In patients with non-resectable and transectable epileptogenic regions, focal radiation can be helpful. Due to this increase in surgical feasibilities for treatment, and thus a considerable increase in treatable patients with pharmacoresistant epilepsies, a rationally based decision requires an assessment of the patient's individual characteristic condition as well as the diagnosis of an epileptic syndrome. For the early recognition and decision, several factors have to be assessed: the influence on cerebral development; plasticity of the epilepsy;[5] psychosocial consequences and the risk of epilepsy surgery.

References

1. Stefan H. *Epilepsien: Diagnose und Behandlung. 3. Auflage.* Stuttgart: Georg Thieme Verlag, 1990.

2. Engel J. ed. *Surgical treatment of the epilepsies* 2nd edn. New York: Raven Press, 1993.

3. Pawlik G, Stefan H. *Focus localization.* Berlin: Ligaverlag, 1996.

4. Wyllie E. *The treatment of epilepsy: principles and practice.* Philadelphia: Lea & Febiger, 1993.

5. Stefan H, Andermann F, Chauvel P, Shorvon S. Plasticity in epilepsy: dynamic aspects of brain function. *Advances in Neurology, Vol. 81.* Philadelphia: Lippincott-Raven, 1999.

11

Rational and cost-effective presurgical evaluation

Donald L Schomer

Introduction

The ability to provide a cost-effective means for the presurgical evaluation of a patient with medically intractable epilepsy is critical if surgical therapies are to be made widely available. Considerable data exist that show that several surgical procedures can be efficacious in treating specific forms of medically intractable epilepsy. Matching the patient to the right surgical procedure requires the combined experience of a team of specialists. The evaluation process itself, while showing some variation dependent on the specific surgical approach under consideration, is for the most part rather straightforward. Problems arise in approaching the difficult-to-manage patient with epilepsy, primarily when it comes to our ability to provide the various tests necessary for a clinical surgical decision on a timely and cost-effective basis. As will be discussed in this chapter, most of these studies, tests and consultations can be provided on an outpatient basis that helps, at least, to reduce the overall expense of an operative approach.

Types of epilepsy surgery and their related clinical indications

When the topic of epilepsy surgery arises, at least five operative procedures can be considered.

Hemispherectomy is the most dramatic of the surgical procedures. Either an anatomical procedure can be performed in which all of the neocortex from one hemisphere is removed down to the level of the basal ganglia or a functional procedure can be performed. In the latter procedure, considerable lateral neocortex is removed but the anterior and posterior portions of the hemisphere are preserved. The remaining neocortex in these two areas is then under-cut, effectively de-afferenting them. This procedure leaves the neocortex in those two areas in place and viable, but non-functional. Their presence seems to reduce the likelihood for development of cerebral hemosiderosis, a common long-term complication of the anatomical procedure.

A corpus callosotomy—the sectioning of the corpus collosum without actually removing it—also may be accomplished by one of two surgical techniques. In one case, only the anterior two thirds of the callosum is transected during the initial operative approach. The remaining one third is transected at a later time only if there has been little or no clinical response to the initial operation. In the alternative surgical approach, the entire corpus callosum is sectioned during the initial operation. Patients seem to have fewer problems neuropsychologically following the partial sectioning. However, the surgical success rate, as measured by a decrease in frequency of atonic drop seizures, is not as high with partial sectioning as it is with single complete transectioning.

Subpial cortical transection is performed as a surgical treatment for seizures that are shown to originate in eloquent cortex such as Broca's speech area or the primary motor strip.

Lesionectomy is the preferred operative procedure for patients whose seizures arise from an area immediately surrounding a tumor that does not involve eloquent cortex. A variation of lesionectomy is the focal cortical excision, which includes lobectomy. In such cases, areas of cortex are targeted for removal based on their involvement in the generation of a seizure. In most cases, these seizures originate in the temporal lobe, particularly in the more anterior, basal and mesial regions, often with no accompanying lesion. These syndromes were addressed in the previous chapter.

The different techniques noted above are appropriate for the treatment of different types of seizures. The hemispherectomy is the preferred approach for seizures that are widely distributed within one hemisphere in the setting of severe neurological impairment involving the same hemisphere. Conditions such as Rasmussen's encephalitis—a progressive inflammatory childhood disorder with multifocal, medically refractory, severe seizures—are often successfully treated through this approach. Other disorders such as a congenital middle cerebral artery infarct with associated porencephaly and recurrent, medically intractable epilepsy are occasionally cured by this procedure.

The corpus callosotomy is reserved to treat the atonic, drop-type seizures seen in patients with widespread, bi-hemispheric disorders such as Lennox–Gastaut syndrome.

The subpial transection is a potential form of surgical intervention in patients with medically unresponsive seizures, whatever their etiology, originating in regions of the brain that retain functional significance despite the presence of seizures. Postoperatively, these areas can preserve most of their functional abilities that are dependent on the columnar organization of the cortex, while the ability of these brain regions to generate a focal seizure is inhibited. The epileptic phenomenon is more dependent on column-to-column excitatory neural transmission. This procedure severs the column-to-column connections in the subpial plane, thus producing its anticonvulsant effect.

Focal removal of neocortex, whether in the form of a lesionectomy or corticectomy, is dependent on demonstrating that seizures originate in the region of the planned removal and that the removal will not be associated with additional unbearable neurological deficits.

While all of these surgical strategies involve very detailed clinical and radiological evaluations, each requires the recording of the patient's typical seizures in order to come to a surgical decision. EEG telemetry is a technique that allows the treating physician to extend the standard EEG recording session sufficiently to record as many seizures as are necessary in order to evaluate the best form of treatment. While EEG is not the lone diagnostic tool for the appraisal of a patient with epilepsy, it is considered to be the standard for the evaluation of a patient considered for focal surgical removals. Ambulatory EEG telemetry is a technique that allows the physician to further extend the recording studio from the EEG laboratory into the home environment, and can markedly reduce costs if used successfully, by avoiding expensive inpatient hospitalizations. Advances in this area of neurophysiology have principally moved extremely sophisticated recording devices that were only found in some inpatient-based EEG laboratories into the patient's home environment.

Evaluation process for partial epilepsy

Incidence

Epilepsy affects between 0.5 and 1 per cent of the population in Western countries. The incidence is considerably higher in Third World countries. Approximately 60 per cent of all patients with epilepsy have focal onset of partial epilepsy. This type of epilepsy is more likely to be amenable to a surgical approach than are other forms of epilepsy. It is estimated that 30 per cent of those patients with partial epilepsy have seizures that are medically refractory by standard criteria. Many more patients feel that they have unacceptable medication side effects. Conservatively, of this group, 15 per cent are felt to be good surgical candidates, if they could be identified. Therefore, in the US alone, over 75,000 people have a form of epilepsy that, if properly evaluated, could lead seizure-free or markedly improved life styles. This group is the one that will be highlighted in the remainder of this chapter.

History and physical/neurological examinations

The evaluation of a patient for epilepsy surgery begins with a detailed history and physical and neurological examinations. The history and examinations are best performed by someone well versed in the surgical evaluation process, looking for risk factors for epilepsy that include prior injury to the central nervous system, birth complications, prolonged febrile convulsions, intracranial infections and head trauma. The seizure-specific history should enquire about both 'ictal' and 'interictal' phenomena. The discussion should detail the nature of the subjective symptoms, which may include feelings, emotions, hallucinatory experiences, etc. that would suggest seizures of temporal lobe, particularly limbic, origin. Additionally, in such cases, detailing a relationship to triggers such as the menstrual cycle, stress and sleep deprivation should be explored. An attempt to define whether one or multiple seizure types exist is important in thinking about whether a single focus or multiple foci of seizure activity exists. The history must detail the patient's exposure to anticonvulsant medications and often this requires input from family members and other physicians who have cared for the person in the past. Emphasis is placed on the reasons for therapeutic failure. Most of the time, patients' seizures prove to be truly resistant to the anticonvulsant properties of multiple drug medication. On the other hand, treatment failure may be the result of serious or unacceptable side effects to the medications that may also justify consideration as a surgical candidate. However, problems with compliance *per se* due to personality disorders may not justify the time and expense of a surgical approach, since medications have not been given an adequate trial.

The clinical examination should focus on subtle developmental anomalies such as growth asymmetries and focal neurological deficits that would suggest an underlying structural abnormality. Additionally, if prior examinations exist, repeating one at this time often helps determine if there is the potential for an underlying progressive disorder.

Radiological testing

The presurgical imaging study should be a magnetic resonance image (MRI). This outpatient-based study is very useful for identifying lesions in the 1–2 mm level.[1] With specialized sequences, small cortical migration abnormalities can be identified. These are now proving to be a fairly common underlying cause for seizures.[1] Once complete MRI scans of a patient are obtained, the radiologist can reconfigure the data to show the 3-D features of the hippocampi. These volume determinations may help localize the side of seizure onset, especially in the condition where one hippocampus is atrophic.[1] If that side is also the one where the EEG ictal focus resides, there is a good likelihood for a positive surgical outcome with little additional neurological deficit. Hippocampal volume determination can also help the physician to predict any additional cognitive problems that might result from the planned surgery. If the operative side is normal in volume, the patient is likely to have additional cognitive problems related to the area removed.

Functional imaging using either single photon emission tomography (SPECT) or positron emission tomography (PET) can be obtained on an outpatient basis when evaluating the interictal state. These images show the metabolic condition of the brain either directly or indirectly. The area of decreased metabolic activity often correlates with the area that initiates the seizure.[1] The electrical focus for the seizure event onset, however, resides within this area of metabolic abnormality as a smaller, more restricted region. Obtaining an ictal SPECT or PET may prove to be confounding. Patients need to be carefully monitored for a seizure if the clinician is going to get useful information. In the case of SPECT, the tracer material needs to be administered within a few moments of the onset of the seizure in order to be helpful. The scan itself can be postponed for up to several hours after the injection, but the injection must be given close to the time of the seizure onset. Ictal SPECT can be obtained on an outpatient basis if the seizure frequency is high. The imaging facility also needs to be flexible enough to incorporate the needs of such patients. In the case of ictal PET imaging,

the patient should be inside the machine with a constant infusion of ^{18}F-flurodeoxyglucose (FDG) at the time of the seizure onset. For practical reasons, this should not be an essential component of the surgical evaluation.

Neuropsychological, neuropsychiatric, pharmacological and nursing evaluations

The neuropsychological and psychiatric assessments of potential epilepsy surgical cases are ideally obtained in the outpatient environment. In the case of the neuropsychological evaluation, several days of difficult and demanding testing often are required in order that the treating neurologist can feel comfortable that the test results are reproducible and accurate. Test results can be skewed if they are obtained during a period when the patient is experiencing more seizures than usual, such as during medication withdrawal. As the outpatient psychiatric assessment is not under the influence of the pressures of the inpatient environment and frequent seizures, it is likely to best reflect the patient's true mental state.

The neuropsychological evaluation is used to determine what parts of the brain are impaired by administering a series of standardized tests designed for those purposes. There are tests that relate primarily to higher cognitive functioning and assess executive functions, while other tests relate to various aspects of memory. The neuropsychologist must be able to differentiate congenital learning disabilities and the effects of medication on test performance as well as being able to take into account the effects of recent seizures on cognition. Testing the higher cognitive functional abilities helps determine whether surgery is required or not. The identifiable cognitive deficits must be explainable in light of the evidence for focal abnormalities found on the neuroimaging tests and on EEG. There must be agreement between these tests before the clinician can advocate surgery. Also, the cognitive testing helps in counseling the patient about possible short- and long-term difficulties that he or she may experience postoperatively. For further details on the specific tests that are used in evaluating patients with epilepsy see Chapter 21.

A formal neuropsychiatric evaluation preoperatively identifies pre-existent major affective disorders, personality disorders and disorders of mood. These conditions need to be addressed in order to improve the postoperative recovery. In some cases, the psychiatrist may feel that an underlying or co-existent psychiatric condition may preclude surgery and, thus identified, save the patient, the patient's family and the medical team time and resources. This evaluation also focuses on helping the patient realize that, if the surgery is successful, there are many adaptive concerns that will need to be addressed. These include the role the patient has in the family, changes in employment, and the general level of independence and self-reliance. Therefore, the psychiatrist involved in such presurgical evaluations needs to be fully informed and aware of the effects that seizures and anticonvulsants have on cognition, attention, sense of control and independence as well as the psychosocial impact of epilepsy.

The nursing staff's evaluation plays a critical role in the entire approach to the potential surgical patient. Nursing assessments often lead to a clearer understanding of how or why a medication may have failed. These findings often allow the clinician to retry medications successfully and avoid the entire presurgical process. Alternatively, if the patient continues as a candidate for surgery, the nursing staff can provide educational information directly or through printed material. This educational process helps the patient to deal more ably with the various tests. The nursing staff, in the process of providing education, discovers the patient's expectations of the surgery. These expectations, if unrealistic, must be dealt with in advance of the surgery taking place.

A preoperative neuropharmacological evaluation is rare but invaluable. Advice often centers around drug–drug interaction and drug metabolism idiosyncrasies. The neuropharmacologist is also helpful in intraoperative and postoperative management because of the various drugs required during these rather unique conditions.

Electro-encephalographic testing

Routine EEG is easily acquired in most patients and can be obtained on an outpatient basis. The recording does not take place in anticipation of a seizure being recorded, but rather to look for interictal epileptiform transients and focal or generalized disturbances of underlying background activity. The recording yield is improved by adding basal temporal electrodes. These include standard sphenoidals,[2,3,11] minisphenoidals, T1–T2 electrodes or nasopharyngeal electrodes. Prior to a recording patients are often deprived of sleep over night to enhance the likelihood of detecting interictal epileptic discharges.[4] If the EEG gives evidence of more diffuse brain disturbances, manifested by encephalopathic changes, or shows focal change, related to structural pathology, those findings may need to be addressed separately from the seizure localization issue.

What is left in the investigative process of the patient for epilepsy surgery is the recording of multiple seizures that reflect the types of spells that the patient routinely experiences.[5-7] This does not imply that the process of investigating a patient for epilepsy surgery follows the order that has been presented. Rather, each case is individualized with respect to the sequencing of the tests. Additionally, the technical quality of the seizure recording must be such that the clinician can confidently localize the seizure onset and document the physiology of the spread of the seizure and its associated behavior. These events need to be identical to the patient's typical events. Often the patient has a basal temporal electrode inserted, typically the standard sphenoidal electrode. The patient can be withdrawn from some or all anti-seizure drugs in a safe inpatient environment monitored by nursing staff in an attempt to increase the likelihood and frequency of seizure events. The patient is usually attached to a videorecording system that is either time-locked to the EEG equipment or is an integral part of the acquisition device.[8] Patients may be subjected to environmental triggers such as sleep deprivation or have their recording sessions timed to their menstrual cycle, if that is a factor.

Recent technological advances allow nearly all of the available technology from the inpatient unit to be used on an outpatient basis.[9–13] The clinician, therefore, decides which patients are better suited to which environment (home or hospital). Patients certainly can go home with the minor invasive electrodes such as the sphenoidals. However, these need to be monitored daily for irritation and infection. Patients who need to have their studies timed to their menstrual cycle, or require other activating procedures, can have those easily arranged with outpatient telemetry. Video equipment can now be taken home by the patient, which requires that either the patient or a family member be conversant with the technology so that it can be set up at home. Since most people have VCRs at home, this problem rarely arises. Therefore, the technical aspects of video monitoring should not be considered a deterrent to home monitoring. The behavior that results from a seizure may be a limiting factor, and if it is so unusual or physically demanding that monitoring at home becomes impractical, that patient is better managed in the hospital. However, the behaviors that are seen in most patients with temporal lobe seizures are usually not so disruptive. These patients tend to lend themselves to home-based recording. If the patient requires medication withdrawal in order to increase the frequency of seizures sufficiently to enable them to be recorded within a limited time period, then EEG recording should be carried out in the hospital. In this situation, the risk for serious injury during a seizure or the risk for developing status epilepticus is considerable. For patients who have undergone invasive electrode placement, such as depth or grid electrodes, the telemetry studies are best done in an inpatient unit. The risk of status epilepticus and infection preclude an outpatient work-up. In fact, many of the patients who are referred with medically refractory complex partial seizures can be evaluated through outpatient means. Patients with infrequent seizures requiring medicine tapers, or those with very disruptive behaviors or significantly invasive electrodes, are the exceptions to this guideline.

Computer-based telemetry methodology

Electrodes and pre-amplifier

The current systems that are used in both the inpatient and outpatient environment are the same. In either location, the physician can choose 16-, 18-, 27- or 32-channel recordings. The 16-channel device, for all intent and purposes, has joined the ranks of historical equipment. The 18-channel unit allows for selective recording from 16 EEG channels and two non-EEG leads, such as cardiac monitor or a pulse-based recording of finger levels of oxygenation (SpO2).[13-15] The 16 EEG channels are bipolar and the physician can choose from three standard montages: classical double banana (Queens Square), sphenoidal–temporal or the sphenoidal–parasagittal. The choice must be made before the recording starts. The 27- and 32-channel systems include all of the standard electrodes in the 10–20 system plus two basal temporal electrodes arranged in a remontagable bipolar fashion. Additionally, there are several channels available for non-EEG recordings. In the 32-channel unit, additional EEG channels can be integrated into the standard montages at the discretion of the electro-encephalographer. The electro-encephalographer can display the recorded data in any number of pre-selected choices or design a montage that best shows what he or she wishes to demonstrate.

An ultralight pre-amplifier, multiplexor and A–D converter weighing a few ounces is wrapped on top of the patient's head with cling gauze (Figures 11.1 and 11.2). This placement and wrapping serves several purposes. It allows the electrode wire leads to be kept fairly short. This reduces the amount of artifact that is seen related to wire movement during a seizure and reduces the antenna-like effect that is seen from time to time in recorders where there are long lead wire lengths. The electrodes themselves exhibit less movement artifact during seizures. Additionally, the bipolar recording technique reduces the amplitude of the recorded signal relative to the amplitudes seen on a referential recording. All in all, the recordings of seizures using a remontagable bipolar technique with on-the-head pre-amplification and multiplexing makes for remarkably artifact-reduced recordings, especially around a seizure event.

Waist-worn recorder and power supply

The patient has a waist belt fitted with a compact rectangular box containing replaceable batteries that power an A–D converter, multiplexor and solid state memory recorder based on a high-end Motorola processor (Figures 11.1 and 11.2). This recorder acquires the EEG data from the patient and channels it through a two-minute delay loop. The current system has sufficient memory to allow for five 4-min records to be stored, therefore, if the patient is ambulating, there is enough memory to record five 4-min duration 'events'. Each event has 2 min of EEG activity recorded that is acquired before the activation signal is seen and 2 min of subsequent activity. This is usually sufficient recording time to allow the EEG reader to observe the beginnings of the seizure and progression into a clinically relevant event. The newest design has 220 or 500 megabytes of flash card-based disk space. This modification allows for virtually unlimited numbers of events to be recorded or to convert the entire system into a low-powered, solid-state, completely ambulatory device.

Computer with automated detection algorithms

This device is an Intel 486 or Pentium-based computer with a large hard-drive capacity. This unit takes the multiplexed signals from the waist-worn recorder and performs on-line analysis. The system can operate in either a continuous or intermittent record mode. In the former, all incoming data is stored along with the time of day. The duration of the recording is determined by the capacity of the hard drive. In the intermittent mode of recording, the data is stored in one of four different files. One file relates to routinely stored segments of time. These time samples can be preprogramed to occur at various intervals. For instance, one can chose to record and save 30 s of EEG every 20 min throughout the recording session. This will allow the reader to evaluate the background activity, the transitions between different stages of sleep and the general activity level of the patient.[12,16]

Another file contains the 'push-button' events. As with the waist-worn device, there is a 2-min delay buffer that holds all of the EEG data in a time loop. If the patient has a symptomatic event, and someone pushes the 'button' on the recorder to identify the time of the event, a file similar to the waist-worn recorder will be put into this file. This unit

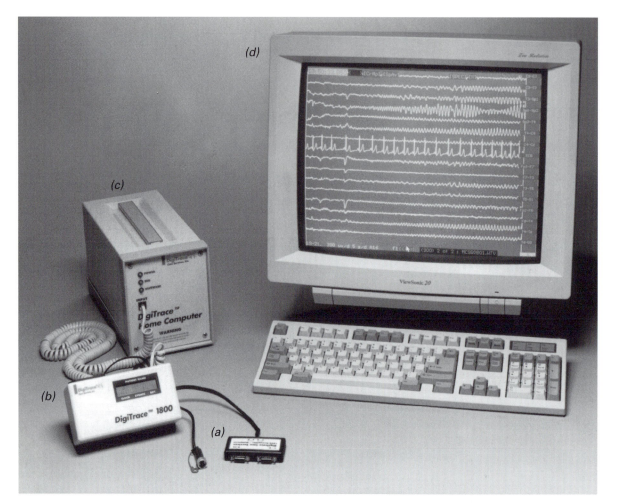

Figure 11.1

The commercialized equivalent of the system described in the chapter. The equipment is displayed prior to attachment to the patient. (a) The preamplifier. This is, in turn, attached to pre-wired electrode arrays after they are glued to the patient's scalp and wrapped onto the patient's head. (b) The waist-worn recorder and power supply. The batteries are internal and are changed daily. (c) The take-home computer which houses a large hard drive and all the data acquisition software. (d) The computer display (CRT), which is either attached to the take-home computer when the patient returns the device to the laboratory or is attached to its own computer. In the latter case, the data is downloaded to that a second computer system can either read directly from the CRT or have the information printed.

does not have a limit on the number of push-buttons because of the amount of storage capacity on the hard drive.

A third type of file is for automatically detected seizures. In this subroutine, the incoming EEG activity is subjected to on-line analysis that looks for sustained rhythmic activity.[17-19] This program is proprietary to the Telefactor

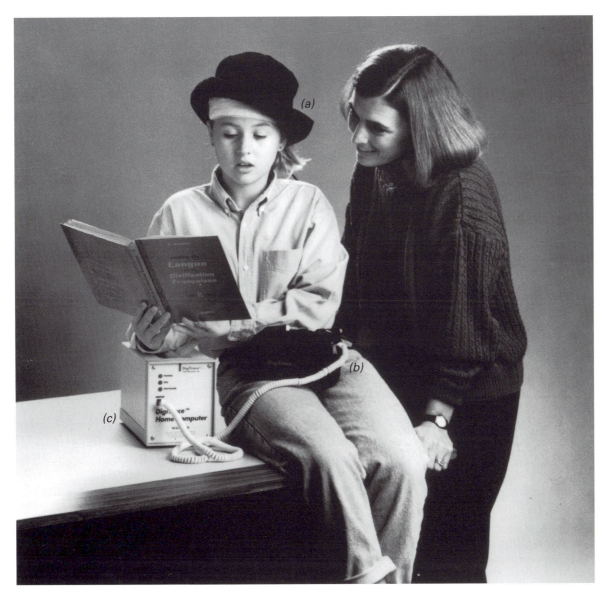

Figure 11.2

This shows the device attached to a patient. The letters identify those components described in Figure 11.1. (a) The preamplifier. (b) The waist-worn recorder. (c) The take-home computer.

Corp. and is based on an algorithm originally devised by Jean Gotman. This routine is usually turned off during the day but programmed to go on-line in the evening as the patient goes to bed. Therefore, most of the detection for clinically unrecognized seizures will occur during the night while the patient sleeps. The last subroutine that is active is the one that does automated interictal epileptiform detection.[20-22] This is also a Telefactor Corp. owned product based on algorithms of Jean Gotman. The current program stores 2 s of EEG data plus the time of day at each detection. The parameters for the detection software can also be manipulated by the electro-encephalographer in advance of the recording session. Other spike and seizure detection algorithms can also be made to run in this environment. Such programs could run in isolation or as a parallel routine.

If the patient is taking home the recording device, he or she should be instructed on electrical safety. The patient should place the computer in the room where most time is spent. Then the waist-worn recorder cable should be plugged into the computer, at which time a green light comes on indicating that the system is acquiring data. The patient can be unplugged from the unit at any time but must carry the waist-worn recorder with them at all times. At night, the computer should be placed alongside the bed and the patient should be attached to it. When the patient returns to the laboratory the next day, the take-home computer and waist-worn recorder are interrogated by the laboratory-based computer system and the data made available for either LaserJet paper printout or high resolution CRT review. If the patient is hospitalized, the patient plugs the waist-worn recorder into a wall box that serves as a link to the computer and VCR, which are housed in the EEG laboratory.

Additional devices are also occasionally employed. One of the more useful instruments

has been a blood oxygenation monitor unit that uses a commercially available device that is interfaced with the computer. It measures the partial pressure of oxygen in the fingernail bed (SpO_2) during every heartbeat.[14,15] This is recorded, stored and played back, time-locked to the EEG. This is useful both in the differential diagnosis of epilepsy and in the presurgical evaluations of cases when assessing for additional factors that may adversely affect the medical treatment or surgical outcome.

Videorecording

Videorecording can be adapted relatively easily for home use and most commercially available units can be fitted for such use. The device is put onto a mobile cart similar to a small piece of luggage. The camera is attached to a tripod and placed at a distance from the patient. The cabling is all color-coded for easy assembly in the home. Most patients feel comfortable setting up the video or seek help from a friend or relative. The videorecorder itself is attached to the home computer through a cable and linked to the EEG through the common time signal. The videorecording system is a 24-h recorder that avoids the need to change tapes but it does compromise the resolution detail that may otherwise be available on the inpatient unit.[8] The camera has a wide-angle lens so that, once focused, it can be left alone. Patients and others who attend the patient are encouraged to speak loudly about their feelings or observations during events so that this information can also be recorded.

Future telemetry direction

The future of home-based EEG monitoring is currently being hastened by the medical insurance industry. As this technology becomes more widely distributed, treating physicians will have to provide sound arguments for inpatient recording. Currently, if the equipment is not available locally or regionally, there is no alternative to an inpatient stay whether for diagnostic or for treatment purposes. In regions where home-based telemetry exists, inpatient stays need to be justified as discussed earlier. Besides the expense related concerns, home-based telemetry has developed to the point where the technology used in the home environment is basically the same as that used in the inpatient unit. This situation will continue into the future as long as the financial concerns surrounding inpatient units exist.

Future technological changes will develop probably along the lines of software analysis and software-based simplification of results. However, with regards to hardware, newer systems will be easily capable of recording 64 or more channels of EEG with variable sampling frequency. Currently, the commercial standard of 100 Hz per channel frequency response will be expanded to allow for 1000–5000 Hz per channel. This will allow for not only the standard recording but also provide a basis for undertaking detailed research-based investigations that require higher levels of frequency resolution. Also, electrodes and electrode arrays that will allow for considerable processing to be done at that level are currently under development. This may allow for electrode array designs that can be permanently implanted. This has already occurred in the field of ECG monitoring and will probably be available in the EEG world soon. This concept also allows for recording of other types of data. For example, EEG arrays could be linked to temperature recorders or ion-specific sensors. Additionally, the take-home computer is being designed to be pushed into the waist-worn recorder. This will provide for a fully ambulatory EEG device with all of the software applications running live. The take-home computer could then be used as a medium for digital video recording,

eliminating the need for a portable VCR system.

More importantly, perhaps, will be the ability to enable EEG data recorded in the home environment to be linked with advanced software. Links to 3-D MRI images and to other radiographic information already exist but need further deployment and testing.

Discussion

The recording of seizures during a presurgical work-up serves several purposes. In the case of a relatively straightforward patient with medically unresponsive seizures, the recordings of several seizures reassures the treating physician that the electrical onset of a typical seizure has origin in the region of planned surgery. In order to accomplish this task, the recording must include a sufficient number of recording sites to enable the reader to easily visualize the origin in three dimensions.[23,24] This requires at least 16–20 scalp-based electrodes. It also assures the physician that the planned approach is likely to remove the area of seizure onset, and provides him with data that can be used to predict the long-term outcome.

In these recording sessions, it is also important to note the time of onset of the first electrical evidence of the seizure and to compare that with the first behavioral correlate or the time when the patient feels the first sensation of the event. In the best situation, the electrical activity is seen before there is a clinical change in behavior. If the behavior correlate of the seizure occurs before the EEG shows a reproducible change, then the chances are that the recording electrodes are not very close to the area of seizure onset. In such cases, the physician may chose to go further and use invasive techniques to localize the area of onset. This is another important potential outcome of a recording session.

The surgical decision to operate depends on the clinician's judgment regarding all available data.[25,26] The neuroimaging studies should confirm the presence of either a convincing or subtle abnormality in or around the area that, on EEG investigation, is felt to be the seizure focus.[25,26] The neuropsychological data should also suggest cognitive deficits that relate to that same area of seizure onset.[25,26] The patient should be realistic about the surgical outcome studies and be fully informed regarding the surgical risks. The psychiatrist should be comfortable that, in his or her opinion, the patient is stable and ready to proceed.

As noted in the introduction, there are different surgical approaches for different types of seizures. Occasionally, a recording session reveals that the seizure appearance on EEG is not what was expected based on the seizure history. In such cases, the seizure semiology may need to be reassessed based on the recordings and a different surgical, or possibly medical, approach may be indicated.

Additionally, the recording of 'seizures' may reveal them to be other events. For example, the patient may experience cardiac arrhythmias that masquerade as seizures.[27-30] The patient may have sleep apnea that produces behavioral changes that previously were felt to be related to a seizure disorder.[31,32,39] In such a case, the antiseizure medications may also contribute to the sleep apnea.[33]

Studies that attempt to compare directly the inpatient and outpatient recordings of seizures find that few differences now exist in the technology. In many laboratories, as in ours, the systems are the same. In those few studies where data exist, patients on stable doses of medication experience more seizures in the outpatient environment.[34-38] Therefore, the major distinguishing factor between the two recording environments is linked to patient safety. If the physician feels that the patient can be as safely recorded as an outpatient as they could be as an inpatient, then the study should be carried out on an outpatient basis because of the cost savings. If the physician feels otherwise, then the study should take place in an inpatient unit.

In most cases of medically intractable complex partial epilepsy of temporal lobe origin, the patients can undergo most, if not all, of their presurgical evaluation as outpatients. In most cases, the frequency of seizures is sufficient to allow for a reasonable chance to record 4–6 typical events over a fairly short period of time. Also the behaviors are usually not too difficult to control in the home situation. Short of using implanted electrodes, the cost savings for such a non-invasive evaluation could save thousands of dollars and potentially make it a more widely utilized treatment modality.

References

1. Moshe SL, Pedley TA. Diagnostic evaluation. In: Engel J Jr, Pedley TA, eds. *Epilepsy: a comprehensive textbook*. New York: Lippincott-Raven, 1998:799–1098.

2. Ives JR, Gloor P. New sphenoidal electrode assembly to permit long-term monitoring of the patient's ictal and interictal EEG. *Electroenceph Clin Neurophysiol* 1977;**42**:575–80.

3. Ives JR, Schomer DL. The significance of using chronic sphenoidal electrodes during the recording of spontaneous ictal events in patients suspected of having temporal lobe seizures. *Electroencephal Clin Neurophysiol* 1986;**64**:23.

4. Mattson RH, Pratt KL, Caverly JR. Electroencephalogram in epileptics following sleep deprivation. *Arch Neurol* 1965;**13**:310–15.

5. Gotman J, Ives JR, Gloor P, eds. *Long-term monitoring in epilepsy (EEG Suppl. 37)*. Amsterdam: Elsevier Science Publishers BV, Biomedical Division, 1985.

6. Gumnit RJ, ed. *Intensive neurodiagnostic monitoring: advances in neurology*. Vol. 46. New York: Raven Press, 1987.

7. Ives JR, Thompson CJ, Gloor P. Seizure monitoring: a new tool in electroencephalography. *Electroenceph Clin Neurophysiol* 1976;**41**:422–7.

8. Ives JR, Gloor P. A long-term time-lapse video system to document the patient's spontaneous clinical seizures synchronized with the EEG. *Electroenceph Clin Neurophysiol* 1978;**45**:412–16.

9. Ives JR, Woods JF. The contribution of ambulatory EEG to the management of epileptic patients. In: Little WA, ed. *Clinical ambulatory monitoring*. London: Chapman & Hall, 1980:122–47.

10. Ives JR. A completely ambulatory 16-channel recording system. In: Stefan H, Burr W, eds. *Mobile long-term EEG monitoring*. Stuttgart: Gustav Fischer, 1982:205–17.

11. Ives JR, Schomer DL. Recent technical advances in long-term ambulatory outpatient monitoring. *Electroenceph Clin Neurophysiol* 1986;**64**:37.

12. Ives JR, Mainwaring NR, Gruber LJ, Schomer DL. Home computing: a remote intelligent EEG data acquisition unit for monitoring epileptic patients in the home environment. *Electroenceph Clin Neurophysiol* 1988;**69**:49.

13. Ives JR, Mainwaring NR, Schomer DL. An 18-channel solid-state ambulatory event recorder for use in the home and hospital environment. *Epilepsia* 1992;**33**:63.

14. Ives JR, Mainwaring NR, Krishnamurthy KB, et al. The contribution of continuous SaO$_2$ recording during long-term EEG monitoring (LTM). *J Clin Neurophysiol* 1995;**12**:520.

15. James MR, Marshall H, Carew-McColl M. Pulse oximetry during apparent tonic-clonic seizures. *Lancet* 1991;**337**:394–5.

16. Ives JR, Gloor P. Automatic nocturnal sleep sampling: a useful method in clinical electroencephalography. *Electroenceph Clin Neurophysiol* 1977;**43**:880–4.

17. Gotman J. Automatic recognition of epileptic seizures in the EEG. *Electroenceph Clin Neurophysiol* 1982;**54**:530–40.

18. Ives JR, Thompson CJ, Gloor P, et al. The on-line computer detection and recording of temporal lobe seizures from implanted depth electrodes via a radio telemetry link. *Electroenceph Clin Neurophysiol* 1974;**37**:205.

19. Koffler D, Gotman J. Automatic detection of spike and wave bursts in ambulatory EEG recordings. *Electroenceph Clin Neurophysiol* 1985;**61**:165–80.

20. Gotman J, Gloor P. Automatic recognition and quantification of interictal epileptic activity in the human scalp EEG. *Electroenceph Clin Neurophysiol* 1976;**41**:513–29.

21. Gotman J, Ives JR, Gloor P. Automatic recognition of interictal epileptic activity in prolonged EEG recordings. *Electroenceph Clin Neurophysiol* 1979;**46**:510–20.

22. Ives JR, Schomer DL. Preliminary technical experience using a portable computer (PC-AT) for on-line data analysis of epileptic spike activity on 16 channels of telemetric EEG data. *Epilepsia* 1986;**27**:626.

23. Lesser RP, Luders H, Dinner DS, Morris H. An introduction to the basic concepts of polarity and localization. *J Clinical Neurophysiol* 1985;**2**:45–61.

24. Sharbrough FW. Electrical fields and recording

techniques. In: Daly DD, Pedley TA, eds. *Current practice of clinical electroencephalography.* 2nd ed. New York: Raven Press, 1990:29–49.

25. Rasmussen T. Localization aspects of epileptic seizure phenomena. In: Thompson RA, Green JR, eds. *New perspectives in cerebral localization.* New York: Raven Press, 1982: 177–203.

26. Spencer D, Weiser HG, Engel J Jr, eds. Surgical Therapy. In: Engel J Jr, Pedley TA. *Epilepsy: a comprehensive textbook.* New York: Lippincott-Raven, 1998:1671–910.

27. Frysinger RC, Harper RM. Cardiac and respiratory correlation with unit discharges in human amygdala and hippocampus. *Electroenceph Clin Neurophysiol* 1989;**72**:463–70.

28. Keilson MJ, Magrill JP. Simultaneous ambulatory cassette EEG/ECG monitoring. In: Ebersole JS, ed. *Ambulatory EEG monitoring.* New York: Raven Press, 1989:171–93.

29. Lai CW, Ziegler DK. Syncope problem solved by continuous ambulatory simultaneous EEG/ECG. *Neurology* 1981;**31**:1152–4.

30. Singh B, Al Shahwan SA, Al Deeb SM. Partial seizures presenting as life-threatening apnea. *Epilepsia* 1993;**34**:901–3.

31. Devinsky O, Ehrenberg B, Barthlen GM, et al. Epilepsy and sleep apnea syndrome. *Neurology* 1994;**44**:2060–4.

32. Kaada BR, Jasper HH. Respiratory responses to stimulation of temporal pole, insula and hippocampal and limbic gyri in man. *Arch Neuro Psychiatry* 1952;**68**:609–19.

33. Krieger JR. Obstructive sleep apnea: clinical manifestations and pathophysiology. In: Thorpy MJ, ed. *Handbook of sleep disorders.* New York: Marcel Dekker Inc., 1990:259–84.

34. Foley CM, Miles DK, Chandler D, et al. Role of computerized outpatient long-term monitoring (CO-LTM) in the diagnosis and treatment of pediatric epilepsy. *Epilepsia* 1994;**35**(Suppl 8):147.

35. Liporace J, Tatum W, Morris GL, French J. Clinical utility of sleep-deprived versus computer-assisted ambulatory 16-channel EEG in epilepsy patients: a multi-center study. *Epilepsy Research* 1998;**32**:357–62.

36. Miles DK, Foley CM, Legido A, et al. A comparative study of the efficacy of inpatient video-EEG and computerized outpatient EEG monitoring in a pediatric population. *Epilepsia* 1994;**35**(Suppl 8):48.

37. Morris GL, Galezowshka J, Leroy R, North R. The results of computer-assisted ambulatory 16-channel EEG. *Electroencephal Clin Neurophysiol* 1994;**91**:229–31.

38. Morris GL. The clinical utility of computer-assisted ambulatory 16-channel EEG. *J Med Engin Technol* 1997;**21**:47–52.

39. Nashef L, Walker F, Sander JWAS, et al. Apnea and bradycardia during epileptic seizures: relation to sudden deaths in epilepsy. *Neurology* 1995;**45**:938.

12

Interictal focus localization

Christian E Elger, Klaus Lehnertz and Guido Widman

Introduction

Surgical treatment of focal epilepsies requires exact localization and delineation of the epileptic focus. Apart from the application of neuroimaging techniques to identify potential morphological correlates, to date, this task requires electrophysiological recordings (electro-encephalography, chronic electrocorticography and/or stereoelectro-encephalography) of the patients' habitual seizures. However, because this procedure is time-consuming and expensive and, in addition, comprises a certain risk for the patient, reliable techniques would be desirable to lateralize and localize the epileptogenic focus both non-invasively and during the interictal state. In this chapter we first give a short introduction to conceptual and methodological problems associated with defining the epileptic focus and then concentrate on methods of interictal focus localization, including electrophysiological and imaging techniques as well as recent non-linear analysis tools for electro-encephalographic data.

Defining the epileptic focus

An epileptic focus is an area of the brain in which a critical amount of neurons has the potency to give rise to epileptic seizures. However, this theoretical definition is not suffi-

cient to base successful epilepsy surgery on. Pathologically discharging neurons may be dispersed over a large area and, depending on localization, complete removal of the affected area may lead to considerable neurological and neuropsychological deficits.

Lüders and Awad's approach,[1] which is based on the identification of different zones and lesions in the epileptogenic brain, is suitable to demonstrate the problem of defining the epileptic focus (Table 12.1). The *epileptogenic zone*—a hypothetical construct generated by results of different investigations—is the brain area, the proper resection of which is necessary and sufficient for complete seizure control. The exact definition of this zone is difficult and may even be impossible in special cases. Thus, the epileptogenic zone and its boundaries have to be defined as closely as possible in order to maximize benefit for the surgical candidate and, at the same time, minimize possible functional deficits.

To define the construct *epileptogenic zone* it is necessary to delineate several brain areas in relation to the epileptic process that are assessable by clinical methods. It is important to note, however, that the result of these delineations merely approximates the epileptogenic zone (Table 12.1).

During the ictal state, two zones may be identified that are of high relevance for defining the epileptogenic zone. The *pacemaker zone* is the area of the brain from which actual

		Table 12.1
Pacemaker zone	brain area from which seizures arise	*Zones and lesions of the epileptogenic brain that have to be assessed for definition of the construct epileptogenic zone (according to Ref. 1).*
Ictal symptomatogenic zone	brain area from which ictal symptoms arise	
Epileptogenic lesion	brain area that initiates seizure disorder	
Functional deficit zone	brain area exhibiting metabolic, neurological and neuropsychological deficits during the interictal state	
Irritative zone	brain area that generates interictal potentials	

seizure activity originates. Several methods can be used to define this zone, although all have significant limitations. The electrophysiological definition requires sensoring electrodes to be placed as closely as possible to the pacemaker zone, in order to pick up the primary start of a seizure. However, this presupposes a sound hypothesis of the most likely location of the pacemaker zone. This hypothesis can be based on clinical semiology, scalp electro-encephalogram (EEG) recordings or functional imaging techniques such as ictal single photon emission computed tomography (SPECT) (see below).

The *ictal symptomatogenic zone* is the area of the brain that, when activated, initiates symptoms characteristic for the patient's seizure onset. Despite the fact that initial symptoms of a seizure are very important to define the epileptogenic zone, the detection of this phenomenon can be very difficult. Seizures may produce symptoms that are visible only when, during spread of seizure activity, a large region of the brain is involved. In contrast, involvement of small areas of the brain, sometimes associated with auras, may not be recognized by the patient or may be impossible for him or her to describe.

During the interictal state three zones and/or a possible lesion can be defined: the *epilepto-*

genic lesion, if it exists, is defined as the brain lesion that is thought to be the original cause of seizure disorder. Epileptogenic lesions can be determined using neuroimaging techniques such as cranial computed tomography (CCT) or magnetic resonance imaging (MRI) (see below). The main problem, however, is to determine whether a lesion is epileptogenic or not and whether a lesion is identical—both functionally and spatially—with the epileptogenic zone. Indeed, there are cases in which a lesion is not related to a nevertheless existing epilepsy.

The *functional deficit zone* is the area of the brain that shows abnormal functioning during the interictal state, as determined by neurological examination, neuropsychological testing or possibly by functional neuroimaging such as positron emission tomography (PET)/SPECT. This zone may result from a morphological destruction of the underlying brain tissue or it can reflect functional deficits due to interictal discharges. Moreover, effects of anticonvulsive drugs can produce a functional deficit zone or enlarge an already existing one. Determination of the functional deficit zone is of considerable value for the definition of the epileptogenic zone. For example, neuropsychological deficits of temporal lobe functions may be ipsi- and contralateral to the primarily assumed pacemaker zone. In these cases, surgical removal of ipsilateral temporal lobe for seizure control has limited success. Thus, the definition of the epileptogenic zone in the case of a widespread functional deficit zone is different from the definition in which the latter is almost non-existent (as in the case of mesial temporal lobe epilepsy). This uncertainty in defining the epileptogenic zone holds true even in patients in whom the pacemaker zone and the so-called *irritative zone* are almost identical. The latter zone can be defined by non-invasive, semi-invasive and invasive recordings of interictal discharges. However, the irritative zone is usually larger than the epileptogenic zone because interictal discharges—as recorded in the EEG or the electrocorticogram—are always generated from a rather extensive area of the cortex. Even the differentiation between steep potentials of quite physiological character and specific epileptiform events can be problematic, especially in invasive recordings, where exact definitions are still lacking. Moreover, spatial sampling using invasive electrodes is always limited so that the definition of exact boundaries of epileptogenic tissue is restricted and in some cases not possible. Defining potentially epileptogenic regions via scalp electrode recordings seems more unequivocal compared with intracranial recordings. However, the former is poor in delineating boundaries and defining the exact location of the epileptogenic area, which holds true particularly in medial and basal parts of the brain. Thus, irritative zones defined by invasive and non-invasive recordings are not identical. Because interictal epileptiform discharges provide a good overview for the possible existence and approximate boundaries of the epileptogenic zone, scalp recordings of interictal activity contribute to the generation of a hypothesis concerning boundaries of the epileptogenic zone. However,

the discriminative value strongly depends on the constancy of occurrence and location of the discharge.

Neuroimaging techniques

Neuroimaging in epilepsy (see Refs 2 and 3 for a review) comprises techniques such as magnetic resonance imaging (MRI), functional MRI (fMRI), magnetic resonance spectroscopy (MRS), positron emission tomography (PET) and single photon emission computed tomography (SPECT). The principle role of MRI is in the definition of a morphological correlate that might be related to seizure disorders.[4–6] Hippocampal sclerosis, as well as other structural abnormalities associated with either neoplastic or non-neoplastic focal lesions in temporal lobe epilepsy, may be identified reliably and thus are of high relevance for presurgical work-up during the interictal state. The same holds true in extratemporal lobe epilepsy, provided that a morphological lesion is indeed identifiable. However, although MRI can demonstrate a structural correlate of epilepsy in many situations, both imaging and clinical (neurophysiological and psychological) data need consideration to prove the epileptogenicity of these abnormalities and to reach a final consensus for individual patients. Moreover, rare patients, particularly with certain tumors, cortical dysgenesis and dual pathology, still require EEG for accurate localization.[7–9]

Functional MRI (fMRI) is thought to localize the seizure focus during the ictal state by observing cerebral blood flow (CBF) changes[10–12] and during the interictal state by tracking spikes via EEG-triggered echoplanar scanning.[13] Moreover, it is used increasingly to identify cerebral areas that are responsible for specific sensory and cognitive processes and is thus of importance in planning resections close to eloquent cortical areas.[14,15] Although, at present, the clinical use of fMRI in epilepsy needs substantially more study, it is none the less a very promising technique that may change the presurgical evaluation.[16]

Magnetic resonance spectroscopy (MRS) takes advantage of the magnetic resonance of specific nuclei such as ^{1}H, ^{31}P or [13]C (see Ref. 17 for details) and allows non-invasive investigation of cerebral metabolites and neurotransmitters associated with these nuclei, such as N-acetyl-aspartate, creatine, choline, gamma-aminobutyric acid (GABA), glutamate or adenosine triphosphate (ATP). In several studies, it was shown that the latter are significantly altered in or near epileptic foci.[18–21] Although there are still limitations in MRS, recent hardware and software developments promise further improvement of this method. Thus, MRS is expected to have significant consequences for the medical and surgical treatment of patients with epilepsy.[3]

Positron emission tomography (PET) has been in clinical use for longer than MRI. Several tracers are available to map cerebral blood flow (^{15}O-labelled water) or regional cerebral glucose metabolism ([^{18}F]-2–deoxyglucose ([^{18}F]DG)) or to demonstrate receptor binding of specific ligands (e.g. [^{11}C]flumazenil to the central benzodiazepine–GABA$_A$ receptor complex; [^{11}C]diphrenorphine or [^{11}C]carfentanil to opiate receptors; [^{11}C]deuterium deprenyl to monoamineoxidase (MAO) B receptors). Although PET has a higher spatial resolution compared with SPECT for example, this technique is none the less costly and entails a certain risk for the patient due to radiation exposure. In focal epilepsies, interictal PET studies can provide more useful information. Since the early 1980s the epileptogenic focus is known to be associated with an area of reduced glucose metabolism and reduced blood flow.[22–24] This area, as defined by [^{18}F]DG or

H$_2$[^{15}O] PET scans, however, is usually considerably larger than the pathological abnormality. This enlargement is thought to be related to inhibition or deafferentiation of neurons around an epileptogenic focus and thus does not contribute to a precise localization of the epileptogenic zone. Moreover, numerous studies have shown [^{18}F]DG PET data to be unspecific with regard to etiology. Thus, it is expected that both [^{18}F]DG and H$_2$[^{15}O] PET investigations will be replaced by MRI and fMRI investigations. In contrast, studies with specific ligands were shown to identify neurochemical abnormalities associated with epilepsy, both static interictal derangements and dynamic changes in ligand–receptor interaction that may occur at the time of seizures. For example, the area of neuronal loss, as defined by a reduced [^{11}C]flumazenil binding to central benzodiazepine receptors, is confined to a more restricted area than the region of reduced metabolism and is thought to be closely related to the epileptogenic zone.[25] Numerous studies have shown [^{11}C]flumazenil PET scans to be good markers for neuronal integrity in both the hippocampus and neocortex. Although the underlying pathological basis of reduced [^{11}C]flumazenil binding is still under study, [^{11}C]flumazenil PET is likely to be important in the interictal presurgical evaluation of patients in whom MRI is not definitive.

Single photon emission computed tomography (SPECT) allows imaging of the cerebral blood flow and specific receptors in the brain. Cerebral blood flow tracers include [^{99m}Tc]hexamethylpropylenamine oxime ([^{99m}Tc] HMPAO), [^{123}I]-N-isopropyl-p-iodoamphetamine and [^{99m}Tc]ethyl cysteinate dimer (ECD). Receptor tracers currently in use are [^{123}I]iomazenil (a derivative of the central benzodiazepine receptor antagonist flumazenil) and [^{123}I]iododexetimide used to label muscarinic acetylcholine receptors). A principal advantage of SPECT over PET is that the former is much less expensive and the equipment is more widespread. Moreover, SPECT provides the possibility to obtain images of cerebral blood flow at the time of seizures. However, although ictal SPECT data contribute to build a hypothesis of the most likely location of the pacemaker zone, these data are non-quantitative and need careful and cautious interpretation. Initial interictal SPECT studies provided evidence of an area of reduced cerebral blood flow associated with the epileptogenic focus. However, numerous studies revealed that this result is not always reliable. As a consequence of the inferior spatial and temporal resolution and the poor sensitivity and specificity, interictal SPECT studies have little place in the routine investigation of patients with epilepsy.[26–29] In a recent meta-analytic study it was thus concluded that institutions using SPECT imaging in epilepsy should perform ictal, preferably, or post-ictal scanning in combination with interictal scanning.[30] By analogy to the above-mentioned PET studies, SPECT receptor studies using high-resolution cameras and optimal scan orientation also suggested that the area of reduced specific binding of [123I]iomazenil is more restricted than the defect of cerebral blood flow and is of greater sensitivity for localization of the epileptogenic focus.[31] [123I]Iododexetimide binding was also found to be reduced at epileptic foci.[32] The clinical utility of these findings, however, remains to be established.

Analysis of interictal electromagnetic epileptiform activity

As mentioned before, recording interictal epileptiform discharges such as spikes or sharp waves is of high value for definition of the irritative zone. For this purpose, several recording techniques with varying degrees of invasiveness are available. These comprise non-invasive techniques such as scalp EEG or its magnetic counterpart the magneto-encephalogram (MEG), semi-invasive electrophysiological recordings using sphenoidal,[33] Peg or foramen ovale electrodes[34,35] as well as the invasive electrocorticogram (ECoG) and the stereoelectro-encephalogram (SEEG) using implanted subdural strip or grid electrodes[36] and stereo-tactically placed depth electrodes.[37] However, because epileptiform discharges represent a highly variant spatio-temporal phenomenon, sufficient sampling both in time and space is required. The number of recording channels usually does not represent a limiting factor because the currently available acquisition devices are capable of handling up to 256 channels simultaneously. To date, electrophysiological recording of patients' habitual seizures is still the *gold standard* for defining the epileptogenic zone, so capturing seizure events often necessitates long-term recordings over several days. Thus, a huge amount of interictal data is collected during presurgical evaluation.

Scoring long-term multi-channel recordings is often supplied by *computer-assisted EEG analysis systems* (see refs 38–40 for a comprehensive overview). In particular, automatic spike detection systems provide quantitative parameters such as spike rates at different recording sites and amplitude, duration and temporal variances of discharge rates (see Refs 41–43 and references therein for an overview). Although these systems allow diagnostically relevant information to be extracted and condensed from interictal electrophysiological long-term recordings, system accuracy is still regarded as not sufficient. Moreover, especially in invasive recordings, it is problematic to differentiate between steep potentials of quite physiological character and specific epileptiform events because exact definitions are still lacking. Thus, in order to increase the reliability of automated spike detection systems, which might provide a means to reduce the necessity of recording seizures, substantially more study is needed at present.

Instead of investigating spontaneously occurring or triggered epileptiform discharges (e.g. via hyperventilation, sleep or photostimulation[44, 45]), an alternative approach is based on the well-known *activating properties of specific barbiturates and narcotics*. Short-acting barbiturates have been used for a long time to identify the epileptogenic zone during preoperative evaluation for epilepsy surgery[46,47]. In several studies, different short-acting barbiturates and narcotics (e.g. methohexital, amobarbital, thiopental and propofol) were shown to have distinct activating and suppressive effects on epileptiform discharges in EEG and ECoG recordings. Hufnagel et al showed that methohexital increases spike density and, in addition, activates spike–burst suppression patterns, which are characterized by a high-amplitude spike burst followed by suppression in the EEG/ECoG consisting of isoelectrical or sub-delta background activity.[46] Both EEG and ECoG alterations are known to be of good localizing value concerning the epileptogenic zone.

Magneto-encephalography (MEG) permits non-invasive evaluation of magnetic fields associated with neuronal activity. Because MEG is a very costly technique and, moreover, requires advanced signal analysis techniques (i.e. development and meaningful application of physical–mathematical source and volume conductor models), at present only a few groups have the requisite equipment at their disposal. Nevertheless, due to the fact that neuromagnetic fields are affected very little by the tissue between generators within the brain and sensoring coils outside the head, and because there is no need for a reference, MEG-based localization of neuronal sources is believed to be highly advantageous to EEG.[48] However, the value of MEG-based localization of the epileptogenic zone is still discussed controversially.[49-54] Because movement artifacts—such as those during seizures—render reliable MEG recordings almost impossible and because the significance of interictally recorded spikes in the MEG with respect to the irritative and the primary epileptogenic zone has not been established fully until now, diagnostically relevant information is needed within short MEG acquisition times.

In a recent study,[53] MEG source imaging of methohexital-induced spike activity (see above) was carried out in 15 patients suffering from unilateral temporal lobe epilepsy. Indeed, after methohexital administration an unequivocal increase of spike activity in the MEG was observed, allowing the epileptogenic zone to be lateralized with an accuracy similar to ECoG recordings. However, from the findings of source localization it was concluded that this method does not, at present, permit non-invasive localization of epileptogenic zones in temporal lobe epilepsy with an accuracy comparable with invasive evaluation techniques. Moreover, methohexital-induced changes in the spectral power of neuromagnetic signals also allowed only the epileptogenic zone to be lateralized.[55] This disadvantage can be attributed in part to an attenuated sensitivity of the MEG to deeper foci, as in the case of temporal lobe epilepsy. Conversely, Smith et al reported on additional spatial localizing data in the presence of convexity foci.[52] A further disadvantage of MEG relies on inadequate models for generators of epileptiform activity and the volume conductor head currently in use for localization procedures.[56] However, ongoing improvements in developing refined models, as well as recently available whole-head neuromagnetometer systems, are expected to increase the importance of MEG as a non-invasive presurgical evaluation tool.

Non-linear time series analysis of interictal electrophysiological data

During latter years non-linear time series analysis (NTSA, colloquially often termed *chaos theory*) has become a growing field of research. Within this physical–mathematical framework, methods are available that allow highly complex dynamic systems to be characterized (see Ref. 57 for a comprehensive overview). Owing to its high versatility, NTSA has already gone beyond the physical sciences and, at present, is being applied successfully in a variety of disciplines, including neurology and psychiatry. In contrast to the aforementioned analysis methods that solely rely on single interictal—spontaneous or induced—epileptiform events, NTSA provides a means to analyze integratively long-lasting recordings of brain electrical activity. In particular, non-linear measures such as the correlation dimension or the Lyapunov exponents were shown to allow reliable characterization of different pathological activities.

Non-linear time series analysis of EEG data recorded in animals with experimental epilepsies led to a better understanding of basic mechanisms.[58-60] Its application to EEG data recorded in patients undergoing presurgical evaluation promises to be important for clinical practice because non-linear measures were shown to provide additional and relevant information about spatio-temporal dynamics of the primary epileptogenic area.[61-64] By extracting the so-called neuronal complexity loss L^* from intracranial EEG recordings of 20 epilepsy patients, we showed that L^* unequivocally localizes the primary epileptogenic area even during interictal states.[65] The discriminative power of this measure was still preserved when semi-invasive EEG recording techniques were applied.[66] Although the latter findings were obtained solely from analyses of patients suffering from temporal lobe epilepsy with seizure onset in mesial parts of the temporal lobe, a recent study[67] provides evidence of an extended applicability of NTSA beyond this well-defined syndrome.[68] On analyzing the interictally recorded ECoG of patients with neocortical lesional epilepsy, we showed circumscribed areas of reduced neuronal complexity (*arc*) to coincide with a favourable postoperative seizure control. In contrast, no clear *arc* was found in patients who experienced only a reduction of seizure frequency or had no benefit from the resection. Apart from an improvement of the topological diagnosis, the neuronal complexity loss L^* also turned out to be helpful for investigating the influence of anticonvulsive drugs on the epileptogenic process[69] and for estimating possible functional disturbances in mesial temporal structures contralateral to the focal side.[70] Moreover, preliminary findings in patients with temporal lobe epilepsy indicate that L^* indexes the spatio-temporal recruitment potency of neurons within or close to the primary epileptogenic area during specific verbal memory tasks.[71] Besides its possible relevance for guiding tailored instead of standard resections within mesial temporal structures, NTSA was also shown to bear potential capabilities of extracting features from EEG activity that can be regarded as long-lasting (up to 25 min) precursors of impending seizures.[72,73] Recent preliminary findings of other research groups also showed different non-linear measures changing characteristically during the pre-ictal state.[74-76] Although NTSA of brain electrical activity is still at its beginning, results achieved up to now are promising. Recent optimizations of algorithms underlying the computation of specific non-linear measures[77] and the development of suitable monitoring systems[78] already allow temporary changes of non-linear measures to be tracked in real time. Thus, NTSA is expected to contribute significantly to an interictal focus localization.

In conclusion, it still remains difficult to achieve unequivocal localization and delineation of the epileptogenic zone during the interictal state. Despite considerable improvements in neuroimaging techniques and analyses of brain electromagnetic activity, current focus localization methods are not convincing enough for ictal electroclinical data to be avoided completely. This holds especially true for patients in whom structural abnormalities are missing or multifocal lesions exist.[79] Moreover, in order to minimize further the risk associated with surgical therapy, as well as to counsel patients individually as to their postoperative quality of life, exact delineation of boundaries of epileptogenic tissue is still required and, in many cases, necessitates invasive evaluation.

Nevertheless, the presented methods for interictal focus localization indisputably contribute, though to a varying degree, to reach a consensus for the individual patient. Moreover, a growing number of candidates admitted to presurgical evaluation, as well as efforts towards further reduction of costs and duration of monitoring, emphasize the high relevance of appropriate interictal focus localization techniques that hopefully will improve further in the near future. In special syndromes of focal epilepsy these improvements may eventually even make seizure recordings dispensable, thus minimizing potential risks associated with drug withdrawal. Converging neurophysiological, neuropsychological, metabolic and anatomic data summarizing multimodal information from interictal investigations in epilepsy patients entering an epilepsy surgery programme are necessary, as a complement to ictal electroclinical data, in the presurgical evaluation. In principle, such a synthesis opens up the possibility to balance the shortcomings of one method by the strengths of another.

References

1. Lüders HO, Awad I. Conceptual considerations. In: Lüders H, ed. *Epilepsy surgery*. New York: Raven Press, 1991:51–62.
2. Theodore WH. Structural neuroimaging. In: Lüders H, ed. *Epilepsy surgery*. New York: Raven Press, 1992:221–30.
3. Duncan JS. Imaging and epilepsy. *Brain* 1997; **120**:339–77.
4. Cascino GD. Commentary: how has neuroimaging improved patient care? *Epilepsia* 1994; 35:S103–7.
5. Spencer SS. The relative contribution of MRI, SPECT and PET imaging in epilepsy. *Epilepsia* 1994;35:S72–89.
6. Zentner J, Hufnagel A, Wolf HK et al. Surgical treatment of temporal lobe epilepsy: clinical, radiological, and histopathological findings in 178 patients. *J Neurol Neurosurg Psychiatry* 1995;**58**:666–73.
7. Fish DR, Spencer SS. Clinical correlations: MRI and EEG. *Magn Reson Imaging* 1995;**13**: 1113–17.
8. King D, Spencer SS, McCarthy G, Luby M, Spencer DD. Bilateral hippocampal atrophy in

Methohexital-induced changes in spectral power of neuromagnetic signals: beta augmentation is smaller over the hemisphere containing the epileptogenic focus. *Brain Topogr* 1997;**10**: 41–7.

56. Alarcon G, Guy CN, Binnie CD, Walker SR, Elwes RD, Polkey CE. Intracerebral propagation of interictal activity in partial epilepsy: implications for source localisation. *J Neurol Neurosurg Psychiatry* 1994;**57**:435–49.

57. Kantz H, Schreiber T. *Non-linear time series analysis*. Cambridge: Cambridge University Press, 1997.

58. Pijn JP, van Neerven J, Noest A, Lopes da Silva FH. Chaos or noise in EEG signals: dependence of state and brain site. *Electroencephalogr Clin Neurophysiol* 1991;**79**:371–81.

59. Beldhuis HJ, Suzuki T, Pijn JP, Teisman A, Lopes da Silva FH, Bohus B. Propagation of epileptiform activity during development of amygdala kindling in rats: linear and non-linear association between ipsi- and contralateral sites. *Eur J Neurosci* 1993;**5**:944–54.

60. Lopes da Silva FH, Pijn JP, Wadman WJ. Dynamics of local neuronal networks: control parameter and state bifurcations in epileptogenesis. *Prog Brain Res* 1994;**102**:359–70.

61. Iasemidis LD, Sackellares JC, Zaveri HP, Williams WJ. Phase space topography and the Lyapunov exponent of electrocorticograms in partial seizures. *Brain Topogr* 1990;**2**:187–201.

62. Elger CE, Lehnertz K. Ictogenesis and chaos. In: Wolf P, ed. *Epileptic seizures and syndromes*. London: J Libbey & Co., 1994:547–52.

63. Pijn JP, Velis DN, van der Heyden MJ, DeGoede J, van Veelen CW, Lopes da Silva FH. Nonlinear dynamics of epileptic seizures on basis of intracranial EEG recordings. *Brain Topogr* 1997;**9**:249–70.

64. Casdagli MC, Iasemidis LD, Savit RS, Gilmore RL, Roper SN, Sackellares JC. Non-linearity in invasive EEG recordings from patients with temporal lobe epilepsy, *Electroencephalogr Clin Neurophysiol* 1997;**102**:98–105.

65. Lehnertz K, Elger CE. Spatio-temporal dynamics of the primary epileptogenic area in temporal lobe epilepsy characterized by neuronal complexity loss. *Electroencephalogr Clin Neurophysiol* 1995;**95**:108–17.

66. Weber B, Lehnertz K, Elger CE, Wieser HG. Neuronal complexity loss in interictal EEG recorded with foramen ovale electrodes predicts side of primary epileptogenic area in temporal lobe epilepsy: a replication study. *Epilepsia* 1998;**39**:922–7.

67. Widman G, Lehnertz K, Elger CE. Spatiotemporal distribution of neuronal complexity loss in neocortical epilepsy. *Epilepsia* 1997; **38**:46 (abstract).

68. Gloor P. Mesial temporal sclerosis: historical background and an overview from modern perspective. In: Lüders H, ed. *Epilepsy surgery*. New York: Raven Press, 1991:689–703.

69. Lehnertz K, Elger CE. Neuronal complexity loss in temporal lobe epilepsy: effects of carbamazepine on the dynamics of the epileptogenic focus. *Electroencephalogr Clin Neurophysiol* 1997;**103**:376–80.

70. Lehnertz K, Elger CE. Neuronal complexity loss in temporal lobe epilepsy: influence of the duration of the disease on the contralateral hippocampus. *J Neurol* 1994;**242**:272 (abstract).

71. Lehnertz K, Weber B, Helmstaedter C, Wieser HG, Elger CE. Alterations in neuronal complexity during verbal memory tasks index recruitment potency in temporo-mesial structures. *Epilepsia* 1997;**38**:238 (abstract).

72. Elger CE, Lehnertz K. Prediction of epileptic seizures in humans from nonlinear dynamics analysis of brain electrical activity. *Eur J Neurosci* 1998;**10**:786–9.

73. Lehnertz K, Elger CE. Can epileptic seizures be predicted? Evidence from nonlinear time series analyses of brain electrical activity. *Phys Rev Lett* 1998;**80**:5019–23.

74. Adam C, Martinierie J, Le Van Quyen M, Renault B, Baulac M, Varela F. Anticipation of seizure onset with non-linear analysis of intracerebral EEG. *Epilepsia* 1997;**38**:217 (abstract).

75. Moser HR, Weber B, Moser S, Meier PF, Wieser HG. Intracranial EEG of mesial temporal lobe characterized by Lyapunov spectra and related measures of complexity: preictal changes. *Epilepsia* 1997;**38**:224 (abstract).

76. Sackellares JC, Iasemidis LD, Gilmore RD, Roper SN. Epileptic seizures as neural resting mechanisms. *Epilepsia* 1997;**38**:189 (abstract).

77. Widman G, Lehnertz K, Elger CE. CPLXMON, a system for real-time, on-line monitoring of

neuronal complexity loss in the ECOG of patients with temporal lobe epilepsy. *Epilepsia* 1995;**36**:5 (abstract).

78. Widman G, Lehnertz K, Jansen P, Meyer W, Burr W, Elger CE. A fast general purpose algorithm for the computation of auto- and cross-correlation integrals from single channel data. *Physica D* 1998; **121**:65–75.

79. Lorenzo NY, Parisi JE, Cascino GD, Jack CR Jr, Marsh WR, Hirschorn KA. Intractable frontal lobe epilepsy: pathological and MRI features. *Epilepsy Res* 1995;**20**:171–8.

V
DIAGNOSIS OF ASSOCIATED BEHAVIORAL DISABILITIES

13

Psychiatric issues

Bettina Schmitz

Psychiatric complications of epilepsy are neither rare nor benign. Interictal disturbances of cognition, memory, personality and affect may interfere with relationships and professional performance, thus being potentially more disabling than ictal events in some patients. The etiology of psychiatric disorders in epilepsy is highly complex, including psychosocial stress, the nature and localization of structural brain lesions, seizure-related brain dysfunction and psychotropic effects of antiepileptic drugs. The identification of patients at risk for developing psychiatric disorders is important for prophylaxis, and the treatment of such complications depends on differentiating psychiatric syndromes based on psychopathology and course, and identifying epilepsy-specific causative factors such as the relationship to seizure activity or treatments. This chapter focuses on four major areas: psychoses, depression, suicide and syndromes related to antiepileptic drugs.

Psychoses

In the mid-19th century, European psychiatrists noted the high incidence of psychotic episodes in institutionalized patients with epilepsy. Several authors described the specific psychopathology of psychiatric complications occurring in the context of epilepsy, using terms like *epilepsie larvée*, *grand mal intel-*lectuel, *epileptoid states*, *transformed epilepsy*, *epileptic rudiments* and *epileptic equivalents*.[1] Samt put forward the idea that the pathophysiology of certain psychoses occurring in the context of epilepsy, especially episodic twilight states, was identical to the pathophysiology of convulsive seizures.[2] He suggested that, in the absence of true seizures, such psychotic epileptic equivalents justified a diagnosis of epilepsy.

With progress in diagnosis and treatment of epilepsy, epileptology shifted away from psychiatry to neurology. Psychiatric aspects were neglected until they were rediscovered in the 1950s and 1960s.[3-6] American and English authors noted an excess of schizophrenia-like psychoses in epileptic patients and especially in those with temporal lobe epilepsy.[7,8] Slater and co-workers published a detailed analysis of 69 patients from two London hospitals who had epilepsy and interictal psychoses.[9] On the basis of this case series, the authors challenged the older antagonism theory[10] and postulated a positive link between epilepsy and schizophrenia. Although Slater was criticized for drawing conclusions on the basis of insufficient statistics,[11] the temporal lobe hypothesis soon became broadly accepted and stimulated extensive research into the role of temporal pathology in schizophrenia.

The spectrum of psychotic syndromes in patients with epilepsy is wide and psychotic complications are not restricted to patients with temporal lobe epilepsy.

Epidemiology

There are only four population-based studies of the frequency of mixed psychoses in epilepsy. Krohn, in a population-based survey in Norway, found a 2 per cent prevalence of psychoses with epilepsy.[12] Zielinski, in a field study of the Warsaw population, found prevalence rates for psychoses in epilepsy of 2–3 per cent.[13] In a field study of 2635 registered epilepsy patients in a district in Poland, only 0.5 per cent were diagnosed with schizophrenia, but 19.5 per cent suffered from post-ictal twilight states.[14] Gudmundsson, in a study on the frequency of mixed psychoses in epilepsy in the population of Iceland, found prevalence rates of 6 per cent for males and 9 per cent for females.[15] These figures can be compared with the findings of an earlier study by Helgason,[16] who looked at the risk of psychosis in the general population of Iceland using the same diagnostic criteria as Gudmundsson. Helgason found prevalence rates of 7 per cent for males and 5 per cent for females. The comparison of Helgason's and Gudmundsson's results suggests a similar risk for psychoses in people with and without epilepsy, being only slightly higher in females but slightly lower in males with epilepsy.

Most figures in the literature on the frequency of psychosis in epilepsy derive from clinical case series and are therefore likely to be biased by unknown selection mechanisms. Prevalence rates range between 4 and 60 per cent, with the highest figures reported in psychiatric series, followed by neurological inpatients and epilepsy outpatients and the lowest figures in patients attending general practice.[17] These data suggest that psychoses are highly over-represented in specialized centres. Although there is no epidemiological evidence for an excess of psychosis in people with epilepsy in general, the numerous clinical case series clearly indicate that psychosis is a significant problem for patients attending specialized centres, suggesting that there are risk factors for psychosis that are related to complicated epilepsy and/or chronic illness.

Classification

There is no internationally accepted syndromic classification of psychoses in epilepsy, and psychiatric aspects are not considered in the international classification of epilepsies.

Most of the previously proposed classification systems for psychosis in epilepsy are based on a combination of psychopathological, aetiological, longitudinal and electro-encephalogram (EEG) parameters.[18-21] In epileptic psychoses, diagnostic criteria are not strictly intercorrelated. Dongier concluded from her detailed analysis of 536 psychotic episodes in 516 patients that it was not possible to deduce the type of epilepsy from the type of psychosis, or vice versa.[5] 'Atypical' syndromes are not unusual, such as ictal and post-ictal psychoses in clear consciousness.[22]

For pragmatic reasons, psychoses in epilepsy can be grouped according to their temporal relationship to seizures as ictal, post-ictal, parictal and alternative. However, such a classification does not necessarily imply fundamental differences in terms of pathophysiology.

Syndromes of psychoses in relation to seizure activity (Table 13.1)

Ictal psychoses

Prolonged focal and generalized non-convulsive epileptic activity—when lasting over several hours or days—may present with psychotic symptoms. Generalized non-convulsive status, also called absence status, petit mal status or spike–wave stupor, is characterized by altered or narrowed consciousness.[23] Patients are

	Ictal psychosis	Post-ictal psychosis	Par-ictal psychosis	Alternative psychosis	Interictal psychosis
Relative frequency	~10%	~50%	~10%	~10%	~20%
Consciousness	Impaired or fluctuating	Impaired or normal	Impaired	Normal	Normal
Special features	Mild motor seizure symptoms	Lucid interval between seizures and psychosis	Gradual development, often during presurgical monitoring	Protracted onset with prepsychotic dysphoria	Schizo-phrenia-like psycho-pathology
Duration	Hours to days	Days to weeks	Days to weeks	Weeks	Months
EEG	Status epilepticus	Increased epileptic and slow activity	Increased epileptic and slow activity	Normalized	Unchanged
Treatment	Antiepileptic drugs i.v.	Benzodiaze-pines or short-term neuroleptic medication	Seizure control	Sleep control in early stages, reduction of antiepileptic drugs, neuroleptics	Long-term neuroleptic medication

Table 13.1
Clinical characteristics of psychoses in relation to seizure activity.

disorientated and apathetic. Contact with the environment is partially preserved and patients are often able to perform simple tasks. Positive psychotic symptoms such as delusions and hallucinations occur only in some patients. The EEG shows generalized bilateral synchronous spike–wave complexes of variable frequency between 1 and 4 Hz. In prolonged generalized status, however, the EEG patterns may become more irregular and lose their symmetric synchrony, which makes it difficult or impossible to distinguish from complex focal status.

The status may be terminated by spontaneous generalized tonic–clonic seizures. Absence status typically occurs in patients with a known history of generalized epilepsy, but 'atypical absence status' may occur as a first manifestation of epilepsy, especially in later life.[24]

Two types of complex focal status (synonyms: status psychomotoricus, epileptic twilight state) have been distinguished: a continuous form and a discontinuous or cyclic form. The latter consists of frequently recurring complex partial seizures. Between seizures, patients may or may not experience simple focal seizure symptoms and consciousness may recover to nearly normal states. Non-cyclic forms of complex partial status consist of prolonged confusional episodes or psychotic behaviour. The EEG during complex partial status shows focal or bilateral epileptiform patterns and slowed background activity. Subtle rudiments of motor seizure symptoms, such as lid fluttering and bursts of myoclonic jerks in absence status or mild oral activity automatisms in continuous complex partial status, may point to the underlying epileptic activity. Mutism, paucity of speech or even speech arrest occurs in both absence status and complex partial status.

Complex partial status may arise from any part of the brain. In discontinuous complex partial status, seizure phenomenology may help to localize the status origin in the mesial or lateral temporal lobe or extratemporally. Continuous complex partial status is more often of frontal or extratemporal origin than cyclic status.[25] Non-convulsive status epilepticus requires immediate treatment with intravenous antiepileptic drugs.

Simple focal status or aura continua may cause complex hallucinations, thought disorders and affective symptoms. The continuous epileptic activity is restricted and may escape scalp EEG recordings. Insight usually is maintained and psychoses emerging from such a state have not been described.

Post-ictal psychoses

Most post-ictal psychoses are precipitated by a series, or status, of generalized tonic–clonic seizures. More rarely, psychoses occur after single grand mal seizures or following a series of complex partial seizures.[26] Post-ictal psychosis is the most common manifestation of psychosis in epilepsy.[5,32]

The relation to the type of epilepsy is not clear: Dongier described a preponderance of generalized epilepsies,[5] Logsdail and Toone[27] noted a higher frequency of post-ictal psychosis in patients with focal epilepsies and complex focal seizures.

In most patients there is a characteristic lucid interval lasting from one to six days between the epileptic seizures and onset of psychosis,[28] which may lead to an incorrect diagnosis. The psychopathology of post-ictal psychosis is polymorphic, but most patients present with abnormal mood and paranoid delusions.[27] Some patients are confused throughout the episode, others present with fluctuating impairment of consciousness and orientation and sometimes there is no confusion at all. The EEG during post-ictal psychosis shows increased epileptic as well as slow wave activity.

Psychotic symptoms remit within days or weeks, often without the need for additional neuroleptic treatment. However, in some cases chronic psychoses develop from recurrent or even a single post-ictal psychosis.[22,27]

Par-ictal psychosis

Many authors do not distinguish between par-ictal and post-ictal psychoses.[26] In par-ictal psychosis,[22] psychotic symptoms develop gradually with an increase in seizure frequency. The relation to seizures is easily overlooked if seizure frequency is not carefully documented over a prolonged period. Rapid development of par-ictal psychoses can be seen especially during the presurgical assessment of patients with intractable epilepsy, when a series of epileptic seizures may be provoked by withdrawal of antiepileptic drugs. Impairment of consciousness is more frequent than in post-ictal psychosis. Treatment of par-ictal psychoses requires improvement of seizure control.

Alternative psychoses

In the 1950s, Landolt[3,29] published a series of papers on patients who had epilepsy and whose behaviour deteriorated when their EEG improved. He defined forced normalization thus: 'Forced normalisation is the phenomenon characterised by the fact that, with the recurrence of psychotic states, the EEG becomes more normal, or entirely normal as compared with previous and subsequent EEG findings'. Forced normalization is essentially an EEG phenomenon. The clinical counterpart of patients becoming psychotic when their seizures became under control, and their psychosis resolving with return of seizures, was referred to as alternative psychoses by Tellenbach.[6]

The existence of forced normalization has often been questioned. It is certainly a rare complication of epilepsy. However, it is easily overlooked because the psychopathology is variable and does not necessarily reach the extent of a psychotic state, and the EEG correlate is transient.

The pathogenesis is unclear but it seems justifiable to postulate a hypothesis based on converging clinical and experimental data. Alternative psychosis is a phenomenon that occurs almost exclusively when a long-lasting epileptic process is suddenly destabilized or switched off. Chronic active epilepsy has become much less frequent these days because of the range of effective drugs available plus epilepsy surgery, which is one explanation for the decreasing incidence since Landolt's days.

Looking back, those at risk for the development of forced normalization have changed. in the 1960s it was adults with idiopathic generalized epilepsies who responded to the newly introduced ethosuximide who were most at risk; nowadays it is patients with long-standing partial epilepsies who respond to one of the new antiepileptic compounds. A particularly vulnerable group of patients are those with 'secondary psychomotor seizures'.[30] This might indicate a secondary limbic involvement and links clinical observations with experimental data which suggest a role for mesolimbic kindling and dopaminergic sensitization in the pathogenesis of forced normalization.[31]

Interictal psychoses

Interictal psychoses occur between seizures and cannot be linked directly to the ictus. They are less frequent than peri-ictal psychoses and account for 10–30 per cent of diagnoses in unselected case series.[5,32] Interictal psychoses are, however, clinically more significant in terms of severity and duration than peri-ictal psychoses, which usually are short-lasting and often self-limiting.

Slater stated that, in the absence of epilepsy, the psychoses in their study group would have been diagnosed as schizophrenia,[9] but they also mentioned distinct differences between process schizophrenia and the schizophrenia-like psychoses associated with epilepsy. They highlighted the preservation of a warm affect and a high frequency of delusions and religious mystical experiences. Other authors stressed the rarity of negative symptoms and the absence of formal thought disorder and catatonic states.[19] McKenna et al pointed out that visual hallucinations were more prominent than auditory hallucinations.[33] Tellenbach[6] stated that delusions were less well organized and Sherwin[34] remarked that neuroleptic treatment was necessary less frequently.

There have been other authors, however, who denied any psychopathological differences between epileptic psychosis and schizophrenia.[35,36] Using the Present State Examination and the CATEGO computer program—which is a semi-standardized and validated method for quantifying psychopathology—it has been possible to compare the presentation of psychosis in epilepsy with process schizophrenia. Very few significant differences emerged from such studies,[37,38] which suggests that, assuming that the patients were representative, a significant number will have a schizophrenia-like presentation indistinguishable from schizophrenia in the absence of epilepsy.

Slater argued that the long-term prognosis of psychosis in epilepsy was better than in process schizophrenia. In a follow-up study he found that psychotic symptoms, although chronic, tended to remit and personality deterioration was rare.[39] Other authors also described outcome to be more favourable and long-term institutionalization to be less frequent than in schizophrenia.[19,34] Unfortunately, there have been no longitudinal studies comparing the long-term outcome of psychosis in epilepsy and process schizophrenia.

Gender	Bias to females
Age of onset	Early adolescence
Interval	Onset of seizures to onset of psychosis: 14 years
Epileptic syndrome	Temporal lobe epilepsy
Seizure type	Complex focal
Seizure frequency	Low, diminished
Neurological findings	Sinistrality
Pathology	Gangliogliomas, hamartomas
EEG	Mediobasal focus, especially left-sided

Table 13.2
Risk factors associated with interictal psychoses of epilepsy.[110]

Risk factors

The pathogenesis of interictal psychotic episodes in epilepsy is likely to be heterogeneous. In most patients a multitude of chronic and acute factors can be identified that are potentially responsible for the development of a psychiatric disorder. These factors are difficult to investigate in retrospect and the interpretation as either causally related or simply intercorrelated is arguable.

The literature on risk factors is highly controversial; studies are difficult to compare because of varying definitions of the epilepsy, the psychiatric disorder and the investigated risk factors. Most studies are restricted to interictal psychoses. Table 13.2 summarizes factors that frequently have been described to be associated with psychosis in epilepsy.

Genetic predisposition
With few exceptions,[40] most authors have not found any evidence for an increased rate of psychiatric disorders in relatives of epilepsy patients with psychoses.[9,37,41]

Gender distribution
There has been a bias towards female gender in several case series,[42] which has not been confirmed in controlled studies.[43–45]

Duration of epilepsy
The interval between age at onset of epilepsy and age at first manifestation of psychosis has been remarkably homogeneous in many series, being in the region of 11–15 years.[21] This interval has been used to postulate the aetiological significance of the seizure disorder and a kindling-like mechanism. Some authors have argued that the supposedly specific interval is an artifact, noting the wide range, being significantly shorter in patients with later onset of epilepsy.[11,18] They also point out that anybody whose psychosis did not succeed their epilepsy

was excluded in most series, and that there is a tendency in the general population for the age of onset of epilepsy to peak at an earlier age than that of schizophrenia.

Type of epilepsy

There is a clear excess of temporal lobe epilepsy in almost all case series of patients with epilepsy and psychosis. Summarizing the data of ten studies, 217 (or 76 per cent) of 287 patients suffered from temporal lobe epilepsy.[21] The preponderance of this type of epilepsy, however, is not a uniform finding; in Gudmundsson's epidemiological study, for example, only 7 per cent suffered from 'psychomotor' epilepsy.[15]

The nature of a possible link of psychoses to temporal lobe epilepsy is not entirely clear,[46] partly due to ambiguities in the definition of temporal lobe epilepsy in the literature, based on seizure symptomatology (psychomotor epilepsy), involvement of specific functional systems (limbic epilepsy) or anatomical localization as detected by depth EEG or neuroimaging (amygdalo-hippocampal epilepsy). Unfortunately, most authors have not differentiated sufficiently between frontal and temporal lobe epilepsy.

The temporal lobe hypothesis, although widely accepted, has been criticized for being based on uncontrolled case series, such as in the studies by Gibbs[7] and Slater et al.[9] It was argued that temporal lobe epilepsy is the most frequent type of epilepsy in the general population, and that there is an over-representation of this type of epilepsy in patients attending specialized centres. There is a general consensus that psychoses are very rare in patients with neocortical extratemporal epilepsies.[5,7,11,18,32,47,48]

The findings are less unequivocal regarding temporal lobe epilepsy and generalized epilepsies. In fact, with only three exceptions,[48–50] the majority of controlled studies failed to establish significant differences in the frequency of psychoses in generalized as compared with temporal lobe epilepsy.[4,11,32,51–54] However, many patients with generalized epilepsy show pathology of temporal structures, making classification difficult.

There are several studies showing that psychoses in generalized epilepsies differ from psychoses in temporal lobe epilepsy.[21] The former are more likely to be short-lasting and confusional.[5,11,53] Alternative psychoses, which are especially common in generalized epilepsy, are usually relatively mild and often remit before the development of paranoid-hallucinatory symptoms. Schneiderian first-rank symptoms and chronicity are more frequent in patients with temporal lobe epilepsy.[32,37] This has considerable significance for psychiatrists attempting to unravel the underlying 'neurology' of schizophrenia.

Type of seizures

There is evidence from several studies that focal seizure symptoms, which indicate ictal, mesial, temporal or limbic involvement, are over-represented in patients with psychosis. Hermann and Chabria noted a relationship between ictal fear and high scores on paranoia and schizophrenia scales of the Minnesota Multiphasic Personality Inventory (MMPI).[55] Kristensen and Sindrup found an excess of dysmnesic and epigastric auras in their psychotic group.[43,44] They also reported a higher rate of ictal amnesia. In another controlled study, ictal impairment of consciousness was related to psychosis but simple seizure symptoms indicating limbic involvement were not.[32] Most patients with psychosis and generalized epilepsies have absence seizures.[32]

Severity of epilepsy

The strongest risk factors for psychosis in

epilepsy are those that indicate the severity of epilepsy: long duration of active epilepsy,[9] multiple seizure types,[18,32,48,56-59] history of status epilepticus[32] and poor response to drug treatment.[59] Seizure frequency, however, is reported by most authors to be lower in patients with psychotic epilepsy than in non-psychotic patients.[41,48,60,61] It has not been clarified whether seizure frequency was low before or during the psychotic episode. This may represent a variant of forced normalization.

Laterality

Left lateralization of temporal lobe dysfunction or temporal lobe pathology as a risk factor for schizophreniform psychosis was originally suggested by Flor-Henry.[41] Studies supporting the laterality hypothesis have been made using surface EEG,[59] depth electrode recordings,[34] computed tomography,[62] neuropathology,[63] neuropsychology[37] and positron emission tomography.[64] The literature has been summarized by Trimble.[21] In a synopsis of 14 studies with 341 patients, 43 per cent had left, 23 per cent had right and 34 per cent had bilateral abnormalities. This is a striking bias towards left lateralization. However, lateralization of epileptogenic foci was not confirmed in all controlled studies.[5,43,44,65] Again, it may be that certain symptoms, e.g. some first-rank psychotic symptoms, are associated with a specific side of focus.

Structural lesions

The literature on brain damage and epileptic psychosis is very controversial. Some authors have suggested a higher rate of neuropathological examinations, diffuse slowing on the EEG and mental retardation,[43,44] whilst others could not find an association with psychosis.[40,41] Neuropathological studies from resected temporal lobes from patients with temporal lobe epilepsy have suggested a link between

psychosis and the presence of cerebral malformations such as hamartomas and gangliogliomas as compared with mesial temporal sclerosis.[42] These findings have been seen as consistent with recent findings of structural abnormalities found in the brains of patients with schizophrenia but no epilepsy that arise during fetal development.

Depression

Affective changes are well recognized in patients with epilepsy. Mania is rare, but most studies agree that both anxiety and depression are more common in epilepsy than in the general population.[66] Blumer has pointed out that there is a specific affective syndrome predominant in epilepsy, called 'interictal dysphoric disorder' that is characterized by labile depressive symptoms (depressive mood, anergia, pain, insomnia), labile affective symptoms (fear, anxiety) and distinctive symptoms (paroxysmal irritability, euphoric moods).[67]

Classification

Like psychoses, depressive disorders in epilepsy may be classified according to their relationship to seizures. Pre-ictally rising tension and dysphoria are not uncommon in epilepsy. Patients often experience an immediate relief or even elation following grand mal seizures. Affective symptoms—anxiety more often than depression—may be part of simple seizures especially when arising in the limbic system, and non-convulsive status may present with prominent affective symptoms,[68,69] which may be difficult to diagnose when seizure activity is restricted to subcortical regions.[70] Post-ictal depression may be severe, including psychotic ideation. Most studies have focused on interic-

	Number of studies showing association	Number of studies showing no association
Epilepsy variables		
Seizure type	1	4
Temporal focus	3	1
Left-sided focus	3	7
High seizure frequency	1	4
Long duration of epilepsy	1	4
Treatment variables		
Polytherapy	3	3
Barbiturates	3	–
Low folate	3	–
Demographic and psychiatric variables		
Male gender	2	3
Loss of control	1	1
Hereditary predisposition	1	1

Table 13.3
Risk factors for depression in epilepsy in 19 studies.[111]

tal depression;[71] its biological and psychological links to epilepsy are discussed in the following.

Risk factors

The risk factors are summarized in Table 13.3.

Seizure variables

Although the majority of studies suggest an excess of depression in temporal lobe epilepsy,[57,58,72] some authors could not find differences between generalized and temporal lobe epilepsies when using standardized rating scales. Whitman et al conducted a literature search to locate all published MMPI investigations, including ten studies of epilepsy patients.[73] Results suggested that there is an increased risk for psychopathology in epilepsy compared with the general population. There

was, however, no difference between people with temporal lobe epilepsy and those with generalized epilepsy.

Localization and lateralization

Flor-Henry was the first to suggest a link between non-dominant epilepsy and depression. However, in his original study on psychopathogy in surgical candidates there were only nine patients with depression: four had right-sided, three had bilateral and two had left-sided temporal lobe epilepsy.[41]

There are several studies suggesting a link between left temporal lobe epilepsy, frontal dysfunction and depression. Hermann et al studied frontal functions using the Wisconsin Card Sorting Test.[74] There were no differences between right- and left-sided temporal lobe epilepsy with respect to measurements of depression. In the left temporal lobe epilepsy group there was a significant correlation between the degree of depression and frontal dysfunction, as indicated by the level of perseverance on the Wisconsin Card Sorting Test. These results were confirmed by a single photon emission computed tomography study using [99mTc]hexamethylpropylenamine oxime (HMPAO). Again, patients with right or left temporal lobe epilepsy did not differ with respect to depression as measured by the Beck inventory. But in patients with left-sided epilepsies, depression was significantly associated with frontal hypoperfusion.[75] These data are consistent with the broader psychiatric literature, which suggest a hypofrontality in depression. These data also suggest that the epileptic focus may cause functional disturbances in remote regions that are connected to the epileptogenic region, for example, via the limbic system.

Epilepsy surgery

Prospective studies have shown an increased risk for affective problems in the first months following epilepsy surgery.[76] In a study of 60 patients there was a 42 per cent prevalence of anxiety six weeks following surgery and a 35 per cent prevalence of depression three months after surgery despite good clinical outcome with respect to seizures (87 per cent had at least 90 per cent reduction in seizure frequency).[77]

Psychological models

Inappropriate restrictions due to stigma as well as justified restrictions in everyday activities due to real dangers of seizures may contribute to the development of depression in epilepsy. According to the model of learned helplessness, clinical depression develops secondary to unavoidable frustrations. This helps to explain depression in epilepsy, a disorder characterized by seizures that are largely unpredictable and unavoidable.[78]

The seemingly paradoxical psychiatric problems that arise in some patients when seizures are controlled by medication or surgery have been referred to as 'burden of normality',[79] a phenomenon that has also been described in patients who were cured from other chronic illnesses, e.g. congenital blindness.

Suicide

Classification

The spectrum of suicidal behaviour includes the following phenomena listed in order of severity: thoughts of death, a wish to be dead, consideration of suicide, plans to commit suicide, parasuicidal acts with the predominating motivation of provoking a break or a reaction in relatives rather than self-harm, the failed 'serious' suicide attempt with the intended self-destruction and, finally, the completed suicide. Patients with epilepsy who ignore seizure-related risks and do not comply with antiepileptic drugs may be parasuicidal. If such behaviour leads to death by way of overdose, fatal accidents or convulsive status epilepticus, it is impossible to prove the suicidal background in retrospect; this is just one methodological problem of mortality studies in epilepsy.

Epidemiology

Chronic physical illness, especially neurological illness, is an accepted risk factor for completed suicide. This has been shown for chronic pain, multiple sclerosis, AIDS, Huntington's chorea, spinal cord injury and tinnitus.[80] A recent meta-analysis of epidemiologically suitable case series suggests a fivefold increased suicide rate in patients with epilepsy as compared with the general population.[81] However, the highest

Patients	Suicides observed	Suicides expected	SMR	95% CI
Surgically treated	7	0.1	87.5	35.2–18.0*
Temporal lobe epilepsy	4	0.5	8.0	2.2–20.5*
Institutionalized	21	4.3	4.9	3.0–7.5 *
Outpatients	25	6.1	4.1	2.7–6.1*
'Petit mal' epilepsy	2	0.5	4.2	0.5–1.5 n.s.
General practice	1	0.3	3.3	0.1–1.9 n.s.
Total	60	11.7	5.1	3.9–6.6*

CI, Confidence interval; *, significantly increased SMR (lower CI is >1); n.s., not significant.

Table 13.4
Standardised mortality ratio (SMR) in different epilepsy groups.[81]

suicide rate is seen in selected patient groups such as postsurgical series and patients with temporal lobe epilepsy, being 88-fold and 8-fold increased, respectively (Table 13.4).

Population-based data on the suicide risk in epilepsy are rare. In a recent study on mortality in 9061 epilepsy patients from Stockholm, suicides accounted for 53 of all deaths ($n = 4001$), resulting in a statistical mortality ratio of 3.5, which was significantly increased compared with the general population of Sweden.[82] However, although this study has the advantage of a uniquely large cohort, there are the disadvantages of selection bias and inaccuracy with respect to establishing the cause of death. Patients were selected through hospital admissions, thus causing a bias towards symptomatic and severe epilepsies. The cause of death was established by death certificate in half of all cases: only 48 per cent had a post-mortem examination. There were 64 unexplained violent deaths, which may or may not have been suicides.

Risk factors

Risk factors for suicides in general, which are also relevant for epilepsy patients (Table 13.5), include male gender and living alone, previous suicide attempts, self-destructive behaviour and a family history of suicide. Ninety per cent of suicides occur in the context of psychiatric diseases, especially depression, schizophrenia, addiction and antisocial or borderline personality disorders. In epilepsy, schizophreniform psychoses may carry a higher suicide risk than depression. Mendez et al compared psychiatric diagnoses of epileptic and non-epileptic persons who attempted suicide.[83] In the epilepsy group psychotic disturbances were more frequent than in the non-epilepsy group, (32 per cent versus 9 per cent), as were borderline personality disorders (46 per cent versus 24 per cent), whereas the rate of depression was lower in the epilepsy group (14 per cent versus 25 per cent; difference not significant). In our series of 25 patients with schizophreniform psychoses and

In general	In epilepsy
Male, living alone	Chronic illness, stigmatization, discrimination
Suicidal ideation, previous suicide attempts, self-destructive behaviour, suicides in the family	Peri-ictal suicidal impulses
Psychiatric disorders: depression, schizophrenia, substance dependence, borderline personality	Epilepsy surgery, depressogenic antiepileptic drugs
Life events	Availability of drugs in large quantities

Table 13.5
Risk factors for suicide.

25 patients with major depression, a history of suicide attempts was noted in 28 per cent and 20 per cent, respectively.[84]

Peri-ictal suicide attempts most often occur in patients with temporal lobe epilepsy and are related to post-ictal depression or paranoid-hallucinatory psychosis.[67] The danger of these is easily underestimated. The post-ictal psychosis may be very brief—some patients are amnesic for post-ictal self-destructive impulses—and the psychopathological status may be competely normal between seizures.

Despite international efforts to fight discrimination against people with epilepsy, stigmatization still exists, which, in addition to social disadvantages due to persisting seizures, may contribute to suicidal reactions. Availability of potentially lethal drugs in large quantities is a recognized risk for suicides. This is of specific relevance with respect to barbiturates, which are implicated in the aetiology of depression in epilepsy.[66,85] Overdose of barbiturates was the most common mode of suicide in one cohort of people with epilepsy.[86] Brent et al compared the prevalence of psychopathology in 15

patients treated with phenobarbital to 24 patients treated with carbamazepine.[87] Patients did not differ over a wide range of demographic and biological variables, but those treated with barbiturates not only showed a higher prevalence of depressive disorder (40 per cent versus 4 per cent) but also a higher prevalence of suicidal ideation (47 per cent versus 4 per cent).

The alarming 88-fold increase in suicides in surgical patients (Table 13.4) relates to early series from the 1960s[88,89] when there was little awareness of the need for presurgical counselling and postsurgical psychiatric care, irrespective of success or failure of operation. Taylor and Falconer studied 100 consecutive cases who underwent temporal lobectomy and followed them for 2–12 years. Eleven had died by the time of follow-up, five by suicide. Jensen reviewed mortality in 2282 patients who had temporal lobe resections between 1928 and 1973.[90] The total number of deaths was 50, with suicide being the most common cause (*n* = 14). The more recent series suggest lower suicide rates, possibly due to improved psychiatric care.

	Positive psychotropic effects	Negative affective effects	Psychoses and other complications
Barbiturates, primidone	Sedative	Aggression, depression, withdrawal syndromes	Attention deficit hyperactivity disorder (ADHD) in children
Benzodiazepines	Anxiolytic, sedative	Withdrawal syndromes	Psychoses possible, disinhibition
Ethosuximide	–	Insomnia	Alternative psychoses
Phenytoin	–	–	Toxic schizophreniform psychoses
Carbamazepine	Mood stabilizing, impulse control	Rarely mania and depression	–
Valproate	Mood stabilising, antimanic	–	Acute and chronic encephalopathy
Vigabatrin	–	Aggression, depression, withdrawal syndromes	ADHD, acute and chronic encephalopathy, alternative psychoses
Lamotrigine	Antidepressive	Insomnia	Rarely psychoses (alternative ?)
Felbamate	Stimulating ?	Agitation ?	Psychoses possible
Gabapentin	Anxiolytic, antidepressive ?	Rarely aggression in children	–
Tiagabine	–	Depression	Non-convulsive status epilepticus
Topiramate	–	Depression (dose-related ?)	Psychoses (dose-related ?)

?, Minimal information.

Table 13.6
Psychotropic effects of antiepileptic drugs.

In the study by Ring et al of 60 patients who had been operated on at the National Hospital for Neurology and Neurosurgery in London, there was no suicide and no suicide attempt within one year of follow-up.[77] In Bladin's follow-up study of 115 surgical patients, three patients had died after a mean observation period of four years, one by suicide.[79]

In accordance with the increased risk of depression in the first months following surgery, suicide attempts are also most common in the early postoperative period. In a follow-up study by Jensen and Larsen, 14 of 74 patients had attempted suicide on one or more occasions; all attempts were made in the first month after operation.[40]

Some of the patients reported in the literature who committed suicide following surgery had been seizure-free (e.g. five of nine cases published by Taylor and Marsh[91]). This is in agreement with the general impression that suicides are not specifically related to severe epilepsy. Janz concluded from his analysis of 19 cases who died from suicide: 'Patients at risk for suicide are not characterised by a particularly severe course of epilepsy. In their biography, suicide marks a point of cumulating critical personal and social decisions, which often have become urgent by way of an effective therapy (*Biographisch steht er (der Selbstmord) auf halbem Wege der Lebensbahn, allerdings meist im Schnittpunkt kritischer persönlicher und sozialer Entscheidungen, die oft durch eine wirksame Therapie unaufschiebbar geworden sind)*'.[30]

Syndromes related to antiepileptic drugs

All antiepileptic drugs may have positive or negative psychotropic effects in individual patients. Mechanisms related to psychiatric adverse effects are polytherapy, drug toxicity, withdrawal and forced normalization. Our knowledge on dose-independent or idiosyncratic psychotropic side effects is limited (Table 13.6). With respect to the older antiepileptic drugs, there are few systematic data. With respect to the new generation of antiepileptics, there are data on psychiatric side effects from drug trials. However, these data are not always entirely transparent to the interested epileptologist. Further, in most trials psychiatric adverse events are not reported systematically, so the severity and psychopathological nature of behavioural problems remain unclear.

In addition to depression[67,85,87] the side effects of barbiturates are increased aggressive behaviour and, in children, an attention-deficit hyperactivity syndrome. Phenytoin may provoke schizophrenia-like psychoses at high dose levels.[92] Valproate is associated with acute[93] and chronic encephalopathies.[94,95] Psychiatric complications of carbamazepine may be depression and, rarely, mania, the latter being explained as a paradoxical effect due to the antidepressant properties of carbamazepine, which is chemically related to tricyclic antidepressants. The link between ethosuximide and forced normalization has already been mentioned.

Of the new drugs, affective problems are significantly increased with the gamma-aminobutyric acid (GABA)-ergic substances: vigabatrin, tiagabine and topiramate. It seems that patients with a previous history or a familial predisposition are specifically prone to affective side effects.[96] Forced normalization or alternative psychoses have been reported with all new drugs but may be particularly common with the more effective substances, such as vigabatrin. There have been some reports on forced normalization secondary to treatment with zonisamide. Zonisamide influences thalamic calcium channels, similar to ethosuximide.[97]

The positive psychotropic effects of carbamazepine and valproate are used in psychiatric praxis, particularly in the treatment and prophylaxis of affective disorders and in the management of episodic dyscontrol. The antidepressive effect of lamotrigine has been recently established in controlled studies of patients with depression.[98] Gabapentin has been anecdotally tried in the treatment of anxiety disorders and depression. Negative psychotropic effects have not been demonstrated in the drug trials of this generally well-tolerated drug, but there have been case reports of the provocation of aggressive behaviour in children.[99,100] One study has suggested that felbamate may be stimulating and that this effect may be positive in some children and negative in others, depending on the pre-existing psychopathology.[101] A specific problem with tiagabine, in addition to the increased risk of 'depressed mood',[102] is the paradoxical provocation of *de novo* non-convulsive status epilepticus due to a narrow therapeutic window, making EEG registrations necessary when behavioural problems arise. The high incidence of depression with topiramate[103] may be related to cognitive side effects, which are particularly common with this drug, but this has not been studied systematically.

Therapy of psychiatric disorders in epilepsy

Psychotherapy

The role of psychotherapy in the management of psychiatric problems (other than pseudo-seizures) in epilepsy is under-researched. Considering psychological models of the development of depression in epilepsy based on the learned helplessness paradigm, cognitive behavioural therapy seems promising and has been shown to be effective in one study of 13 depressed patients with epilepsy.[104] A personal impression is that patients with epilepsy have little access to behavioural and psychoanalytic therapy the reason for this is not entirely clear but it may be a combination of the patient's defence, the epileptologist's ignorance of psychotherapy and the psychotherapist's ignorance of seizures. Systemic approaches may be appropriate and family therapy is of particular use in early onset epilepsy.[105] Supportive psychotherapy is a useful adjunct also in interictal psychosis. For all forms of psychotherapy the therapist's understanding of epilepsy is crucial for its success.

Psychopharmacotherapy

Psychosis

If an acute psychosis cannot be controlled sufficiently with benzodiazepines, haloperidol is the preferred neuroleptic drug. For long-term neuroleptic management sulpiride, pimozide and flupenthixol are the drugs most commonly used because of their relatively mild impact on seizure threshold. Clozapine, a highly effective D_4-antagonist, should be avoided because of its strong proconvulsive effects with seizures occuring in 1–4 per cent of patients treated. Interestingly, there is evidence for a positive relationship between seizures and the antipsychotic effect of clozapine, suggesting that seizures may be therapeutic in schizophrenia.[106] There is limited clinical experience with the new 'atypical' neuroleptics, such as risperidone and olanzapine, although their proconvulsive effects seem relatively low. Because the long-term prognosis of interictal schizophreniform psychosis in epilepsy may be better than in 'endogeneous' schizophrenia, the need for chronic neuroleptic treatment with all the risks of long-term side effects is arguable and should only be prescribed when other procedures, such as improved seizure control, psychosocial support, etc. have failed.

Depression

There is a risk of seizures as an adverse effect with most, if not all, antidepressants. However, the danger of increased seizures in patients with epilepsy is generally overestimated.[107] In the only placebo-controlled study in patients with epilepsy, seizures were not provoked by nomifensine or amitriptyline.[108]

In mild depression, St John's wort may be used without risking any adverse effects except photosensitization. Monoamine oxidase inhibitors (MAOIs) have no effect on the seizure threshold. Moclobemide is a reversible inhibitor of monoamine oxidase that has fewer problems with drug interactions than the irreversible MAOIs. There is no evidence for problems arising with co-medication of carbamazepine, which is contraindicated with irreversible MAOIs because of its tricyclic structure. Selective serotonin reuptake inhibitors (SSRIs) have little impact on seizures. Both SSRIs and MAOIs are therefore generally preferred to tricyclic antidepressants. Among the older antidepressants the tetracyclic maprotiline should be avoided. If a tricyclic drug is believed to be indicated, doxepin has been suggested to have the lowest proconvulsive effect.[109]

In addition to pharmacodynamic problems, pharmacokinetic interactions need to be considered. With fluoxetine, but not with other SSRIs such as paroxetine, there may be an increase in serum concentrations of anti-epileptics. In order to avoid intoxication (proconvulsive effects of antidepressants are dose-dependent) and to recognize pseudo-resistance (when antidepressants are combined with enzyme-inducing antiepileptics) and non-compliance (often there is a warning of seizures in information leaflets of antidepressants), drug levels (of anticonvulsants and antidepressants) should be monitored. General advice is that antidepressive drugs should only be increased slowly without exceeding moderate dosages.

Electroconvulsive therapy

Electroconvulsive therapy (ECT) is effective in the treatment of schizoaffective psychosis and depression and should be used in cases where conventional drug treatment has failed. Epilepsy is neither a contraindication nor a specific reason to treat a co-existing psychiatric disorder with ECT.[109] This also applies to those rare cases of forced normalization or depression following successful surgery and ECT.

If I had a psychiatric problem in addition to epilepsy ...

If I had epilepsy as well as a psychiatric problem, I would hope to find a doctor who: takes his or her time to listen to my history and to my actual problems; knows about psychiatric complications of epilepsy; does not accept such problems as inevitable and irreversible in epilepsy; is familiar with the specific prophylaxis and treatment of psychiatric disorders in the context of epilepsy; and, works with a multidisciplinary team that provides psychological and social support if necessary. I would hope that anticonvulsants prescribed for my epilepsy are not just effective with respect to seizure control but also have positive psychotropic effects. If there was a risk for psychiatric adverse effects of antiepileptic drugs I would like to be informed, in order to be prepared when such problems arise. If I had a psychiatric disorder I would hope that this would not cause therapeutic nihilism and that I would still be given the chance of optimal antiepileptic treatment, including new drugs and epilepsy surgery.

References

1. Schmitz B. Forced normalisation. The history of a concept. In: Trimble MR, Schmitz B, eds. *Forced normalisation*. Petersfield: Wrightson Biomedical Publishing, 1998:7–24.
2. Samt P. Epileptische Irreseinsformen. *Arch Psychiat* 1875;**5**:393–444.
3. Landolt H. Some clinical EEG correlations in epileptic psychoses (twilight states). *EEG Clin Neurophysiol* 1953;**5**:121.
4. Gastaut H. Colloque de Marseille, 15–19 Octobre 1956. Compte rendu du colloque sur l'etude electroclinique des episodes psychotiques qui surviennent chez les epileptiques en dehors des crises cliniques. *Rev Neurol* 1956;**95**:587–616.
5. Dongier S. Statistical study of clinical and electroencephalographic manifestations of 536 psychotic episodes occuring in 516 epileptics between clinical seizures. *Epilepsia* 1959/60;**1**:117–42.
6. Tellenbach H. Epilepsie als Anfallsleiden und als Psychose. Über alternative Psychosen paranoider Prägung bei 'forcierter Normalisierung' (Landolt) des Elektroencephalogramms Epileptischer. *Nervenarzt* 1965;**36**:190–202.
7. Gibbs FA. Ictal and non-ictal psychiatric disorders in temporal lobe epilepsy. *J Nerv Ment Dis* 1951;**113**:522–8.
8. Pond DA. Discussion remark. *Proc R Soc Med* 1962;**55**:316.
9. Slater E, Beard AW, Glithero E. The schizophrenia-like psychoses of epilepsy. *Br J Psychiatry* 1963;**109**:95–150.
10. Meduna L von. Versuche ueber die bioogische Beeinglussung des Ablaufes der Schizophrenie. I. Campher- und Cadiazolkraempfe. *Z gesante Neurol Psychiatr* 1935;**152**:235–62.
11. Stevens JR. Psychiatric implications of psychomotor epilepsy. *Arch Gen Psychiatry* 1966;**14**:461–71.
12. Krohn W. A study of epilepsy in northern Norway, its frequency and character. *Acta Psychiatr Scand Suppl* 1961;**150**:215–25.
13. Zielinski JJ. *Epidemiology and medical–social problems of epilepsy in Warsaw*, Final report on Research Program No. 19-P-58325-F-01 DHEW. (Social and Rehabilitation Services). Washington, DC: US Government Printing Office, 1974.
14. Bilikiewicz A, Matkowski K, Przybysz K, Dabkowski M, Ksiazkiewicz-Cuwinska J, Jakubowska M. Untersuchungen zur Epidemiologie und Psychopathologie der zwischen 1976 und 1980 in der Woiwoidschaft Bydgoscz registrierten Epileptiker. *Psychiatr Neurol Med Psychol (Leipzig)* 1988;**40**:9–15.
15. Gudmundsson G. Epilepsy in Iceland. *Acta Neurol Scand Suppl* 1966;**25**:1–124.
16. Helgason T. Epidemiology of mental disorders in Iceland: psychoses. *Acta Psychiatr Scand* 1964;**40**:67–95.
17. Trimble MR, Schmitz B. The psychoses of epilepsy/schizophrenia. In: Engel J Jr, Pedley TA, eds. *Epilepsy: a comprehensive textbook*. Philadelphia: Lippincott-Raven, 1997:2071–82.
18. Bruens JH. Psychoses in epilepsy. In: Vinken PJ, Bruyn GW, eds. *Handbook of clinical neurology*. Vol 15. Amsterdam: Elsevier, 1974:593–610.
19. Köhler GK. Epileptische Psychosen - Klassifikationsversuche und EEG-Verlaufsbeobachtungen. *Fortschr Neurol Psychiat* 1975;**43**:99–153.
20. Fenton GJ. Psychiatric disorders of epilepsy: classification and phenomenology. In: Reynolds E H, Trimble MR, eds. *Epilepsy and psychiatry*. Edinburgh: Churchill Livingstone, 1981:12–26.
21. Trimble M. *The psychoses of epilepsy*. New York: Raven Press, 1991.
22. Wolf P. *Psychosen bei Epilepsie. Ihre Bedingungen und Wechselbeziehungen zu Anfällen. Habilitationsschrift*, Berlin: Freie Universität, 1976.
23. Lennox WG. The treatment of epilepsy. *Med Clin North Am* 1945;**29**:1114–28.
24. Lee SI. Nonconvulsive status epilepticus. *Arch Neurol* 1985;**42**:778–81.
25. Delgado-Escueta AV. Status epilepticus. In: Dam M, Gram L, eds. *Comprehensive epileptology*. New York: Raven Press, 1990:375–83.
26. Savard G, Andermann F, Olivier A, Remillard

GM. Post-ictal psychosis after partial complex seizures: a multiple case study. *Epilepsia* 1991;**32**:225–31.

27. Logsdail SJ, Toone BK. Postictal psychoses. A clinical and phenomenological description. *Br J Psychiatry* 1988;**152**:246–52.

28. Sommer W. Postepileptisches Irresein. *Arch Psychiatr Nervenkr* 1881;**11**:549–612.

29. Landolt H. Serial electroencephalographic investigations during psychotic episodes in epileptic patients and during schizophrenic attacks. In: Lorentz de Haas AM, ed. *Lectures on epilepsy*. Amsterdam: Elsevier, 1958: 91–133.

30. Janz D. *Die Epilepsien. Spezielle Pathologie und Therapie*, Vol. 2. Stuttgart: Thieme, 1998.

31. Trimble MR, Schmitz B, eds. *Forced normalisation*. Petersfield: Wrightson Biomedical Publishing, 1998.

32. Schmitz B, Wolf P. Psychosis with epilepsy: frequency and risk factors. *J Epilepsy* 1995;**8**: 295–305.

33. McKenna PJ, Kane JM, Parrish K. Psychotic symptoms in epilepsy. *Am J Psychiat* 1985; **142**:895–904.

34. Sherwin I. Differential psychiatric features in epilepsy; relationship to lesion laterality. *Acta Psychiatr Scand* 1984;**69**:92–103.

35. Helmchen H. Zerebrale Bedingungkonstellationen psychopathologischer Syndrome bei Epileptikern. In: Helmchen H, Hippius H, eds. *Entwicklungstendenzen biologischer Psychiatrie*. Stuttgart: Thieme, 1975:125–48.

36. Kraft AM, Price TRP, Peltier D. Complex partial seizures and schizophrenia. *Compr Psychiatry* 1984;**25**:113–24.

37. Perez MM, Trimble MR. Epileptic psychosis - diagnostic comparison with process schizophrenia. *Br J Psychiatry* 1980;**137**: 245–9.

38. Toone B. Psychoses of epilepsy. In: Reynolds EH, Trimble MR, eds. *Epilepsy and psychiatry*. Edinburgh: Churchill Livingstone, 1981: 113–37.

39. Glithero E, Slater E. The schizophrenia-like psychoses of epilepsy. IV. Follow-up record and outcome. *Br J Psychiatry* 1963;**109**: 134–42.

40. Jensen I, Larsen JK. Mental aspects of temporal lobe epilepsy. *J Neurol Neurosurg Psychiatry* 1979;**42**:256–65.

41. Flor-Henry P. Psychosis and temporal lobe epilepsy. a controlled investigation. *Epilepsia* 1969;**10**:363–95.

42. Taylor DC. Ontogenesis of chronic epileptic psychoses. A reanalysis. *Psychol Med* 1971;**1**: 247–53.

43. Kristensen O, Sindrup HH. Psychomotor epilepsy and psychosis. I. Physical aspects. *Acta Neurol Scand* 1978;**57**:361–9.

44. Kristensen O, Sindrup HH. Psychomotor epilepsy and psychosis. II. Electroencephalographic findings. *Acta Neurol Scand* 1978; **57**:370–9.

45. Bash KW, Mahnig P. Epileptiker in der psychiatrischen Klinik. Von der Däemmerattacke zur Psychose. *Eur Arch Psychiatr Neurol Sci* 1984;**234**:237–49.

46. Schmitz B. Psychosis in epilepsy. The link to the temporal lobe. In: Trimble MR, Schmitz B, eds. *Forced normalisation*. Petersfield: Wrightson Biomedical Publishing, 1998: 149–67.

47. Onuma T. Limbic lobe epilepsy with paranoid symptoms: analysis of clinical features and psychological tests. *Folia Psychiatr Neurol Jpn* 1983;**37**:253–8.

48. Sengoku A, Yagi K, Seino M, Wada T. Risks of occurrence of psychoses in relation to the types of epilepsies and epileptic seizures. *Folia Psychiatr Neurol Jpn* 1983;**37**:221–6.

49. Gureje O. Interictal psychopathology in epilepsy—prevalence and pattern in a Nigerian clinic. *Br J Psychiatry* 1991;**158**:700–5.

50. Shukla GD, Srivastava ON, Katiyar BC, et al. Psychiatric manifestations in temporal lobe epilepsy. A controlled study. *Br J Psychiatry* 1979;**135**:411–7.

51. Small JG, Milstein V, Stevens JR. Are psychomotor epileptics different? *Arch Neurol* 1962;**7**:187–94.

52. Mignone RJ, Donnelly EF, Sadowsky D. Psychological and neurological comparisons of psychomotor and non-psychomotor epileptic patients. *Epilepsia* 1970;**11**:345–59.

53. Bruens JH. Psychoses in epilepsy. *Psychiatr Neurol Neurochir* 1971;**74**:174–92.

54. Standage KF, Fenton GW. Psychiatric symptom profiles of patients with epilepsy: a controlled investigation. *Psychol Med* 1975;**5**:152–60.

55. Hermann BP, Chabria S. Interictal psychopathology in patients with ictal fear. *Arch Neurol* 1980;**37**:667–8.

56. Ounsted C. Aggression and epilepsy. Rage in children with temporal lobe epilepsy. *J Psychosomat Res* 1969;**13**:237–42.

57. Hermann BP, Dikmen S, Schwartz MS, Karnes WE. Psychopathology in patients with ictal fear: a quantitative investigation. *Neurology* 1982;**32**:7–11.

58. Rodin EA, Collomb H, Pache D. Differences between patients with temporal lobe seizures and those with other forms of epileptic attacks. *Epilepsia* 1976;**17**:313–20.

59. Lindsay J, Ounsted C, Richards P. Long-term outcome in children with temporal lobe seizures. II. Psychiatric aspects in childhood and adult life. *Dev Med Child Neurol* 1979; **21**:630–6.

60. Standage KF. Schizophreniform psychosis among epileptics in a mental hospital. *Br J Psychiatry* 1973;**123**:231–2.

61. Slater E, Moran PAP. The schizophrenia-like psychoses of epilepsy: relation between ages of onset. *Br J Psychiatry* 1969;**115**:599–600.

62. Toone B, Dawson J, Driver MV. Psychoses of epilepsy. A radiological evaluation. *Br J Psychiatry* 1982;**140**:244–8.

63. Taylor DC. Mental state and temporal lobe epilepsy. A correlative account of 100 patients treated surgically. *Epilepsia* 1972;**13**:727–65.

64. Trimble MR. PET-scanning in epilepsy. In: Trimble MR, Bolwig TG, eds. *Aspects of epilepsy and psychiatry*. Chichester: Wiley, 1986:147–62.

65. Shukla GD, Katiyar BC. Psychiatric disorders in temporal lobe epilepsy: the laterality effect. *Br J Psychiatry* 1980;**137**:181–2.

66. Robertson MM, Trimble MR, Townsend HRA. Phenomenology of depression in epilepsy. *Epilepsia* 1987;**28**:364–72.

67. Blumer D, Altshuler LL. Affective disorders. In: Engel J Jr, Pedley TA, eds. *Epilepsy: a comprehensive textbook*. Philadelphia: Lippincott-Raven, 1997:2083–100.

68. Tucker WM, Foster FM. Petit mal epilepsy occurring in status. *Arch Neurol* 1950;**64**: 823–7.

69. Wells CE. Transient ictal psychosis. *Arch Gen Psychiatry* 1975;**32**:1201–3.

70. Wieser HG. Simple status epilepticus. In: Engel J Jr, Pedley TA, eds. *Epilepsy: a comprehensive textbook*. Philadelphia: Lippincott-Raven, 1997:709–22.

71. Robertson M. Mood disorders associated with epilepsy. In: McConnell HW, Snyder PJ, eds. *Psychiatric comorbidity in epilepsy*. Washington DC: American Psychiatric Press, 1997:133–67.

72. Dikmen S, Hermann BP, Wilensky AJ, et al. Validity of the Minnesota Multiphasic Personality Inventory (MMPI) to psychopathology in patients with epilepsy. *J Nerv Ment Dis* 1983;**171**:114–22.

73. Whitman S, Hermann BP, Gordon AC. Psychopathology in epilepsy: how great is the risk? *Biol Psychiatry* 1984;**2**:213–36.

74. Hermann BP, Seidenberg M, Haltiner A, Wyler AR. Mood state in unilateral temporal lobe epilepsy. *Biol Psychiatry* 1991;**30**:1205–18.

75. Schmitz B, Trimble MR, Moriarty J, Costa DC, Ell PJ. Psychiatric profiles and patterns of blood flow in patients with focal epilepsies. *J Neurol Neurosurg Psychiatry* 1997;**62**:458–63.

76. Chovaz CJ, McLachlan RS, Derry PA, Cummings AL. Psychosocial functioning following temporal lobectomy: influence of seizure control and learned helplessness. *Seizure* 1994;**3**:171–6.

77. Ring HA, Moriarty J, Trimble MR. A prospective study of the early post-surgical psychiatric associations of epilepsy surgery. *J Neurol Neurosurg Psychiatry* 1998;**64**:601–4.

78. Hermann BP, Trenerry MR, Colligan RC. The Bozeman Epilepsy Surgery Consortium, learned helplessness, attributional style, and depression in epilepsy. *Epilepsia* 1996;**37**: 680–6.

79. Bladin PF. Psychosocial difficulties and outcome after temporal lobectomy. *Epilepsia* 1992;**33**:898–907.

80. Robertson MM. Suicide, parasuicide, and epilepsy. In: Engel J Jr, Pedley TA, eds. *Epilepsy: a comprehensive textbook*. Philadelphia: Lippincott-Raven, 1997:2141–52.

81. Harris C, Barraclough B. Suicide as an outcome for mental disorders. *Br J Psychiatry* 1997;**170**:205–28.

82. Nilsson L, Tomson T, Farahmand BY, Diwan V, Persson PG. Cause-specific mortality in

epilepsy: a cohort study of more than 9,000 patients once hospitalized for epilepsy. *Epilepsia* 1997;**38**:1062–8.

83. Mendez MF, Lanska DJ, Manon-Espaillat R, Burnstine TH. Causative factors of suicide attempts by overdose in epileptics. *Arch Neurol* 1989;**46**:1065–8.

84. Schmitz B, Trimble MR. Schizophrenia and depression in epilepsy. *Epilepsy Research*, in press.

85. Victoroff JI, Benson DF, Grafton ST, Engel J, Mazziotta JC. Depression in complex partial seizures. Electroencephalography and cerebral metabolic correlates. *Arch Neurol* 1994;**51**: 155–63.

86. Samant JM, Desai AD. Suicides in epileptic patients—a retrospective social study. *Neurol India* 1976;**24**:110–11.

87. Brent DA, Crumrine PK, Varma RR, Allan M, Allman C. Phenobarbital treatment and major depressive disorder in children with epilepsy. *Pediatrics* 1987;**80**:909–17.

88. Taylor DC, Falconer MA. Clinical, socio-economic, and psychological changes after temporal lobectomy for epilepsy. *Br J Psychiatry* 1968;**114**:1247–61.

89. Stepien L, Bidzinski J, Mazurowski W. The results of surgical treatment of temporal lobe epilepsy. *Pol Med J* 1969;**8**:1184–90.

90. Jensen I. Temporal lobe epilepsy: late mortality in patients treated with unilateral temporal lobe resections. *Acta Neurol Scand* 1975;**52**:374–80.

91. Taylor DC, Marsh SM. Implications of long-term follow-up studies in epilepsy: with a note on the cause of death. In: Penry JK, ed. *Epilepsy: the 8th International Symposium.* New York: Raven Press, 1977:27–34.

92. Schmitz B, Wolf P. Epilepsy and psychosis. *Front Clin Neurosci*, 1991;**12**:97–128.

93. Pakalnis A, Drake ME, Denio L. Valproate-associated encephalopathy. *J Epilepsy* 1989;**2**: 41–4.

94. Zaret BS, Cohen RA. Reversible valproic acid-induced dementia: a case report. *Epilepsia* 1986;**27**:234–40.

95. Schöndienst M, Wolf P. Zur Möglichkeit neurotoxischer Spätwirkungen von Valproin-säure. In: Krämer G, Laub M, eds. *Valproinsäure*. Berlin: Springer, 1992:259–65.

96. Thomas L, Trimble MR, Schmitz B, Ring HA. Vigabatrin and behaviour disorders: a retrospective study. *Epilepsy Res* 1996;**25**:21–7.

97. Trimble MR. Anticonvulsant drugs and forced normalisation. In: Trimble MR, Schmitz B, eds. *Forced normalisation.* Petersfield: Wrightson Biomedical Publishing, 1998:169–78.

98. Kasumakar V, Yatham LN. An open study of lamotrigine in refractory bipolar depression. *Psychiatry Res* 1997;**72**:145–8.

99. Lee DO, Steingard RJ, Cesena M, Helmers SL, Riviello JJ, Mikati MA. Behavioral side effects of gabapentin in children. *Epilepsia* 1996;**37**: 87–90.

100. Wolf SM, Shinnar S, Kang H, Balaban Gil K, Moshé SL. Gabapentin toxicity in children manifesting as behavioural changes. *Epilepsia* 1996;**36**:1203–5.

101. Ketter TA, Malow BA, Flamini R, Ko D, White SR, Post RM, Theodore WH. Felbamate monotherapy has stimulant-like effects in patients with epilepsy. *Epilepsy Res* 1996;**23**:129–37.

102. Novo Nordisk. *Tiagabine.* Product monograph, undated.

103. Janssen-Cilag. *Topamax.* Product monograph, 1996.

104. Davis GR, Armstrong HE, Donovan DM, Temkin NR. Cognitive behavioural treatment of depressed affect among epileptics. *J Clin Psychol* 1984;**40**:930–5.

105. Ferrari M, Verbanac A, Kane V. Family systems theory: an approach to therapy for families of patients with epilepsy. In: McConnell HW, Snyder PJ, eds. *Psychiatric comorbidity in epilepsy.* Washington DC: American Psychiatric Press, 1997:363–89.

106. Stevens JR. Clozapine: the yin and yang of seizures and psychosis. *Biol Psychiatry* 1995;**37**:425–6.

107. Dailey JW, Naritoku DK. Antidepressants and seizures: clinical anecdotes overshadow neuroscience. *Biochem Pharmacol* 1996;**52**:1323–9.

108. Robertson MM, Trimble MR. The treatment of depression in patients with epilepsy. a double-blind trial. *J Affect Disord* 1985;**9**: 127–36.

109. McConnell HW, Duncan D. In: McConnell HW, Snyder PJ, eds. *Psychiatric comorbidity in*

epilepsy. Washington DC: American Psychiatric Press, 1997:245–361.

110. Trimble MR, Schmitz B. On the psychoses of epilepsy. A neurobiological perspective. In: McConnell HW, Snyder PJ, eds. *Psychiatric comorbidity in epilepsy.* Washington DC:

American Psychiatric Press, 1997:169–86.

111. Trimble MR, Ring H, Schmitz B. Epilepsies and epileptic syndromes. In: Fogel BS, Schiffer RB, Rao SM, eds. *Neuropsychiatry.* Williams & Wilkins, Baltimore: 1996:771–803.

14

Neuropsychological assessment of memory functions in epilepsy

Mark Hendriks, Albert P Aldenkamp and Harry van der Vlugt

Introduction: memory complaints in epilepsy

Memory dysfunction is the most frequently reported cognitive complaint in the general population and in patients with epilepsy. Clinical experience corroborates this finding. In Chapter 22, Aldenkamp et al estimate that 15–20 per cent of patients with refractory epilepsy suffer from memory impairment.

However, memory complaints do not necessarily involve memory deficits. In fact, only moderate correlations (i.e. 0.30–0.40) are found between self-reported memory complaints and objective neuropsychological test results.[1] Several reasons have been suggested for this discrepancy. First, the 'ecological' validity of most neuropsychological tests may not be sufficient. Second, it is suggested that this discrepancy reflects the fact that memory problems are easy to recognize in daily living. Thus other cognitive dysfunctions, such as attentional deficits or language disorders, may go unnoticed, whereas the consequences may be experienced subjectively as memory impairment. For instance, a frequently reported memory complaint in the general population and in patients with epilepsy is the 'tip of the tongue' phenomenon.[2] It is still unclear whether such difficulties in word-finding are the result of language or memory dysfunction. Consequently, patients may overestimate their memory impairment in daily life.

Vermeulen et al[3] found that patients with epilepsy have more memory complaints than actual deficits on memory tests and suggest that this may be related to personality factors. Of course it is well known that the emotional context in which information is encoded influences memory functioning. This may also be related to the clinical observation that some patients complain about forgetting emotionally loaded episodes more easily. Deutsch et al[4] suggested that depression plays an important role in so-called metamemory in patients with temporal lobe epilepsy. They reported more depression than controls, but there were no differences in the level of depression or the accuracy of metamemory between patients with right or left temporal lobe epilepsy. If patients were reported to be more depressed then they underestimated their memory, but their actual memory performances with neuropsychological testing did not differ.

At the level of the individual patient this implies that in clinical practice it is almost impossible to give a good judgement of a patient's memory complaints. Research is mostly based on group comparisons, whereas clinical decisions have to be made on individual test data and on what the patient reports.

In this chapter we explore further the relation between epilepsy and memory deficits. Cognitive models of memory functions, and the cerebral systems that mediate them, will be described. It will be shown that these factors implicate a complex research design and have consequences for the neuropsychological assessment of the memory functions of patients with epilepsy.

Cognitive models of memory functions

The concepts of learning and memory are closely related. Learning may be seen as the process of acquiring information, whereas memory is the persistent consequence of this process.[5] The term memory is usually used to refer to a unitary, passive unit. However, research in cognitive and neuropsychology has shown that memory is the collection of a number of active cooperating functional subsystems that encode, store and reproduce information.[6] These subsystems are differentiated by:

1. The length of time for which information is stored.
2. Their storage capacity.
3. The type of information that is stored.

The most influential 'time-based' structure of memory was that proposed by Atkinson and Shiffrin.[7] They described memory as consisting of three memory systems: sensory, short-term and long-term memory. However, clinical observations showed that patients with a deficient short-term memory can learn and consolidate information. This indicates that these processes act in parallel, leading Baddeley and Hitch[8] to hypothesize that short-term memory is not a unitary store but a multi-component working memory. They propose that working memory consists of at least three subsystems: a phonological loop and a visuo-spatial scratchpad, for verbal and non-verbal material, and a central executive that acts as an interface between the subsystems.[9] Another characteristic of short-term memory is that it has limited storage capacity.

Like short-term memory, the structure of long-term memory consists of many cooperating subsystems. Squire and Zola-Morgan[10] propose a distinction between declarative and non-declarative memory. Non-declarative or procedural memory consists of all kinds of motor skills and is preserved in patients with the amnesic syndrome. Declarative memory contains semantic and episodic knowledge. In semantic memory our knowledge of the world is collected. It refers to the meaning of words and other facts that we gradually learn in school. With episodic memory we store and recollect personal events and experiences and it is this system that is very vulnerable to brain damage. The functional structure of the long-term storage systems is highly organized and is based on association. It is assumed that by the association of information our knowledge accumulates, and in this respect the capacity of the long-term memory system is not measurable.

The most frequent distinction in type of information is between verbal and non-verbal information.

Memory functions and the brain

Most of these memory systems are involved during cognitive function. Thus, the entire brain is involved in most memory processing but it is becoming apparent that some structures have a more important role than others. Squire[5] concluded that memory is distributed in a localizable and non-localizable way. He states that memory cannot be assigned to one specific brain location. The total amount of information is stored in many cooperating cerebral areas that are functionally similar.

Clinical neuropsychological research has provided much of our current knowledge about the neural basis of human memory.[11] Prolonged alcohol abuse may result in damage of the diencephalic structures, such as the dorsomedial nuclei of the thalamus, and causes severe memory deficits as part of the Korsakoff syndrome. The most well-known and intensively studied patient in neuropsychology is H.M., who received a bilateral resection of the mesial temporal lobes to control his epileptic seizures in 1953. The extraordinary aspect of H.M.'s amnesia is that it is very profound, pervasive and selective, affecting only certain facets of his memory and preserving others. Since these initial studies, the involvement of the temporal cortex and the mesial temporal structures (e.g. the hippocampal complex) has been proven, even though this involvement sometimes may be overestimated. The hippocampal complex plays a crucial role in the acquisition of new episodic knowledge, and any damage to it results in anterograde memory deficits. When the hippocampal complex in the left hemisphere is damaged it mostly leads to the reduced learning of verbal information. Damage of the right hippocampal complex causes specific problems in acquiring non-verbal knowledge.

Damage of the lateral temporal cortex affects the retrieval of previously learned information, which results in retrograde amnesia. Analogous to the functional lateralization of the mesial temporal structures, the temporal cortex of the left hemisphere is specialized in the retention of verbal semantic information and the right temporal cortex is involved in non-verbal knowledge such as the storage of faces.

Frontal brain structures also play an important role in memory. There is some debate about whether the frontal lobes have an additional function or participate directly in memory. Lesions to the frontal cortex produce an impairment in the strategic capacities that may result in deficits of prospective memory (i.e. remembering to do something).[12] As a consequence, patients have problems with tasks requiring memory for temporal order: they know what, but not in what order.[13] Also, so-called source memory is affected.[14] The recall of the source of information is disturbed because contextual aspects are not associated with the actual information. Finally, the basal forebrain associates different aspects of the material that has to be remembered. The functioning of this cerebral region combines the name, the face and all other different aspects in the memory of a particular person.[11]

Memory problems and epilepsy: is there a relation?

As early as 1885, Gowers[15] stated that memory deficit is one of the most frequent cognitive dysfunctions associated with epilepsy. Nevertheless, only during the last decade has special attention been paid to memory problems. In the past, most investigations were oriented at the global intellectual capacities and based on institutionalized patients, which has biased the conclusions. The development of neuropsychological tests for memory functions and the increasing emphasis on neurosurgical treatment for epilepsy have led to more comprehensive assessment procedures. However, in our opinion we have to be aware of the fact that the conclusions about cognitive function in people with epilepsy are determined by investigations on neurosurgical candidates, and this specific subpopulation is not representative of the patient with epilepsy in general. Knowledge in neuropsychology has probably gained more from pre-/postoperative studies on patients with epilepsy who have undergone surgery than otherwise.

The literature shows a number of epilepsy-related factors that may influence memory function in patients with epilepsy:

1. The presence and the localization of lesions.
2. The type of epilepsy and the electroclinical localization of the epileptic focus.
3. The age at onset of the epileptic seizures and the duration of active epilepsy.
4. Seizure frequency.
5. The cognitive side effects of antiepileptic medication.

Presence and localization of cerebral lesions

Epilepsy may be the symptom of many different types of brain pathology, such as trauma, brain infections, brain tumours or haemorrhages. All these pathological processes may, by themselves, cause memory deficits without the presence of epileptic seizures. In fact, they are assumed to be the most potent factor for the presence of memory problems. As early as the 1960s it was known that the cognitive abilities of people with symptomatic epilepsy were often less than those with idiopathic epilepsies.[16] The differentiation between symptomatic and idiopathic epilepsy is not as clear as it seems, in this respect. With symptomatic epilepsy there is a definite lesion. With idiopathic epilepsy the lesion is, in fact, unknown. The development of neuroimaging techniques such as magnetic resonance imaging (MRI) will increase the number of patients diagnosed as having a symptomatic epilepsy. For instance, many patients who now are diagnosed with the syndrome of mesial temporal sclerosis used to be considered to have a functional lesion.

It is still not determined whether sclerosis of the hippocampus is a cause or consequence of epileptic activity. Dam[17] concludes that neuron loss is related to the frequency of tonic–clonic seizures and the duration of the active epilepsy (more than 30 years). Neuron loss was not related to a certain type of epilepsy and in his opinion it must be regarded as an accumulating and continuous process. Additionally, brain damage preceding the onset of epileptic seizures can also be an influence.[18] Bertram et al[19] investigated these two models in an animal study. The results showed that hippocampal damage may be rather acute and the expected accumulating effect of seizures was in fact quite small. It was concluded that the hypothesis of progressive neuron loss in the hippocampus as an accumulated result of recurrent seizures could not be supported.

Unilateral damage of the hippocampal structures results in material-specific memory deficits. Some studies have examined the relationship between hippocampal sclerosis and memory function. Sass et al[20] investigated the correlation between neuron loss in specific areas of the hippocampus and different verbal functions. No correlation was found between verbal intelligence, other language functions and immediate and delayed story recall. Significant correlations were found between the retention of logical coherent verbal information and neuronal loss in the areas CA3 and CA4 of the hippocampus for patients with a left temporal focus. In a later study they used a verbal learning task because these tasks are better in distinguishing between patients with left or right hippocampal sclerosis.[21] The left temporal group was more impaired in verbal learning than those with right temporal hippocampal sclerosis. Again, the correlation was found in those with neuron loss in the areas CA3 and CA4. Jones-Gotman[22] used self-developed verbal and non-verbal learning tasks in patients with left or right hippocampal sclerosis. The advantage of her technique is that it follows the same procedure in both tests and she found the expected dissociations between left and right patient groups.

In general, the correlation between right hippocampal neuron loss and non-verbal memory deficits seems less strong. To our knowledge only in a recent study by Matkovic et al[23] was a significant correlation found between right hippocampal neuron loss and test performances in a test for the reproduction of geometric designs.

Type of epilepsy and the electroclinical localization of the epileptic focus

An epileptic focus in the absence of an established cerebral lesion may indicate a functional impairment rather than a lesion and disactivate local cerebral systems that are of importance for memory functioning. Most of the research on this factor is based on patients who are candidates for surgery for their pharmacologically intractable epilepsy. The well-described localization of the electroclinical epileptic activity in these patients makes it possible to study correlations between local dysfunctions in the brain and the pattern of neuropsychological deficits. However, this is a selected group within the total population of patients with epilepsy, and there is a risk of sample selection bias. Another problem with pre-/postoperative studies may be that cognitive function is influenced more by the cortical resection itself than by the epileptic focus.

An epileptic seizure or epileptic discharges can disrupt all kinds of functions, including memory. Epileptic activity in the hippocampal formation can disrupt the process of long-term potentiation *in vitro*.[24] Long-term potentiation is crucial for the neuronal plasticity that is

responsible for the storage of episodic information. The process of long-term potentiation can last a few minutes to several days, so an epileptic seizure or discharge may influence memory more than just during the actual episode with discharges. Halgren et al[25] found that the performance of patients with an episode of partial seizures was much more impaired on memory tests two days afterwards than two weeks later. Of course, this does not mean that a disturbance in long-term potentiation is the cause of these deficits, but it illustrates that it is not just the epileptic seizure that is of importance.

Some studies found evidence for transient memory deficits as a consequence of subclinical activity in the temporal brain structures during the execution of memory tasks.[26] Left-sided discharges caused deficits in verbal learning, and discharges in the right hemisphere resulted in deficits of non-verbal learning.

Support for a direct relation between epileptic activity and memory deficits can be found in case studies that describe subjects with so-called amnesic epileptic attacks,[27,28] transient memory deficits being the only clinical symptom. Electro-encephalogram registrations show discharges from the hippocampus and medial temporal brain areas, without exception. When antiepileptic drugs are used, the amnesic attacks disappear in most cases. The methodological problem with these case reports is that these studies are done retrospectively and are based on subjective complaints. Brigman et al[29] tested two patients during subclinical hippocampal seizures and concluded that these seizures were responsible for the memory deficits.

When seizure type is analysed, more cognitive impairment is found in patients with tonic–clonic generalized seizures when compared with partial seizures.[30,31] However, studies that reported these findings rarely use adequate examination of memory functions. Already in 1955, Quadfasel and Pruyser[32] found that memory was specifically impaired in a group with partial seizures when compared with a group of patients with generalized seizures. In several recent studies the specific memory problems in patients with complex partial seizures have been confirmed, and these investigations have consistently documented material-specific memory deficits equally to those found with cerebral lesions.[33,34] However, this finding cannot be interpreted in isolation because most of these patients will have temporal lobe dysfunctions.

Age at onset of the epileptic seizures and the duration of active epilepsy

Matthews and Kløve[35] found that in patients with tonic-clonic seizures of early onset, intellectual functioning was more impaired. Also, Dikmen et al[36] described lower intelligence scores for adult patients with a seizure onset of tonic–clonic seizures before 5 years of age, compared with a group of patients in whom seizures started between the age of 10 and 15 years. It is hypothesized that cerebral dysfunction before the age of 5 years may influence lateralization patterns of cognitive function. In more than 96 per cent of the right-handed population and 67 per cent of the left-handed population, the left hemisphere predominantly mediates language functions and the right hemisphere mediates visual spatial abilities. This lateralization process can be disrupted by a left-sided focus before the age of 5 years. Children may develop pathological left-handedness and the mediation of language functions may consequently shift from the left to the right hemisphere. As a consequence, visual spatial abilities may not develop to their full potential; the so-called 'crowding effect'.[37]

Van der Vlugt and Bakker[38] found support for this hypothesis in a study with adult epileptic patients.

Dodrill[39] suggests that age at onset may be more strongly related to cognitive function than to other seizure-related variables. An early onset of seizures increases the risk of brain damage, developmental problems, lesser education, the early prescription of medication with negative side effects on cognitive functioning and the possibility of an accumulating effect of seizure frequency on cerebral organization.

Additionally, duration of active epilepsy might also be an influential variable with respect to cognitive decline.[40] This factor is of course correlated with age at onset. Delaney et al[41] investigated the memory functions of patients with localization-related epilepsies and concluded that those with a longer duration showed more deficits. However, Dodrill[39] concludes that the duration of epilepsy compared with other factors 'tends to be somewhat weaker than others'. Farwell et al[42] concluded that there was a stronger causal relation between cognitive function and the number of years in which seizures actually occurred. Herman and Whitman[43] agree with these authors and suggest that duration be defined as the number of years in which the epilepsy was active.

Seizure frequency

One might argue that if seizures cause cognitive deficits then more seizures will cause more severe cognitive deficits.[44] The literature, however, does not always support this relationship, possibly because of the plethora of methodological problems related to this factor. First, seizure frequency at one particular moment in time is often the only parameter available, and not the total amount of seizures in the patient's life. Yet this latter factor may be more important for explaining cognitive impairment. If the total amount of seizures is taken into account, it is always estimated. Second, seizure severity may be important, but a clear estimation of severity is not always available. Third, a high seizure frequency may simply reflect the severity of the underlying cerebral pathology.

Yet data do suggest that the effect of seizure frequency is important. Loiseau et al,[45] for example, did not find memory impairment in patients with seizure remission or in patients with low seizure frequency, and Dodrill[46] found positive evidence for cognitive impairment in patients with high seizure frequency. In particular, patients who had more than 100 tonic–clonic seizures in their lives showed most impairments. Interestingly, patients who experienced one or more episodes of status epilepticus in their lives showed even more cognitive impairment. It therefore seems important to consider status epilepticus as a separate seizure-related factor when studying cognitive deficits.

Cognitive side effects of antiepileptic medication

The relationship between memory deficits and epilepsy was described long before the introduction of current antiepileptic drugs. However, since the development of a variety of antiepileptics it has been indicated that some of these drugs may cause cognitive side effects, including memory problems. In particular, high serum levels or toxic doses will impair cognitive functioning. In clinical practice most concern should be given to possible cognitive deficits caused by antiepileptic medication within the therapeutic range. Another more general finding is that the negative effects of polytherapy are more profound than of monotherapy.[47]

Recent reviews and meta-analyses[48] have found most evidence of drug-induced cognitive impairments for phenobarbitone and phenytoin, and information processing speed and memory are found to be the critical areas. For valproate and carbamazepine, minimal adverse cognitive effects are reported.

Implications for clinical practice

Memory must be considered as a complex of active cooperating functional subsystems that cannot be assigned to one specific cerebral localization. Also, epilepsy must be regarded as a multifactorial condition. These many different aspects implicate a plethora of possible relationships between 'epileptic factors' (i.e. seizures, frequency, age at onset) and memory systems. As a consequence, most researchers have concentrated on one or a few different aspects, and systematic research of the prevalence, manifestation and aetiology of memory problems in patients with epilepsy has been sparse. Ossetin[49] therefore suggests the use of multiple neuropsychological tests in order to investigate memory functions.

Based on these arguments, research has to focus on the relative contribution of each separate 'epilepsy-related' factor. However, these factors are often associated, e.g. the duration of epilepsy is associated with a longer duration of the use of medication and also with age at onset.

Neuropsychological assessment in epilepsy

Neuropsychological assessment is a standardized way of enhancing observations. With this, self-reports by the patients or their relatives and clinical observations by the neurologist can be confirmed psychometrically. To do so, we use an individualized, hypothesis-testing assessment approach.[50] We use composite batteries of tests that are presented in a formalized way but with qualitative interpretations of performances; the pattern of test results being just as important as the test scores. Test results must be interpreted within the context of the relationships between behaviour and cerebral functioning.

The initial goal of neuropsychological assessment was the differential diagnosis of organic versus functional disorders. At present, the development of neuroimaging techniques such as functional magnetic resonance imaging (fMRI), positron emission tomography (PET), magneto-encephalography (MEG), etc. has had a significant impact on clinical neuropsychology. Nevertheless, the most sensitive measure of cerebral dysfunction is still behaviour, especially in epilepsy, so neuropsychological assessment remains an important diagnostic tool. Secondly, a neuropsychological assessment is used to direct patient care and rehabilitation, providing information about the possible effects of treatment, e.g. the effects of antiepileptic medication or surgical interventions.

Neuropsychological assessment of memory functions in patients with epilepsy

The measurement of memory functions must firstly reflect the theoretical structure of memory. This implicates that a neuropsychological battery for memory should include measurements of verbal and non-verbal information and tests of short- and long-term recall, learning and recognition. An international, widely used test battery for memory functions is the revised Wechsler Memory Scale (WMS-r).[51] The WMS-r consists of several subtests and provides a broad evaluation of short-term verbal and non-verbal memory and attentional skills. Furthermore, a compound index for long-term memory is provided. Moore and Baker[52] investigated the psychometric properties of the WMS-r in

patients with epilepsy who were candidates for temporal lobe surgery, and identified indications for a verbal memory factor, a visual memory factor and a factor that reflects attentional processes. In time with other reports, they noticed that it is difficult to develop tasks that measure only non-verbal memory.

None the less, there are still a few shortcomings. In the WMS-r there are no tasks for recognition. Also, it is not possible to make a qualitative analysis of learning characteristics such as learning rate, rate of forgetting and semantic clustering. For these reasons in our assessment we included a verbal learning test,[53] which is originally based on the California Verbal Learning Test,[54] recognition tests for words and figures and rhythm discrimination (FePsy).[55] In addition, tests for simple reaction time measurement, finger tapping, vigilance and visual searching task of the FePsy battery are also included. Although computerized tests will never replace the paper and pencil testing procedure, they can have advantages as additive components of a neuropsychological assessment battery. Technically, the stimuli are always presented in the same way and the responses of the patients are scored and stored automatically. This may be of particular importance with testing the effects of antiepileptic drugs. An advantage of FePsy that specifically accounts for the diagnostic procedures in patients with epilepsy is the possibility of linking the presentation of the tests with EEG/video recording and finding out if epileptic discharges have an effect on cognitive function. The most important disadvantage of computerized psychological assessment is that these highly standardized quantitative testing procedures do not analyse the qualitative behavioural aspects of how responses come about. The complexity of the assessment of brain–behaviour relationships requires an integration of the strengths of both techniques

Domain	Aspect[a]	Test[b]
Intelligence		Wechsler Adult Intelligence Scale (WAIS)
Memory functions	Verbal STM	Digit span (WAIS)
		Simultaneous word recognition (FePsy)
		Verbal memory index (WMS-r)
		California verbal learning test (VLGT)
	Verbal LTM	Delayed recall verbal subtests (WMS-r)
		Delayed recall and recognition (VLGT)
		Information (WAIS)
		Vocabulary (WAIS)
	Non-verbal STM	Simultaneous figure recognition (FePsy)
		Seashore rhythm (FePsy)
		Visual memory index (WMS-r)
	Non-verbal LTM	Delayed recall non-verbal subtests (WMS-r)
		Delayed recall CFT
	Metamemory	Memory questionnaire
Language	Word knowledge	Vocabulary (WAIS)
	Verbal fluency	UNKA test
	Lateralization	Dichotic listening
Visual constructive functions	Perception	Picture completion (WAIS)
		Visual searching (FePsy)
	Construction	Block design (WAIS)
		Object assembly (WAIS)
	Drawing	Complex figure test of Rey
Attention and concentration	Attention	Simple auditive reaction time (FePsy)
	Focused attention	Stroop colour word test
	Divided attention	Trail making test
	Sustained attention	Vigilance (FePsy)
Fine motor functions	Tapping	Tapping (FePsy)

[a]STM, short-term memory; LTM, long-term memory.
[b]WMS-r, revised Wechsler Memory Scale; CFT, complex figure test.

Table 14.1
Neuropsychological test battery for memory problems.

and the theoretical contributions. A neuropsychological assessment must adapt to the patient, and not the other way around.

Finally, we included a memory questionnaire to assess the kind of memory problems that occur in everyday life.[3]

Memory functions cannot be assessed in isolation from adjacent cognitive functions, especially those that are also mediated by the temporal lobes, such as language functions in the left hemisphere and visual spatial functions in the right hemisphere. Within the domain of language we examine aspects such as naming, fluency, vocabulary and lateralization. With regard to visual spatial functions, tests for visual spatial perception and scanning are included, as well as tests for visual constructive abilities such as object assembly and drawing.

Concentration or attentional deficits may lead to memory difficulties in daily life. If the attention span is too short, if patients are incapable of processing information in parallel or if they are very susceptible to interference, then information is stored less well. Also, non-cognitive functions such as personality traits and mood may have an impact on memory function or neuropsychological test performance.[4] For this reason we included some personality questionnaires.

In the Netherlands there is agreement on the neuropsychological test battery for patients with epilepsy who are referred for memory problems (Table 14.1).

When discussing the results of neuropsychological assessment with the patients and their relatives, we should consider the worries that patients sometimes have about memory impairment as a first sign of dementia. Moreover, many patients relate or associate their memory problems with their antiepileptic medication. If the conclusions of the neuropsychological tests show that the memory complaints are based on clear memory deficits, then memory training to support these problems can be offered. However, this does not implicate that if the complaints are not caused by a cerebral dysfunction that a treatment is not indicated. Memory complaints should always be taken seriously; the cause just directs the treatment approach. The impact of the memory complaints on daily life also depends on the patient's everyday activities or the demands that the patient faces in a job or at school.

References

1. Berg I. *Memory rehabilitation for closed-head injured patients.* Dissertation, 1993.
2. Thompson PJ, Corcoran R. Everyday memory failures in people with epilepsy. *Epilepsia* 1992;**33** (Suppl 6):18–20.
3. Vermeulen J, Aldenkamp AP, Alpherts WCJ. Memory complaints in epilepsy: correlations with cognitive performance and neuroticism. *Epilepsy Res* 1993;**15**:157–70.
4. Deutsch GK, Saykin AJ, Sperling MR. Metamemory in temporal lobe epilepsy. *Assessment* 1996;**3**:255–63.
5. Squire LR. *Memory and brain.* New York: Oxford University Press, 1987.
6. Baddeley AD. The psychology of memory. In: Baddeley AD, Wilson BA, Watts FN, eds. *Handbook of memory disorders.* Chichester: John Wiley & Sons, 1995.
7. Atkinson RC, Shiffrin RM. Human memory: a proposed system and its control processes. In: Spence KW, ed. *The psychology of learning and motivation: advances in research and theory,* Vol. 2. New York: Academic Press, 1968.
8. Baddeley AD, Hitch G. Working memory. In: Bower GA, ed. *The psychology of learning and motivation,* Vol. 8. New York: Academic Press, 1974.
9. Baddeley AD, Wilson BA, Watts FN, eds. *Handbook of memory disorders.* Chichester: John Wiley & Sons, 1995.
10. Squire LR, Zola-Morgan S. Memory: brain systems and behavior. *Trends Neurosci* 1988;**11**:170–6.
11. Tranel D, Damasio AR. Neurobiological foundations of human memory. In: Baddeley AD, Wilson BA, Watts FN, eds. *Handbook of memory disorders.* Chichester: John Wiley & Sons, 1995.

12. Manich MT. *Neuropsychology: the neural bases of mental function.* Boston: Houghton Mifflin Company, 1997.

13. Shimamura AP, Janowsky JS, Squire LR. What is the role of frontal lobe damage in memory disorder? In: Levin HS, Eisenberg HM, Benton AL, eds. *Frontal lobe function and dysfunction.* New York: Oxford University Press, 1991.

14. Janowski JS, Shimamura AP, Squire LR. Source memory impairment in patients with frontal lobe lesions. *Neuropsychologia* 1989;**27**(8): 1043–56.

15. Gowers WR. *Epilepsy and chronic convulsive disorders.* New York: William Wood, 1885.

16. Kløve H, Matthews CG. Psychometric and adaptive abilities in epilepsy with differential etiology. *Epilepsia* 1966;**7**:330–8.

17. Dam AM. Epilepsy and neuron loss in the hippocampus. *Epilepsia* 1980;**21**:617–29.

18. Dam AM. Hippocampal neuron loss and epilepsy. *Acta Neurol Scand* 1982;**65**:195–6.

19. Bertram EH, Lotham EW, Lenn NJ. The hippocampus in experimental chronic epilepsy: a morphometric analysis. *Annals of Neurology* 1990;**27**(1):43–8.

20. Sass KJ, Sass A, Westerveld M, Lencz T, Novelly RA, Kim JH, Spencer DD. Specificity in the correlation of verbal memory and hippocampal neuron loss: dissociation of memory, language, and verbal intellectual ability. *J Clin Exp Neuropsychol* 1992;**14**: 662–72.

21. Sass KJ, Westerveld M, Buchanan C. Degree of hippocampal neuron loss determines severity of verbal memory decrease after left anteromesiotemporal lobectomy. *Epilepsia* 1994;**35**: 1179–86.

22. Jones-Gotman M. Psychological evaluation for epilepsy surgery. In: Shorvon S, Dreifuss F, Fish D, Thomas D, eds. *The treatment of epilepsy.* Oxford: Blackwell Science, 1996.

23. Matkovic Z, Oxbury SM, Hiorns RW, Morris JH, Carpenter KN. Hippocampal neuronal density correlates with pre-operative non-verbal memory in patients with temporal lobe epilepsy. *Epilepsia* 1995;**36** (Suppl 3):S93.

24. Moore SD, Barr DS, Wilson WA. Seizure-like activity disrupts LTP *in vitro. Neurosci Lett* 1993;**163**:117–19.

25. Halgren E, Stapleton J, Domalshi P, Swartz BE, Delgado-Escueta AV, Walsh GO, Mandelhern M, Blahd W, Ropchan J. Memory dysfunction in epilepsy patients as a derangement of normal physiology. In: Smith D, Treiman D, Trimble M, eds. *Advances in neurology,* Vol. 55. New York: Raven Press, 1991:385–410.

26. Aarts JPH, Binnie CD, Smit AM, Wilkins AJ. Selective cognitive impairment during focal and generalised epileptiform EEG activity. *Brain* 1984;**107**:293–308.

27. Pritchard PB III, Holmstrom VL, Roitzsch JC, Giacinto J. Epileptic amnesic attacks: benefit from antiepileptic drugs. *Neurology* 1985;**35**: 1188–9.

28. Gallasi R, Morreale A, Lorusso S, Pazzaglia P, Lugaressi E. Epilepsy presenting as memory disturbances. *Epilepsia* 1988;**29**:624–9.

29. Brigman PA, Malamut BL, Sperling MR, Saykin AJ, O'Connor MJ. Memory during subclinical hippocampal seizures. *Neurology* 1989;**39**: 853–6.

30. Rausch R, Victoroff JI. Neuropsychological factors related to behavior disorders in epilepsy. In: Devinsky O, Theodore WH, eds. *Epilepsy and behavior.* New York: Wiley–Liss, 1991.

31. Perrien K, Gershengorn J, Brown ER. Interictal neuropsychological function in epilepsy. In: Devinsky O, Theodore WH, eds. *Epilepsy and behavior.* New York: Wiley-Liss, 1991.

32. Quadfasel AF, Pruyser PW. Cognitive deficits in patients with psychomotor epilepsy. *Epilepsia* 1955;**4**:80–90.

33. Hermann BP, Wyler AR, Richey ET, Rea JM. Memory function and verbal learning ability in patients with complex partial seizures of temporal origin. *Epilepsia* 1987;**28**:547–54.

34. Bornstein RA, Drake ME, Pakalnis A. Effects of seizure type and waveform abnormality on memory and attention. *Arch Neurol* 1988;**45**:884–7.

35. Matthews CG, Kløve H. Differential psychological performances in major motor, psychomotor and mixed seizure classification of known and unknown etiology. *Epilepsia* 1967; **8**:117–28.

36. Dikmen S, Matthews CG, Harley JP. The effect of early versus late onset of major motor epilepsy upon cognitive-intellectual performance. *Epilepsia* 1975;**16**:73–81.

37. Spreen O, Tupper D, Risser A, Tuokko H,

Edgell D. *Human developmental neuropsychology*. New York: Oxford University Press, 1984.

38. Van der Vlugt H, Bakker D. Lateralization of brain function in persons with epilepsy. In: Kulig BM, Meinardi H, Stores G, eds. *Epilepsy and behavior '79*. Lisse: Swets & Zeitlinger, 1980.

39. Dodrill CB. Neuropsychological aspects of epilepsy. *Psychiatr Clin North Am* 1992;**15**: 383–94.

40. Rodin EA, Schmaltz S, Twitty G. Intellectual functions of patients with childhood-onset epilepsy. *Dev Med Child Neurol* 1986;**28**: 25–33.

41. Delaney RC, Rosen AJ, Mattson RH, Novelly RA. Memory function in focal epilepsy: a comparison of non-surgical, unilateral and temporal lobe and frontal lobe samples. *Cortex* 1980;**16**:103–17.

42. Farwell JR, Dodrill CB, Batzel LW. Neuropsychological abilities of children with epilepsy. *Epilepsia* 1985;**26**:395–412.

43. Herman HP, Whitman S. Psychopathology in epilepsy: a multietiologic model. In: Hermann BP, Whitman S, eds. *Psychopathology in epilepsy; social dimensions*. New York: Oxford University Press, 1986.

44. Bennett TL. Cognitive effects of epilepsy and anticonvulsant medications. In: Bennett TL, ed. *The neuropsychology of epilepsy*. New York: Plenum Press, 1992; 73–96.

45. Loiseau P, Struber E, Broustet D, Battellochi S, Gauneni C, Morselli PL. Learning impairment in epileptic patients. *Epilepsia* 1983;**24**:183–92.

46. Dodrill CB. Correlates of generalized tonic-clonic seizures with intellectual, neuropsychological, emotional, and social function in patients with epilepsy. *Epilepsia* 1986;**27**:399–411.

47. Trimble MR. Anticonvulsant drugs and cognitive function: a review of the literature. *Epilepsia* 1987;**28** (Suppl 3):s37–45.

48. Vermeulen J, Aldenkamp AP. Cognitive side-effects of chronic antiepileptic drug treatment: a review of 25 years of research. *Epilepsy Res* 1995;**22**:65–95.

49. Ossetin J. Methods and problems in the assessment of cognitive function in epilepsy patients. In: Trimble, M, Reynolds E, eds. *Epilepsy, behaviour and cognitive function*. Chichester: Wiley, 1988.

50. Lezak M. *Neuropsychological Assessment*, 3rd edn. New York: Oxford University Press, 1995.

51. Wechsler D. *Manual for the Wechsler Memory Scale—Revised, 1987*. York: Psychological Corporation, 1987.

52. Moore PM, Baker GA. Psychometric properties and factor structure of the Wechsler Memory Scale–Revised in a sample of persons with intractable epilepsy. *J Clin Exp Neuropsychol* 1997;**19**:897–905.

53. Mulder JL, Dekker R, Dekker PH. *Verbale Leer en Geheugen Test*. Lisse: Swets & Zeitlinger, 1996.

54. Delis DC, Kramer JH, Kaplan E, Ober BA. *California Verbal Learning Test. Research Edition*. New York: Psychological Corporation/Harcourt Brace Jovanovich, 1987.

55. Alpherts WCJ, Aldenkamp AP. Computerised neuropsychological assessment of cognitive functioning in children with epilepsy. *Epilepsia* 1990;**31** (Suppl 3):s35–40.

THERAPEUTIC CHALLENGES

VI

INITIATION AND TERMINATION OF TREATMENT

15

Starting antiepileptic drugs

Anne T Berg and David W Chadwick

Introduction

Antiepileptic drugs (AEDs) are highly effective at suppressing seizures in seizure-prone patients. On the other hand, all of the AEDs are associated with idiosyncratic and dose-related side effects, and some of the more recently approved drugs can be expensive. In addition, the very fact that a patient is taking a drug on a regular basis carries a stigma and may influence that patient's well-being. In the past, concern that seizures might be part of an escalating process (seizures beget seizures)[1] led to the rather aggressive use of AEDs in the hope that suppression of seizures could alter the supposedly malignant process underlying epilepsy.[2] As the natural history of seizures and epilepsy became better understood, it became clear that this was not of paramount concern, especially early in the course of the disorder. Consequently, the rational use of AEDs depends on a thorough understanding and assessment of what AEDs can and cannot do in specific situations, as well as the risks associated with treatment and its alternative—nontreatment.

This chapter discusses three different situations in which a decision to initiate AEDs might be considered: 1) in patients at risk of developing unprovoked seizures and epilepsy who have not yet experienced a first unprovoked seizure; 2) in patients who come to medical attention after having experienced only the first unprovoked seizure; and 3) in patients who have experienced at least two separate unprovoked seizures and therefore meet the accepted definition of epilepsy.[4] In each of these situations, the chapter considers the risks faced by the patient, the potential goals of treatment, what treatment can actually accomplish versus what it cannot based upon available evidence and the problems associated with treatment. Finally we provide some guidelines regarding the selection of AEDs in various scenarios. Ultimately the decision to treat will be based on the interaction of many factors. The decision must be individualized in each instance.

Situations in which treatment might be considered

Patients at risk of developing epilepsy

In certain situations, AEDs have been used prophylactically, before unprovoked seizures have even occurred, in the hope of preventing unprovoked seizures and epilepsy. The primary goal of treating was not just prevention of acute provoked seizures, but alteration of the longer term prognosis associated with the insult or condition, and ultimately, the prevention of epilepsy. This has been subject to study in randomized clinical trials in at least four settings: a) following craniotomy, b) after head trauma, c) in patients with cerebral tumors and d) in children with benign febrile seizures.

Craniotomy

Patients who undergo craniotomy face a number of risks as a result of the indication for surgery and the surgery itself. The incidence of seizures and epilepsy after craniotomy has been reported to be ~20 per cent, although the risk varies considerably with the underlying reason for surgery.[5] In a randomized trial of patients who underwent craniotomy for a variety of neurological conditions, patients were randomized to receive either phenytoin or carbamazepine for either 6 or 24 months.[6] Although the risk of seizures was lower in patients while they were on medication, there were no substantial differences among the different treatment groups in the proportion who were seizure-free after 4 years. Thus treatment suppressed the occurrence of seizures during active treatment. However, it did not result in a long-term benefit in terms of an overall reduction in the risk of unprovoked seizures once treatment was stopped.

Head trauma

One study randomized patients immediately after severe head trauma to 1 year of treatment with either phenytoin or placebo.[7] This study clearly demonstrated that the incidence of acute provoked seizures during treatment was substantially lower in the treatment group compared with the placebo group (4 per cent versus 14 per cent). However, at the end of 2 years, the incidence of unprovoked seizures was actually slightly higher in the treatment group compared with the placebo group (28 per cent versus 21 per cent). Treatment could suppress the expression of seizures, but did not

reduce the risk of later epilepsy which is, in all likelihood, caused by the severity and nature of the brain trauma rather than the occurrence of acute post-traumatic seizures.

A subsequent study by the same investigators examined patients with head trauma who were randomized to one of three groups: 1 week phenytoin, 1 month valproate, 6 months valproate.[8] The risk of late seizures was 14, 16, and 22 per cent in each group, respectively. Mortality was significantly higher in the valproate groups compared with the phenytoin group (14 per cent versus 8 per cent). Overall, longer periods of treatment appeared to be less beneficial. Whether there are true drug differences in the risk of mortality or the differences are due to duration of treatment cannot be determined because of the design of the study.

A recent systematic review of randomized clinical trials (RCTs) of AEDs following head injury concluded that there was no evidence that AEDs reduced the risk of late seizures and epilepsy.[9]

Brain tumors

Three RCTs have investigated the possible effects of AEDs in patients with cerebral tumors. The numbers at risk are too small to exclude beneficial effects, but no obvious reduction in risk was apparent.[10-12]

Febrile seizures

Finally, three randomized trials of children with febrile seizures examined this issue.[13-15] In all three trials, children who experienced at least one febrile seizure were randomized either to some form of AED treatment or to placebo. During each trial, the treated group had a lower risk of recurrent febrile seizures than those in the placebo group. With longer term follow-up, no differences were discernible in the risk of subsequent unprovoked seizures in the treated versus the placebo groups.[16-18]

Summary

Early treatment does reduce the risk of acute provoked seizures in the particular situations that have been studied. At the same time, there is no evidence to support the use of AEDs to improve long-term seizure outcomes. Provoked seizures may be associated with an increased risk of later unprovoked seizures and epilepsy. Provoked seizures are most likely a marker for the severity of brain injury,[19-22] and it is the latter which is then associated with the risk of late seizures. The provoked seizures themselves are not a cause of the late seizures. Treatment can suppress the expression of this marker, but it cannot alter the underlying predisposition to later seizures. All available evidence suggests this is not an attainable goal, at least with the forms of therapy studied to date.

There is increasing interest in neuroprotective agents. Whether sparing more of the marginal tissue after brain injury can result in lower risk of epilepsy is unknown. Commonly used AEDs are not known to have neuroprotective effects in these situations. There is some interest in vigabatrin as a possible neuroprotective agent as well as an AED. Most of this work has been done in experimental models of temporal lobe epilepsy, not in acute trauma, stroke or craniotomy.[23]

Problems associated with treatment

Long-term AED therapy always carries a risk of side effects (idiosyncratic, dose-related, chronic, and teratogenic). These effects may range from relatively mild to serious, and on occasion, potentially fatal. The risks of adverse effects of treatment are much more difficult to quantify than the benefits. In particular, the risk of rare but serious adverse reactions cannot be determined from RCTs. The likelihood that treatment can actually prevent late epilepsy is, at best, so small that hundreds, perhaps thousands, of patients would need to be treated and exposed to drug-related risks to prevent one late case of epilepsy. At a practical level, patient compliance with such a policy is also likely to be very poor. In addition, because the risk of seizures persists for many years, it is unclear how long the physician should recommend that treatment be continued. This, however, does not preclude the short-term use of AEDs in selected cases to prevent acute symptomatic seizures.

The issues surrounding the treatment of febrile seizures have created tremendous controversy in the past.[24,25] Fewer than 10 per cent of children with febrile seizures eventually go on to have unprovoked seizures. However, in these children, there is a risk of recurrent febrile seizures, of about 30–40 per cent during the 2 or more years after the initial febrile seizure. Treatment reduces this risk by up to half, but the cost to the patient and family may be prohibitive. During an illness the commonly used medications are daily phenobarbital or diazepam. The former causes significant behavioral side effects and is often discontinued for these reasons. One RCT found that there was some persistence in cognitive and developmental side effects long after the phenobarbital had been discontinued,[26] suggesting that such treatment does more long-term, and perhaps, permanent, harm than the disorder itself, which is now generally acknowledged to be benign.[27]

Alternatively, diazepam is given only when a child who is prone to febrile seizures is ill. It is effective in lowering the risk of recurrent febrile seizures, but only if the parents recognize the illness and can administer the medication before a seizure occurs. Diazepam is also associated with significant sedative effects. These persist only as long as the child is treated, yet, one of the most important assessments of illness severity in a young child is behavior and state of alertness. Thus, the administration of diazepam may prevent accurate assessment of illness severity, and lead parents to miss a serious illness or lead to excessive diagnostic testing in the face of uncertainty regarding the cause of the lethargy or changes in mental status. The relatively modest effect of treatment coupled with its disadvantages has led one authority in the field to suggest that 'talking is the best medicine for febrile seizures'.[28]

Patients who present with a single unprovoked seizure

This section is limited to those patients who, as best as can be determined, have never previously experienced an unprovoked seizure. By necessity, this tends to focus on patients presenting after their first tonic–clonic seizure and will exclude patients with several forms of epilepsy that are almost never identified at the time of the first seizure (e.g. absence epilepsy, infantile spasms, temporal lobe epilepsy). It will also exclude patients who simply did not seek medical attention for the first seizure episode.

In the not-too-distant past, it was common practice in the US to institute AED therapy in most patients who presented with a first seizure. This practice was driven by two related concerns: 1) the belief that seizure recurrence was inevitable; and 2) the fear that seizure disorders were progressive.

The risk of seizure recurrence in patients who present after their first unprovoked seizure is ~40 per cent during the 2 years after the initial seizure.[29] In those studies with long-term follow-up, the risk continues to rise a little each year, but most recurrences occur within the first 2 years. At the time of a first seizure, there are two or three salient factors that can distinguish patients at especially high (>50 per cent) and fairly low (~20 per cent) risk of recurrence. The best studied factors are the presence of

EEG abnormalities and remote symptomatic etiology. The presence of each of these factors independently increases the risk of a recurrent seizure. Patients with both factors have a higher risk than those with just one. Three studies have also found that patients whose first seizure occurs during sleep are two to three times more likely to have a recurrence than those whose seizures occur during wakefulness.[30–32] In one study, patients with normal EEGs and a cryptogenic etiology, those who had a first seizure while awake had a risk of recurrence at 2 years of ~20 per cent, versus 40 per cent if they had been asleep when the first seizure occurred.[30]

Although patients who have a first seizure while asleep are at higher risk of having a second seizure, they are also most likely (~75 per cent) to have the second seizure while asleep.[30] Thus the higher risk of seizure recurrence is somewhat mitigated by the relatively safer circumstances under which the seizure is most likely to occur.

Status epilepticus represents a neurological emergency.[41] Fortunately, patients who present with status as their first seizure do not seem to have an increased risk for a recurrent seizure. However, should their seizures recur, these patients have a higher risk of having an episode of status than patients whose first seizures were relatively briefer. This was first observed in children with febrile seizures[33] and then in children with unprovoked seizures.[30] Subsequently the tendency for status to recur has been studied in three different groups of adults with epilepsy[34] and another group of children with refractory epilepsy.[35] While treatment cannot eliminate the risk of a seizure recurrence, and of status in particular, the reduction in risk in these patients with chronic AED may be worth while.

Mortality is an important outcome that cannot be overlooked. In studies of patients with first seizures, few if any data have been reported on deaths associated with recurrence. This does not mean that deaths do not occur, but that they are so infrequent as to be rarely reported in the available studies. In general, mortality is not a primary concern in patients who present with a first seizure. The risk of seizure-associated mortality would parallel that for seizure recurrence and perhaps be influenced by prior episodes of status epilepticus as well as seizure type (particularly generalized tonic–clonic seizures). Thus, for most patients with a first seizure, mortality is not an overriding factor in making treatment decisions after a first seizure.

Treatment for a first seizure

Three RCTs that examined the efficacy of treatment after a first unprovoked seizure, each found a reduction (~50 per cent) in the risk of a second seizure.[36–38]

The study from Milan[37] was the largest study and randomized over 400 patients (primarily adults) to immediate treatment after the first seizure or to delayed treatment in the event of a second seizure. The treated group experienced half as many recurrences as the initially untreated group. Prolonged follow-up in this RCT revealed that despite the lower recurrence risk in patients treated after the first seizure, the long-term outcome of remission was identical in the immediate and delayed treatment groups.[39] Because immediate treatment did not alter long-term outcome, improvement in long-term seizure control was not shown to be a valid goal of early institution of therapy. Well-analysed observational data from several large population-based cohorts have also suggested similar conclusions. These studies tend to report that the number of seizures prior to instituting treatment does not influence the long-term chances for achieving remission.[40–43]

As discussed previously, treatment is associated with a number of potential side effects.

Long-term treatment can also be a source of financial and psychosocial strain on the patient and his or her family. While the available evidence supports the use of early treatment for reducing the risk of recurrence, treatment does not prevent all recurrences and patients who are treated still have about half the risk of recurrence as those who are treated. This point should be emphasized to the patient lest he or she be lulled into a false sense of security. For these reasons, the same precautions that are recommended for an untreated patient still apply to one who is treated. These include close supervision of children with seizures, insistence on the use of helmets for some activities (e.g. bicycling), refraining from certain activities (often recreational) that might be especially dangerous if a seizure were to occur, and for adults, refraining from driving for a certain period as dictated by local law.

The decision whether to start treatment after the first seizure depends on the individual patient's risk of recurrence, the consequences of a recurrence, the level of risk that is acceptable to the patient and his or her family, and the patient's attitude towards treatment. In children, the consequences of a recurrence are usually embarrassment and, occasionally, injuries. Most of the AEDs that are used in children have significant behavioural and cognitive side effects that can be as troublesome as a seizure recurrence, if not more so. For the majority of patients, especially children, treatment need not be started after a first seizure. An extremely high predicted risk of recurrence, status epilepticus or perhaps, a generalized tonic–clonic seizure as the initial presentation are factors that would most favor treatment, both to reduce the risk of seizure recurrence and to avoid the consequences of a severe seizure. Improvement in long-term seizure outcome has not been shown to be an achievable goal of early treatment. If treatment is started, a clear reason for treatment must be identified and a goal for duration of treatment should be set. Assuming no further seizures occur, treatment might be tried for 1–2 years. This goal may have to be reassessed as additional information (particularly from subsequent EEGs or imaging studies) accumulates. Stopping AEDs is discussed in greater detail in Chapter 18.

The decision to start treatment does not have to be absolute. If treatment produces intolerable side effects and the balance of the risk–benefit equation only slightly favors treatment, then it may be reasonable to stop treatment early and not try another medication. On the other hand, if the equation highly favors treatment, it may be reasonable to switch to another medication.

Patients with epilepsy

Patients who have had at least two separate unprovoked seizures are considered to have epilepsy.[4] In patients followed from the time of a first unprovoked seizure, the risk of a third seizure after a second is ~70 per cent or higher, and no such patients with a risk <50 per cent can be identified.[44,45] After a third seizure, the risk of a fourth is also ~75 per cent. Most patients with epilepsy tend to present after not just two but many seizures. In some forms of epilepsy, particularly childhood and juvenile absence, the risk of further recurrences is virtually 100 per cent. The risk of subsequent seizures in patients who present with epilepsy is high enough that it can be assumed that most of these patients will have recurrent seizures if untreated. Overall, 70 per cent or more of patients will respond favorably to treatment and eventually, if not immediately, become seizure-free.

Potential suppression of seizures, especially when the risk of further seizures is so great, is highly worthwhile for several reasons. Chief among these is the avoidance of injuries, interruptions in daily activities from the seizures and their after-effects, and restrictions on various activities (both necessary and recreational). Other important factors are the social embarrassment of having seizures in public and all the associated psychosocial pressures. A recent report[46] documented a high rate of accidents and injuries in children with absence seizures as a result of the absence seizures. Thus the risks associated with even relatively mild seizures should be taken seriously.

Another factor favoring treatment is the generally small but significant risk of death associated with seizures. There is an elevated risk of mortality in people with epilepsy from a variety of causes compared with the population at large.[47] Some of this increased risk is attributable to the underlying disorders that cause epilepsy. Another proportion may be due to accidents that occur during a seizure, such as drowning. In recent years, concerted efforts have been made to study the remaining excess mortality in epilepsy. The syndrome of 'sudden unexplained death in epilepsy' or SUDEP has been the focus of recent studies and a symposium.[48] SUDEP refers to deaths that are presumed to have occurred in the context of a seizure that was not witnessed.[49] Population-based studies from Rochester (Minnesota, US) indicate that the rates vary tremendously by age and by severity of epilepsy. In children and young adults with non-intractable epilepsy, the rate is roughly 1 per 10,000 patients per year, roughly twice that in the general population. In those with intractable epilepsy, the rate is >10 times this amount. Through adulthood, the rate rises in the non-intractable group in parallel and very near to the values observed in the general population. By the seventh decade of life, there are only very small differences between population rates and those seen in people with epilepsy. Generally, most of the excess risk in epilepsy is realized during the first several years after diagnosis, most likely attributable to patients with symptomatic epilepsy, although a small elevation in risk persists for decades. The mechanisms by which seizures may cause SUDEP include cardiac arrhythmias and central apnoea, but remain poorly characterized.[50,51]

No data exist on whether treatment effectively reduces the risk of death associated with seizures. To the extent that treatment can prevent seizures, it seems that it should prevent some, although certainly not all, instances of SUDEP or accidental death associated with seizures. Those patients at highest risk of SUDEP, patients with refractory epilepsy or associated neurological conditions, will still remain at high risk even with treatment. Ultimately, the incidence of SUDEP among low-risk new onset patients is so low that it is extremely difficult to study definitively. Given the current absence of useful evidence and considering what is at stake, the risk of SUDEP should be weighed in the decision to initiate treatment. Without causing undue alarm, the physician should discuss SUDEP and accidental injuries and death with patients who have epilepsy so that they can be fully informed about the risks associated with their disorder.

Improvement in long-term seizure outcomes by early aggressive treatment to suppress seizure occurrence is probably not an attainable goal. Data from definitive RCTs regarding the effect of withholding treatment and continued seizures on the course of epilepsy in patients are not yet available. While the epidemiological data on epilepsy in its entirety suggest no benefits from early as opposed to later treatment, it must be remembered that epilepsy is a heterogeneous disorder and that some epilepsy syndromes, as yet undefined, may benefit from early intervention. Currently, however, improvements in social and educational outcomes, quality of life, and probably reduction in injuries and possibly death are strong enough reasons to attempt early treatment in patients with epilepsy.

Although the equation largely favors attempting treatment once epilepsy is established, there are still some selected circumstances where treatment may often be withheld. Benign rolandic epilepsy (BRE) provides the best example. This idiopathic, age-related partial epilepsy syndrome almost always resolves in early to mid-adolescence. The seizures are usually simple partial, although some may present as secondarily generalized tonic–clonic seizures. They tend to occur at night and not with an especially high frequency. Often such children are not treated at the time of initial diagnosis, although treatment may be initiated later if the seizures are frequent or bothersome.

Other factors which may influence the decision to treat include the frequency and severity of seizures. For example, someone with a normal EEG and normal examination who has had three or four simple partial seizures over a 2-year period might elect not to pursue treatment. On the other hand, a patient with an abnormal EEG or neurological impairment who has had two generalized tonic–clonic seizures 2 weeks apart might quite reasonably be encouraged to choose treatment.

Depending on the patient's seizure type and epilepsy syndrome, as well as his or her response to the medication, it may be necessary to reassess the goals of treatment. If after a trial of treatment, the side effects of the AED are intolerable and the patient has a relatively good risk profile in terms of frequency and severity of seizures, some patients may elect to do without medication.

Generalized				Partial	
Absence	Myoclonic	Tonic/atonic	Generalized onset tonic–clonic	Simple partial	Complex partial
					Secondarily generalized
Ethosuximide	Benzodiazepines			Carbamazepine Phenytoin Vigabatrin Gabapentin Topiramate Tiagabine	
			Valproate		
			Lamotrigine Phenobarbital (?)		

Figure 15.1
Spectrum of efficacy of antiepileptic drugs (AEDs) by seizure type.

Choosing a drug

Treatment with a single drug is preferred to treatment with multiple agents.[52,53] Because different drugs have different mechanisms of action and their effectiveness differs for different seizure types and different forms of epilepsy, it is essential that an accurate diagnosis of the type of epilepsy be made first before initiating treatment. Some drugs may not only be ineffective against certain seizure types, but may actually exacerbate the seizures. This is of particular concern with carbamazepine and vigabatrin, which have been shown to exacerbate absence and myoclonic seizures in the generalized epilepsies. The efficacy of different drugs against different seizure types is shown in Figure 15.1.

Many syndromes are associated with more than one seizure type. At the time of diagnosis and the decision to initiate treatment, not all seizure types may yet have been expressed. By recognizing the underlying syndrome, the treating physician can select a medication that is known to be effective not only against the seizures that the patient has manifested, but also those that are associated with the patient's epilepsy syndrome and therefore which may appear at a later time. This accounts, in part, for the wide-spread popularity of valproic acid in the treatment of many forms of primary generalized epilepsy. Valproic acid would be a treatment of choice for juvenile absence epilepsy or juvenile myoclonic epilepsy because of its demonstrated efficacy against both absence and generalized tonic–clonic seizures, as well as myoclonic seizures.

Localization-related epilepsies

With the addition of the most recent drugs to enter the market, there are currently 10 or more that can be used to treat localization-related epilepsy. Several studies have compared monotherapy regimens with various individual drugs.[54–56] Phenytoin and carbamazepine are the best drugs to try first when treating localization-related epilepsy. Both are highly efficacious and both have greater tolerability than do phenobarbital and primidone.[54] Although the basic mechanisms of action are similar for phenytoin and carbamazepine, there are some differences. Relative advantages of phenytoin over carbamazepine are the potential for once-daily dosing and the lower cost. Despite this, phenytoin is not always chosen first because of its complex pharmacokinetics (which require more frequent blood level monitoring), its cosmetic effects, its enzyme-inducing and protein binding properties that result in drug–drug interactions, and its teratogenicity.

Valproate has recently been licensed by the FDA in the US for use with partial seizures, although it has been approved for the treatment of all epilepsies in Europe for many years. Although evidence from some clinical trials suggested that it was less effective than carbamazepine for treatment of partial seizures, it is still clearly very effective. It has a further advantage in that it is also effective against absence seizures. In some children, it may be difficult to distinguish complex partial from atypical absence seizures. Valproate is effective against both kinds of seizures whereas phenytoin and carbamazepine can exacerbate absence seizures. While physicians should not abandon pursuit of an accurate diagnosis, valproate's broad spectrum of action at least allows effective treatment in patients for whom the correct diagnosis of partial versus primary generalized epilepsy is in doubt.

Lamotrigine, a relatively recently approved AED, has been compared with phenytoin and carbamazepine in three RCTs. One study suggested that lamotrigine might be better tolerated than carbamazepine;[57] the other two studies failed to find any advantage of one drug over the other with respect to both efficacy and tolerability.[58,59] Guidelines for the use of other new AEDs as first-line agents will require future monotherapy trials in which the newer drugs are compared with carbamazepine and possibly phenytoin.

Generalized epilepsies

The generalized epilepsies subdivide into two groups, idiopathic (presumed genetic) and symptomatic/cryptogenic. In the International Classification of the Epilepsies,[60] the primary generalized epilepsies correspond to the 2.1 grouping, and the others correspond to the 2.2 and 2.3 groupings. Most generalized forms of epilepsy begin during the first 10–12 years of life with relatively fewer appearing during adolescence and only rare occurrences in adulthood. The idiopathic generalized epilepsies constitute ~20 per cent of all childhood onset epilepsies and ~10 per cent of all epilepsies. In most circumstances, valproate is the drug of first choice for idiopathic generalized epilepsy. As mentioned previously, it is effective against all the seizure types that may occur in these syndromes. Its tolerability is good, although weight gain and hair loss may limit its use in some patients. Ethosuximide may also be used in childhood absence epilepsy, a syndrome in which there is a low risk of generalized tonic–clonic seizures.

The newer antiepileptic drugs have yet to be adequately assessed in the idiopathic generalized epilepsies. Comparative RCTs in the future will help clarify their role in the treatment of these syndromes.

The symptomatic/cryptogenic generalized syndromes are more problematic. These may start in early infancy and may be symptomatic of other underlying disorders. The diagnosis and treatment of most of these forms of epilepsy make up a highly specialized area that deserves separate and extensive discussion.

Summary

For any individual patient, the decision to initiate treatment must take into account the likelihood and severity of drug side effects (reasons not to treat), the risk of further seizures and the consequences if such seizures should occur (reasons that may or may not compel treatment), and what treatment can realistically do to reduce those risks to a significantly different level (factors that may or may not compel treatment). All these factors must be weighed together and the balance for each patient determined (Figure 15.2). As emphasized above, suppression of seizures to improve long-term seizure outcome is not something that current forms of treatment appear able to do and hence this should not be a reason to initiate treatment. The known and documented benefits of treatment in patients with epilepsy are sufficient motivation to encourage a trial of therapy in most patients with epilepsy, but not in most of those patients who present with a single

Do not treat	Do treat
• Risk and severity of AED side effects and toxicity • Psychosocial impact of treatment • Cost of AEDs and concomitant medical treatment • Inability of treatment to alter long-term seizure outcome	• Risk of further seizures • Seizure severity (including status) • Decreased psychosocial and educational impact of seizures • Reduction in injuries from seizures • ?Decreased risk of seizure-associated mortality

Figure 15.2
For each patient, the decision to treat or not to treat must be based on the balance between factors in favor of treatment and against treatment for that particular individual.

seizure, and certainly in very few, if any, of those who have not yet developed unprovoked seizures.

Acknowledgment

Supported by NIH grant RO1-NS31146(ATB).

References

1. Gowers WR. Epilepsy and other chronic convulsive disorders: their causes symptoms and treatment. London: J&A Churchill, 1881.
2. Reynolds E, Elwes R, Shorvon S. Why does epilepsy become intractable? Prevention of chronic epilepsy. *Lancet* 1983;**22**:952–4.
3. Berg AT, Shinnar S. Do seizures beget seizures: an assessment of the clinical evidence in humans. *J Clin Neurophysiol* 1997;**14**:102–10.
4. Commission on Epidemiology and Prognosis, International League Against Epilepsy.

Guidelines for epidemiologic studies on epilepsy. *Epilepsia* 1993;34:592–6.

5. Foy PM, Copeland GP, Shaw MDM. The incidence of postoperative seizures. *Acta Neurochir* 1981;55:253–64.

6. Foy PM, Chadwick DW, Rajgopalan N, Johnson AL, Shaw MDM. Do prophylactic anticonvulsant drugs alter the pattern of seizures after craniotomy? *J Neurol Neurosurg Psychiatry* 1992;55:753–7.

7. Temkin NR, Dikmen SS, Wilensky AJ, Keihm J, Chabal S, Winn R. A randomized, double-blind study of phenytoin for the prevention of post-traumatic seizures. *N Engl J Med* 1990; 323:497–502.

8. Temkin NR, Dikmen S, Anderson G, et al. Valproate for preventing late post-traumatic seizures. *Epilepsia* 1997;38(Suppl 8):102.

9. Schierout G, Roberts I. Prophylactic antiepileptic agents after head injury: a systematic review. *J Neurol Neurosurg Psychiatry* 1998;64: 108–12.

10. Franceschetti S, Binelli S, Casazza M, et al. Influence of surgery and antiepileptic drugs on seizures symptomatic of cerebral tumors. *Acta Neurochir* 1990;103:47–51.

11. Glantz MJ, Cole BF, Friedberg MH, et al. A randomized, blinded, placebo-controlled trial of divalproex sodium prophylaxis in adults with newly diagnosed brain tumors. *Neurology* 1996;46:685–91.

12. North JB, Penhall RK, Hanieh A, Frewin DB, Taylor WB. Phenytoin and postoperative epilepsy: a double blind study. *J Neurosurg* 1983;58:672–7.

13. Wolf SM, Carr A, Davis DC, et al. The value of phenobarbital in the child who has had a single febrile seizure: a controlled prospective study. *Pediatrics* 1977;59:378–85.

14. Knudsen FU. Effective short-term diazepam prophylaxis in febrile convulsions. *J Pediatr* 1985;106:487–90.

15. Rosman NP, Colton T, Labazzo J, et al. A controlled trial of diazepam administered during febrile illnesses to prevent recurrence of febrile seizures. *N Engl J Med* 1993;329:79–94.

16. Knudsen FU, Paerregaard A, Andersen R, Andresen J. Long term outcome of prophylaxis for febrile convulsions. *Arch Dis Child* 1996; 74:13–18.

17. Wolf SM, Forsythe A. Epilepsy and mental retardation following febrile seizures in childhood. *Acta Paediatr Scand* 1989;78:291–5.

18. Rosman NP, Labazzo J. Factors predisposing to afebrile seizures after febrile convulsions and preventive treatment. *Ann Neurol* 1993;34:452.

19. So EL, Annegers JF, Hauser WA, O'Brien PC, Whisnant JP. Population-based study of seizure disorders after cerebral infarction. *Neurology* 1996;46:350–5.

20. Murphy DJ, Hope PL, Johnson A. Neonatal risk factors for cerebral palsy in very preterm babies: case-control study. *BMJ* 1997;314: 404–8.

21. Arboix A, Comes E, Massons J, Garcia L, Oliveres M. Relevance of early seizures for in-hospital mortality in acute cerebrovascular disease. *Neurology* 1996;47:1429–35.

22. Jennet WB. *Epilepsy after non-missile head injuries.* London: Heineman Books, 1975.

23. Pitkanen A. Treatment with antiepileptic drugs: possible neuroprotective effects. *Neurology* 1996;47:S12–S16.

24. Berg AT. Febrile seizures and epilepsy: the contributions of epidemiology. *Paediatr Perinat Epidemiol* 1992;6:145–52.

25. Berg AT, Shinnar S. The contributions of epilepsy to the understanding of childhood seizures and epilepsy. *J Child Neurol* 1994; 9(Suppl)2S19–2S26.

26. Farwell JR, Lee YJ, Hirtz DG, Sulzbacher SI, Ellenberg JH, Nelson KB. Phenobarbital for febrile seizures—effects on intelligence and on seizure recurrence. *N Engl J Med* 1990;322: 364–9.

27. Freeman JM. Febrile seizures: an end to confusion. *Pediatrics* 1978;61:806–8.

28. Freeman JM. The best medicine for febrile seizures. *N Engl J Med* 1992;327:1161–2.

29. Berg AT, Shinnar S. The risk of seizure recurrence following a first unprovoked seizure: a quantitative review. *Neurology* 1991;41:965–72.

30. Shinnar S, Berg AT, Moshe SL, et al. The risk of seizure recurrence after a first unprovoked afebrile seizure in childhood: an extended follow-up. *Pediatrics* 1996;98:216–25.

31. van Donselaar C, Schimsheimer R, Geerts A, Declerk A. Value of the electroencephalogram in adult patients with untreated idiopathic first seizures. *Arch Neurol* 1992;49:231–7.

32. Hopkins A, Garman A, Clarke C. The first seizure in adult life: value of clinical features. *Lancet* 1988:**1**:721–6.

33. Berg AT, Shinnar S. Complex febrile seizures. *Epilepsia* 1996;**37**:126–33.

34. Shinnar S, Berg AT, Hauser WA, et al. Evaluation of the incidence of status epilepticus in association with tiagabine therapy. *Epilepsia* 1997;**38**(Suppl 3):65.

35. Novak G, Maytal J, Alshansky A, Ascher A. Risk factors for status epilepticus in children with symptomatic epilepsy. *Neurology* 1997; **49**:533–7.

36. Camfield P, Camfield C, Cooley J, Smith E, Garner B. A randomized study of carbamazepine versus no medication after a first unprovoked seizure in childhood. *Neurology* 1989;**39**:851–2.

37. First Seizure Trial Group. Randomized clinical trial of the efficacy of antiepileptic drugs in reducing the risk of relapse after a first unprovoked tonic-clonic seizure. *Neurology* 1993;**43**: 478–83.

38. Gilad R, Lampl Y, Gabbay U, Eshel Y, Sarova-Pinhas I. Early treatment of a single generalized tonic-clonic seizure to prevent recurrence. *Arch Neurol* 1996;**53**:1149–52.

39. Musicco M, Beghi E, Solari A, for the First Seizure Trial Group. Treatment of a first tonic-clonic seizure does not improve the prognosis of epilepsy. *Neurology* 1997;**49**:991–8.

40. Camfield C, Camfield P, Gordon K, Dooley J. Does the number of seizures before treatment influence ease of control or remission of childhood epilepsy? Not if the number is 10 or less. *Neurology* 1996;**46**:41–4.

41. Placencia M, Shorvon S, Paredes V, et al. Epileptic seizures in an Andean region of Ecuador: incidence and prevalence and regional variation. *Brain* 1992;**115**:771–82.

42. Collaborative Group for the Study of Epilepsy. Prognosis of epilepsy in newly referred patients: a multicenter prospective study of the effects of monotherapy on the long-term course of epilepsy. *Epilepsia* 1992;**33**:45–51.

43. Cockrell OC, Johnson AL, Sander JWAS, Shorvon SD. Prognosis of epilepsy: a review and further analysis of the first nine years of the British National General Practice Study of Epilepsy, a prospective population-basesd study. *Epilepsia* 1997;**38**:31–46.

44. Hauser WA, Rich SS, Lee J, Annegers JF, Anderson VE. Risk of recurrent seizures after two unprovoked seizures. *N Engl J Med* 1998;**338**:429–34.

45. Shinnar S, Berg AT, Newstein DD, et al. Predictors of multiple seizures in a cohort of children prospectively followed from the time of their first unprovoked seizure. *Epilepsia* 1996;**37**(Suppl 5):84.

46. Wirrell EC, Camfield PR, Camfield CS, Dooley JM, Gordon KE. Accidental injury is a serious risk in children with typical absence epilepsy. *Arch Neurol* 1996;**53**:929–32.

47. Hauser WA, Annegers JF, Elveback LR. Mortality in patients with epilepsy. *Epilepsia* 1980;**21**:399–412.

48. Nashef L, Brown SW (eds). Epilepsy and sudden death. *Epilepsia* 1997;**38**(Suppl 11).

49. Annegers JF. United States perspective on definitions and classifications. *Epilepsia* 1997; **38**(Suppl 11):S9–S12.

50. Jallon P. Arrhythmogenic seizures. *Epilepsia* 1997;**38**(Suppl 11):S43–S47.

51. Walker F, Fish DR. Recording respiratory parameters in patients with epilepsy. *Epilepsia* 1997;**38**(Suppl 11):S41–S42.

52. Shorvon SD, Chadwick D, Galbraith AW, Reynolds EH. One drug for epilepsy. *BMJ* 1978;**1**:474–6.

53. Reynolds EH, Shorvon SD, Galbraith AW, et al. Phenytoin monotherapy for epilepsy: a long-term prospective study, assisted by serum level monitoring, in previously untreated patients. *Epilepsia* 1981;**22**:475–88.

54. Mattson RH, Cramer JA, Collins JF, et al. Comparison of carbamazepine, phenobarbital, phenytoin and primidone in partial and secondary generalized tonic-clonic seizures. *N Engl J Med* 1985;**313**:145–51.

55. Mattson RH, Cramer JA, Collins JF, et al. A comparison of valproate with carbamazepine for the treatment of complex partial seizures with secondarily generalized tonic-clonic seizures in adults. *N Engl J Med* 1992;**327**: 765–71.

56. Heller AJ, Chesterman P, Elwes RDC, et al. Phenobarbitone, phenytoin, carbamazepine or sodium valproate for newly diagnosed adult epilepsy: a randomized comparative monotherapy trial. *J Neurol Neurosurg Psychiatry* 1995;**58**:44–50.

57. Brodie MJ, Richens A, Yeun AWC, for the UK Lamotrigine/Carbamazepine Monotherapy Trial Group. Double-blind comparison of lamotrigine and carbamazepine in newly diagnosed epilepsy. *Lancet* 1995;**345**:476–9.

58. Reunanen M, Dam M, Yuen AWC. A randomized open multicentre comparative trial of lamotrigine and carbamazepine as monotherapy in patients with newly diagnosed or recurrent epilepsy. *Epilepsy Res* 1996;**23**:149.

59. Steiner TJ, Yuen AWC. Comparison of lamotrigine and phenytoin monotherapy in newly diagnosed epilepsy. *Epilepsia* 1994;**35**:31.

60. Commission on Classification and Terminology of the International League Against Epilepsy. Proposal for revised classification of epilepsies and epileptic syndromes. *Epilepsia* 1989;**30**:389–99.

16

Stopping treatment for epilepsy

David W Chadwick and Anne T Berg

Introduction

Both population and cohort studies have demonstrated that 70–80 per cent of patients diagnosed and treated for epilepsy will attain long-term remission in excess of 2 years.[1,2] Most who remit do so immediately or shortly after beginning therapy. Once a patient has been seizure-free for some time it is reasonable to consider stopping antiepileptic drug (AED) therapy to decide whether the epilepsy is cured or whether the patient remains dependent on treatment to suppress seizures.

The decision to start a trial of drug withdrawal should be made by the patient after appropriate advice. This needs to cover difficult areas which include an individual assessment of risk of relapse upon withdrawal of treatment, and indeed, on continued treatment, the timing of any trial of withdrawal and the outlook if seizures recur.

How long seizure-free?

Most commonly, periods of ≥ 2 years are generally considered necessary before consideration of AED withdrawal. Recently, pediatricians have advocated treatment for shorter periods of time (see below). It is usually suggested that achieving longer seizure-free periods results in a lower risk of recurrence. This is most likely to be due to selection bias;

patients who relapse while still on medication after shorter periods of time being excluded. In the Medical Research Council's (MRC's) randomized controlled trial (RCT) one of the major prognostic factors for recurrence was the period of time that patients were seizure-free; however, this applied both to patients continuing their treatment and to those stopping it.[3]

Recent RCTs have examined policies of differing lengths of treatment prior to stopping medication. Peters et al[4] randomized children who entered remission within 2 months of starting treatment to stop medication after 6 months or 12 months. Six months after the first follow-up, 22 per cent of those still on AEDs had relapsed despite treatment compared with 37 per cent who had been withdrawn from their drugs. However, by 24 months after randomization the risk of relapse was 49 per cent and 48 per cent respectively. This study shows higher rates of seizure recurrence than would usually be expected in children staying on treatment for ≥ 2 years (29 per cent by 2 years after withdrawal).[5] Braathen et al[6] came to somewhat different conclusions. They randomized 244 children to treatment for either 1 or 3 years. Randomization took place before treatment was commenced. Drugs were withdrawn in each group only in those patients who were seizure-free for at least 6 months at the end of 1 and 3 years respectively. The primary study outcome was reinstitution of medications, not seizure recurrence as in most studies. A total of 161 children commenced withdrawal, 77 after treatment for 1 year and 84 after treatment for 3 years. The report gives no information about the median period seizure-free in the two groups withdrawing treatment, but the probabilities of reinstitution of treatment were generally higher than might be expected from studies demanding remission of 2 years: a 30 per cent probability in patients treated for 3 years compared with a 50 per cent probability in the group treated for 1 year. The observed outcome is consistent with the effect of longer periods of remission having better outcomes and probably does not indicate a true treatment benefit for 3 years of therapy compared with 1 year.

There are a number of studies from developing countries where patients with a diagnosis of epilepsy remained untreated. One study found that 55 per cent of untreated patients achieved spontaneous remission.[7] This is not dissimilar from rates of remission in the developed world where ~70 per cent of patients become seizure-free on medication, of whom 60–70 per cent can successfully withdraw therapy. This suggests that, regardless of length of treatment or whether treatment is given at all, half of all cases of epilepsy spontaneously remit.

The relationship between the length of time patients remain seizure-free and the risk of seizures in the following year on AED treatment is illustrated in Figure 16.1 using data from the MRC study.[8] This uses data from those patients who had a recurrence of seizures during the course of the study (and who were on treatment after such a seizure), and all those patients randomized to continue treatment at the outset of the study. The risk of a seizure in the next year is about 50 per cent immediately after a seizure and approximately 20 per cent after 1 year seizure-free. By 4–5 years, the risk of a seizure in the next year falls to about 10

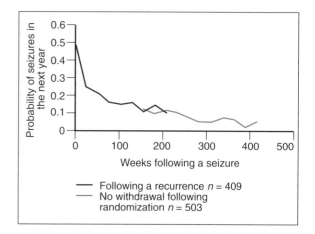

Figure 16.1
Probability of a seizure in the next year after remaining seizure-free for varying periods following a seizure.[8]

per cent. The risk for seizures after this time changes relatively little, so that a policy of considering discontinuation of AEDs after 2–5 years in adults and after only ≥1 year in children seems reasonable.

Risk of relapse

Studies that include a broad mix of patients and that require seizure remission for 2 years before stopping treatment show a risk of relapse, on average, of 25 per cent in the first year and 29 per cent after 2 years.[5] Eighty per cent of all recurrences occur within the first year and 90 per cent within the first 2 years. These estimates are derived from a meta-analysis across several studies and the great majority of these provide individual estimates within about 10 per cent of the summary estimate.

Many factors have been identified that appear to influence the degree of risk.

Epilepsy syndrome

Epilepsy syndromes can be used to define both the prognosis for response to treatment and to treatment withdrawal. The international classification of the epilepsies was first approved after a number of revisions in 1989.[9] Syndromes are identified by age at onset, seizure type, EEG characteristics, the presence or absence of underlying etiology, and sometimes, the diurnal pattern of seizure occurrence. Some syndromes are very clearly associated with a particular risk of relapse after stopping treatment. Benign rolandic epilepsy (BRE) has been shown by a number of investigators to have an excellent response to treatment and relatively rare relapse of seizures when medications are stopped. Absence epilepsy has a more uncertain prognosis for remission. Although in the short term, most patients become seizure-free on treatment, about 25 per cent relapse when medications are withdrawn. The seizures associated with juvenile myoclonic epilepsy (JME) respond extremely well to treatment; however, relapses occur in almost all patients when medications are stopped. The partial epilepsies are less well defined with respect to both response to treatment and the prognosis following withdrawal.

However, epilepsy syndromes may be difficult to identify in patients with mild epilepsies characterized by only a few seizures that respond immediately to treatment. In one study, almost a quarter of cryptogenic cases could not easily be classified as having either generalized or partial epilepsy.[5]

Seizure type

Most studies have examined the outcome of particular types of seizures rather than syndromes. Because a single seizure type may be a characteristic of very differing syndromes, the results of such analyses show some conflict. Thus, tonic–clonic seizures may occur in JME, BRE, juvenile absence epilepsy and many other syndromes as well. Similarly, simple partial seizures occur in both BRE and the more refractory types of temporal lobe epilepsy. Patients with multiple, as compared with single, seizure types have a higher risk of relapse, according to several studies. An equal number of studies, however, failed to find such an effect.[10] Because a number of epilepsy syndromes are characterized by multiple seizure types, it is likely that the underlying epilepsy syndrome may better account for the likelihood of relapsing after stopping AEDs, than the specific seizure types.

Age at onset

Most studies find a favorable prognosis in epilepsy with onset in childhood. Studies including both childhood and adolescent onset epilepsy usually demonstrate a substantially increased risk of relapse in those with adolescent onset. Childhood onset of epilepsy is usually associated with a risk of relapse of ~20 per cent compared with 35–40 per cent for adolescent onset epilepsy. Adult onset epilepsy, on the other hand, is about 30 per cent more likely to relapse than childhood onset epilepsy.[5] Some confusion exists in this literature because of the failure to differentiate between the age of onset of epilepsy and the age at which discontinuation is considered. The former is a function of the underlying biology of the epilepsy, while the latter is a function not only of age of onset but also of the period of time that it took for the epilepsy to be diagnosed and to come under control.

Underlying etiology

Patients with an identifiable etiology associated with their epilepsy (remote symptomatic epilepsy) are less likely to enter remission than those with idiopathic or cryptogenic epilepsy. Once in remission, such patients are about 50 per cent more likely to relapse if medication is stopped.[5] Learning disability, at least in children, may be a stronger predictor of relapse than motor impairments or other neurological disorders that are not associated with impairment of cognitive function.[11] The impact of remote symptomatic epilepsy on prognosis for adult onset epilepsy is rather less dramatic and was not found to be an important factor in the MRC Withdrawal Study[3], which was essentially a study of adults in remission.

The electro-encephalogram

There is considerable controversy over the value of the electro-encephalogram (EEG) in predicting the prognosis for relapse after stopping treatment. Some studies have examined the amount of 'improvement' in the EEG from starting treatment to the time of its cessation. Most studies examine the correlation between an EEG immediately prior to withdrawal and relapse of seizures. Different studies have focused on different types of EEG abnormalities. In one study,[12] children with normal EEGs had an extremely low risk of relapse, those with either epileptiform abnormalities or slowing had a moderate risk, and those with both epileptiform abnormalities and slowing had an almost 100 per cent risk of relapse. Mastropaolo et al[13] reported high rates of relapse in patients with photoconvulsive responses on their EEGs. Overall, the data suggest that the EEG is of greater prognostic significance in children than in adults. It is uncertain if EEG abnormalities are independent

prognostic variables, that is to what degree EEG abnormalities are simply more common in patients already identified to be at high risk by clinical factors such as a diagnosis of symptomatic epilepsy. Because of considerable variation among the studies, we cannot say with any certainty which aspects of the EEG are most important. Certainly, in a study that utilized a multivariate model to predict outcomes, the EEG added little to other more important clinical factors.[3]

Severity of epilepsy

A number of different clinical features that may reflect the severity of epilepsy have been studied and reported in the literature. They include the occurrence of status epilepticus, the duration of epilepsy, the number of seizures before remission, the duration of treatment, the requirement for two or more AEDs for remission and previous failed attempts to stop medication. Most studies indicate that these surrogate measures all adversely affect the risk of recurrence.[10] However, no single indicator or set of indicators is clearly superior to the others as a marker of prognosis after stopping AEDs.

Status epilepticus

Although status epilepticus is associated with poorer response to drug treatment,[14,15] patients with a history of status who become seizure-free do not seem to have a higher risk of relapse. This was the case in adults[8] and in children.[11]

Response to treatment

The duration of epilepsy and the duration of treatment have been examined by a number of studies; these two factors are clearly correlated. There is a consensus that patients with infrequent seizures that respond more rapidly to treatment have a better outcome when medication is withdrawn. In the MRC study, having seizures while on drug treatment and requiring two or more drugs for remission were both associated with an increased risk of relapse.

In studies of children[11] and adults[8] a previous failed attempt to stop treatment was not found, by itself, to be associated with an increased risk of relapse.

The influence of individual drugs

It is often suggested that the risk of seizure recurrence may differ depending on the drug that is to be withdrawn. Withdrawal seizures are particularly said to occur with the discontinuation of phenobarbitone. The subject has rarely been exposed to systematic study. There were large subgroups of patients receiving monotherapy with carbamazepine, valproate, phenytoin or barbiturate drugs (phenobarbitone or primidone) in the MRC study.[8] The temporal pattern of seizure recurrence was similar in the barbiturate group and the other groups. Surprisingly, the withdrawal of carbamazepine was associated with a lower relative risk of seizure recurrence on withdrawal than were other drugs, even after adjustment for other predictors of outcome. The significance of this finding is uncertain (unpublished observations); it may represent as yet unmeasurable or difficult-to-identify differences in patients who are treated with one drug versus another.

Prediction of relapse

The MRC study[3] was sufficiently large to develop and test a predictive model for relapse in patients continuing or stopping their medication. The model gives decreasing weight to the following factors: whether or not treatment is withdrawn, period of time seizure-free, taking two or more AEDs, being 16 years or older at the time of withdrawal, having myoclonic seizures and having tonic–clonic seizures of any type; the final factor was an abnormal EEG. While the model does not include the presence of remote symptomatic epilepsy, factors retained in the model may, singly or in combination, provide surrogate measures for symptomatic epilepsy and capture those aspects of remote symptomatic epilepsy that are most associated with an increased risk of relapse. In addition, since the study was largely in adults, it is possible that the types of underlying etiologies associated with adult onset epilepsy do not carry the same risk for relatively poor prognosis as those factors associated with childhood onset epilepsy. Because of the methods and inclusion criteria, the study was able to recruit a large number of patients from a general population who were highly representative of relevant patients in the population with respect to clinical prognostic factors. Consequently,

Starting score		−175
Age >15 years	add	45
Taking >1 AED	add	50
Seizures after starting treatment	add	35
History of tonic–clonic seizures	add	35
EEG in past year		
not done	add	15
abnormal	add	20
Seizure-free period (years)	add	
200/years		
Total		T
Total/100 and exponentiate	$z = e^{T/100}$	

Probability of recurrence. On treatment: by 1 year 1–0.89 (to power z); by 2 years 1–0.79 (to power z). On withdrawal: by 1 year 1–0.69 (to power z); by 2 years 1–0.60 (to power z).

Figure 16.2
Predictive model for seizure recurrence.

this model should have good generalizability outside the study population from which it was derived, although this has never formally been tested. The resulting predictive equation was well calibrated for risks between 10 and 80 per cent and would correctly identify juvenile myoclonic epilepsy as having a high risk of relapse. Figure 16.2 outlines the use of this model.

Two groups of investigators described relatively simple models to predict relapse in children. Dooley et al[16] developed a model derived from a study of 97 children in whom drugs were withdrawn after 12 months of remission. A point scoring system was devised in which subjects were allocated 1 point for being female; 1 for seizure onset after 10 years, the presence of neurological abnormality, and generalized seizures; and 2 points for partial seizures (other than those of BRE). No subjects with 0 points relapsed (they had BRE by definition). Ninety-five per cent of patients with 1 point, 80 per cent with 2 points, 45 per cent with 3 points and 5 per cent with 4 points remained seizure-free. Shinnar et al[11] determined risk of relapse 2 years after stopping AEDs in 264 children as a function of the number of risk factors for relapse (0–3). This was done separately for those with cryptogenic/idiopathic versus remote symptomatic epilepsy. In the idiopathic group, predictors of relapse were age at onset >12 years, family history of epilepsy, slowing on the EEG and atypical febrile seizures. The risk of relapse after 2 years was 12, 46 and 71 per cent in children with 0, 1 and 2 of these factors, respectively; no child had more than 2 factors. In remote symptomatic cases, predictors were age of onset >12 years, mental disability, absence seizures and atypical febrile seizures. The risk of relapse after 2 years was 11, 35, 51 and 78 per cent in children with 0, 1, 2 and 3 risk

factors respectively; no child had all 4 risk factors. Of note, the lowest risk stratum in the remote symptomatic group had virtually the same risk as the lowest risk stratum in the cryptogenic/idiopathic group. The lowest risk stratum represented only 10 per cent (9 of 99) of the remote symptomatic group, whereas it comprised 59 per cent (97 of 165) of the cryptogenic/idiopathic group.

When discussing the risk of relapse when medication is withdrawn, it is important to recognize that continued treatment with AEDs is not a guarantee of freedom from seizures. Data from the MRC Study[8] indicated a risk of 10 per cent per annum in patients who had a median of 3 years seizure-free at the point of randomization and who continued to take medication (Figure 16.1).

Prognosis after relapse

Most data indicate that the majority of patients who relapse when medication is stopped will regain acceptable control when treatment is reintroduced. In the MRC study,[8] 95 per cent of those who relapsed experienced at least a 1-year remission within 3 years of the initial relapse. By 5 years, 90 per cent had experienced a remission of at least 2 years' duration. Factors associated with a poorer outcome after relapse were having a partial seizure at the time of relapse, having a previous history of seizures while on medication and shorter duration of seizure freedom prior to the relapse. All patients who continued to have seizures were analysed regardless of whether they had been randomized to stop or continue treatment. The outcome was the same following seizure recurrence regardless of whether a patient had discontinued or remained on treatment prior to the recurrence.[17]

Psychosocial consequences of withdrawal and continued treatment

In the MRC study, the impact of the two randomized policies (continued treatment or withdrawal) on psychosocial outcomes was assessed.[18] There was good evidence that seizure recurrence had an adverse effect on psychosocial outcomes, but that this was very much counter-balanced by the effects of continuing to take medication in the group randomized to do so. Thus, even though the group randomized to withdrawal experienced more seizures, psychosocial outcome was similar in the two groups. This indicates that there are significant benefits to the successful withdrawal of AEDs that may relate to the removal of the stigma of diagnosis of epilepsy and the daily burden of taking AEDs.

The practical issues

The decision to withdraw AEDs will be influenced both by the risk of further seizures and also by a personal view of the impact of further seizures on the patient's expectations and the risk of continued AED treatment. These issues demand careful consideration and discussion, and the ultimate decision can only be made by the patient. Personal circumstances may play a very large role in this decision making. For example, a 25-year-old man whose job is dependent on holding a driving licence might well feel that a 40 per cent risk of seizure recurrence on drug withdrawal was unacceptable. However, a similar risk in his 25-year-old wife might be acceptable if it allowed a drug-free pregnancy.

The complexity of these issues is further highlighted by studies of patients' views. Jacoby et al[19] found that 43 per cent of subjects with their epilepsy in remission were undecided as to what to do after a period in remission. This number was considerably reduced (to 9 per cent) by the use of a predictive model which presented the risk of seizure recurrence for policies of continued treatment and withdrawal. The latter policy consistently predicted greater risks of relapse than did the former. Only 10 per cent of subjects (almost entirely adults) decided to withdraw treatment after reviewing the results of the model. In a study of children, Gordon et al[20] found that parents' views of acceptable risk of withdrawal corresponded very poorly with those of their physicians, and in a way that was not easily predicted by clinical factors in the children.

If a decision is taken to withdraw treatment, clear advice should be offered about the speed of withdrawal and the steps to take if seizures recur. Tennison et al[21] found no evidence of a difference in recurrence rates when AEDs were tapered over 6 weeks as opposed to 9 months. From a practical point of view, it seems reasonable to taper most regimens gradually over a 2–3-month period. For children in remission, occasional seizures while remaining off treatment may be acceptable under some circumstances, but for many adults a seizure recurrence will usually require the prompt reinstitution of the AED regimen that was previously successful.

Summary

The decision to stop AEDs requires a careful, individualized assessment of the risks of both seizures and continuing treatment. The physician's role is to provide satisfactory information for the individual patient and their family to help them make a decision. In adults, treatment should usually be continued until there has been a remission of between 2 and 5 years, but in children shorter remission periods of 12 months may be adequate. The benefits of stopping medications in children certainly seem to outweigh their risks in most circumstances. In adults, by contrast, the risks and consequences associated with a relapse are such that the decision to stop medications is more complicated. Overall, the clinical risks of relapse appear to be largely counter-balanced by the psychosocial benefits of discontinuing treatment. Predictive models can be satisfactorily used to identify risks of further seizures. There is no evidence to indicate that withdrawal of treatment and seizure recurrence adversely affects future responsiveness to AED therapy.

References

1. Annegers JF, Hauser WA, Elveback LR. Remission of seizures and relapse in patients with epilepsy. *Epilepsia* 1979;20:729–37.
2. Cockerell OC, Johnson AL, Sander JWAS, Shorvon SD. Prognosis of epilepsy: a review and further analysis of the first nine years of the British National General Practice Study of Epilepsy, a prospective population-based study. *Epilepsia* 1997;38:31–46.
3. Medical Research Council Antiepileptic Drug Withdrawal Study Group. Prognostic index for recurrence of seizures after remission of epilepsy. *BMJ* 1993;306:1374–8.
4. Peters AC, Brouwer OF, Geerts AT, et al. Randomized prospective study of early discontinuation of antiepileptic drugs in children with epilepsy: Dutch study of epilepsy in childhood. *Neurology* 1998;50:724–30.
5. Berg AT, Shinnar S. Relapse following discontinuation of antiepileptic drugs: a meta-analysis. *Neurology* 1994;44:601–8.
6. Braathan G, Andersson T, Gylje H, et al. Comparison between one and three years of treatment in uncomplicated childhood epilepsy: a prospective study. I. Outcome in different seizure types. *Epilepsia* 1996;37:822–32.
7. Placencia M, Shorvon S, Paredes V, et al. Epileptic seizures in an Andean region of Ecuador: incidence and prevalence and regional variation. *Brain* 1992;115:771–82.
8. Medical Research Council Antiepileptic Drug Withdrawal Study Group. Randomised study of antiepileptic drug withdrawal in patients in remission. *Lancet* 1991;337:1175–80.
9. Commission on Classification and Terminology of the International League Against Epilepsy. Proposal for revised classification of epilepsies and epileptic syndromes. *Epilepsia* 1989;30:389–99.
10. Berg AT, Shinnar S, Chadwick D. Discontinuing antiepileptic drugs. In: Engel J, Pedley TA, eds. *Epilepsy: a comprehensive textbook*. New York: Lippincott-Raven, 1998:1275–84.
11. Shinnar S, Berg ST, Moshe SL, et al. Discontinuing antiepileptic drugs in children with epilepsy: a prospective study. *Ann Neurol* 1994;35:534–45.
12. Shinnar S, Vining EPG, Mellits ED, et al. Discontinuing antiepileptic medication in children with epilepsy after two years without seizures. *N Engl J Med* 1985;31:976–80.
13. Mastropaolo T, Tondi C, Carboni F, Manca S, Zoroddu F. Prognosis after therapy discontinuation in children with epilepsy. *Eur Neurol* 1992;32:141–5.
14. Berg AT, Levy SR, Novotny EJ, Shinnar S. Predictors of intractable epilepsy in childhood: a case-control study. *Epilepsia* 1996;37:24–30.
15. Sillanpaa M. Remission of seizures and prediction of intractability in long-term follow-up. *Epilepsia* 1993;34:930–6.
16. Dooley J, Gordon K, Camfield P, Camfield C, Smith E. Discontinuation of anticonvulsant therapy in children free of seizures for 1 year: a prospective study. *Neurology* 1996;46:969–74.
17. Chadwick D, Taylor J, Johnson A. Outcomes after seizure recurrence in people with well-controlled epilepsy and the factors that influence it. *Epilepsia* 1996;37:1043–50.

18. Jacoby A, Johnson A, Chadwick D. Psycho-social outcomes of antiepileptic drug discontin-uation. *Epilepsia* 1992;**33**:1123–31.

19. Jacoby A, Baker G, Chadwick D, Johnson A. The impact of counselling with a practical statistical model on patients' decision-making about treatment for epilepsy: findings from a pilot study. *Epilepsy Res* 1993;**16**:207–14.

20. Gordon K, MacSween J, Dooley J, Camfield C, Camfield P, Smith E. Families are content to discontinue antiepileptic drugs at different risks than their physicians. *Epilepsia* 1996;**37**: 557–62.

21. Tennison M, Greenwood R, Lewis D, Thorn M. Discontinuing antiepileptic drugs in children with epilepsy: A comparison of six-week and a nine-month taper period. *N Engl J Med* 1994;**330**:1407–10.

17

Overtreatment of epilepsy and how to avoid it

Dieter Schmidt

'Don't overdo it. With anticonvulsants less may be more.'

Introduction

In a recent survey, epilepsy experts named overtreatment as one of the most common errors in the medical management of epilepsy.[1] More specifically, three forms of overtreatment were discussed by the experts: (i) inappropriately starting drug therapy, (ii) unnecessarily high dosage of antiepileptic drugs (AEDs), and (iii) adding another drug before monotherapy had failed. Although it is difficult to be certain about the incidence and the impact of overtreatment, there is growing concern about the long-term risks associated with unnecessary AED treatment. In this chapter, a brief overview of overtreatment in epilepsy will be presented, and clinical guidelines for prevention of overtreatment will be discussed. The comments should not be taken as a rigid blueprint for medical practice for each and every patient with epilepsy. Instead they are meant to provide general management principles and recommendations based on the best available clinical evidence.

Erroneous AED exposure in patients misdiagnosed as having epilepsy

Unnecessary treatment with AEDs is common in patients misdiagnosed as having epilepsy.

About 20 per cent of patients referred to specialized epilepsy centers for refractory epilepsy carry a misdiagnosis of epilepsy.[2] Accurate diagnosis of non-epileptic seizures is further complicated because they may co-exist with epileptic seizures in some patients. Syncope (see Chapter 2) and non-epileptic psychogenic seizures are often mistaken for epilepsy (Figure 17.1).

A recent videometric analysis of 56 brief syncopal events showed myoclonic activity in 90 per cent, together with head turns, upward gaze, oral automatism, righting movements, and visual and auditory hallucinations in 60–80 per cent.[3] The following useful factors, if present, usually prevent misdiagnosis of syncope as a tonic–clonic seizure and subsequent erroneous treatment with anticonvulsants:[4] characteristic precipitating factors; premonitory features such as nausea, sweating and palpitation; brief duration of <25 s; absence of paroxysmal electro-encephalographic (EEG) activity; and no evidence for disorientation, exhaustion or sleep following the attack. Clearly, AEDs are not only unhelpful, they may even worsen the non-epileptic attacks. Cardiovascular side effects of carbamazepine, such as bradycardia, may potentially worsen the symptomatology of syncope.

Patients with psychogenic seizures may show a variety of psychopathological symptoms and specific pharmacological treatment including antidepressants may be necessary. AEDs have

Misdiagnosis of absence
- Daydreaming
- Narcolepsy
- Focal cataplexy
- Psychogenic seizures
- Tics

Misdiagnosis of simple partial seizures
- Migraine
- Transient ischemic attacks
- Psychogenic seizures
- Paroxysmal dysfunction in multiple sclerosis
- Focal myoclonus
- Hyperventilation
- Unilateral tic
- Hemifacial spasm
- Cataplexy

Misdiagnosis of complex partial seizures
- Psychogenic seizures
- Narcolepsy
- Sleepwalking
- Paroxysmal medical symptoms (e.g. dislocation of pacemaker electrodes)
- Migraine
- Panic attacks

Misdiagnosis of tonic–clonic seizures
- Syncope
- Psychogenic seizures
- Tetany
- Generalized myoclonus
- Cataplexy

Misdiagnosis of epileptic drop attacks
- Vertebrobasilar vascular disease
- Peripheral vestibular dysfunction
- Hydrocephalus-associated drop attacks
- Parkinson's syndrome
- Orthopedic problems
- Cryptogenic drop attacks
- Psychogenic drop attacks
- Cataplexy

Figure 17.1
Non-epileptic seizures misdiagnosed as epileptic seizures and inappropriately treated with anticonvulsants.

not been shown to be effective in the treatment of psychogenic seizures. Given that depression is one of the many psychopathological features of patients with psychogenic seizures, it is worth noting that a number of AEDs may either cause or contribute to depression in some patients. These drugs include phenobarbital and phenytoin among the older drugs, and tiagabine and vigabatrin among the more recently developed AEDs.

Perhaps the most dramatic and extreme manifestation of psychogenic seizures is pseudostatus epilepticus. The term refers to repeated or continuous seizures which are psychogenic in origin, but resemble (at least superficially) convulsive status epilepticus.[5] The danger of the condition is that misdiagnosis results in mistreatment. A vicious cycle starts when status epilepticus is misdiagnosed and intravenous anticonvulsants are given. Seizures do not stop and more drugs are administered until the patient is comatose. As soon as the patient regains consciousness, seizures recur, and more anticonvulsants are given. Often, the patient ends up in an intensive care unit receiving artificial respiration. The cycle may not stop here. Seizures recur and anesthesia is continued. The large doses of sedative drugs carry a high risk of iatrogenic morbidity and mortality. The drama ends once the psychogenic seizures are recognized or the patient suffers a serious complication of treatment. To the experienced observer the diagnosis is usually straightforward. The bizarre thrashing movements do not have the classic features of convulsive seizures, but fluctuate in intensity, frequency, and distribution as the status proceeds, often influenced by verbal intervention or emotional external factors. In rare cases the patient may use mydriatics to produce dilated, unresponsive pupils, and intentional tongue biting, often involving the tip of the tongue, is not uncommon. It should be kept in mind that tongue bites in the course of convulsive seizures are typically found on the lateral tongue and not on the tip of the tongue. Video-EEG during pseudostatus reveals no paroxysmal changes and sometimes the patient can be observed to purposely fall out of bed. The history typically reveals previous episodes of pseudostatus resulting in hospitalization, and most patients have a long history of psychiatric and personality disorders including, in some cases, Munchausen's syndrome.

The immediate treatment of pseudostatus is quite simple. All anticonvulsants and sedative therapy should be stopped immediately, and supportive but firm verbal encouragement should be given. As soon as the patient realizes that the correct diagnosis has been made, the episode usually ends. A few patients may have co-existing epilepsy, and a tonic–clonic seizure may have started the whole episode of pseudo-seizures. Long-term treatment is less successful—many patients relapse and soon present to another hospital. The mechanisms are often obscure—malingering, depression or abnormal personality are usually diagnosed, but treatment efforts often fail.

Finally, after discussing Munchausen's syndrome in the context of pseudostatus epilepticus, parents (usually the mother), may in rare cases admit to inducing epileptic seizures in the child. This is called Munchausen-by-proxy syndrome. Alternatively, a parent may claim to have witnessed fictitious seizures in her children. Immediate anticonvulsant treatment and elaborate diagnostic evaluation is requested by the parent. Typically, the mother is a nurse or has been working in a medical environment, and insists on taking part in the care of the child at the hospital. The diagnosis is straightforward if the physician considers the possibility, although it may initially meet with opposition from the nursing staff, because the mother is seen as taking particularly good care of the child. Often she does not allow anyone to come close to the child without her being present. Treatment is straightforward. The parents, including the father, are informed about the diagnosis and if the mother is prevented from seeing the child for a while, the

Causes of non-epileptic seizures	Number of patients (n = 298)	%
Syncope	63	21.14
Convulsive syncope	36	12.08
Psychogenic including panic disorders	10	3.36
Vertigo	6	2.01
Transient global amnesia	5	1.68
Transient ischemic attack	4	1.34
Migraine with aura	4	1.34
Other (seen in <4 cases)	29	9.73
Etiology unknown	141	47.32

From Forsgren et al, 1996.[6]

Table 17.1
Situation-related seizures and seizures with medical causes in 298 Norwegian adults.

seizures stop. The long-term treatment is more difficult and separation from the mother by legal restraint may be required. The mechanism of Munchausen-by-proxy syndrome is poorly understood and the incidence, although probably uncommon, is unknown.

Overtreatment of epileptic seizures induced by precipitating or predisposing factors

AEDs may not be necessary to control situation-related or acute symptomatic seizures that are indisputably epileptic in nature. Patients with tonic–clonic seizures that exclusively occur in temporal relationship with well-defined seizure precipitants, such as lack of sleep or alcohol consumption, are very common. Patients with a first tonic–clonic seizure that is clearly related to such a precipitant do not need anticonvulsant medication. However, the causes of so-called situation-

related seizures are identified in only about half of these patients (Table 17.1).

Another large group of patients has seizures due to medical causes and does not truly have epilepsy. The medical causes of epilepsy are manifold and include systemic disease affecting the nervous system, organ failure, ischemia-hypoxia, electrolyte and endocrine disturbances, cancer, medication and medication withdrawal, alcohol, drugs and poisonings, hypertensive encephalopathy and organ transplantation. There is a general consensus that only patients with recurrent seizures due to medical causes who have uncorrectable predisposing factors need long-term treatment with anticonvulsant medication.[7]

Changing life-style may be sufficient for seizure control in individual patients with epilepsy, e.g. some patients with juvenile myoclonic epilepsy (JME) who have exclusively mild and infrequent myoclonic seizures.[8] It has been estimated that 7–17 per cent of patients in hospital and clinic-based series have only myoclonic seizures. The authors of these reports suggest that the percentages may be underestimated because myoclonic jerks alone may not be recognized as epilepsy, often being interpreted as early morning clumsiness or nervousness. In a Norwegian series of 43 patients with JME, 7 per cent were seizure-free without medication.[9] In fact, the efficacy of AEDs in JME was never scrutinized in a controlled trial. The specific antiepileptic effect of medications, such as valproate cannot therefore be distinguished from concurrent reduction of seizure precipitants or spontaneous remission. Although the impact and extent of seizure precipitation in JME is not well known, as many as 50 per cent of patients with JME reported at least one seizure recurrence during drug treatment due to seizure precipitation. In fact, 13 of 25 patients had two or more such recurrences.[10] Accordingly, control of specific seizure precipitants may be important, at least in some patients with JME.[11] In a recent publication, 27 of 213 cases of JME with specific seizure precipitants were unresponsive to standard AEDs.[12] Astonishingly, it is not known to what extent JME can be controlled without drug treatment just by eliminating seizure precipitants. A recent review concluded that both the response to AEDs and the relapse following discontinuation of drugs in patients in remission (requiring re-institution of drug treatment) have been determined by retrospective studies of biased cohorts, and that the general concensus for the need for drug treatment in JME may be, at least in part, a result of selection bias.[13]

Finally, and perhaps most intriguingly, the extent of placebo response in previously untreated epilepsy is unknown. Nevertheless, there is some evidence that AEDs are effective in newly diagnosed epilepsy where, for example, treatment with carbamazepine was better than no treatment in a trial of first seizures.[14] However, in patients with uncontrolled chronic epilepsy, the placebo response is variable and may result in a reduction of seizure frequency by half in 10 to 20 per cent of patients.[15] Given the placebo response in patients with uncontrolled epilepsy, it is difficult to estimate the specific effects of adding a second drug in failures of monotherapy. This aspect will be discussed below.

Overtreatment with unnecessarily high dosages of AEDs

Overtreatment with unnecessarily high dosages of AEDs may, in principle, occur at the start of treatment in previously untreated patients with early epilepsy, and, perhaps more often, in partially responsive patients with chronic epilepsy receiving further dose increments. Ideally, any patient with early epilepsy is treated with the lowest effective dose of an anticonvulsant at the onset of treatment. But two problems emerge. First, the lowest effective dose (which is more effective than placebo) has not been determined for most AEDs, and second, physicians eager to suppress seizures as soon as possible may choose a higher than necessary dose rather than risk another seizure. A study of 500 mg valproate for initial treatment of patients with newly diagnosed JME showed that the dose was sufficient for complete seizure control in many patients, suggesting that the usually recommended effective dose of anticonvulsants may be higher than necessary for some patients. While the impact and incidence of initial overtreatment are unknown, it has been shown that patients with tonic–clonic seizures alone require lower serum concentrations (and lower effective doses) for treatment than patients with simple and partial seizures.[16]

In patients continuing to have seizures, increasing the dosage of the AED may be beneficial. In one report, 31 per cent of patients with previously uncontrolled partial seizures became seizure-free when the dosage of their AED was increased.[17]

Conversely, failure to reach the maximum tolerated dose is a common error in the treatment of epilepsy.[1] Unfortunately, as many as two thirds of patients with uncontrolled seizures do not benefit from treatment with the maximum tolerated dose. In fact, in some patients, seizure frequency may even increase with the further dose increments, as discussed recently in a review on the exacerbation of seizures induced by AEDs.[18] The maximum tolerated dose should be maintained only in those who show a meaningful reduction in seizure frequency or intensity. In all other cases the dose should be reduced to the previous lower dosage that provided a similar benefit. Leaving the patient on the maximum tolerated dose, when a lower dose is equally effective, is a common cause of overtreatment and of chronic AED toxicity. In fact, some patients may even have fewer seizures when the dose is reduced.[17]

Not surprisingly, patients who have not received the appropriate drug will not benefit from dose increments or decrements. Errors in the choice of drugs due to misdiagnosis of the seizure type are among the most common errors in treatment, as discussed in Chapter 23. If the first AED continues to be ineffective at the maximum tolerated dose, two therapeutic options are available: (i) add a second drug or (ii) substitute another drug for the original drug. These options and their inherent risk of overtreatment are covered in the following section (Figure 17.2).

Overtreatment with a second drug in failures of monotherapy

Physicians who prefer to add a second drug (instead of replacing the first drug) justify their practice by the observation that some patients appear to require multiple drug therapy in order to achieve optimal seizure control; yet the proportion of patients requiring multiple drug therapy is unknown. Furthermore, the need for polytherapy has been convincingly demonstrated for only a few drug combinations, most notably valproate and ethosuximide in absence seizures refractory to either drug alone.[19] However, few physicians will deny their patients the chance of trying combinations of drugs when monotherapy has failed. The main advantage of this approach is that seizures in patients requiring combination therapy can be more rapidly controlled than if one AED is substituted for another. Psychologically, adding more drugs seems intuitively the right thing to do, and it may be thought that patients expect to receive more medication when seizures persist. Obviously, one disadvantage is that those who would do well on alternative monotherapy are exposed to overtreatment; but it can be argued that the unnecessary first drug can be removed later after evaluating the effects of combination therapy more fully. As a practical matter, however, removal of the first AED is met with little enthusiasm by those who do well on both drugs. As a consequence, potential overtreatment may remain undetected and uncorrected.

Unfortunately, a rational choice of therapeutic strategies for patients who fail to respond to initial monotherapy is hampered by a lack of useful information from controlled trials. It is largely unknown whether combining AEDs with a different mechanism of action can produce additive therapeutic effects and whether adverse effects may be additive or infra-additive. Indeed, except for a small study, published as an abstract only, that suggested little advantage of combining phenytoin and carbamazepine,[20] no controlled study has yet

- Ensure that the patient has experienced epileptic seizures before starting AED therapy. Patients with syncope and other non-epileptic seizures do not benefit from anticonvulsants and may, in fact, worsen. Consider the diagnosis of pseudostatus in unusual cases of refractory status epilepticus, and of Munchausen-by-proxy syndrome in unresponsive seizures in a child, before embarking on invasive evaluation.
- In patients with indisputable epileptic seizures, identify those with situation-related seizures and seizures of medical cause. Patients with situation-related seizures do not need treatment with AEDs, instead, control of seizure precipitants may be sufficient. Patients with seizures of medical cause do not need long-term treatment with AEDs except for those with recurrent seizures and uncorrectable predisposing factors.
- Seizure precipitation may also play a major role in JME and those with myoclonic seizures alone may not need AEDs if seizure precipitants can be controlled.
- In patients with refractory epilepsy who continue to have disabling seizures despite adequate first-line treatment: (i) review patient compliance, and (ii) ensure that the maximum tolerated dose has been used. If a standard drug continues to be ineffective at the maximum tolerated dose: (i) reduce the dosage until a further dose decrement is precluded by an unacceptable increase in seizure frequency or intensity, and (ii) introduce an alternative drug.
- If the patient responds well to the addition of the second drug, consider slowly withdrawing the original drug. However, if the patient did not benefit from adding the second drug, the original drug should be withdrawn to avoid unnecessary polytherapy before introducing a further drug as described before.
- In patients whose seizures cannot be controlled by monotherapy substitution or add-on drug: (i) review the diagnosis and identify non-epileptic seizures and episodes, and (ii) explore surgical options including vagal nerve stimulation.
- If surgical options are not suitable or have been exhausted, the patient should receive one anticonvulsant only (if possible) at a dose that provided maximum symptom control without intolerable adverse effects (or even better, without any adverse effects) in the past and see the patient regularly until better treatment becomes available. In anticonvulsant treatment of refractory epilepsy, less may be more.

Figure 17.2

Clinical guidelines for treatment with AEDs

evaluated the risk:benefit ratio of add-on therapy versus alternative monotherapy. Complete seizure control following the addition of a second drug was seen in 11 per cent of 82 cases with mostly early epilepsy in the large Veterans Administration Cooperative Study.[21] A similar result on addition of a second drug was reported in 4 of 30 patients

(13 per cent) with refractory partial seizures who failed to respond to monotherapy.[22] The relatively small benefit of adding a second drug prompted an investigation as to how many patients whose seizures were uncontrolled despite combination therapy actually need both drugs to maintain their level of seizure control. The effects of reducing two-drug treatment to single-drug therapy was studied in 36 patients with refractory complex partial seizures. In 30 patients (83 per cent) this was possible without an increase in seizure frequency. In only six patients (17 per cent) the number of seizures increased during single-drug therapy. Surprisingly, a reduction in seizure frequency was noted in 13 patients (36 per cent). The number of patients with side effects was similar with both two-drug and single-drug treatment, probably because single-drug therapy was titrated to the maximum tolerated dose.[17] Clearly, this early report documented unnecessary overtreatment with a second drug in >80 per cent of patients with refractory partial epilepsy treated with polytherapy. The main conclusion of this study was that reduction of polypharmacy may be beneficial for patients with intractable epilepsy.

In patients with refractory Lennox–Gastaut syndrome, reduction of sedative polypharmacy is possible without exacerbation of seizures.[23] In six patients followed for >2 years, the number of sedative drugs, mainly phenobarbital and primidone, dropped from 1.26 to 0.76 at the end of the observation period. There was no relationship between the serum concentrations of phenytoin and phenobarbital and the seizure frequency. The data suggested that reduction of polypharmacy is possible in some patients with Lennox–Gastaut syndrome receiving polytherapy. Surprisingly, none of the first-line anticonvulsants for Lennox–Gastaut syndrome, including valproate, was shown to be effective in a controlled trial, raising the intriguing possibility that because of confounding factors (including placebo response) some patients may, at least in part, be treated by medication without adequate evidence for specific efficacy.

Although the concept of reducing polypharmacy is well accepted, its implementation in clinical practice is much more difficult. The proposal to cancel anticonvulsants in the face of uncontrolled seizures appears counter-intuitive to many patients. The message that fewer drugs do not necessarily mean more seizures and may even mean fewer seizures in some patients needs careful explanation. Intensive counselling about the benefit and the small risk of gradual withdrawal is required. Supplying the relatives or caregivers with rectal benzodiazepine medication is recommended to stop flurries of seizures, if necessary, and will increase the chances that the reduction of polypharmacy will be successful. Patients who have doubts of their own about the effectiveness of their medications are usually interested in reduction. Waiting-room contacts will spread the word and others will follow. A caveat should be introduced, contrary to expectations, that adverse reactions may not necessarily be lower if one of several drugs is discontinued. Often, the dosage of the remaining drug needs to be increased to maintain the previous level of seizure control. This may account for the failure to reduce the side effects of the treatment. Furthermore, discontinuation of sedative drugs such as barbiturates or phenytoin at high doses may lead to an improvement only several months later. This, too, should be discussed prior to the transition to monotherapy.

The alternative approach to adding a further drug is gradual or immediate substitution with another drug. Although the response rate that can be achieved by alternative monotherapy in partial epilepsy has not been evaluated in a controlled trial, the evidence about the effectiveness of alternative monotherapy is suggestive. In one study, 59 patients with chronic partial epilepsy refractory to the maximum tolerated dose of carbamazepine, phenytoin, phenobarbital and primidone were substituted by single-drug treatment with one of the other standard drugs. Alternative monotherapy resulted in a seizure reduction of ⩾75 per cent in 18 patients (31 per cent).[24] In another study, 7 of 48 children (15 per cent) became seizure-free and a further 31 per cent had a reduction of ⩾50 per cent.[25] Unfortunately, no controlled trial has compared the effect of alternative monotherapy and add-on therapy in failures of initial monotherapy. Most surprisingly, the effect of alternative monotherapy in other less common epilepsy syndromes is unknown, raising the concern that the extent of overtreatment remains unknown for many patients with refractory epilepsy.

Summary

Overtreatment with anticonvulsants may, in principle, occur at all stages of treatment. Early in their course, patients may receive anticonvulsants, although their seizures may be controlled without any medication by avoiding seizure precipitants or letting spontaneous remission take its course. Patients with single seizures and those with situation-related seizures or acute symptomatic seizures due to medical conditions do not need long-term medication if the predisposing factors can be corrected. Furthermore, misdiagnosis of non-epileptic seizures and episodes may lead to mistreatment with anticonvulsants. Although dose increments are beneficial for many patients with ongoing partial seizures, failure to reverse the dose increments in those who do not benefit is a common form of overtreatment. Perhaps even more common is the failure to reduce unsuccessful polytherapy and establish alternative monotherapy at an optimum dosage in patients with refractory epilepsy. Although the percentage of patients exposed to the various forms of overtreatment has only been assessed in retrospective studies of biased cohorts, a conservative estimate is that as many as 50 per cent of patients with refractory epilepsy may be either misdiagnosed and given inappropiate treatment (20 per cent) or overtreated with unnecessary polytherapy (30 per cent). In addition, overtreatment may occur (to an unknown extent) during early epilepsy in those who would have entered remission without being exposed to anticonvulsants and in inappropriate long-term overtreatment of situation-related or acute symptomatic seizures. Although not well recognized, overtreatment may significantly contribute to the long-term risks of anticonvulsant treatment in patients with epileptic seizures.

References

1. Schmidt D. The ten most relevant errors in the treatment of epilepsy. *Epilepsia* 1998; **39** (Suppl 6):195.
2. Gates J, Ramani V, Whalen S. Ictal characteristics of pseudoseizures (abst). *Epilepsia* 1983; 24:246.
3. Lempert T, Bauer M, Schmidt D. Syncope: a videometric analysis of 56 episodes of transient cerebral hypoxia. *Ann Neurol* 1994;36:233–7.
4. Schmidt D. Syncopes and seizures. *Curr Opin Neurol* 1996;9:78–81.
5. Shorvon S. *Status Epilepticus. Its clinical features and treatment in children and adults.* Cambridge: Cambridge University Press, 1994:240.

6. Forsgren L, Edvinsson S-O, Nystrom L, Blomquist HK. Influence of epilepsy on mortality in mental retardation: an epidemiologic study. *Epilepsia* 1996;**37**:956–63.

7. Delanty N, Vaughan CJ, French JA. Medical causes of seizures. *Lancet* 1998;**352**:383–90.

8. Jain S, Padma MV, Maheshwari MC. Occurrence of only myoclonic jerks in juvenile myoclonic epilepsy. *Acta Neurol Scand* 1997;**95**:263–7.

9. Kleveland G, Engelsen BA. Juvenile myoclonic epilepsy: clinical characteristics, treatment and prognosis in a Norwegian population of patients. *Seizure* 1998;**7**:31–8.

10. Penry JK, Dean JC, Riela AR. Juvenile myoclonic epilepsy: long-term response to therapy. *Epilepsia* 1989;**30**(Suppl 4):S19–S23.

11. Inoue Y, Seino M, Kubota H, Yamakaku K, Tanaka M, Yagi K. Epilepsy with praxis-induced seizures. In: Wolf P, ed. *Epileptic seizures and syndromes*. London: John Libbey & Co, 1994:81–91.

12. Inoue Y. Praxis induced JME. In: Schmitz B, Sander T, eds. *Janz-syndrome: juvenile myoclonic epilepsy*. Wrighton; 1998.

13. Schmidt D. Response to antiepileptic drugs, and the rate of relapse after discontinuation of drug treatment in patients with juvenile myoclonic epilepsy. 1999; in press.

14. Beghi E, for the REST-1 Group. Morbidity and accidents in patients with epilepsy: a multicenter European study. *Epilepsia* 1997;**38**(Suppl 8):248.

15. Schmidt D. *Drug trials in epilepsy*. London: Martin Dunitz, 1998.

16. Schmidt D, Einicke I, Haenel F. The influence of seizure type on the efficacy of plasma concentrations of phenytoin, phenobarbital, and carbamazepine. *Arch Neurol* 1986;**43**:263–5.

17. Schmidt D. Single drug therapy for intractable epilepsy. *J Neurol* 1983;**229**:221–6.

18. Perucca E, Gram L, Avanzini G, Dulac O. Antiepileptic drugs as a cause of worsening seizures. *Epilepsia* 1998;**39**:5–17.

19. Rowan AJ, Meijer JWA, de Beer-Pawlikowski N, van der Geest P. Valproate ethosuximide combination therapy for refractory absence seizures. *Arch Neurol* 1983;**40**:797–802.

20. Hakkarainen H. Carbamazepine vs diphenylhydantoin vs their combination in adult epilepsy. *Neurology* 1980;**30**:354.

21. Mattson RH, Cramer JA, Collins JF, et al. Comparison of carbamazepine, phenobarbital, phenytoin and primidone in partial and secondary generalized tonic-clonic epileptic seizures. *N Engl J Med* 1985;**313**:145–51.

22. Schmidt D. Two antiepileptic drugs for intractable epilepsy with complex partial seizures. *J Neurol Neurosurg Psychiat* 1982;**45**:1119–24.

23. Schmidt D, Machus B. The use of blood levels in the treatment of patients with Lennox Syndrome. In: Johannessen SI, et al, eds. *Antiepileptic therapy: advances in drug monitoring*.New York: Raven Press, 1980, 279–85.

24. Schmidt D, Richter K. Alternative single anticonvulsant drug drug therapy for refractory epilepsy. *Ann Neurol* 1986;**19**:85–7.

25. Elkis LC, Bourgeois BFD, Wyllie E, et al. Efficacy of second antiepileptic drug after failure of one drug in children with partial epilepsy. *Epilepsia* 1993;**34**(Suppl 6):107.

18

Pregnancy and epilepsy

Dick Lindhout

Introduction

Drug treatment during the pregnancy of a woman with epilepsy frequently poses dilemmas for doctors because of the difficult-to-weigh risks and benefits of treatment versus no treatment. There are two main questions with respect to this issue:

- Do seizures harm the fetus?
- Does antiepileptic drug (AED) treatment harm the fetus?

The well-being of the offspring of mothers with epilepsy is also influenced by many other factors that may relate indirectly to specific treatment decisions, e.g. aetiology of the mother's epilepsy, seizure and treatment history, her concomitant disease and previous maternal adverse drug reactions. Therefore, treatment decisions are always made on an individual basis, and the outcome of pregnancy will depend on more factors than the relatively simple answers to the two questions addressed here. This complex background of pregnancy and epilepsy also has implications for the design of clinical epidemiological studies of pregnancy and epilepsy and the interpretation of their results. Lack of human evidence concerning the safety of many of the AEDs, especially the new drugs, of which there are more than 10 available, severely hampers evidence-based treatment decisions. This situation may improve consider-

ably with ongoing international multi-centre prospective population-based studies of pregnancy outcome.

Drug treatment in epilepsy is usually chronic. This adds another problem for doctors involved in the care of teenagers and women of reproductive age who have no immediate plans for pregnancy. Specifically, when should doctors begin to educate and counsel women of reproductive potential? Is before puberty too soon?

Effect of seizures on the unborn child

The answer to the question of whether seizures during pregnancy are harmful to the fetus commonly refers to the effects on the fetus from status epilepticus or severe, protracted generalized convulsions. There is a definite association between such seizures and fetal reactions, ranging from change in fetal cardiovascular function (e.g. rate decelerations) that may be interpreted as signs of fetal distress, to fetal death and to (subsequent) stillbirth.[1,2] Fetal lactic acidosis probably occurs during long-standing generalized seizures as a result of insufficiency of feto-maternal exchange and possibly also as a direct effect of maternal lactic acidosis secondary to generalized tonic–clonic seizures.[3] From a theoretical point of view, seizure-induced compromise of fetal circulation might also disrupt fetal development, but most if not all studies do not demonstrate an embryonic stage-specific (temporal) association between the occurrence of seizures and fetal malformations or deformities. Several studies do show a more general association between occurrence or frequency of generalized (non-absence) seizures, but this may reflect an association with type(s) and dose(s) of the antiepileptic medication(s) used during pregnancy.

Seizures during pregnancy and delivery not only present risks to the fetus but also impact the mother's well-being, indirectly affecting the fetus. Pre-pregnancy counselling should include information on the risk of generalized seizures provoked by suddenly stopping medication, e.g. when the patient unexpectedly finds out about her pregnancy and is concerned about possible teratogenic side effects of AEDs. This possibility alone is a good reason to discuss these issues long before pregnancy occurs, and to make optimal use of information leaflets if available. If printed information is not available, try to develop these for your own region in collaboration with other medical disciplines, the local chapter of the International League against Epilepsy and the local representatives of the International Bureau for Epilepsy.

Seizure frequency may change during pregnancy. Over the past 30 years, variable figures have been put forward with respect to the proportion of women experiencing an increase, decrease, or no change at all during successive stages of pregnancy.[4] These studies usually demonstrate nearly equal probabilities for these three possible outcomes, even in the same women in successive pregnancies. The results are very much dependent on uncontrolled factors like patient selection, seizure registration methods, and the proportion of patients who achieved complete seizure control before they became pregnant, as reviewed by Tomson.[5] Unfortunately, there is no good predictor for the change in seizure frequency

during pregnancy compared with pre-pregnancy.

Pregnancy is also associated with many changes in pharmacokinetic parameters. For the first generation AEDs, these changes tend to decrease total blood levels. Extended volume of distribution, changes in gastrointestinal absorption, induction of hepatic drug metabolism, and altered renal clearance are some of the factors that lower drug levels. At the same time, pregnancy is also associated with lower protein binding and therefore, free plasma AED concentrations tend to stay unchanged or decrease only slightly. There is no clear relationship between lower plasma concentrations of AEDs and increased seizure frequency. Consequently adjustment of AED dosages or change of AED should be carried out on clinical grounds in order to control seizures or decrease toxicity and not on the basis of plasma drug concentrations alone.

During pregnancy, medication compliance may decrease because of maternal concern about the teratogenic side effects of the drugs. The extent to which this plays a role in loss of seizure control during pregnancy is not well known, because of the lack of prospective studies monitoring both serum drug concentrations and seizure frequency during pregnancy.

Special attention is needed in the case of termination of pregnancy because of prenatally diagnosed fetal abnormalities. This can be illustrated by a retrospective case analysis of a woman who participated in a prospective prenatal cohort study of pregnancy outcome.[6] Three days after hearing about the diagnosis of spina bifida aperta in her monozygous twin-fetuses, she decided to terminate her pregnancy. During prostaglandin-induced labour, she experienced generalized tonic–clonic seizures. Literature review suggested that the prostaglandin might be the precipitating factor.[7] However, later analysis of the maternal serum, fetal blood, and amniotic fluid samples collected at amniocentesis and termination of pregnancy showed AED serum concentrations that were, at the time of termination of pregnancy, only a fraction of what they had been at the time of the initial amniocentesis. However, the amniotic fluid levels at termination of pregnancy in this case were much higher than maternal and fetal serum levels. This indicated that the amniotic fluid compartment is a deep compartment, and that the measured levels were compatible with the mother stopping medication shortly after she learned of the adverse outcome of the prenatal diagnostic procedures. Proper counselling about the need for medication compliance, and adequate drug-level monitoring when the fetal diagnosis is communicated is required and may help to prevent or eliminate such additional risks.

The risk of major generalized seizures during labour and delivery and immediately thereafter is probably between 2 and 5 per cent.[5] Taking into account the duration of labour and delivery, this risk is estimated to be about 10 times higher than during the rest of pregnancy.[8] Adequate facilities for seizure control and for artificial termination of delivery will help to avoid serious complications in most cases.

Stillbirth and neonatal death rates are increased by a factor of two to three compared with various control populations.[9,10]. However, there has been no single cause identified, which limits possibilities for targeted prevention.

Effects of AEDs on the unborn

Chemically-induced congenital abnormalities include a wide range of effects, from abnormal pre- and postnatal growth and development to major malformations.[11] The four main features of chemical-induced birth defects are:

- The teratogenic effect is related to the *structure of the chemical agent*. This explains why subtle differences in the structure of the chemical may be related to large differences in teratogenic effects, such as demonstrated by two thalidomide stereoisomers—one is strongly teratogenic and the other not—and by the enantiomers of teratogenic valproic acid derivatives.[12]

- The teratogenic effect occurs only in a *sensitive susceptible organism*. Its sensitivity is partly determined by its genetic make up, which explains species and strain differences in teratogen sensitivity under similar conditions.[13] This also explains why teratogenic effects in humans may occur despite negative pre-clinical testing for teratogenicity in a number of animal species. The genetic predisposition may also be mediated through pharmacogenetic differences (pharmacokinetics, metabolism), but may also be active at the pharmacodynamic level (cellular teratogen end-points). The aforementioned frequently noticed stereo-isomer-dependent differences in teratogen activity suggests that many compounds do indeed exert their effect through a kind of receptor–ligand interaction, where the drug, or one of its metabolites, is specifically bound to a receptor involved in the primary teratogenic process.[12]

- The teratogenic effect is related to the *dose* of the compound administered or exposed to. In this respect, there is some academic discussion as to whether there really is a dose dependency in the individual organism, since frequently the teratogenic endpoint is an all or none effect, i.e. a specific major malformation is either present or absent. Its occurrence may then depend only on the degree of the exposure and the chance that it goes beyond a certain threshold for that specific organism. When studying a heterogeneous population of individuals from the same species or strain, each with its own threshold, the results may reflect a dose-response curve. The relationship between dose and teratogenic effects also depends on the mode of administration. It has to be borne in mind that under certain circumstances, e.g. general anaesthesia for surgery, the occurrence of protracted generalized seizures or status epilepticus will often prompt non-oral administration of anticonvulsant medications. Depending on drug and species, the total daily dose, the dose per administration, the peak blood levels, or the area under the curve of blood levels may be some of the more relevant parameters determining teratogenicity.[14,15]

- The teratogenic effect is dependent on the *embryonic stage of development*. If a sensitive organism is exposed to a teratogenic agent outside the period of teratogen sensitivity, then no side effects occur. In combination with the inter-individual differences in teratogen sensitivity, this also implies that there may be considerable variation in the type of defect related to chronic AED exposure. Some fetuses may be more prone to a teratogenic effect in an early phase of embryonic development and others more to effects that occur in later stages. Only a few exposed fetuses will show susceptibility to the complete spectrum of drug-specific teratogenic effects.

The possible endpoints of teratogenesis in general are:

- Prenatal growth abnormalities—usually growth failure, but excessive growth may

also occur, as is illustrated with the influence of maternal diabetes on fetal growth.
- Stillbirth and neonatal death.
- Impaired perinatal adaptation.
- Major congenital anomalies.
- Minor abnormalities or so-called dysmorphic features.
- Postnatal growth abnormalities (length or height, weight, head circumference).
- Disturbed postnatal psychomotor and cognitive development.
- Permanent changes in functions.
- Induction of new mutations during early embryogenesis, which may lead to gonadal or somatic mozaicism in the offspring, and subsequent occurrence of neoplasia, or transmission of genetic defects to the third generation.
- Other third-generation effects, including effects on fertility (compare the effects of diethylstilboestrol on the reproductive capability of prenatally exposed offspring).

Many of these outcome parameters are also dependent on genetic and environmental factors like:

- Genetic factors causing or predisposing to maternal epilepsy and possibly also responsible for (a predisposition to) specific adverse fetal outcomes.
- Genetic factors that predispose for a specific malformation, but that are not related to the maternal epilepsy or the fetal sensitivity to side effects of the AED(s).
- Genetic factors that predispose the fetus to the side effects of the AEDs; pharmacogenetic or pharmacodynamic predispositions that may be effective in the maternal organism, the placenta or the fetus itself, and therefore are also under the influence of paternally inherited genes.
- Nutritional factors, such as folic acid

status, which may interact with both folate-dependent genetic factors and drugs to which the mother and the fetus are exposed.

- Other environmental factors, partly related to socio-economic status.

Several of these factors are not independent from partner choice, which in fact implies that partner choice—because of its relevance for the genetic and environmental background of the fetus—may have considerable influence on the outcome of pregnancy and postnatal development.[16,17]

Rather than dealing superficially with all the topics listed above, the following will focus on some major issues and discuss several aspects in more detail. It has to be borne in mind, however, that similar points of discussion can be raised with each of the other topics. The evaluation of some of the other endpoints, such as growth parameters (continuous values), is facilitated by the fact that measurements from each individual are equally contributing to the analysis as opposed to discrete parameters reflecting low frequency of adverse outcome. On the other hand, analysis of such parameters frequently provides statistically significant differences between exposed and non-exposed pregnancies, but the absolute difference in measurement outcome may be relatively so small that its clinical relevance *per se* remains totally unclear. In such cases the only conclusion may be that there is an effect which in combination with other effects, e.g. on psychomotor or cognitive development, is indicative of a teratogenic potential of the drug under analysis.

A second aspect of each endpoint analysis is the role of genetic factors and the need to control for these as much as possible. This can be done by family history (major malformations, epilepsy, febrile seizures), examination of parents and siblings exposed to similar or different drugs or non-exposed (dysmorphic features, growth and other quantifiable parameters) and molecular genetic analysis of predispositions (future risk).

The currently available AEDs may be subdivided into:

- first-generation (phenobarbitone, primidone, phenytoin and ethosuximide),
- second-generation (carbamazepine, valproate and many benzodiazepines including clobazam, clonazepam, clorazepate, lorazepam, and nitrazepam), and
- third-generation (oxcarbazepine, lamotrigine, felbamate, topiramate, gabapentin, losigamone, piracetam, progabide, remacemide, stiripentol, tiagabine, vigabatrin, and zonisamide).

In 1997, some third-generation AEDs were still undergoing clinical trials, but during the mid-1990s the majority of these compounds had been released for prescription in many countries on several continents. Of primary and immediate concern is whether any of these drugs might cause major congenital malformations.

The first-generation AEDs were mainly associated with an increased risk of congenital heart anomalies and cleft lip and palate as well as many other types of defects.

The two major AEDs of the second generation, valproate and carbamazepine, were predominantly associated with neural tube defects and hypospadias. Whereas valproate is especially associated with spina bifida aperta, usually of the lumbosacral type and frequently complicated by hydrocephalus, the spectrum of neural tube defects that occur with carbamazepine seems to be more diverse and possibly includes isolated hydrocephalus and encephalocele.[18] The overall risk of major malformations is more or less the same for the major compounds of the first and second generation, approximately two-to-three times the general population risk. Several studies point towards a relatively higher than average risk with valproate and a relatively lower than average risk with monotherapy in general. The risk of neural tube defects is about 1–2 per cent with valproate, 0.5–1 per cent with carbamazepine and about 0.35 per cent with AEDs from the first generation.

Several studies also found a relationship between daily dose of some of the drugs and overall risk of major malformation or adverse pregnancy outcome. With regard to specific malformations, a significant dose-effect relationship is found between valproate and spina bifida aperta, indicating that daily doses >1500 mg/day are associated with much higher risk of spina bifida aperta than the average risk given by most authors (1–2 per cent).[6,19,20]

These risk figures justify the need for prenatal diagnosis by ultrasound examination in the 16–20th week of pregnancy for a patient taking any kind of AED, and amniotic fluid analysis during the first trimester when the pregnant woman is taking valproate or carbamazepine. In some countries, maternal serum α-fetoprotein (msAFP) screening may be available and also offered to pregnant women with epilepsy taking AEDs. However, this screening is not as reliable as AFP analysis of amniotic fluid (afAFP), and missing the diagnosis may cause extreme disappointment in couples who were already aware of the increased risk of neural tube defect associated with maternal AED. Furthermore, there are strong indications that msAFP screening may be even less reliable in cases of valproate-induced neural tube defects. In a prospective cohort study of women referred for prenatal diagnosis, Omtzigt et al evaluated the value of msAFP analysis as compared with routine afAFP

analysis. They found that four out of six cases of neural tube defect would have been missed or diagnosed only much later in pregnancy by ultrasound examination if only msAFP screening had been used.[21]

There is only limited, if any, information about the third-generation AEDs regarding their safety for the human fetus. The companies that market lamotrigine and vigabatrin have set up drug-specific registries in an attempt to recruit information from all countries were the drug is released for prescription use. When using the data in these registries or reading the registry reports, it should be taken into account that such information is retrieved through selective reporting. Even the prospective series may have selectively enrolled patients because of additional risk factors. Also, these drug-specific registries do not allow for comparison between different drugs marketed by different companies. Furthermore, most new drugs are initially released for prescription as add-on medication for patients with difficult-to-control seizures, so that most pregnancy experience is confounded by the indication for its prescription as well as by the co-medication and the possible drug interactions. This clearly demonstrates the need for population-based prospective studies conducted by independent third parties that will allow performance of the most clinically relevant analysis and that may form a basis for evidence-based prescription.

The main advantage of drug-specific registries is the possibility that a signal of a potentially significant teratogenic side effect will be recognized, as early as possible, by the emergence of a more or less specific pattern of defects in a number of registered pregnancy outcomes. For this reason, the companies keeping such registries should not hesitate to make their retrospectively ascertained and analysed case series available for external evaluation as well as their prospectively registered case series. If such a signal of a potentially teratogenic effect occurs, this should not automatically lead to 'conviction' of the drug, but rather to subsequent case-comparison or case-control studies and prospective studies that may provide an independent confirmation.

A difficult problem in daily clinical practice is the question of when to use a new third-generation drug with unknown teratogenic profile instead of drugs from the first or second generation, which have more or less proven risks of teratogenic side effects. A cautious approach would be to avoid prescribing third-generation AEDs to fertile women of reproductive age until the following is known:

- Does the drug have no effect on oral contraception efficacy?
- Does the drug show therapeutic advantages over other drugs with greater available pregnancy experience?

As soon as the answer to both questions is positive, one may decide to try the drug for patients in whom seizures are uncontrolled or who have severe side effects, still recommending to the patient that pregnancy be avoided. If, subsequently, the drug indeed proves to be superior in seizure control and shows no or a favourable pattern of maternal side effects, one may discuss the possibility of pregnancy with the patient under the new treatment. If pregnancy occurs, both doctor and mother should be prepared to share relevant information with registries evaluating pregnancy outcome on a population basis.

This guideline would prohibit doctors from taking women whose seizures are completely controlled with an older drug off their treatment in order to try a new compound, under the assumption that the new drug is more safe for the unborn child than the older one. In cases like these, the basis for change from an old to a new drug is only the balance between the known teratogenic side effects of the old drug versus the unknown teratogenic profile of a new drug. Such an approach is in fact a clinical drug trial, with the pregnancy outcome as an endpoint and the unborn embryo as the patient, taking risks that are difficult to calculate and providing data that may only be significant with denominators of several hundred exposed pregnancies. Such an approach would obviously need prior evaluation by a medical ethics body.

In general, polytherapy during pregnancy should be avoided for two reasons:

- By addition of effects of each of the drugs, and moreover through metabolic or pharmacodynamic interactions between drugs, the risk of teratogenic side effects may unpredictably increase by elevating levels of the teratogenic agent, whether one of the parent drugs or one or more of their metabolites. In fact, each specific drug combination should be regarded as a new therapeutic agent being marketed without preclinical testing. It is predominantly a 'back-to-the-wall' situation in an epilepsy patient that must justify the application of polytherapy during pregnancy.
- The teratogenic potential of some specific drug combinations is already known: such as phenobarbitone, primidone and phenytoin,[22] phenobarbital, carbamazepine and valproate,[23] and possibly, valproate and some of the benzodiazepines.[24,25]

Nutritional factors play an important role in the occurrence of major malformations in the general population. Several prospective controlled trials have demonstrated a significant reduction in the risk of neural tube defects when women were taking folic acid supplementation from before conception until at least the third month of pregnancy. The lowering effect on recurrence was demonstrated with 4–5 mg of folic acid per day (*high dose* folic acid) given to women who had at least one previous child with an open neural tube defect.[26] On first occurrence of neural tube defects, the lowering effect was demonstrated with 0.4–1.0 mg of folic acid (low dose) given to women in the general population.[27,28] As women on AEDs had been excluded in the study of the effect of *high dose* folic acid, there is no basis of evidence for prescribing high dose folic acid to epileptic women without a previous child with a neural tube defect. Furthermore, the relationship between folic acid and AED-induced birth defects is at least paradoxical if not unclear. Drugs that are most significantly associated with lower folate levels, like barbiturates and phenytoin, are least associated with neural tube defects and vice versa for valproate and carbamazepine. The identification of genetic factors that are dependent on folate levels and possibly predispose to neural tube defects, like the thermolabile variant of methylene-tetrahydrofolate reductase,[29] may help to elucidate this complex issue further.

Despite precautions, such as reduction of polytherapy, reduction of daily doses, and reduction of dose per administration (i.e. dividing the daily dose over more administrations per day), a child with a major malformation may be born. Parents will then be more concerned about the risk of recurrence of any kind of defect to a subsequent child. Although some studies indicate that indeed the recurrence risk is proportionally increased after the birth of a prenatally AED-exposed child with a major malformation, the available data are too scarce and heterogeneous to draw general conclusions. The best approach would be to refer the family to a clinical genetics centre with expertise in both genetic and teratogenic causes of congenital handicaps, in order to provide the parents with appropriate individual risk assessment and counselling.[30]

Summary

Maternal epilepsy is associated with increased risks for the human fetus. The general principles of teratogenesis and its possible endpoints are reviewed. Main-risk factors in maternal epilepsy are the use of antiepileptic drugs, the occurrence of seizures during pregnancy and possibly genetic factors, whether related to the maternal epilepsy or not. The large heterogeneity among the epilepsies, the large number of different treatment regimens, the increasing number of new and different antiepileptic drugs, the interaction between drugs, and uncertainty about the role of genetic factors all limit the power of epidemiological studies. Known risk factors are high dose levels and specific polytherapies. Antiepileptic drug use during the first trimester of pregnancy is an indication for structural prenatal ultrasound examination and, in case of an increased risk for neural tube defects such as with carbamazepine and valproate, also for amniotic fluid analysis of α-1-fetoprotein level. Unknown risk factors are presented by the new antiepileptic drugs of the third generation that have recently become available. Low-dose (daily 0.4–0.5 mg) folic acid supplementation is advised. Pre-pregnancy counselling should start early enough, maybe during puberty, to enable risk-factor reduction whenever possible.

Multicentre prospective and population-based studies are needed to evaluate the safety of the new drugs, and to further unravel the aetiological factors in adverse pregnancy outcome with treated maternal epilepsy.

References

1. Sabers A, Dam M. Pregnancy, delivery and puerperium. In: Dam M, Gram L, eds. *Comprehensive epileptology*. New York: Raven Press, 1990:299–307.

2. Hiilesma VK, Bardy AG, Teramo K. Obstetric outcome in women with epilepsy. *Am J Obstet Gynecol* 1985;**152**:499–504.

3. Orringer CE, Eustace JC, Wunsch CD, Gardner LB. Natural history of lactic acidosis after grand-mal seizures: a model for the study of an anion-gap acidosis not associated with hyperkalemia. *N Engl J Med* 1977;**297**:796–9.

4. Schmidt D. The effect of pregnancy on the natural history of epilepsy: a review of the literature. In: Janz D, Dam M, Richens A, Bossi L, Helge H, Schmidt D, eds. *Epilepsy, pregnancy, and the child*. New York: Raven Press, 1982:3–14.

5. Tomson T. Seizure control during pregnancy and delivery. In: Tomson T, Gram L, Sillanpää M, Johannessen SI. *Epilepsy and pregnancy*. Petersfield: Wrightson Biomedical, 1997:113–23.

6. Omtzigt JGC, Nau H, Los FJ, Pijpers L, Lindhout D. The disposition of valproate and its metabolites in the late first and early second trimesters of pregnancy in maternal serum, urine and amniotic fluid: effect of dose, comedication and the presence of spina bifida. *Eur J Clin Pharmacol* 1992;**43**:381–8.

7. Brandenburg H, Yahoda MGJ, Wladimiroff JW, Los FJ, Lindhout D. Convulsions in epileptic women after administration of prostaglandin E_2 derivative. *Lancet* 1990;**2**:1138.

8. Bardy AH. Incidence of seizures during pregnancy, labour and puerperium in epileptic women: a prospective study. *Acta Neurol Scand* 1987;**75**:356–60.

9. Källén B. A register study of maternal epilepsy and delivery outcome with special reference to drug use. *Acta Neurol Scand* 1986;**73**:253–9.

10. Martin PJ, Milac PAH. Pregnancy, epilepsy, management, and outcome: a 10–year prospective study. *Seizure* 1993;**2**:227–80.

11. Wilson JG. *Environment and birth defects*. New York: Academic Press, 1973.

12. Andrews JE, Ebron-McCoy MT, Bojic U, Nau H, Kavlock RJ. Stereoselective dysmophogenicity of the enantiomers of the valproic acid analogue 2-N-propyl-4-pentynoic acid (4-yn-VPA): cross-species evaluation in whole embryo culture. *Teratology* 1997;**55**:314–8.

13. Finnell RH, Wlodarczyk BC, Craig JC, Piedrahita JA, Bennett GD. Strain-dependent alterations in the expression of folate pathway genes following teratogenic exposure to valproic acid in a mouse model. *Am J Med Genet* 1997;**70**:303–11.

14. Nau H. Teratogenic valproic acid concentrations: infusion by implanted minipumps vs conventional injection regimen in the mouse. *Toxicol Appl Pharmacol* 1985;**80**:243–50.

15. Nau H. Species differences in pharmacokinetics and drug teratogenesis. *Environ Health Perspect* 1986;**70**:113–29.

16. Dansky LV, Andermann E, Andermann F. Marriage and fertility in epileptic patients. *Epilepsia* 1990;**21**:261–71.

17. Schupf N, Ottman R. Reproduction among individuals with idiopathic/cryptogenic epilepsy: risk factors for reduced fertility in marriage. *Epilepsia* 1996;**37**:833–40.

18. Lindhout D, Omtzigt JG. Pregnancy and the risk of teratogenicity. *Epilepsia* 1992;**33**(Suppl 4):S41–S48.

19. Lindhout D, Omtzigt JG, Cornel MC. Spectrum of neural-tube defects in 34 infants prenatally exposed to antiepileptic drugs. *Neurology* 1992;**42**(Suppl 5):111–18.

20. Samren EB, van Duijn CM, Koch S, et al. Maternal use of antiepileptic drugs and the risk of major congenital malformations: a joint European prospective study of human teratogenesis associated with maternal epilepsy. *Epilepsia* 1997;**38**:981–90.

21. Omtzigt JG, Los FJ, Hagenaars AM, Stewart PA, Sachs ES, Lindhout D. Prenatal diagnosis of spina bifida aperta after first-trimester valproate exposure. *Prenat Diagn* 1992;**12**:893–7.

22. Dansky LV, Finnell RH. Parental epilepsy, anticonvulsant drugs, and reproductive outcome: epidemiologic and experimental findings spanning three decades: 2 Human studies. *Reprod Toxicol* 1991;**5**:301–35.

23. Lindhout D, Höppener RJ, Meinardi H. Teratogenicity of antiepileptic drug combinations with special emphasis on epoxidation (of carbamazepine). *Epilepsia* 1984;**25**:77–83.

24. Laegreid L, Kyllerman M, Hedner T, Hagberg B, Viggedahl G. Benzodiazepine amplification of valproate teratogenic effects in children of mothers with absence epilepsy. *Neuropediatrics* 1993;**24**:88–92.

25. Samrén B. Maternal epilepsy and pregnancy outcome: a population-based study. Academic Thesis, Erasmus University Medical School, Rotterdam, 1998.

26. MRC Vitamin Study Research Group. Prevention of neural tube defects: results of the Medical Research Council Vitamin Study. *Lancet* 1991;**338**:131–7.

27. Czeizel AE, Dudas I, Metneki J. Pregnancy outcomes in a randomised controlled trial of periconceptional multivitamin supplementation. Final report. *Arch Gynecol Obstet* 1994;**255**:131–9.

28. Czeizel AE. Periconceptional folic acid containing multivitamin supplementation. *Eur J Obstet Gynecol Reprod Biol* 1998;**78**:151–61.

29. van der Put NM, van den Heuvel LP, Steegers-Theunissen RP, et al. Decreased methylene tetrahydrofolate reductase activity due to the 677c–>T mutation in families with spina bifida offspring. *J Mol Med* 1996;**74**:691–4.

30. Lindhout D, Omtzigt JG. Teratogenic effects of antiepileptic drugs: implications for the management of epilepsy in women of childbearing age. *Epilepsia* 1994;**35**(Suppl 4):S19–S28.

VII

REFRACTORY EPILEPSY

19

Effective treatment for status epilepticus
David M Treiman

Introduction

All epileptic seizures are frightening to patients, lay observers, and even to physicians and other health care professionals. When seizures are continuous or rapidly repetitive without recovery between them there is cause for even more alarm, and many families have described fear that a loved one was dying after observing an episode of status epilepticus (SE). Because of this reaction, and especially because of the neuronal damage prolonged seizure activity can cause, SE is recognized as a medical emergency that must be treated aggressively and effectively to stop the seizures and to prevent seizure-induced neuronal damage.

Definition

Operationally, SE is defined as recurrent epileptic seizures without complete recovery of all neurologic function between seizures or as more-or-less continuous seizure activity for a period of 3 min or more. In the first International Classification of Epileptic Seizures[1] Gastaut defined SE as a term '...used whenever a seizure persists for a sufficient length of time or is repeated frequently enough to produce a fixed and enduring epileptic condition...'. This definition, which lacks the precision to be a useful operational definition, captures the essence of the pathophysiology of

SE—that the subject continually experiences either the direct physiological effects of the seizure activity or post-ictal alterations in brain physiology, which do not completely clear before the next seizure once again alters brain physiology. Thus there is a continuous pathophysiological effect of the recurrent seizures.

Classification

Effective treatment of SE begins with accurate classification. Generalized convulsive status epilepticus (GCSE) is the most common and the most dangerous type of SE. However, the operational definition discussed above makes it clear that any of the nine types of epileptic seizures described in the International Classification[2] can recur frequently enough or be prolonged sufficiently to present as SE. Although a detailed discussion of the classification of SE is beyond the scope of this chapter, there are several issues of classification that have a direct impact on treatment decisions, and thus need to be considered. There is considerable controversy and confusion regarding the terms overt GCSE, subtle GCSE, myoclonic SE, and non-convulsive SE. Treiman[3] has argued GCSE is a dynamic condition that, if untreated or inadequately treated, progresses over time from overt to subtle convulsive activity to eventually complete cessation of all movements, even though ictal discharges persist on the

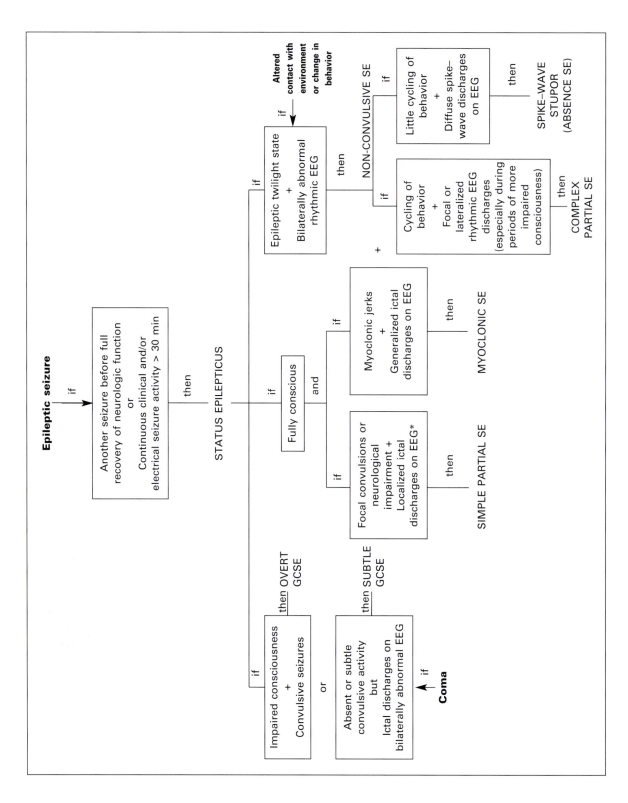

electroencephalogram (EEG). This suggests that GCSE is one entity, with different clinical presentations, depending on whether the patient is observed early or late in the episode. Thus Treiman has argued against the use of terms such as non-convulsive SE and myoclonic SE being applied to late GCSE.[3] In his opinion the term non-convulsive SE should be applied only to SE of non-convulsive seizure types, e.g. complex partial seizures and absence seizures, and that the term myoclonic SE be applied only to SE which is a complication of myoclonic epilepsy. Figure 19.1 presents an algorithm for the diagnosis and classification of various types of SE.

Diagnosis and initiation of therapy

A critical question that must be addressed with regard to treatment is when to initiate therapy. Clearly if a patient is having recurrent epileptic seizures and remains comatose between seizures then aggressive therapy should be initiated. However, what should be done if recovery of consciousness is apparent but the patient is not fully alert and completely back to his or her baseline when another seizure occurs? This patient is also in GCSE and should thus be treated aggressively because without aggressive therapy the seizures are likely to become more frequent and more difficult to stop. Most clinicians would also initiate therapy if a single seizure persisted for more than 10 min and some have argued more recently for only 5 min of continuous convulsive activity before initiating intravenous treatment. This is based on two observations: animal studies have detected histopathological damage after less than 15 min of continuous SE; and almost all isolated discrete generalized convulsions last less than 120 s.[4]

The observation in animal and human studies that prolonged seizure activity can result in neuronal damage is an important principle that emphasizes the need for very rapid control of the episode of SE to complete cessation of all epileptiform activity. There is now abundant evidence that the neuronal damage that occurs after prolonged SE is primarily the direct result of the ongoing seizure activity rather than a complication of secondary systemic changes.[5] Continuing seizure discharges result in release of large amounts of glutamate from presynaptic terminals, which then cause N-methyl-D-aspartate (NMDA) receptors to open cation channels to calcium. The influx of excessive amounts of calcium then sets up a cascade of intracellular neurochemical events, which are toxic to the cell, causing injury or cell death.[6-9] This phenomenon is now known as the excitotoxic mechanism of neuronal death, and has been implicated in neuronal damage in a number of neuronal diseases. However, systemic factors, especially hyperpyrexia,[10] can exacerbate seizure-induced neuronal injury and thus need to be monitored and quickly corrected.

It is also increasingly clear that rapid control of seizure activity during SE is correlated with

Figure 19.1

Algorithm for the diagnosis of various types of status epilepticus. Clinical presentations that start the diagnostic process are in bold at the top and sides. Decision parameters are in boxes. Specific types of status epilepticus are capitalized. SE = status epilepticus; GCSE = generalized convulsive status epilepticus.

*Scalp EEG may be normal during a simple partial seizure if the seizure activity remains sufficiently localized.

Modified from Treiman (1994).[60]

more successful treatment. Just as there is a progression from overt to increasingly subtle motor manifestations, at least during GCSE, there is also a predictable sequence of progressive EEG changes that occur during GCSE.[11] GCSE starts with discrete seizures, that then merge together in a waxing and waning pattern before becoming continuous and relatively monomorphic. Ultimately, the continuous discharges begin to be punctuated by periods of relative flattening, which lengthen as the ictal discharges shorten, until finally only periodic epileptiform discharges (PEDs) on a relatively flat background are seen. Treiman[3,12] has argued that in the context of coma, especially when preceded by other evidence of SE, PEDs are ictal and should be treated aggressively until eliminated from the EEG. There is now evidence that the longer the episode of SE,[13] the more subtle the clinical presentation,[14] and the later the EEG stage,[15] the less responsive to treatment the episode of SE will be. The mechanism of this progressive refractoriness to treatment is not known, but may be related to the progressive attenuation of GABA-mediated inhibition observed in experimental SE.[16,17]

Goals of therapy

From these observations it follows that the goals of effective management of SE are simple: to stop seizure activity as quickly as possible, to protect neurons from seizure-induced damage, and to then allow full recovery from the episode of SE.

General measures

The initial management of SE is that of any medical emergency: establish an airway, ensure oxygenation by supporting respiration if necessary, gain access to circulation and monitor blood pressure. Then blood samples for hematology and serum chemistry assessment and determination of antiepileptic drug serum concentrations should be obtained. If hypoglycemia is suspected, the plasma glucose level should be confirmed by finger stick. If significant hypoglycemia is present, a bolus of glucose should be given by intravenous push. In adults the dose is 50 ml of 50 per cent glucose. In children, 2 ml/kg of 25 per cent glucose is given. A bolus of glucose should not be administered without confirming hypoglycemia, because hyperglycemia may exacerbate neuronal damage caused by GCSE.[18–20] If thiamine deficiency is a concern (in chronic substance abusers, etc.), 100 mg thiamine should be given intravenously before or simultaneously with the glucose to avoid precipitating or exacerbating Wernicke's encephalopathy. The blood pH should be assessed. However, bicarbonate should not be used unless serum pH is so low as to be immediately life-threatening. There is little evidence that GCSE-induced acidosis results in permanent injury. Administration of large amounts of bicarbonate may result in metabolic alkalosis once GCSE is controlled. Muscle paralysis is never indicated in the management of GCSE (except in certain postoperative situations) and should never be used without ongoing EEG monitoring to ensure the continuing absence of cerebral seizure activity. The value of supplemental oxygen, steroids (to reduce cerebral edema) and monitoring for increased cerebral pressure in the management of GCSE has not been proven. Once SE is controlled, the underlying cause of the episode of GCSE needs to be evaluated and treated.

Pharmacotherapy

Effective pharmacotherapy requires prompt administration of enough antiepileptic drug to stop ongoing seizure activity and to ensure it does not recur. This is best accomplished by establishing a treatment protocol that specifies drug(s), dose(s) and rates of administration.

An ideal anti-status drug would have the following properties:

- rapid intravenous administration possible (potent, so low volume required; no adverse reactions from rapid administration);
- rapid brain entry;
- rapid antiepileptic effect;
- prolonged effective duration of action against SE;
- rapid elimination from the body;
- non-sedating.

No currently available drugs fulfil all of these criteria, but the benzodiazepines come closest. In general, drugs that enhance GABA-mediated inhibition appear to be most often effective at controlling epileptiform activity in SE.

A number of drugs have been reported to be effective in the initial intravenous management of SE, including the barbiturates phenobarbital, amobarbital, pentobarbital and thiopental; phenytoin (and fosphenytoin); the benzodiazepines diazepam, lorazepam, midazolam and clonazepam; chlormethiazole; paraldehyde; lidocaine; propofol and valproic acid. Success rates of 40–100 per cent have been reported from various series, mostly based on retrospective chart reviews. Only a few comparative trials of anti-SE drugs have been completed. Leppik et al[21] found no difference in the efficacy of lorazepam and diazepam in 79 cases of various types of SE. Shaner et al[22] compared diazepam followed by phenytoin with phenobarbital in 36 patients with GCSE. There was no statistically significant difference in the frequency of success between treatments, although phenobarbital stopped SE somewhat more quickly than diazepam followed by phenytoin. In the only large-scale randomized blinded direct compari-

son of first line drugs used in the treatment of GCSE, Treiman et al[14] compared the efficacy of lorazepam (0.1 mg/kg), phenobarbital (15 mg/kg), diazepam (0.15 mg/kg) followed by phenytoin (18 mg/kg), and phenytoin (18 mg/kg) in the initial management of overt and subtle GCSE in a multicenter VA Cooperative trial. In the overt group, 384 patients had evaluable data. Lorazepam stopped GCSE in 65 per cent of the patients randomized to that group, phenobarbital in 58 per cent, diazepam followed by phenytoin in 56 per cent and phenytoin in 44 per cent. Lorazepam was more often effective than phenytoin, other paired comparisons were not statistically significant. In the 134 subtle patients with evaluable data there were no statistically significant differences among treatment groups.

Treatment protocol

The treatment protocol outlined in Table 19.1 is useful in the management of GCSE and, with some modifications, in other types of SE as well. The choice of lorazepam as the initial treatment is based on several considerations: it has many of the characteristics of an ideal anti-status drug discussed above; it was the most effective drug in the VA study[14] and there are no reports of other drugs being more effective than lorazepam in the initial management of SE; and it has favorable pharmacokinetics compared with diazepam.[23] Although diazepam may stop SE slightly faster than lorazepam, lorazepam has a much longer effective duration of action. This is because diazepam is so lipid soluble that there is a rapid redistribution of diazepam into body lipid stores so that by 20 min after bolus intravenous infusion, serum (and brain) concentrations fall to 20 per cent of their initial concentrations.[24] Lorazepam is less lipid soluble and also appears to be actively retained in the brain so over the first hour after administration there is an increase in the brain–blood concentration ratio.[25] This results in a much longer effective duration of protection against recurrence of SE. In the VA study,[14] lorazepam had no greater incidence of recurrence of GCSE than phenobarbital or phenytoin. If diazepam is used as the initial intravenous treatment for GCSE it must be followed immediately by administration of phenytoin (or fosphenytoin) to avoid recurrence of SE. There is, however, one negative consequence of the greater effective duration of action exhibited by lorazepam, which is that there is also a prolonged period of sedation. If the ability to monitor level of consciousness is essential in the management of a patient with GCSE (as in a neurosurgical emergency) lorazepam may not be the treatment of choice.

If lorazepam is not successful at stopping seizure activity within 15–20 min, phenytoin (20 mg/kg) should be administered. Phenytoin is a sodium channel blocker, and thus has a different mechanism of action from lorazepam (an enhancer of GABA-mediated inhibition). Rational polytherapy suggests that the combination of drugs with different mechanisms of action may enhance efficacy without simultaneously increasing toxicity. In the VA study,[14] the addition of phenytoin when lorazepam failed resulted in control of GCSE in 7 per cent additional patients. There is a significant risk of cutaneous complications when phenytoin is given intravenously, including phlebitis, tissue sloughing after extravasation and, most devastating, purple glove syndrome, a delayed soft-tissue injury which may result in severe edema that results in arterial occlusion, tissue necrosis and sometimes requires amputation. O'Brien et al[26] recently reported a 6 per cent incidence of purple glove syndrome in 152 consecutive patients at the Mayo Clinic to whom intravenous phenytoin was administered in the arm or hand during a three-month period. The proposed reason for the high incidence of cutaneous complications from intravenously administered phenytoin is that it must be dissolved in 40 per cent propylene glycol and 10 per cent ethanol at a pH of 12.2. Fortunately, cutaneous complications of intravenous phenytoin can now be avoided because of the availability of fosphenytoin, a phosphate ester of phenytoin that is enzymatically converted to phenytoin by serum phosphatases. Fosphenytoin is dissolved in Tris buffer, at a pH of 8–9, and thus does not cause the tissue complications that phenytoin does. Seventy-five mg fosphenytoin results in 50 mg phenytoin after enzymatic conversion, which is complete.

Unfortunately, the current labeling of fosphenytoin in the US is confusing. Fosphenytoin (Cerebyx™) is labeled in phenytoin equivalents (PE), so that 75 mg fosphenytoin is labeled 50 mg PE. This labeling has resulted in considerable confusion, and there is now a consideration of labeling fosphenytoin in actual milligram amounts, rather than in phenytoin equivalents. If 20 mg/kg is not effective then the dose should be increased by 5 or 10 mg/kg, up to a total of 30 mg/kg. This will result in a serum concentration of 30–40 μg/ml, which may be necessary to stop pharmacoresistant SE.

If SE still persists then intravenous general anesthesia must be initiated. This can be achieved by administration of a fixed dose of phenobarbital of 15 to 20 mg/kg or by starting a continuous intravenous infusion of a short-acting barbiturate, benzodiazepine, or propofol. Although a fixed dose of phenobarbital has the advantage that it does not require monitoring of a continuous intravenous infusion, there is little evidence for significant additional improvement in seizure control when used as a third drug. However, large doses may substantially delay recovery of consciousness because of phenobarbital's 3–5-day half-life. Therefore, some clini-

Time (min)	
0	Make the diagnosis by observing one additional seizure in a patient with a history of recent seizures or impaired consciousness or by observing continuous behavioral and/or electrical seizure activity for more than 10 min. Call EEG technician and start EEG as soon as possible, but do not delay treatment while waiting for the EEG unless necessary to verify diagnosis.
5	Establish intravenous catheter with normal saline (dextrose solutions may precipitate phenytoin)—with fosphenytoin either dextrose or saline is OK. Draw blood for serum chemistries, hematology studies and AED concentrations. If hypoglycemia is suspected, confirm by finger stick. Then administer 100 mg of thiamine (if indicated) followed by 50 ml of 50 per cent glucose by direct push into the intravenous line.
10	Administer lorazepam (0.1 mg/kg) by intravenous push (<2 mg/min).
25	If status does not stop, start phenytoin (20 mg/kg) by slow intravenous push (<50 mg/min) directly into intravenous port closest to patient (fosphenytoin can be given at the fast i.v. push rate of 150 mg PE/min). Monitor BP and ECG closely during infusion. If status does not stop after 20 mg/kg phenytoin, (or 20 mg PE/kg of fosphenytoin) administer an additional 5 mg/kg and, if necessary, another 5 mg/kg, to a maximum dose of 30 mg/kg.
60	If status persists, give phenobarbital (20 mg/kg) by intravenous push (<100 mg/min) or start barbiturate coma. Support respiration by endotracheal intubation. Give pentobarbital (5–15 mg/kg) slowly as an initial intravenous dose to suppress all epileptiform activity. Continue 0.5–5 mg/kg/h to maintain suppression of all epileptiform discharges. Slow the rate of infusion periodically to see if seizure has stopped. Monitor BP, ECG and respiratory function closely. If unable to suppress all epileptiform activity change to continuous infusions of propofol or midazolam.

Modified from Treiman (1993).[59]

Table 19.1
Treatment protocol. Generalized convulsive status epilepticus.

cians have advocated going directly to intravenous infusion anesthesia if lorazepam followed by phenytoin fails to control seizures.[27] Whatever drug is used, the airway and respiratory drive must be protected, and this almost always requires endotracheal intubation and respiratory support. The management of refractory SE is discussed below.

The protocol in Table 19.1 is also appropriate and effective for the management of complex partial SE. For simple partial SE, where, by definition there is no impairment of consciousness, sedating drugs should be avoided. Therefore, diazepam (0.15 mg/kg) should be substituted in place of lorazepam, and phenytoin administration should be initiated as soon as diazepam infusion has been completed, whether or not seizures have stopped. If necessary, the phenytoin dose can be increased up to 30 mg/kg, as discussed above. If diazepam, followed by high-dose phenytoin does not completely control simple partial SE, then the relative risk of allowing SE to continue must be weighed against the risk of heavily sedating or inducing coma in a conscious patient.

The protocol is not appropriate for absence SE (spike–wave stupor), where phenytoin and possibly even phenobarbital may exacerbate the situation. For absence SE a single dose of diazepam 0.15–0.25 mg/kg administered by slow intravenous push is usually effective, unless the episode of absence SE has gone undiagnosed for days before treatment. Lorazepam can be given in place of diazepam, but will cause significant sedation for at least several hours after a 0.1 mg/kg intravenous dose. If a benzodiazepine is not effective, valproic acid can be given intravenously. There is no established dose for valproate for absence SE, not even from animal studies. Data from experimental GCSE in rats suggest a serum concentration of 270 µg/ml may be necessary to control GCSE in humans.[28] Therefore, it is likely that concentrations of at least 100–200 µg/ml may be necessary to control absence SE that is not responsive to benzodiazepines. Because the volume of distribution of valproic acid is approximately 0.25 l/kg, a dose of 25 mg/kg will be necessary to achieve an acute serum concentration of 100 µg/ml.

Pediatric considerations

Management of SE in children is similar to that in adults, although there are no controlled clinical trials that provide proof of efficacy for any of the antistatus drugs in children. In general, however, children tolerate higher rates of infusion than do adults. Intravenous access is sometimes difficult, especially in the vigorously convulsing child, and rectal administration of diazepam should be considered if there is likely to be a delay of more than 10–15 min in establishing an intravenous line, because peak diazepam concentrations are achieved within 10–15 min after insertion of a diazepam suppository. Rectal administration of diazepam has been used for years in Europe and there is now a commercially available preparation of diazepam for rectal administration (Diastat™). The dose for rectal administration in children is 0.5 mg/kg to a maximum of 20 mg. Rectal diazepam can be valuable both for hospital use when intravenous access is difficult and for home use, when patients have frequent flurries of seizures, which may progress into SE if not quickly stopped.

Role of EEG monitoring

Continuous EEG monitoring while managing SE can be extremely helpful and sometimes is essential. It is not always possible to be certain that treatment has been successful by clinical observation alone. Certainly, if convulsions stop completely and then the patient progressively regains consciousness, EEG monitoring is not necessary to confirm successful treatment. However, if convulsive movements stop but coma persists without progressive recovery of consciousness, then EEG monitoring is essential to verify cessation of all epileptiform activity. In the VA study,[14] 20 per cent of the patients in whom all convulsive movements stopped after treatment had persistent ictal discharges on the EEG.[29] In another recent study,[30] 14 per cent of 164 patients in GCSE had persistent ictal discharges after cessation of convulsive movements. In this study PEDs were not considered ictal.

Management of refractory status epilepticus

The majority of patients in SE respond to initial therapy and many patients who are treated aggressively with a benzodiazepine, phenytoin and/or phenobarbital experience complete cessation of all behavioral and electrical seizure activity. In the VA study[14] GCSE was successfully treated with one to three drugs in 74 per cent of the overt patients in whom lorazepam was the first drug, phenytoin the second and phenobarbital the third. However, a substantial number of patients do require intravenous general anesthesia to eliminate all ictal discharges on the EEG. As the longer SE persists the more difficult it is to treat, some investigators have suggested that treatment for refractory SE should be initiated if a benzodiazepine followed by phenytoin or fosphenytoin is not successful.[27] There have been no prospective randomized comparative studies of the treatment of refractory SE upon which to base choice of drug. However, in retrospective reviews of clinical experience, pentobarbital[31-37], propofol[37], midazolam[38-40], diazepam[41-43], lorazepam[44] and chlormethiazole[45-47] continuous infusions have been reported to have efficacy in the management of refractory SE. Choice of treatment should be based on clinical experience, ease of use and cost. If aggressive treatment with one agent is not successful, another should be tried. Management of refractory GCSE requires continuous EEG monitoring. The rate of administration of whatever drug is used must be increased until there is a cessation of all epileptiform activity. This usually requires that the EEG become nearly flat. Increasing evidence suggests that achievement of a burst–suppression pattern is not sufficient. Frequently what are interpreted to be bursts are actually epileptiform discharges, which must be suppressed completely if SE is to be controlled. The persistence of even periodic epileptiform discharges predicts the return of earlier SE ictal patterns when the rate of infusion is reduced. Once all epileptiform activity has been eliminated from the EEG, the patient should be continued in this state for 24–96 h before attempting to slow the infusion rate and allow the level of anesthesia to lighten. However, there are no data on which to determine how long the epileptiform discharges must be suppressed. In general, the longer SE has persisted, the longer the patient should be kept free from all epileptiform activity before reducing the infusion rate and lightening the level of anesthesia. If ictal activity returns, repeat the process by increasing the infusion rate and again eliminating all epileptiform discharges from the EEG. Patients in refractory GCSE with continuing epileptiform activity on their EEG do not recover. Some patients, in whom all epileptiform activity is suppressed, remain free from epileptiform discharges as the level of anesthesia is lightened, even after being maintained under anesthesia for four to six weeks.

Follow-up management

Lorazepam, phenobarbital and phenytoin are all equally effective at preventing recurrence of SE over at least 12 h.[14] During this period the patient can be started on a maintenance antiepileptic drug, if this is indicated. Patients with a previous history of epilepsy or with structural brain lesions need chronic antiepileptic drug therapy.[48-50] When SE is caused by a transient metabolic disturbance, chronic anti-epileptic therapy is not indicated. When SE is the first seizure then the decision to initiate chronic antiepileptic therapy should be based on the probability of further seizures. The presence of epileptiform abnormalities on the EEG is a good predictor of further seizures.[51–53] Adults are usually started on antiepileptic therapy after an episode of SE, regardless of etiology, because of the social consequences of recurrent seizures. However, children who develop SE as a complication of febrile seizures should not be started on maintenance antiepileptic therapy in the absence of neurological abnormalities[50,54–58], even though there is a sixfold increased risk of subsequently developing epilepsy.[56,58] There is no evidence that chronic antiepileptic drug therapy reduces this risk.

Phenytoin is most commonly used to initiate maintenance therapy, because this is the only currently available antiepileptic drug that can be loaded to rapidly achieve a therapeutic drug concentration. However, if the patient has been taking another antiepileptic drug, or if rapid achievement of steady state concentrations is not paramount, other antiepileptic drugs are appropriate. When phenytoin is loaded to rapidly achieve therapeutic concentrations, it is sometimes necessary to re-administer a partial loading dose in order to increase the steady-state concentration of the drug. The appropriate dose for such a 'mini-load' can be easily calculated using the following formula:

$$D = V_d \times (C_1 - C_0)$$

where D = dose, V_d = volume of distribution, C_1 = the desired concentration and C_0 = the starting concentration. For a drug with a V_d of 1 l/kg it can be seen that a loading dose in mg/kg is equal to the desired increase in serum concentration in mg/l. As most antiepileptic drugs have a V_d of about 1 l/kg or slightly less, a rule of thumb close enough for clinical

purposes is to give a mini-loading dose of 1 mg/kg for each mg/l (μg/ml) increase in serum concentration that is desired. Thus, if a patient is found to have a phenytoin serum concentration of 12 μg/ml and the physician wishes to maintain the phenytoin concentration at 17 μg/ml, the mini-loading dose that should be given to achieve this concentration is 5 mg/kg. In either case the calculations are the same for fosphenytoin, as long as PE units are used (see discussion above).

If I had status epilepticus...

If I developed an episode of SE I would want it to be recognized rapidly and aggressive treatment initiated immediately. I would not expect the recognition of overt GCSE to be difficult, but if I had even a single convulsion I would want GCSE to be considered if I did not begin to recover consciousness within a few minutes after termination of the seizure. Furthermore, if I developed an episode where I became even a little confused or mildly lethargic, I would hope that I would be quickly brought for neurological evaluation in an emergency room and that non-convulsive SE would be considered. I would want to be treated at a hospital where an EEG could be recorded quickly at any hour I might arrive and that neurologic expertise would be available immediately to interpret the EEG and to manage my case.

Once the diagnosis of SE was made, and the ABCs of emergency measures addressed, I would want to be treated with lorazepam, 0.1 mg/kg and I would want success of treatment confirmed by EEG, unless I was clearly recovering neurologic function. If lorazepam was not successful, and I had GCSE, I would like to be given fosphenytoin, 20 mg P.E./kg, by rapid intravenous infusion (< 150 mg P.E./min) and I would want my blood pressure and cardiogram to be monitored during the infusion. If SE still persisted, I would want intravenous general anesthesia to be initiated. I would want an expert in SE treatment to manage my case if I failed to respond to lorazepam and fosphenytoin, but with no delay in treatment while awaiting the expert. I personally have the most experience with pentobarbital in refractory SE. However, I would want the treating epileptologist to use whichever intravenous general anesthetic agent he or she is most confident in using. I would want careful attention paid to systemic support, with close monitoring of blood pressure and respiratory status. Most importantly, I would want aggressive pharmacotherapy of my SE, with rapid elimination of all epileptiform discharges, including periodic epileptiform discharges. I would want the rate of drug infusion to be fast enough so that my EEG remained free from all epileptiform discharges for 24–96 hours. Then I would like the rate of infusion to be slowly decreased, with close monitoring of the EEG, so that if any ictal discharges reappeared that rate of infusion would be increased again to eliminate them for another 24–96 hours. I would want this process repeated until either SE stopped or I died during the effort to stop it. I would ask that my physicians not give up, no matter how long the process might continue, because if they have been aggressive in my management from the very beginning, I would expect that I might be able to return to a useful and meaningful life.

References

1. Gastaut H. Clinical and electroencephalographic classification of epileptic seizures. *Epilepsia*, 1970;**11**:102–13.
2. Commission on Classification and Terminology of the International League Against Epilepsy. Proposal for revised clinical and electroencephalographic classification of epileptic seizures. *Epilepsia*, 1981;**22**:489–501.
3. Treiman DM. Generalized convulsive status epilepticus in the adult. *Epilepsia*, 1993; **34** (Suppl 1):S2–S11.
4. Theodore WH, Porter RJ, Albert P et al. The secondarily generalized tonic–clonic seizure: A videotape analysis. *Neurology* 1994; **44**: 1403–7.
5. Meldrum BS, Vigouroux RA, Brierley JB. Systemic factors and epileptic brain damage: Prolonged seizures in paralyzed artificially ventilated baboons. *Arch Neurol* 1973;**29**:82–7.
6. Lipton SA, Rosenberg PA. Mechanisms of disease: excitatory amino acids as a final common pathway for neurologic disorders. *N Engl J Med* 1994; **330**:613–22.
7. Meldrum B. Excitotoxicity and epileptic brain damage. *Epilepsy Res* 1991;**10**:55–61.
8. Meldrum BS. Excitotoxicity and selective neuronal loss in epilepsy. *Brain Pathol* 1993; 3:405–12.
9. Rothman SM, Olney JW. Excitotoxicity and the NMDA receptor. *Trends Neurosci* 1993;3: 405–12.
10. Simon RP. Management of status epilepticus. *Recent Adv Epilep* 1985;2:137–60.
11. Treiman DM, Walton NY, Kendrick C. A progressive sequence of electroencephalographic changes during generalized convulsive status epilepticus. *Epilepsy Res* 1990;5:49–60.
12. Treiman DM. Electroclinical features of status epilepticus. *J Clin Neurophysiol* 1995;**12**:343–62.
13. Treiman DM, Meyers PD, Walton NY, DVA Status Epilepticus Cooperative Study Group. Duration of generalized convulsive status epilepticus: relationship to clinical symptomatology and response to treatment. *Epilepsia* 1992;33(Suppl. 3): 66 (abstract)
14. Treiman DM, Meyers PD, Walton NY, et al. A comparison of four treatments for generalized convulsive status epilepticus. *N Engl J Med* 1998;**339**:792–8.

15. Treiman DM, Meyers PD, DVA Status Epilepticus Cooperative Study Group: utility of the EEG pattern as a predictor of success in the treatment of generalized convulsive status epilepticus. *Epilepsia* 1991; **32**(Suppl. 3):93 (abstract).
16. Kapur J, Lothman EW. NMDA receptor activation mediates the loss of GABAergic inhibition induced by recurrent seizures. *Epilepsy Res* 1990;**5**:103–11.
17. Kapur J, Lothman EW, DeLorenzo RJ. Loss of GABAA receptors during partial status epilepticus. *Neurology* 1994;**44**:2407–8.
18. Blennow G, Brierley JB, Meldrum BS, Siesjö BK. Epileptic brain damage: the role of systemic factors that modify cerebral energy metabolism. *Brain* 1978;**101**:687–700.
19. Melamed E. Reactive hyperglycemia in patients with acute stroke. *J Neurol Sci* 1976;**29**:267–75.
20. Pulsinelli WA, Levy DE, Sigsbee B, et al. Increased damage after ischemic stroke in patients with hyperglycemia with or without established diabetes mellitus. *Am J Med* 1983;**74**:540–4.
21. Leppik IE, Derivan AT, Homan RW, et al. Double-blind study of lorazepam and diazepam in status epilepticus. *JAMA* 1983;**249**:1452–4.
22. Shaner DM, McCurdy SA, Herring MO, Gabor AJ. Treatment of status epilepticus: a prospective comparison of diazepam and phenytoin versus phenobarbital and optional phenytoin. *Neurology* 1988;**38**:202–7.
23. Greenblatt DJ, Divoll M. Diazepam versus lorazepam: relationship of drug distribution to duration of clinical action. In: Delgado-Escueta AV, Wasterlain CG, Treiman DM, Porter RJ, eds, *Status epilepticus: mechanisms of brain damage and treatment* 487–91. New York: Raven Press, 1983 (*Adv Neurol* **34**:487–91).
24. Bleck TP. Convulsive disorders: Status epilepticus. *Clin Neuropharmacol* 1991;**14**:191–8.
25. Walton NY, Treiman DM. Lorazepam treatment of experimental status epilepticus in the rat: relevance to clinical practice. *Neurology* 1990;**40**:990–4.
26. O'Brien TJ, Cascino GD, So EL, Hanna DR. Incidence and clinical consequence of the purple glove syndrome in patients receiving intravenous phenytoin. *Neurology* 1998;**51**:1034–9.
27. Bleck TP. Advances in the management of refractory status epilepticus. *Crit Care Med* 1993;**21**:955–7.
28. Walton NY, Treiman DM. Valproic acid treatment of experimental status epilepticus. *Epilepsy Res* 1992;**12**:199–205.
29. Craven W, Faught E, Kuzniecky R, et al. Residual electrographic status epilepticus after control of overt clinical seizures. *Epilepsia* 1995;**36**(Suppl. 4):46 (abstract)
30. DeLorenzo RJ, Waterhouse EJ, Towne AR, et al. Persistent non-convulsive status epilepticus after the control of convulsive status epilepticus. *Epilepsia* 1998;**39**:833–40.
31. Fischer JH, Raineri DL. Pentobarbital anesthesia for status epilepticus. *Clin Pharm* 1987;**6**:601–2.
32. Mirski MA, Williams MA, Hanley DF. Prolonged pentobarbital and phenobarbital coma for refractory generalized status epilepticus. *Crit Care Med* 1995;**23**:400–4.
33. Rashkin MC, Youngs C, Penovich P. Pentobarbital treatment of refractory status epilepticus. *Neurology* 1987;**37**:500–3.
34. Van Ness PC. Pentobarbital and EEG burst-suppression in treatment of status epilepticus refractory to benzodiazepines and phenytoin. *Epilepsia* 1990;**31**:61–7.
35. Yaffe K, Lowenstein DH. Prognostic factors of pentobarbital therapy for refractory generalized status epilepticus. *Neurology* 1993;**43**:895–900.
36. Young GB, Blume WT, Bolton CF, Warren KG. Anesthetic barbiturates in refractory status epilepticus. *Can J Neurol Sci* 1980;**7**:291–2.
37. Stecker MM, Kramer TH, Raps EC, et al. Treatment of refractory status epilepticus with propofol: clinical and pharmacokinetic findings. *Epilepsia* 1998;**39**:18–26.
38. Kumar A, Bleck TP. Intravenous midazolam for the treatment of refractory status epilepticus. *Crit Care Med* 1992;**20**:483–8.
39. Parent JM, Lowenstein DH. Treatment of refractory generalized status epilepticus with continuous infusion of midazolam. *Neurology* 1994;**44**:1837–40.
40. Rivera R, Segnini M, Baltodano A, Perez V. Midazolam in the treatment of status epilepticus in children. *Crit Care Med* 1993;**21**:991–4.
41. Bertz RJ, Howrie DL. Diazepam by continuous intravenous infusion for status epilepticus in

anticonvulsant hypersensitivity syndrome. *Ann Pharmacother* 1993;**27**:298–301.

42. Walker MC, Smith SJ, Shorvon SD. The intensive care treatment of convulsive status epilepticus in the UK. Results of a national survey and recommendations. *Anaesthesia* 1995;**50**:130–5.

43. Delgado-Escueta AV, Wasterlain C, Treiman DM, Porter RJ. Current concepts in neurology: management of status epilepticus. *N Engl J Med* 1982;**306**:1337–40.

44. Labar DR, Ali A, Root J. High-dose intravenous lorazepam for the treatment of refractory status epilepticus. *Neurology* 1994;**44**:1400–3.

45. Bentley G, Mellick R. Chlormethiazole in status epilepticus—three cases. *Med J Aust* 1975;**1**:537–8.

46. Harvey PK, Higenbottam TW, Loh L. Chlormethiazole in treatment of status epilepticus. *Br Med J* 1975;**2**:603–5.

47. Martin PJ, Millac PA. Status epilepticus: management and outcome of 107 episodes. *Seizure* 1994;**3**:107–13.

48. Hauser WA, Hesdorffer DC. *Epilepsy: frequency, causes and consequences.* New York: Demos, 1990.

49. Driscoll SM, Towne AR, Pellock JM, et al. Recurrent status epilepticus in children. *Neurology* 1990;**40**(Suppl. 1):297 (abstract)

50. Shinnar S, Maytal J, Krasnoff L, Moshe SL. Recurrent status epilepticus in children [published erratum appears in *Ann Neurol* 1992;**32**:394]. *Ann Neurol* 1992;**31**:598–604.

51. Berg AT, Shinnar S. The risk of seizure recurrence following a first unprovoked seizure: a quantitative review. *Neurology* 1991;**41**:965–72.

52. Shinnar S, Berg AT, Moshe SL, et al. Risk of seizure recurrence following a first unprovoked seizure in childhood: a prospective study. *Pediatrics* 1990;**85**:1076–85.

53. Van Donselaar CA, Schimsheimer R-J, Geerts AT, Declerck AC. Value of the electroencephalogram in adult patients with untreated idiopathic first seizures. *Arch Neurol* 1992;**49**:231–7.

54. Maytal J, Shinnar S, Moshe SL, Alvarez LA. Low morbidity and mortality of status epilepticus in children. *Pediatrics* 1989;**83**:323–31.

55. Dunn DW. Status epilepticus in children: etiology, clinical features, and outcome. *J Child Neurol* 1988;**3**:167–73.

56. Annegers JF, Hauser WA, Shirts SB, Kurland LT. Factors prognostic of unprovoked seizures after febrile convulsions. *N Engl J Med* 1987;**316**:493–8.

57. Nelson KB, Ellenberg JH. Prognosis in children with febrile seizures. *Pediatrics* 1978;**61**:720–7.

58. Maytal J, Shinnar S. Febrile status epilepticus. *Pediatrics* 1990;**86**:611–16.

59. Treiman DM. Current treatment strategies in selected situations in epilepsy. *Epilepsia* 1993;**34**(Suppl 5):S17–S23.

60. Treiman DM. Generalized convulsive, nonconvulsive, and focal status epilepticus. In: Feldman E, ed, *Current diagnosis in neurology*, 11–18. St Louis: Mosby Yearbook, Inc., 1994.

20

Non-responsive partial epilepsy: what should be done?

Jørgen Alving and Lennart Gram

Introduction

In adults with epilepsy, partial seizures with or without secondary generalization are the most frequent seizure types. This applies especially to complex partial seizures, which are seen in about 40 per cent of adult patients attending specialized epilepsy clinics.[1,2] This has also been found in population studies, although complex partial seizures are somewhat less frequent.[3]

Diagnostic and therapeutic re-evaluation

The key areas of a comprehensive diagnostic and therapeutic re-evaluation are: diagnosis, drug history, psychosocial problems and other options.

Diagnosis
- Does the patient really have epilepsy?
- Are there other causes for the observed seizures?
- What type of epileptic seizures/syndrome does the patient have?

Drug history
Previous treatment
- Which drugs?
- Are they appropriate for the seizures/syndrome in question?
- What are dosage/drug levels?

- What is the compliance?
- Are the observation times on a stable regimen sufficient?
- Is there seizure monitoring?

Remaining drug options
- Have higher doses of drugs already been tried?
- Which relevant drugs have not been tried?
- Which new drugs and which relevant (rational) drug combinations have not been investigated?

Psychosocial problems
- Are there any disorders?
- Are there problems with work, leisure time and other everyday activities?

Other therapeutic options
- Non-marketed drugs
- Surgery
- Vagal nerve stimulation

Each of these points will now be discussed.

Re-evaluating the diagnosis

There is extensive coverage of this essential subject in other chapters of this book, so it is mentioned only briefly here.

As many patients referred for refractory epilepsy (42 per cent in our patient population) have epilepsy that has been imprecisely or incorrectly classified, it is often important to admit the patient to hospital for seizure observation, including long-term EEG monitoring if necessary. These procedures not only allow simplification of a drug regimen, but also make possible a more goal-directed choice of drugs. Furthermore, in 10–30 per cent of patients, these procedures will show the existence of non-epileptic seizures, either on their own or as a complicating feature of intractable epilepsy.

Several studies have shown that it is possible to obtain a significant reduction in seizure frequency through this comprehensive diagnostic and therapeutic re-evaluation.[4] However, the follow-up periods in these studies vary in length (there are no true cohorts), and possible associated psychosocial benefits have not been addressed precisely, although one study[5] has demonstrated a significant reduction in toxicity of antiepileptic drugs at follow-up. Clearly, there is a need for more systematic prospective studies.

Previous treatment

In our experience, it is often difficult to obtain exact information about the extent to which these problems have been addressed from the referral case notes. Many patients (42 per cent) do not use a seizure diary, and an astonishing number (30 per cent) have not been offered this simple, indispensable tool for optimal epilepsy treatment. As most partial seizures (in contrast to, for example absences and myoclonic seizures) are easily recognized, every patient should use a seizure calendar. Equally important, the physician should inspect the diary at every visit, otherwise the patient soon loses interest. Compliance is difficult to evaluate if a drug dispenser is not used, and this simple item should also be offered to the patient. Checking

serum levels of antiepileptic drugs gives only a crude estimate of compliance.[6] Not infrequently, more than one change in drug regimen has been done at the same time, making it difficult or impossible to evaluate the efficacy of individual measures.

The individual antiepileptic drugs have often been tried at dosages that are too low, partly because of misunderstanding about so-called 'therapeutic levels'. Testing one drug at a time until toxicity symptoms emerge has been undertaken only infrequently. It is not unusual to see a patient with epilepsy that is difficult to control, when that patient has reached 'therapeutic blood levels' for all the drugs tried so far, but has never experienced toxicity symptoms from any of the drugs. There are other patients who have tried only a few drugs at limited amounts even though they have had uncontrolled seizures for several years.

Therapeutic options that have not been considered

When patients with non-responsive partial epilepsy present, the first task is to evaluate whether there are any possibilities that have not been exploited in the previously administered drug regimens. Quite a number (about 33 per cent) of patients seen in our hospital have been managed successfully by us through the simple measure of increasing the dosage of the drug that the patient received on referral. This increase is made in steps until the seizures stop or clinical side effects emerge, regardless of serum drug levels. Only if clinical toxicity develops is the dosage reduced again. This approach ensures that the full potential of the drug for each individual patient has been obtained. Some patients may actually need 'toxic' serum levels of the drug, e.g. phenytoin levels at 150–200 µmol/l.[7] We have successfully treated selected patients by pushing carba-mazepine levels up to 60–65 µmol/l. In his study Løyning[8] found that 40 per cent of patients with refractory epilepsy had plasma levels of antiepileptic drugs that were below 'therapeutic' ranges. These data agree with our own experience.

It is well known that optimum serum levels for the individual patient depend upon the severity of the epilepsy, as well as the seizure type in question, with partial seizures requiring higher levels than primary generalized seizures.[9–11] When undertaking this type of 'aggressive' drug titration, it is important to be aware of the phenomenon of paradoxical intoxication, which refers to situations in which an increase in seizure frequency is observed at high doses/plasma levels compared with lower ones. This has been described mainly with phenytoin and carbamazepine,[11] but it may also occur with other antiepileptic drugs. Most reports have been anecdotal, and systematic studies of the phenomenon have not been carried out.

Alternative monotherapy versus polytherapy

In about half of our patients, more radical changes are necessary, i.e. new drugs have to be used.[12] This poses the problem of whether combination therapy or alternative monother-apy should be tried.

Alternative monotherapy has only occasion-ally been systematically investigated.[13–15] Combination therapy (two-drug treatment) has been studied much more extensively. However, the benefits of one versus two drugs are ambiguous in the literature,[16] and a strictly scheduled transition from combination therapy to monotherapy may pose practical difficulties.

It is our policy that, if one drug does not provide seizure control, a second one is added while maintaining a stable dosage/plasma level of the first. If this approach renders the patient seizure-free and there are no side effects, a dilemma arises. Should the first drug be tapered off in order to clarify whether it was the combination or the second drug that worked? In our opinion, as always in epilepsy treatment, the patient's point of view is decisive, and it is necessary to weigh the risks of seizure recurrence against the potentially increased risk of drug toxicity and the slightly more complicated drug schedule.

However, this discussion applies to well-controlled patients. What happens if the seizures continue despite using two drugs? It is still quite common for patients to take three or

Persistent seizures on treatment with	Score
Other than primary drug in any dose	0
Primary drug below recommended daily dose	1
Primary drug within recommended daily dose	2
Primary drug with plasma levels within 'therapeutic' range	3
Primary drug with maximal tolerated daily dose	4
More than one drug with maximal tolerated daily dose in subsequent single-drug treatment	5

From Schmidt (1986).

Table 20.1
Intractability score.

more drugs. To avoid this situation, careful seizure monitoring and evaluation of the efficacy of each drug against its side effects are essential, although frequently neglected.

In the evaluation of our short-stay patients,[12] polypharmacy was not a major issue, with the average number of antiepileptic drugs at admission being 1.9 and with no one receiving more than three drugs. This number of drugs was virtually unaltered at discharge.

A graduated spectrum of intractability (Table 20.1) has been proposed by Schmidt.[7] Although this approach may seem logical and attractive, curiously enough we are not aware of any study that has used it. As seen from Table 20.1, this rating scale could be extended to, for example, combinations of more than two drugs in maximally tolerated dosages.

Duration of a diagnostic and therapeutic re-evaluation

Long-term admissions are usually necessary when carrying out extensive changes in antiepileptic drug treatment, mainly because of two frequently encountered problems.

The first is the well-known risk of seizure exacerbation (including status epilepticus) that occurs when drugs are tapered off.

The second is a much less known, or frequently neglected, problem—the so-called '2-week honeymoon'. This term refers to the fact that admission itself often results in a transient, but profound, reduction in seizure frequency (and, in some a total abolition) for the first few weeks in spite of no change in dosage/serum levels of antiepileptic drugs.[17] With ever-increasing pressure to reduce the length of hospital admissions, this phenomenon often makes seizure observation very difficult in an ordinary hospital setting, and results in a false impression of the seriousness of the

seizure disorder. However, from a resource–economical point of view, this short-admission policy is not rational. Patients can have many repetitive short hospital stays, which cumulate a large number of bed-days, with the essential diagnostic problems remaining unsolved. In the long run, a structured and well-planned admission of 3 or 4 weeks (or until the problem has been solved) would probably be less costly. The same applies to management in the outpatient clinic: if the patient is not allotted sufficient time, the visit will often be a waste of time for both patient and physician.

Surgery

New drugs and resective surgery: miracle makers?

How much can new drugs be expected to achieve and, in particular, to what extent can they fulfill the expectations of patients with intractable seizures, and their relatives?

In controlled trials and post-marketing studies, the key figure is the percentage of responders, i.e. patients with more than a pre-set reduction (usually ≥ 50 per cent) in seizure frequency in association with treatment. Rarely mentioned is what patients think about such proof of effect. In our experience, for some patients a reduction of less than 50 per cent may represent a clear benefit, especially if seizure severity is markedly reduced or if the patient's warning signs come sufficiently in advance to provide protection. In other patients, a 50 per cent reduction in seizure frequency makes absolutely no difference to the quality of their lives.

What really makes the big difference is total freedom from seizures, although the percentage of patients attaining this goal is often almost impossible to find in trial reports of antiepileptic drugs.[18] When this information is supplied, the figures are usually between 2 and 5 per cent, although sometimes they go up to 10 per cent. This is far below the results obtained with resective surgery. Temporal lobectomy leads to freedom from seizures in about two thirds of carefully selected patients.[19] The words 'carefully selected' highlight the problem here, because only a minority of intractable patients will be candidates for surgery. Many patients with refractory epilepsy suffer from extratemporal, mainly frontal lobe, seizures. In this condition, the surgical prognosis is less favourable, and less that half become seizure-free. Perhaps the technique of multiple subpial transections could increase the number of surgical candidates in the future, once the problem of bilateral epileptogenic lesions extending into eloquent cortical areas can be dealt with safely.[20]

In Denmark, as in many other countries, surgical treatment is still underused. Since 1993, sixteen of our patients have been operated on, with nine (56 per cent; 95% confidence limits of 29–80%) being totally seizure-free (Engel class 1), seven in class 2–3, and three in class 4 (with no worthwhile improvement). Thirteen were temporal lobectomies and three extratemporal resections were performed in the USA. In about one third of patients considered for surgery, an operation is declined for various reasons (uncertain EEG seizure localization with no convincing lesion on magnetic resonance imaging (MRI); seizures that are different from expected; dementia or personality disorder; insufficient social network, etc.).

Most publications about the outcome of epilepsy surgery do not mention confidence limits, and this omission makes comparison between different centres difficult, especially as many study populations are very small. Taking the wide confidence limits into consideration,

our results are in line with what is reported elsewhere.

We still need the development of new AEDs, as well as advances in surgical techniques, as shown in the following lists.

Why epilepsy surgery?
- Long-standing intractable epilepsy in adults rarely remits spontaneously.
- Refractory epilepsy carries a poor social prognosis and is associated with significant excess mortality (seizures/accidents, sudden unexplained death, suicide).
- New drugs will give freedom from seizures in a maximum of 5–10 per cent.
- In carefully selected cases, 50–70 per cent of patients will become seizure-free from a temporal lobectomy, and will often experience considerable social benefit.

Why new antiepileptic drugs?
- Twenty to thirty per cent of patients still have seizures despite optimum treatment.
- Adverse effects are seen in half the patients, even on monotherapy with new antiepileptic drugs.
- Surgical treatment is possible in only a limited percentage of all patients.

How many drugs should be tried before surgery?

Clearly, with the excellent results obtained, particularly with temporal lobectomy in 'good' candidates (e.g. mesial temporal sclerosis or indolent tumours), surgery is not the last resort in such patients; they should be referred for presurgical evaluation after a few years of insufficient seizure control with three to five major antiepileptic drugs, as either monotherapy or a two-drug combination. The following is our preferred list of drugs for non-responsive partial seizures:

The pros	The cons
No exact seizure localization required	Chronic nuisance from stimulator
(Almost) reversible	In principle, not a cure
Can be switched on optionally (in patients with a warning)	No predictive knowledge at present about efficacy
	No MRI studies possible after implantation

Table 20.2
Vagal nerve stimulation.

- Lamotrigine
- Benzodiazepines (clobazam preferred to clonazepam because of fewer side effects)
- Topiramate
- Vigabatrin
- Tiagabine
- Valproate
- Phenytoin
- Gabapentin

In less suitable cases, e.g. patients with no MRI pathology, or with extratemporal seizures, a larger number of antiepileptic drugs must be tried, because there is a decrease in the difference between medical and surgical prognosis, i.e. the decision is highly individual.

What should be done if surgery is refused?

One option is vagal nerve stimulation (VNS), a treatment that was introduced in the late 1980s.[21] The pathophysiological background to this treatment comes from animal experiments, which demonstrate a 'desynchronization' effect on diverse hemispherical brain structures via the stimulation of the vagus nerve(s), probably as a result of that nerve's massive afferent connections. Human data from implantation of VNS in patients with therapy-resistant partial seizures (by implanting electrodes) confirm this hypothesis, although the efficacy is by no means spectacular. Very few become seizure-free, and a response (> 50 per cent seizure reduction) is seen in about one third of patients, which is comparable with the results obtained with the new antiepileptic drugs. Interestingly, the maximal effect may have a delay of up to 18 months, in contrast to antiepileptic drugs, from which some early decline in seizures is often seen.

Vagal nerve stimulation requires a minor operative procedure similar to a cardiac pacemaker, but no preoperative focus localization is needed (Table 20.2).

There is no evidence of any permanent change in the clinical status after removal of the stimulator. VNS is reversible but the electrodes surrounding the vagus nerve cannot be removed because of the risk of damaging the nerve. As strong magnetic fields generate currents that can heat the electrodes, MRI should be discouraged. Neuroimaging studies must therefore be carried out with appropriate caution after VNS implant. An advantage of VNS is that there are no sedative and cognitive effects. In addition to the chronic repetitive stimulation, the patient can, optionally (during an aura), activate the stimulator by placing a magnet over the stimulator and removing it immediately. This sometimes results in abortion of a seizure.

The most frequent problems encountered are local and related to the stimulation itself: hoarseness, spasms in the laryngeal muscles, borborygmi, etc. all of which are attributable to stimulation. Bradycardia is rarely of clinical significance. The left vagus nerve is used because it has fewer cardiac and more numerous afferent fibres.

We have had experience in VNS in only a limited number of patients, and the results have not been very encouraging. It must be borne in mind that our candidates for VNS have been treated with a large number of antiepileptic drugs, so their intractibility may not be entirely comparable with that of patients in the published literature on VNS.

Do the drugs work?

Understandably this question is sometimes posed by frustrated patients and relatives. It has been claimed that some patients might indeed have the same seizure frequency, regardless of medication, and that only half the patients admitted for intensive monitoring have more seizures during drug withdrawal.[22] Unfortunately, no systematic controlled study of this obviously important issue has been undertaken. However, it is common experience that, when patients are tapered off antiepileptic drugs for presurgical monitoring, they experience a major increase in seizures when they have almost finished the medication, rather than during the withdrawal phase itself.[23] The interpretation of this observation, which we have made in a substantial number of presurgical monitoring situations, is not, however, without problems. Patients who are subjected to presurgical evaluation usually have a very high level of vigilance because they are obviously concerned to see when they develop seizures. This 'hypervigilance', which is probably at its peak during the first days of video-EEG monitoring, may temporarily suppress seizures.

A prudent and stepwise removal of antiepileptic drugs may be justified in patients who are extremely refractory, especially those on polytherapy, and also for those whose treatment has been successfully converted to a one-drug regimen. In contrast to the high-dose strategy mentioned above, this approach could be termed a 'defensive' treatment. A gradual tapering off all treatment should include a sufficiently long observation period at each drug level to allow for proper monitoring of seizure frequency. If seizures become more frequent or severe, further drug reduction should be stopped immediately. The risk of status epilepticus must always be borne in mind, so ethical concerns may pose difficulties, but the perspective is still interesting and intriguing. Sometimes it is worthwhile considering whether our therapeutic efforts are, in fact, of any value.

In our experience, most patients and relatives find it easy to understand the rationale behind this defensive strategy: namely, to ascertain what amount of medication is really needed to maintain an endurable state.

Drug	Seizure type/syndrome
Carbamazepine/Oxcarbazepine	Partial seizures ± GTCS
Valproate	All seizure types, generalized syndromes, photosensitive epilepsy
Vigabatrin	Partial seizures ± GTCS; infantile spasms (especially in tuberous sclerosis)
Benzodiazepines	All seizure types/syndromes
Lamotrigine	Generalized syndromes; partial seizures ± GTCS
Topiramate	Probably as for lamotrigine
Tiagabine	As for carbamazepine/oxcarbazepine

GTCS, generalized tonic–clonic seizures.

Table 20.3
Range of efficacy of newer antiepileptic drugs against different seizure types/syndromes.

Partial seizures: are they all the same?

Transferring data from controlled studies to the individual patient is not straightforward.[24] Statistical analyses describe group differences, which are not applicable to individuals, and the index population may have a different level of severity of epilepsy to that of the patient in question. The seizure classification, which forms the basis for selecting patients for drug trials, does not take the aetiology and pathogenesis of epilepsy in the individual patient into consideration. Furthermore, our basic knowledge of the pathophysiology of epilepsies and the action(s) of the antiepileptic drugs are still too limited to be of great value in treating individual patients. Consequently, the often-mentioned 'cookbook' approach to treatment of different types of epilepsy (Table 20.3) clearly represents an oversimplification.

Partial seizures may be pathophysiologically different according to the site of origin as well as to the underlying cause. An interesting and potentially important example is given by Engel.[25] Frequently, the initial seizure activity in hippocampal sclerosis is not one of repetitive depolarization firing; instead, it shows a hypersynchronous pattern with alternating hyperpolarization and depolarization, giving an EEG appearance (using depth electrodes) that resembles the spike–wave pattern of an absence seizure. Later in the seizure, the pattern changes to the repetitive discharging neuronal activity that is usually encountered. Does this observation mean that such seizures can be expected to respond to ethosuximide and other specific anti-absence antiepileptic drugs? This option has never been tried, but could be worth considering, because hippocampal sclerosis is one of the most frequent pathologies associated with intractable temporal lobe epilepsy. However, from this hypothesis, we should perhaps expect valproate to be more efficient in this situation than is actually the case, although valproate and ethosuximide are not strictly comparable from the point of view of mode of action.

Other novel and individualized approaches to different types of epilepsy may emerge in the years to come. On consideration of the rapidly growing number of new and efficacious antiepileptic drugs, the possibilities for developing true 'rational polytherapy' may increase correspondingly, especially if drugs with different mechanisms of action can be used. Until now, however, no convincing proof of this assumption has emerged, except for the synergism that exists between valproate and ethosuximide,[26] and perhaps between lamotrigine and valproate.[27]

Other options: psychological and psychosensory treatment of epilepsy

The relationship between epileptic seizures and various psychosocial events has been recognized for many years, and different approaches have been made in order to evaluate their significance and how to use them therapeutically.[28,29] However, it is even more difficult, to blind patients and investigators, for example, than with, for example, VNS, especially in treatment strategies that depend on a personal relationship between the patient and therapist (an aspect that even the most rigorously controlled study can never totally circumvent). One study[30] has shown a significant effect of a progressive relaxation programme; this uses a control group who are allowed to sit quietly, i.e. non-specific relaxation. More specific behaviour modification strategies, which are 'tailored' to the individual patient, have been used in selected patients.[28,29] These behavioural modification techniques demand high levels of resources and their place in the treatment armamentarium has still not been established. The main feature of the treatment is to teach the patient to perform some specific act whenever an aura or a prodrome emerges. This is combined with teaching the patient how to identify seizure-provoking situations. The method is based on the description/analysis of seizures, seizure-precipitation and seizure abolishing situations, experiences with aborting seizures and seizure monitoring. In our hospital, we employ simpler methods that need fewer resources; methods based on different non-specific sensory (including painful) stimuli, which the patient applied as the seizure began. The drawback of such strategies is that not only is an aura (i.e. start of a simple partial seizure beginning) or some other warning signal necessary, but the patient must also be able to act on it. Of 15 patients who were possible candidates for this technique, six could not use them. In the remaining nine, however, five benefited from it – not only succeeding in aborting seizures, but also in giving them a better feeling of control over their disability.[31] More systematic studies, using larger patient groups, are necessary to evaluate the efficacy of this treatment strategy, but as a supplement to medical and surgical treatment, these relatively simple behavioural strategies seem to be promising because they can be applied on a larger scale.

Summary

A substantial proportion of patients with refractory partial seizures may benefit from a diagnostic and therapeutic work-up in the setting of a comprehensive epilepsy care programme. In our experience, the most frequent problems regarding drug treatment are: not enough drugs tried, suboptimal dosages, insufficient evaluation of the efficacy of each drug regimen, and lack of or insufficient seizure monitoring. When admitted to ordinary hospitals, the admission time is usually far too short for a proper evaluation of the condition.

In spite of major progress in the development of AEDs, only 5–10 per cent of patients with refractory epilepsy can expect to become seizure-free as a result of taking the new drugs. Many of these patients could also obtain significant benefit if currently available drugs were used optimally.

Besides these problems, psychological and social issues that influence the seizure frequency are often unrecognized or not dealt with. Epilepsy surgery is still an underused but very effective option—the only potentially curative treatment for this patient group.

References

1. Alving J. Classification of the epilepsies. *Acta Neurol Scand* 1978;58:205–12.
2. Sabers A, Alving J, Gram L. Evaluation of the Danish Epilepsy Center: Adults. *Seizure* 1992; 1(Suppl A):P13/34.
3. Sander JWAS, Hart YM, Johnson AL, Shorvon SD. National general practice study of epilepsy: newly diagnosed epileptic seizures in a general population. *Lancet* 1990;336: 1267–71.
4. Alving J. What is intractable epilepsy? In: Johannessen SI, Gram L, Sillanpää M, Tomson T, eds. *Intractable epilepsy*. Bristol, PA: Wrightson, 1995: 1–12.
5. Theodore WH, Schulman EA, Porter RJ. Intractable seizures: long-term follow-up after prolonged inpatient treatment in an epilepsy unit. *Epilepsia* 1983;24:336–43.
6. Cramer JA. Optimizing long-term patient compliance. *Neurology* 1995;45(Suppl 1): S25–8.
7. Schmidt D. Diagnosis and therapeutic management of intractable epilepsy. In: Schmidt D, Morselli PL, eds. *Intractable Epilepsy*, LERS Monograph Series No. 5. New York: Raven, 1986:237–57.
8. Løyning Y. Comprehensive epilepsy service. In: Dam M, Johannessen SI, Nilsson B, Sillanpää M, eds. *Epilepsy: progress in treatment.* Chichester: Wiley, 1987:225–45.
9. Schmidt D, Haenel SF. Therapeutic plasma levels of phenytoin, phenobarbitone and carbamazepine. Individual variation in relation to seizure frequency and type. *Neurology* 1984;4:1252–6.
10. Goggin T, Casey C, Callaghan N. Serum level of sodium valproate, phenytoin and carbamazepine and seizure control in epilepsy. *Irish Med J* 1986;79:150–6.
11. Perucca E, Gram L, Avanzini G, Dulac O. Antiepileptic drugs as a cause of worsening seizures. *Epilepsia* 1998;39:5–17.
12. Alving J, Brunbech L, Meinild H. Comprehensive epilepsy care in a short-stay adult department. *Epilepsia* 1996;37(Suppl 4):11 (abstract).
13. Hakkarainen H. Carbamazepine versus diphenylhydantoin versus their combination in adult epilepsy. *Neurology* 1980;30:354 (abstract).
14. Kälviäinen R, Aikiä M, Saukkonen AM, et al. Vigabatrin versus carbamazepine monotherapy in patients with newly diagnosed epilepsy: a controlled study. *Arch Neurol* 1995;52:989–96.
15. Tanganelli P, Regesta G. Vigabatrin versus carbamazepine monotherapy in newly diagnosed epilepsy: a randomized response

conditional cross-over study. *Epilepsy Res* 1996:**25**:257–62.

16. Schmidt D, Gram L. Monotherapy versus polytherapy in epilepsy: a reappraisal. *CNS Drugs* 1995;**3**:194–208.

17. Riley T, Porter RJ, White BG, Penry JK. The hospital experience and seizure control. *Neurology* 1981;**31**:912–5.

18. Walker MC, Sander JWAS. The impact of new antiepileptic drugs on the prognosis of epilepsy: seizure freedom should be the ultimate goal, *Neurology* 1996;**46**:912–4.

19. Engel J, Jr. Update on surgical treatment of the epilepsies. *Neurology* 1993;**43**:1612–7.

20. Patil A-A, Andrews R. Surgical management of independent bihemispheric seizure foci. *J Epilepsy* 1997;**10**:203–7.

21. McLachlan RS. Vagus nerve stimulation for intractable epilepsy: a review. *J Clin Neurophysiol* 1997;**14**:358–68.

22. Schmidt D. Medical intractability in partial epilepsies. In: Lüders HO, ed. *Epilepsy Surgery* New York: Raven, 1991:83–90.

23. Marks DA, Katz A, Scheyer R, Spencer SS. Clinical and electrographic effects of acute anticonvulsant withdrawal in epileptic patients. *Neurology* 1991;**41**:508–12.

24. Walker MC, Sander JWAS. Difficulties in extrapolating from clinical trial data to clinical practice: the case of antiepileptic drugs. *Neurology* 1997;**49**:333–7.

25. Engel J Jr. Introduction to temporal lobe epilepsy. *Epilepsy Res* 1996;**26**:141–50.

26. Rowan AJ, Meijer JWA, Beer-Pawlikowski N, et al. Valproate-ethosuximide combination therapy for refractory absences. *Arch Neurol* 1983;**40**:797–802.

27. Brodie MJ, Yuen AWC. Lamotrigine substitution study: evidence for synergism with sodium valproate? *Epilepsy Res* 1997;**26**:423–32.

28. Fenwick PBC, Brown SW. Evoked and psychogenic epileptic seizures. I. Precipitation. *Acta Neurol Scand* 1989;**80**:535–40.

29. Brown SW, Fenwick PBC. Evoked and psychogenic epileptic seizures: II. Inhibition. *Acta Neurol Scand* 1989;**80**:541–7.

30. Puskarich CA, Whitman S, Dell J, et al. Controlled examination of effects of progressive relaxation training on seizure reduction. *Epilepsia* 1992;**33**:675–80.

31. Brunbech L, Hermansen H, Sahlholdt L. Patients' evaluation of behavioural seizure management. *Epilepsia* 1997;**38**(Suppl 3):87 (abstract).

21

Neuropsychology and epilepsy surgery: optimizing the timing of surgery, minimizing cognitive morbidity, and maximizing functional status

Bruce P Hermann, Michael Seidenberg, Gary Wendt and Brian Bell

Introduction

This chapter addresses the issue of the optimal timing of consideration for epilepsy surgery, a significant practical clinical problem. The topic is considered primarily from the perspective of neuropsychology and health-related quality of life, but an important component of the discussion involves the characterization of surgically treatable and curable syndromes of temporal lobe epilepsy and pertinent neuroradiological findings. While brief and selected reviews of the pertinent literature are provided, the clinical issues and implications will be made clear.

The NIH Consensus Conference on Surgery for Epilepsy[1] noted that surgery is beneficial for selected patients but that, unfortunately, potential candidates typically suffer from the effects of medically resistant epilepsy for 10–20 years prior to surgical consideration because of current referral patterns. They concluded that research pertaining to the optimal timing of surgery was needed. The current chapter addresses this issue among the most common group of epilepsy surgery candidates—those with complex partial seizures of temporal lobe origin. Within this group, we will focus on those patients for whom the issue of optimal timing is least clear—those with intractable seizures not associated with foreign tissue lesions (tumors). Optimal surgical timing refers not only to

maximizing the degree of seizure control, but avoiding potential cumulative adverse consequences of epilepsy and maximizing life-long health and quality of life.[1] The optimal timing of surgery will be addressed here by reviewing whether there are detectable neuroradiological, cognitive and health-related quality of life consequences associated with increasing duration and/or severity of epilepsy. If an increased incidence of abnormal neuroradiological findings (e.g. atrophy), cognitive impairments or compromised quality of life are found to be associated with longer duration and/or increases severity of epilepsy, then an empirical rationale for earlier surgical consideration will result. If, on the other hand evidence of cumulative impairment is weak compared with the impact of immutable factors (e.g. age at onset), then modification of current practice may not be necessary. Further, there are distinct syndromes of localization-related temporal lobe epilepsy, and the risk of postoperative cognitive (memory, language) morbidity varies among these groups and needs to be considered and avoided in surgical planning. The material to follow will develop these theses.

First, recent evidence will be reviewed that characterizes the syndrome of mesial temporal lobe epilepsy, a surgically treatable syndrome of typically early age of onset. Second, findings related to the neuroradiological, neuropsychological and health-related quality of life status of patients at the conventional time of presentation for consideration of surgery (adulthood) will be reviewed briefly. As will be discussed, there appears to be evidence of more diffuse adverse neuroradiological and neuropsychological effects than would be anticipated on the basis of a focal (temporal lobe/hippocampal) pathology, with considerable quality of life impairments. Fourth, the degree to which these neuroradiological, neuropsychological and health-related quality of life impairments are associated with increasingly severe and/or prolonged epilepsy will be reviewed. The possibility that poorly controlled epilepsy of long duration has added to the patient's neurobehavioral burden will be examined. Fifth, literature will be reviewed which suggests that *postoperative* cognitive and psychosocial adequacy is strongly related to patients' *preoperative* cognitive and psychosocial status. The implication of this relationship is that in order to maximize postoperative quality of life and functional status it may be important to consider surgical intervention before chronic, intractable epilepsy has exerted increasingly adverse effects on cognitive and behavioral status. Finally, there is differential postoperative neuropsychological morbidity associated with the various localization-related syndromes of temporal lobe epilepsy, least in mesial temporal lobe epilepsy and highest in other syndromes. This relative cognitive morbidity will be examined.

Characterizing the syndrome of mesial temporal lobe epilepsy

As readers of this volume know, epilepsy is a common disorder, and complex partial seizures are a particularly common seizure type, about 80 per cent of such seizures originate in the temporal lobes, and patients with this seizure type represent the largest group of potential surgical candidates.[1] Advances have been made in characterizing surgical candidacy, the emphasis shifting from attempting to define 'intractable epilepsy' to identifying surgically remediable syndromes,[2-4] the most prominent of which is the syndrome of mesial temporal lobe epilepsy (MTLE).[2,4,5] This disorder is possibly the most common form of epilepsy and among the most refractory to medical treatment, often intractable by adolescence.[4] Its defining features include an early age of onset (primarily in the first decade), underlying hippocampal sclerosis reflected on magnetic resonance imaging (MRI) as unilateral hippocampal atrophy, commonly with a history of complicated febrile convulsions or other early etiological insults.[2,4-7] Other defining symptom complexes (e.g. clinical semiology, interictal/ictal EEG characteristics) associated with MTLE have been described.[4,6,7] The report of the NIH Consensus Conference on Surgery for Epilepsy,[1] as well as reports from contemporary surgical epilepsy centers,[8,9] indicate that at the time of surgery, patients with complex partial seizures of temporal lobe origin have a modal chronological age of 30 years with 10–20 years of epilepsy. The same modal features characterize MTLE patients at the time of surgery.[6-8] For instance, in our Memphis surgical series, patients with MTLE had an average age at onset of epilepsy of 7.2 years, but did not present for surgery until age 31 years, thus having approximately 24 years of typically poorly controlled epilepsy.

There are two other localization-related epilepsies of temporal lobe origin which will be discussed as this chapter proceeds. These include so-called idiopathic, cryptogenic or MRI-negative temporal lobe epilepsy (here called MRI-negative TLE) and lesional (e.g.

tumor, stroke) epilepsy of temporal lobe origin.[4,10] However, the emphasis will remain on MTLE.

In summary, MTLE is a surgically remediable syndrome of characteristically early age of onset (primarily in the first decade). By the time of referral for surgical consideration, patients with MTLE have typically experienced prolonged duration of intractable epilepsy (10–20 years), the consequences of which are poorly understood and are directly related to the issue of optimal surgical timing. Given the early onset of MTLE, the possibility for earlier surgical consideration is obviously present.

Neuroradiological, neuropsychological, and health-related quality of life status at the time of surgery

Neuroradiology

Neuroradiological/MRI investigations of anterior temporal lobectomy (ATL) candidates have focused largely on the hippocampus/mesial structures, particularly the to-be-resected (ipsilateral) hippocampus. These data have been shown to have important implications for patient selection and surgical outcome.[11] Whether there is evidence of progressive damage to other neuronal regions has been investigated very infrequently. The available reports and abstracts, several of modest sample size and involving heterogenous patient groups, have reported abnormalities in contralateral hippocampus,[12] cerebellum,[13] ipsilateral thalamus,[14,15] cingulate gyrus,[15] bilateral frontoparietal gray matter, temporal lobe white matter,[16] ventricular volumes in general[12] and frontal horn volumes in particular.[17] Some have suggested that extrahippocampal MRI volumet-

ric abnormalities may be associated with poorer surgical outcome as well as greater preoperative neuropsychological impairment.[13,18] A recent study reported that abnormalities of contralateral hippocampus on magnetic resonance spectroscopy predicted poorer postoperative memory status.[19] The degree to which these findings are secondary to the effects of chronic and intractable epilepsy versus the effects of an initial etiological insult (or a combination of the two) will be discussed in further detail below. It should be noted that because the average MTLE surgical patient (30 years old at surgery) has yet to face the neuropathological and neuropsychological consequences of normal aging, it would appear important to better understand the factors that adversely affect the contralateral hippocampus in particular.[20]

Neuropsychology

Results of neuropsychological testing in patients with chronic MTLE have focused primarily on memory functioning and recently it was emphasized that at the time of surgery there is evidence of more diffuse and generalized cognitive impairment than can be explained by the primary focal hippocampal neuropathology.[21] Specifically, these patients often show attenuated performance on measures of general intellectual functioning,[22] neuropsychological evidence of co-existing frontal lobe compromise[23,24] and contralateral memory impairments.[25]

More specifically, recent conceptualizations of MTLE have suggested that it is characterized primarily by material-specific memory impairments (left MTLE→verbal memory impairment, right MTLE→visual memory impairment), with generalized cognitive deficits thought to be uncharacteristic and inconsistent with MTLE.[2] However, very few studies have actually examined the status of cognitive functions other than memory in MTLE. We recently investigated the overall neuropsychological status of adult patients with MTLE (*n* = 66) versus MRI-negative TLE patients (*n* = 41) using a broad and representative battery of neuropsychological measures.[21] As proposed, material-specific memory impairments were indeed found to be associated with MTLE, the impairments more pronounced for verbal memory measures in left MTLE patients. However, the more striking finding was that MTLE patients (irrespective of laterality of seizure focus) exhibited generalized impairment across diverse domains of higher cognitive functioning. The affected cognitive domains included intelligence (Wechsler Adult Intelligence Scale-Revised (WAIS-R) Verbal and Performance IQ), academic achievement, language function and visual-perceptual/spatial ability. Thus, among this group of typical ATL candidates presenting after a prolonged history of poorly controlled epilepsy, patients with MTLE exhibited generalized neuropsychological impairment, an unexpected finding given the primary neuropathology (hippocampal sclerosis).[21] It is our hypothesis that this generalized neuropsychological impairment represents either the accumulated neurobiological consequences of prolonged exposure to MTLE or is a static encephalopathy secondary to the effects of the initial etiological insult.

Further, as reviewed above, a substantial proportion of patients with temporal lobe epilepsy presenting for surgical consideration have MRI abnormalities outside the to-be-resected hippocampus, e.g. cerebellar atrophy. In the broader neuroscience community there is now considerable evidence to suggest that the cerebellum makes distinct contributions to discrete higher cognitive functions, and previous neuropsychological investigations of epilepsy patients with cerebellar atrophy suggested that this neuroradiological finding would be of significance. To investigate this

issue further, we identified a consecutive series of 14 patients scheduled for ATL with MRI evidence of concomitant cerebellar atrophy detected on routine review of preoperative MRI, and subsequently confirmed via blinded review by a second board certified neuroradiologist.[26] Patients with unilateral temporal lobe epilepsy and cerebellar atrophy were matched to 28 ATL candidates without cerebellar atrophy in regard to laterality of seizure onset, gender, education, chronological age and age at onset of epilepsy. The groups were then compared across conventional domains of neuropsychological status including intelligence, academic achievement, language, visual-perceptual/spatial ability, memory and learning, attention, problem solving and sensorimotor function. Patients with cerebellar atrophy exhibited a tendency to perform worse on a diversity of neuropsychological measures, the most significant effects of which were obtained on WAIS-R Performance IQ.

Maguills and collaborators carried out a more rigorous investigation using quantitative MRI volumetrics when examining relationships between cerebellar atrophy and neuropsychological status among patients with temporal lobe epilepsy.[27] Again, they reported a significant relationship between cerebellar atrophy and poorer performance on measures of higher cognitive functioning. These findings indicate that neuroradiological evidence of anatomical abnormality outside the primary epileptogenic region (i.e. cerebellar atrophy) is a concomitant finding in some patients with chronic and long duration temporal lobe epilepsy, and this MRI finding carries additional neuropsychological consequences. The same might be true of atrophic lesions in other neuronal regions as well: i.e. such lesions probably contribute to the pattern of more generalized neuropsychological dysfunction often seen in this patient population.

Health-related quality of life

Health-related quality of life, including depression,[32-35] is widely appreciated to be adversely affected by intractable seizures[28-31] and indeed one of the major objectives of surgical intervention is to improve subsequent quality of life status.[29]

In summary, by the time MTLE patients are typically referred for surgical consideration the available literature suggests that a proportion of patients exhibit MRI evidence of volumetric abnormalities in contralateral hippocampus and extrahippocampal regions, neuropsychological impairments that extend beyond material-specific memory findings, and compromised quality of life. The frequency, severity and determinants of these abnormalities have not been comprehensively examined in a large and well-characterized cohort of MTLE patients. The degree to which such findings are attributable to adverse neurobiological consequences of increasingly prolonged exposure to MTLE remains to be clarified.

Potential causes of neuroradiological, neuropsychological, and quality of life findings at surgery

A basic question raised in this chapter is whether the duration and severity of MTLE is associated with extrahippocampal and contralateral MRI abnormalities, generalized cognitive impairment and adverse quality of life. Literature to support these points is now reviewed.

Neuroradiological studies

A limited number of studies have examined the relationship of the duration of severity of MTLE to MRI abnormalities outside the ipsilateral hippocampus. These studies have reported positive findings including reduced contralateral hippocampal volumes with increased seizure frequency,[17] increased cerebellar atrophy with a history of secondarily generalized tonic–clonic seizures[13] and reduced frontoparietal volumes with increasing years of seizures.[16]

Neuropsychological findings

The broader (non-surgical) epilepsy literature has suggested a link between the severity of epilepsy and neuropsychological status, but formal study of potential surgical candidates has yet to be conducted. Retrospective studies have linked lower IQ and/or more impaired neuropsychological status with an increasing number of estimated lifetime generalized tonic–clonic seizures,[36,37] episodes of status epilepticus,[36,38] or other markers of prolonged and intractable epilepsy (longer duration of poorly controlled seizures).[39-41] Farwell et al[42] reported that years of active epilepsy (subtracting years of inactive epilepsy from the overall duration of the seizure disorder) was a significant predictor of cognitive impairment among children and adolescents with epilepsy. Prospective studies are relatively few in number, and a careful and often cited investigation[43] demonstrated cognitive deterioration over a 4-year period in 15 per cent of newly diagnosed children. This deterioration was associated with a more severe and complicated/difficult-to-treat course. Ounsted and Lindsay[44] reported significant neuropsychological and psychosocial deterioration in a subset of 100 children with temporal lobe epilepsy with mixed etiologies. While this very brief review cannot do justice to this complicated topic, it should be noted that there are findings to suggest that duration and/or severity of epilepsy has a deleterious impact on cognitive status.

Health-related quality of life

Increasingly chronic and intractable epilepsy has long been hypothesized to lead to progressively impaired quality of life,[45] but this field could benefit from additional prospective controlled investigations. Consistent with this thesis, more favorable postsurgical outcomes (vocational, psychiatric, general psychosocial status) have been reported with earlier age at surgery,[46,47] but controlled trials have yet to be undertaken. In this regard it has been reported recently that a significant predictor of *postoperative* health-related quality of life is the adequacy of *preoperative* quality of life.[34,48] This relationship applies to vocational outcome,[49,50] emotional-behavioral status[51–54] and adequacy of cognitive functioning.[55–59] Thus, quality of life outcome of epilepsy surgery appears to be highly linked to functional status prior to surgery, and the degree to which neurobehavioral status itself may be associated with the duration and severity of epilepsy is an important topic for prospective investigation.

In summary, reports from studies of human epilepsy suggest that the duration and/or severity of epilepsy may be related to MRI anatomic abnormalities *outside* the ipsilateral hippocampus, generalized neuropsychological impairment and impaired health-related quality of life. The strong relationship of presurgical status to postoperative status makes it imperative to determine whether increasing duration or severity of MTLE is associated with progressive MRI, neuropsychological and quality of

life impairments. The relationship of MRI, neuropsychological and health-related quality of life impairments to increasingly prolonged and/or severe MTLE has yet to be comprehensively investigated and these findings will have direct relevance for the optimal timing of epilepsy surgery.

The importance of preoperative neurobehavioral status

The degree of seizure relief provided by ATL is associated with improved quality of life and psychosocial outcomes.[60] As would be predicted, better (seizure-free) surgical outcomes were generally associated with significant pre- to postoperative improvements in self-reported depression,[61] and self-reported emotional and psychosocial function.[48] These reports demonstrated a relationship between significant improvements in behavioral and psychosocial status with completely seizure-free surgical outcomes. More pertinent to the theme of this review, we found evidence to support Taylor's[34] hypothesis that the adequacy of postoperative neurobehavioral status was strongly predicted by preoperative status. Examining 97 ATL patients pre- and postoperatively, patients with poor preoperative psychosocial status, increased psychopathology and reduced health-related quality of life tended to remain that way postoperatively. Interestingly, preoperative health-related quality of life status was a stronger predictor of health-related quality of life outcome than was seizure outcome,[48] and this association was maintained 5 years after surgery.[62]

In summary, the adequacy of neuropsychological and neurobehavioral status of patients prior to surgery is a major predictor of the adequacy of postoperative psychosocial and health-related quality of life outcomes. To the degree that greater duration or severity of MTLE has adverse neurobiological, neuropsychological and neurobehavioral effects, then more optimal neurodevelopmental timing of epilepsy surgery would serve both to avoid the potential adverse effects of intractable epilepsy as well as to maximize postoperative capacity.

ATL outcomes: MTLE versus MRI-negative TLE

Considerable efforts have been expended recently by neuropsychologists to better understand the preoperative relationship between markers of mesial temporal lobe/hippocampal integrity and memory function.[63-67] As noted previously, another major localization-related epilepsy of temporal lobe origin is so-called cryptogenic,[10] idiopathic,[68] or MRI-negative temporal lobe epilepsy.[69] Like MTLE, this syndrome is not associated with macroscopic mass lesions on either pathological examination or neuroimaging. It differs from MTLE in that it is without MRI hippocampal atrophy or underlying hippocampal sclerosis,[70,71] has different etiological and clinical features (e.g. later age at onset, decreased incidence of early etiological insults such as febrile convulsions), and a poorer surgical outcome[8,72] and increased neuropsychological morbidity.[9,24,73-75] The latter is attributable to resection of a more structurally and functionally intact mesial temporal region.[56,77] This syndrome is recognized as being distinct from MTLE and is relatively poorly understood.[10]

Considerable efforts have been devoted to characterizing the neuropsychological morbidity associated with ATL and identifying the responsible factors so as to avoid or minimize such adverse outcomes.[78] As noted above, the factor most strongly associated with minimal risk of surgically-induced neuropsychological morbidity is the presence of unilateral hippocampal sclerosis, that is, MTLE. Significant adverse outcomes are associated with ATL for patients with MRI-negative TLE, which underscores the importance of distinguishing between these two epileptic syndromes. More optimal surgical intervention could pose significant advantages for the patient with MTLE by avoiding the adverse consequences of continuing intractable epilepsy. However, earlier consideration for non-MTLE would not appear to be beneficial given the neuropsychological morbidity to be briefly reviewed below.

MRI-negative TLE patients exhibit significantly greater pre- to postoperative decline in verbal learning and memory function following left ATL compared with MTLE patients,[79,80] a reliable finding detected across multiple measures of declarative verbal memory function including recall of prose passages,[79] paired-associate learning[81] and supraspan list learning.[80] This psychometric finding has been shown to be of day-to-day clinical significance.[82] MTLE patients show minimal adverse memory outcomes, most probably because an already structurally damaged (sclerotic) and functionally compromised hippocampal formation is resected. The characteristic post-surgical memory impairment noted among MRI-negative TLE patients is a decreased ability to encode/consolidate new information into long-term memory,[83] reflected in adverse effects on classic markers of secondary memory (e.g. serial position effects).[52] It should be appreciated that memory function is surely moderated by a distributed neuronal system including not only hippocampus but temporal lobe neocortex and other regions. In fact, very elegant work has demonstrated the relative contributions of lateral temporal versus mesial temporal regions to a variety of memory and learning tasks.[84-86]

In a randomized prospective clinical trial of partial versus total hippocampectomy for complex partial seizures of temporal lobe origin, it has been demonstrated that the extent of hippocampal resection was unrelated to the degree of neuropsychological morbidity, but was associated with significantly improved seizure control. The risk of adverse cognitive outcome was associated with operation for MRI-negative TLE,[9] reinforcing and extending the findings reviewed above.

In summary, MRI-negative TLE patients constitute a sizable minority of ATL patients at surgical centers, and have less favorable surgical outcome and increased cognitive morbidity. Earlier consideration might convey particular advantage to MTLE patients if more prolonged duration and severity of MTLE results in progressive neuroanatomic, neuropsychological or health-related quality of life impairments. In contrast, similar operations on patients with MRI-negative TLE result in a reliable pattern of cognitive morbidity that is of day-to-day significance along with significantly poorer surgical outcome compared with MTLE. Therefore earlier surgical intervention (ATL) would not be of apparent major benefit to MRI-negative TLE patients.

Summary

The following are what we believe to be the essential clinical ramifications of the literature reviewed above.

First, patients with MTLE (a surgically treatable syndrome) typically have an early age of onset of recurrent seizures, but on average surgery is typically not seriously considered and performed until well into adulthood.

Second, by the time of surgical presentation in adulthood, subsets of MTLE patients present with evidence of diffuse neuropsychological impairment indicative of dysfunction to neural regions outside the epileptogenic hippocampus, and MRI evidence of abnormal extrahippocampal anatomy (e.g. cerebellar atrophy) for which there appears to be additional cognitive morbidity. Whether these findings are a consequence of prolonged exposure to severe and intractable epilepsy versus the effects of the initial etiological insult (or a combination of both) remains to be determined conclusively, but there is some evidence to suggest that the former is an important consideration.

Third, from a postoperative quality of life standpoint, presurgical neuropsychological and behavioral status appears to be a powerful predictor (determinant) of postoperative cognitive and behavioral ability. As such, if cognition, neuroanatomy and quality of life are progressively impaired secondary to increasing duration and severity of MTLE, then prolonged delay of surgical consideration will compromise postoperative functional status and quality of life.

Fourth, both in pediatric and adult samples the adequacy of neuropsychological status is associated with factors reflecting the severity of epilepsy, with increasing cognitive impairment associated with previous episodes of status epilepticus, increasing number of secondarily generalized tonic–clonic seizures and fewer periods of seizure remission.

Fifth, the neuropsychological morbidity associated with ATL for MTLE is generally minimal as opposed to the possible considerable cognitive morbidity following surgery among patients with MRI-negative TLE. The fundamental nature and day-to-day impact of this surgically-induced cognitive morbidity has been studied in some detail and clarified. Thus, there should be greater consideration for earlier surgical intervention for patients with MTLE given the minimal degree of postoperative neuropsychological morbidity and the possibility of avoiding cumulative adverse effects of intractable epilepsy. The neuropsychological morbidity associated with ATL for MRI-negative TLE is of significant concern.

Acknowledgment

This publication was supported in part by NIH grant RO1 NS37738–01.

References

1. Surgery for Epilepsy. NIH Consensus Conference, 1990;**8**:1–20.
2. Engel J. Update on surgical treatment of the epilepsies: summary of the Second International Palm Desert Conference on the Surgical Treatment of the Epilepsies. *Neurology* 1993; **43**:1612–17.
3. Engel J. *Surgical treatment of the epilepsies*. 2nd edn. New York: Raven Press, 1993.
4. Engel J. Surgery for epilepsy. *N Engl J Med* 1996a;**334**:647–52.
5. Wieser HG, Engel J, Williamson PD, et al. Surgically remediable temporal lobe syndrome. In: Engel J, ed. *Surgical treatment of the epilepsies*. New York: Raven Press, 1993:49–63.
6. French JA, Williamson PD, Thadani VM, et al. Characteristics of medial temporal lobe epilepsy: I. Results of history and physical examination. *Ann Neurol* 1993;**34**:774–80.
7. Williamson PD, Spencer DD, Spencer SS et al. Complex partial seizures of frontal lobe origin. *Ann Neurol* 1985;**18**:497–504.
8. Davies KG, Hermann BP, Dohan FC, et al. Relationship of hippocampal sclerosis to duration and age at onset of epilepsy and childhood febrile seizures in temporal lobectomy patients. *Epilepsy Res* 1996;**24**:119–26.
9. Wyler AR, Hermann BP, Somes G. Extent of medial temporal resection and outcome from anterior temporal lobectomy: a randomized prospective study. *Neurosurgery* 1995;**37**: 982–91.
10. Engel J. Introduction to temporal lobe epilepsy. *Epilepsy Res* 1999;**26**:141–50.
11. Cascino GD, Jack CR. *Neuroimaging in epilepsy: principles and practice*. Boston, MA: Butterworth-Heinemann.
12. Quigg M, Bertram EH, Jackson T, Laws E. Volumetric magnetic resonance imaging: evidence of bilateral hippocampal atrophy in mesial temporal lobe epilepsy. *Epilepsia* 1997;**38**:588–94.
13. Specht U, May T, Rohde M, et al. Cerebellar atrophy and prognosis after temporal lobe resection. *J Neurol Neurosurg Psychiatry* 1997; **62**:501–6.
14. Hatta J, Fazilat S, Theodore WT, DeCarli C. Hippocampal and thalamic volumes in patients with complex partial epilepsy of left temporal origin. *Ann Neurol* 1995;**38**:296 (abst.).
15. Pennell PB, Beckham JS, Henry TR, et al. Hippocampal and extrahippocampal MRI volumetric abnormalities in patients with mesial temporal lobe epilepsy. *Neurology* 1997;**48**:42–3.
16. Marsh L, Morrell MJ, Shear PK, et al. Cortical and hippocampal volume deficits in temporal lobe epilepsy. *Epilepsia* 1997;**38**:576–87.
17. Barr WB, Ashtari M, Schaul N. Bilateral reductions in hippocampal volume in adults with epilepsy and a history of febrile seizures. *J Neurol Neurosurg Psychiatry* 1997;**63**:461–7.
18. Sisodiya SM, Moran N, Free SL, et al. Correlation of widespread preoperative magnetic resonance imaging changes with unsuccessful surgery for hippocampal sclerosis. *Ann Neurol* 1997;**41**:490–6.
19. Incisa della Rocchetta A, Gadian DG, Connelly A, et al. Verbal memory impairment after right temporal lobe surgery: role of contralateral damage as revealed by 1H magnetic resonance spectroscopy and T2 relaxometry. *Neurology* 1995;**45**:797–802.
20. Rausch R. Neuropsychological and psychosocial follow-up of patients with temporal lobe surgery for intractable epilepsy: results at 1-year and 10-years. *Epilepsia* 1995;**36**(Suppl 1):S138.
21. Hermann BP, Seidenberg M, Schoenfeld J, Davies K. Neuropsychological characteristics of the syndrome of mesial temporal sclerosis. *Arch Neurol* 1994;**54**:369–76.

22. Glosser G, Cole LC, Saykin AJ, Sperling M. Predictors of intellectual performance in adults with temporal lobe epilepsy. *J Int Neuropsychol Soc* 1997;9:252–9 (abst.).

23. Corcoran R, Upton D. A role for the hippocampus in card sorting? *Cortex* 1993;29:293–304.

24. Trenerry MR, Jack CR, Ivnik RJ, et al. MRI hippocampal volumes and memory function before and after temporal lobectomy. *Neurology* 1993;43:1800–5.

25. Helmstaedter C, Hufnagel A, Elger CE. Preoperative memory profiles in patients with temporal lobe epilepsy are related to postoperative seizure control. *J Epilepsy* 1992;5:17–23.

26. Hermann BP, Paradiso S, Seidenberg M, et al. Neuropsychological correlates of cerebellar atrophy in temporal lobe epilepsy. *Epilepsia* 1997;38 (Suppl 8):158.

27. Maguills C, Abou-Khahil B, Welch L, *et al.* Cerebellar volume in patients with epilepsy correlates with cognitive measures. *Epilepsia* 1997;38 (Suppl 8):141.

28. Hermann BP. Quality of life in epilepsy. *J Epilepsy* 1992;5:153–65.

29. Vickrey BG, Hays RD, Hermann BP, et al. Quality of life outcomes. In: Engel J, ed. *Surgical treatment of the epilepsies*. New York: Raven Press, 1992.

30. Vickrey BG, Perrine K, Hays RD, et al. *Quality of Life in Epilepsy (QOLIE-89) Inventory: Manual* (Version 1.0). Santa Monica, CA: Rand Corporation, 1993.

31. Vickrey BG, Perrine K, Hays RD, et al. *Quality of Life in Epilepsy (QOLIE-31) Inventory: Manual* (Version 1.0). Santa Monica, CA: Rand Corporation, 1993.

32. Altshuler L. Depression and epilepsy. In: Devinsky O, Theodore W, eds. *Epilepsy and behaviour*. New York: Wiley-Liss, 1992:47–65.

33. Blumer D, Montouris G, Hermann BP. Psychiatric morbidity in seizure patients on a neurodiagnostic monitoring unit. *J Neuropsychiatry* 1995;7:445–56.

34. Taylor DC. Psychiatric and social issues in measuring input and output of epilepsy surgery. In: Engel J, ed. *Surgical treatment of the epilepsies*. New York: Raven Press, 1987:485–503.

35. Victoroff J. DSM-III-R psychiatric diagnoses in candidates for epilepsy surgery: lifetime prevalence. *Neuropsychiatry Neuropsychol Behav Neurol* 1994;7:87–97.

36. Dodrill C. Correlates of generalized tonic-clonic seizures with intellectual, neuropsychological, emotional, and social function in patients with epilepsy. *Epilepsia* 1986;27:299–411.

37. Lennox W, Lennox M. *Epilepsy and related disorders*. Vol 1 and 2. Boston: Little, Brown and Co, 1960.

38. Dodrill CB, Wilensky AJ. Intellectual impairment as an outcome of status epilepticus. *Neurology* 1990;40(Suppl 2):23–7.

39. Dikmen S, Matthews CG, Harley JP. The effect of early versus late onset of major motor epilepsy upon cognitive-intellectual performance. *Epilepsia* 1975;16:73–81.

40. Dikmen S, Mathews CG, Harley JP. Effect of early versus late onset of major motor epilepsy on cognitive-intellectual performance: further considerations. *Epilepsia* 1977;18:31–6.

41. Dikmen S. Neuropsychological aspects of epilepsy. In: Hermann BP, ed. *A multidisciplinary handbook of epilepsy*. Springfield, IL: Charles C Thomas, 1980:36–73.

42. Farwell JR, Dodrill C, Batzel LW. Neuropsychological abilities of children with epilepsy. *Epilepsia* 1985;26:295–400.

43. Bourgeois BFD, Prensky AL, Palkes HS, et al. Intelligence in epilepsy: a prospective study in children. *Ann Neurol* 1983;7:438–44.

44. Ounsted C, Lindsay J. The long-term outcome of temporal lobe epilepsy in childhood. In: Reynolds E H, Trimble MR, eds. *Epilepsy and psychiatry*. Edinburgh: Churchill Livingstone, 1981:185–215.

45. Glaser GH. Natural history of temporal lobe-limbic epilepsy. In: Engel J, ed. *Surgical treatment of the epilepsies*. New York: Raven Press, 1987:13–30.

46. Duchowney M. Identification of surgical candidates and timing of epilepsy surgery: an overview. In: Wyllie E, ed. *The treatment of epilepsy: principles and practice*. Philadelphia: Lea & Febiger, 1993.

47. Lindsay J, Ounsted C, Richards P. Long-term outcome in children with temporal lobe seizures. V. Indications and contraindications for neurosurgery. *Dev Med Child* 1984;26: 25–32.

48. Hermann BP, Wyler AR, Somes G. Preoperative psychological adjustment and surgical outcome

are determinants of psychosocial status after anterior temporal lobectomy. *J Neurol Neurosurg Psychiatry* 1992;**55**:491–6.

49. Fraser RT, Gumnit R, Thorbecke R, Dobkin B. Psychosocial rehabilitation: a pre- and postoperative perspective. In: Engel J, ed. *Surgical treatment of the epilepsies.* New York: Raven Press, 1992.

50. Novelly RA, Augustine EA, Mattson RH, et al. Selective memory improvement and impairment in temporal lobectomy for epilepsy. *Ann Neurol* 1984;**15**:64–7.

51. Chovaz C, McLachlan R, Derry P, Cummings A. Psychosocial function following temporal lobectomy: influence of seizure control and learned helplessness. *Seizure* 1994;**3**:171–6.

52. Hermann BP, Austin J. Psychosocial status of children with epilepsy and the effects of epilepsy surgery. In: Wyllie E, ed. *The treatment of epilepsy: principles and practice.* Philadelphia: Lea & Febiger, 1993:1141–48.

53. Rose KJ, Derry PA, McLachlan R. Neuroticism in temporal lobe epilepsy: assessment and implications for pre- and postoperative psychosocial adjustment and health-related quality of life. *Epilepsia* 1996;**37**:484–91.

54. Rose KJ, Derry PA, Wiebe S, McLachlan RS. Determinants of health-related quality of life after temporal lobe epilepsy surgery. *Quality of Life Res* 1996;**5**:395–402.

55. Chelune GJ. Using neuropsychological data to forecast postsurgical cognitive outcome. In: Luders H, ed. *Epilepsy surgery.* New York: Raven Press, 1991.

56. Chelune GJ, Naugle RI, Luders H, et al. Individual change after epilepsy surgery: practice effects and base-rate information. *Neuropsychology* 1993;**7**:41–52.

57. Chelune GJ. Hippocampal adequacy versus functional reserve: predicting memory functions following temporal lobectomy. *Arch Clin Neuropsychol* 1995;**10**:413–32.

58. Hermann BP, Wyler AR, VanderZwagg R, et al. Predictors of neuropsychological change following anterior temporal lobectomy: the role of regression toward the mean. *J Epilepsy* 1991;**4**:139–48.

59. Hermann BP, Seidenberg M, Haltiner A, Wyler AR. The relationship of age at onset, chronological age, and adequacy of preoperative performance to verbal memory change following anterior temporal lobectomy. *Epilepsia* 1995;**36**:137–45.

60. Vickrey BG, Hays RD, Engel J, et al. Outcome assessment for epilepsy surgery: the impact of measuring health-related quality of life. *Ann Neurol* 1995;**37**:158–66.

61. Hermann BP, Wyler AR. Depression, locus of control, and the effects of epilepsy surgery. *Epilepsia* 1993;**30**:332–8.

62. Petersen J, Hermann BP, Wyler AR, et al. Long term outcome of anterior temporal lobectomy, unpublished observations. *Epilepsia* 1997;**38** (Suppl 8):150.

63. Miller LA, Munoz DG. Hippocampal sclerosis and human memory. *Arch Neurol* 1993;**50**: 391–4.

64. Rausch R, Babb TL. Hippocampal neuron loss and memory scores before and after temporal lobe surgery for epilepsy. *Arch Neurol* 1993;**50**:812–17.

65. Saling MM, Berkovic S, O'Shea MF, et al. Lateralization of verbal memory and unilateral hippocampal sclerosis: evidence of task specific effects. *J Clin Exp Neuropsy* 1993;**15**:608–18.

66. Sass KJ, Spencer DD, Kim JH, et al. Verbal memory impairment correlates with hippocampal pyramidal cell density. *Neurology* 1990;**40**: 1694–7.

67. Sass KJ, Sass A, Westerveld M, et al. Specificity in the correlation of verbal memory and hippocampal neuron loss: dissociation of memory, language, and verbal intellectual ability. *J Clin Exp Neuropsy* 1992;**14**:662–72.

68. Mathern GW, Pretorius JK, Babb TL. Influence of the type of initial precipitating injury and at what age it occurs on course and outcome in patients with temporal lobe seizures. *J Neurosurg* 1995;**82**:220–7.

69. Van Paesschen W, Connelly A, King MD, et al. The spectrum of hippocampal sclerosis: a quantitative magnetic resonance imaging study. *Ann Neurol* 1997;**41**:41–51.

70. Bruton CJ. *The neuropathology of temporal lobe epilepsy.* New York: Oxford University Press, 1988.

71. Mathern GW, Babb TL, Vickrey BG, et al. The clinical-pathogenic mechanisms of hippocampal neuron loss and surgical outcomes in temporal lobe epilepsy. *Brain* 1995;**118**:105–18.

72. Spencer DD, Inserni J. Temporal lobectomy. In: Luders H, ed. *Epilepsy surgery*. New York: Raven Press, 1991:533–45.

73. Oxbury JM, Oxbury SM. Neuropsychology, memory and hippocampal pathology. In: Reynolds E H, Trimble MR, eds. *The bridge between neurology and psychiatry*. Edinburgh: Churchill Livingstone, 1989.

74. Sass K, Westerveld M, Spencer SS, et al. Degree of hippocampal neuron loss mediates verbal memory decline following left anteromedial temporal lobectomy. *Epilepsia* 1994;35:1179–86.

75. Saykin AJ, Stafiniak P, Robinson LJ, et al. Language before and after temporal lobectomy: specificity of acute changes and relation to early risk factors. *Epilepsia* 1995;36:1071–7.

76. Wolf RL, Ivnik RJ, Hirshorn KA, et al. Neurocognitive efficiency following left temporal lobectomy: standard versus limited resection. *J Neurosurg* 1998;79:76–83.

77. Seidenberg M, Hermann BP, Wyler AR, et al. Neuropsychological outcome following anterior lobectomy in patients with and without the syndrome of mesial temporal lobe epilepsy. *Neuropsychology* 1997;12:303–16.

78. McMillan TJ, Powell GE, Janota I, Polkey CE. Relationships between neuropathology and cognitive functioning in temporal lobectomy patients. *J Neurol Neurosurg Psychiatry* 1987;50:167–76.

79. Hermann BP, Wyler AR, Somes G, et al. Pathological status of the mesial temporal lobe predicts memory outcome from left anterior temporal lobectomy. *Neurosurgery* 1992;31:652–7.

80. Hermann BP, Wyler AR, Somes G, et al. Declarative memory following anterior temporal lobectomy in humans. *Behav Neurosci* 1994;108:3–10.

81. Rausch R. Anatomical substrates of interictal memory deficits in temporal lobe epileptics. *Int J Neurol* 1987;21–22:17–32.

82. Hermann BP, Seidenberg M, Dohan FC, et al. Patient and family report of memory change following left anterior temporal lobectomy: relationship to degree of hippocampal sclerosis. *Neurosurgery* 1995;36:39–45.

83. Seidenberg M, Hermann BP, Dohan FC, et al. Neuronal density in human hippocampus and verbal encoding ability following anterior temporal lobectomy. *Neuropsychologia* 1995;34:699–708.

84. Helmstaedter C, Elger CE. Functional plasticity after left anterior temporal lobectomy: reconstitution and compensation of verbal memory functions. *Epilepsia* 1998;39:399–406.

85. Helmstaedter C, Gleissner U, DiPerna M, Elger CE. Relational verbal memory processing in patients with temporal lobe epilepsy. *Cortex* 1997;33:667–78.

86. Helmstaedter C, Grunwald T, Lehnertz K, et al. Differential involvement of left temporolateral and temporalmesial structures in verbal declarative learning and memory: evidence from temporal lobe epilepsy. *Brain Cogn* 1997;35:110–31.

22

Cognitive deficits in epilepsy: is there a treatment?

Albert P Aldenkamp, Mark Hendriks and Jan Vermeulen

Introduction

People who have refractory epilepsies frequently complain about cognitive impairments. Memory impairment is the dominant complaint in clinical practice.[1-3] In our own studies, we demonstrated memory complaints in approximately 20 per cent of the outpatients of an epilepsy centre (all diagnosed as suffering from a localization-related epilepsy with an average duration of >10 years).[4,5] This estimate is also reported in a number of other studies.[1,3,6]

Nevertheless this estimate cannot be taken at face value. Several studies mention discrepancies between subject memory complaints and the results of neuropsychological testing.[7] Thompson[3] concludes that many patients who complain often perform within normal limits on standardized memory tests. Spontaneous complaints may thus overestimate the incidence of actual impairment. In our own study, memory impairment could be confirmed in approximately 80 per cent of the patients who had persistent memory complaints.[8] Such discrepancies may simply reflect inadequacies of the neuropsychological test repertoire. Thus, a patient may rightly complain of 'having trouble remembering things', but the problem eludes detection with the psychologists' standard repertory of tests if these do not tap the specific aspect of memory that the patient is complaining about.[7] An example would be that most standard clinical memory testing involves fairly short retention intervals,

i.e. minutes to hours.[9] Retention and forgetting over the long term, as in a person's own memory for events long past, are obviously much more difficult to test.[10] Conversely, there is evidence that some patients overestimate their capacities and do not complain, although their memory scores reveal impairment.

By combining these findings, we reach a practical estimate of 15–20 per cent of the patients with refractory epilepsy having memory impairment, which demonstrates that this is a serious problem in clinical practice.

Concerning the type of complaints, most patients (57 per cent) report problems in reproducing information after a long time or difficulties in learning new information. Retrieval complaints (such as the 'tip of the tongue' phenomenon) are reported only in a minority of patients (7 per cent). This contrasts with the studies on memory loss in, for example, elderly patients, where such retrieval complaints are the most frequent complaint;[11] this suggests that there may be specific types of memory impairment in epilepsy.

Although the immediate and prolonged effects of seizures[12] or the side effects of antiepileptic drugs[13,14] have serious impact on cognitive function, memory impairment is rarely seen as a consequence of these factors. Localized dysfunction, related to epileptic focal activity in specific areas of the brain, is probably one of the key factors for memory impairment.[2] Memory disorders occur more frequently in temporal lobe epilepsy[6] than in forms of epilepsy that originate elsewhere in the brain. Verbal and visuospatial memory loss are more often associated with an epileptogenic focus in the left and right hemisphere respectively.[2,15,16] The evidence for lateralization of dysfunction has been confirmed to some extent in the course of preoperative invasive procedures.[17] The association between memory impairment and temporal lobe epilepsy is not unexpected. The importance of structures that lie deep and medial in the temporal lobe (e.g. the hippocampus) in mnemonic processes, and particularly in the registration of new information, is well established,[18,19] and epileptic seizures often originate in these structures. For example, complex partial seizures are the most common type of epilepsy, they are often not controlled by medication[20] and they often originate in mesiotemporal structures that are important to memory.

Changes in drug treatment or improvements of seizure control will, thus, normally have limited influence on memory impairment. We therefore need methods to treat memory impairment in clinical practice. This chapter evaluates the possibilities of such treatment. Potentially, two methods for memory treatment are available: behavioural methods (i.e. 'training memory') and the pharmacological approach.

Models for memory training

In general, it is crucial to distinguish the literature on improving memory skills from the studies that focus on the treatment of memory impairment. Improving memory skills has been studied in normal individuals for several decades.[21-23] In addition, there is now a considerable body of scientific literature on programmes for the treatment of memory

impairment.[24-26] In this chapter, only studies on treatment of memory impairment are analysed. Two broad approaches to memory treatment have been utilized: reconstruction of the impaired function using stimulation and activation, and training compensation strategies to bypass the deficit, without necessarily producing an improvement in memory capacity.[26]

Reconstruction approach

The reconstruction approach, which is probably the one used most often in practice,[27] relies heavily on repetitive drilling. The tasks used in this form of training can easily be computerized, and there are commercially available software packages requiring patients to practise remembering letters, digits, words, pictures, shapes and stories. The stimuli that are used in such programmes do not necessarily have any inherent practical value. The aim is to improve memory in general, by drill and practise, as if memory were a kind of mental muscle that can be conditioned by systematic exercise. Another related assumption underlying this approach is that the repeated stimulation and activation of a target process, memory in this case, will somehow force the brain to consider new pathways or utilize new structures,[24] i.e. guide the neuronal reorganization of function. It would be beyond the scope of this chapter to examine the validity of the theoretical basis of this approach. From a practical point of view, however, it is more interesting to consider the efficacy of this 'muscle building' approach to memory training.

The general picture emerging from studies carried out on the efficacy of this approach is that it does *not* produce any general improvements in memory functioning. There are studies, for example, that report only minimal or no improvement on untrained tasks or on functional memory outside the clinic, even after hundreds of hours of practise.[28,29] Apparently, memory is not a mental muscle; it will not get stronger simply by exercising it. The drill and practise method may have beneficial effects, however, in the sense that memory-impaired patients can learn very specific pieces of useful new information, e.g. a medication schedule or the most adequate method to perform a job.

Compensatory approach

The compensatory approach to memory training involves the training of techniques to circumvent difficulties that arise as a result of memory impairment. One way to compensate for memory difficulties is to use external aids; the other involves the use of internal aids. Most normal people use such memory aids at some time or another in order to compensate for the normal failures of everyday memory.[30] External memory aids can be subdivided into three types.[26] First, there are various means to organize and store information — a diary, for example. A second type of aid is intended to remind a memory-disordered person to perform a particular activity at a specified future time. Alarms and watches fall this into category. A third type of external aid is environmental modification: the restructuring of the environment to decrease the impact of memory deficit on daily life. A specially structured work environment or a posted reminder on a mirror would both be examples of this type of aid.

There is little systematic research on the effectiveness of external memory aids.[25,31] One problem with external memory aids is that, in order to use them, a minimal number of instructions must be learned and remembered, and even this may be a problem for people who have memory impairment. The problem with using an agenda or a notebook, for example, is not so much in writing down things to

remember, but in learning a routine for looking them up at the right moment. However, learning to use external aids may well be the only effective form of treatment in patients with severe memory impairment.

There are a fair number of internal strategies that have been developed; these involve verbal as well as visual imagery techniques, which can be used for memorizing information and may be helpful in compensating for memory failure. A common principle behind such 'mnemonic strategies' is that they focus on deliberately organizing the things to be memorized so that they can be found again more easily when they are needed. Organization is the key to any large database, of course, and our memory is no exception. Learning mnemonic strategies has been a popular form of memory training since at least the time of the ancient Greeks. Only a few illustrative examples of mnemonics are given here.[24,25] Visual imagery takes advantage of the fact that information can often be dually coded, i.e. as images or as words. If recall from one representational system fails, recall from the other may still be successful. Adding mental pictures is thus one way to remember information more easily. Imagery can be used, for example, to learn people's names.[25] One technique is to turn the name to be learned into a picture. With 'Mike' one can imagine a man holding a microphone, and 'Carrie' may be pictured as a woman carrying a basket. Verbal techniques typically involve imposing structure on unstructured material, or associating meaningless information that has to be remembered with meaningful information. For example, a string of digits such as 16111991 is easier to remember as a date — 16 November 1991 — than as a meaningless number sequence.

There can be no doubt that such mnemonic techniques can improve memory performance. Professional memory artists use them, they have beneficial effects for normal subjects in experimental situations, and there are indications that they can improve memory performance in memory-disordered patients as well.[24,25] One potential advantage of these internal strategies is that they might have generalized effects, in the sense that a strategy taught to help with one problem, such as learning names, may also be used to help with another problem, such as remembering a shopping list. However, in practice not many patients will do this spontaneously. Also, it is difficult to persuade patients to use such strategies beyond the training period and to put them into practice in natural settings outside the laboratory.[32,33] In fact, it is hard to imagine how internally generated strategies such as imagery or various verbal techniques could begin to be used to store and retrieve the huge amounts of information about events or people that are important to daily life. Also, these techniques require a good deal of concentrated effort and creativity and they often seem somewhat unnatural, so that it is not surprising that memory-impaired people do not apply them spontaneously in daily life. Internal strategies may be useful, of course, in the acquisition of specific small bodies of information. For example, visual imagery techniques have been used with some success for teaching memory-impaired patients the names of people in their immediate environment.[25]

In the neuropsychological departments of our epilepsy centres, we use several methods of memory training, mostly in the form of group training. These training sessions aim at teaching patients to use external memory aids, and specific bits of information, skills and behaviour that are important to their daily needs.

A group approach is used, because most patients find that this is more motivating than individual training sessions. To give an example, one form of group training is divided into three

subsequent steps: after extensive neuropsychological assessment and monitoring of memory deficits in daily life (also using reports from partners), the patients are invited for an introductory session. The group size is kept to a maximum of five patients, and the patient's partner is also invited for this session to stimulate support. After the introduction, memory training is given in six subsequent sessions: half of these sessions are used for training specific skills using the reconstruction approach and half to train memory aids. Each session is concluded with practical advice about the use of trained skills in daily life. Each new session starts with an evaluation of the use of these skills over the preceding period. The interval between the training sessions is 2 weeks. Besides teaching memory aids and specific information/skills, the sessions aim at assisting the patients and their partners in reorganizing their lives and preventing ineffective compensatory methods.

A relatively short training period appears to be critical for several reasons. First, a ceiling effect emerges after four or five sessions. Longer training periods are reported to be stressful for the patients as they are constantly confronted with their failures. Moreover, after the first sessions, the function of the group changes gradually to a social-supportive group. As this could interfere with forms of individual treatment, we choose to stop the training after the sixth session. After an interval of 2 months we reinvite the patients for two additional sessions and finally the neuropsychological assessment is repeated.[34]

Neuropharmacological models

The neuropharmacological approach to memory treatment starts from the axiom that drug treatment is not likely to give a positive response when used in cases with structural damage, i.e. stroke, and it cannot replace degenerated neurons in syndromes such as multi-infarct dementia.[35] Some efficacy may be expected, theoretically, when used for functional impairment.[36] Thus, it may hasten neuronal recovery, improve the function of surviving neuronal structures in chronic disease and prevent further neuronal damage.[37] As early as the 1930s,[38,39] it was suggested that some types of drug treatment might also be helpful to treat cognitive impairment. However, it appeared to be difficult to confirm this assumption, partly caused by the methodological difficulties that are inherent in such trials.[40]

Neuropharmacological models for memory treatment can be classified into four major classes.

Non-specific CNS stimulation

Non-specific central nervous system (CNS) stimulation with amphetamines or caffeine is found to have a positive effect on cognitive functions, particularly in the presence of fatigue.[41] Most positive results have been found for speed factors, arousal and activation, and associated short-term effects, mostly using *d*-amphetamines.[37] Special attention has to be paid to the inversed U-shaped relationship between task level, attentional factors and drug effects, causing, at some point, negative results. A special target for this drug may be the reversible effects on CNS depressants in elderly people. This approach was not considered useful for the treatment of memory in epilepsy as none of the trials has reported a specific role as memory modulator.

Replacement of depleted neurotransmitters

Replacement of depleted neurotransmitters may have important future therapeutic potential. Until now, this approach has met with variable

success and only in specific syndromes such as compounds reinforcing the cholinergic system in Alzheimer-type dementia.[37] The rationale for this approach is that memory defects produced by anticholinergic compounds mimic some of the anterograde memory deficits in Alzheimer's disease.[42] Memory impairment may therefore be related to dysfunction in the cholinergic transmission. In line with dopamine supplementation in Parkinson's disease, choline or lecithin is given, so far without convincing results. In epilepsy, the role of exhaustion of specific neurotransmitters is still under study and therefore this approach is not yet open for therapeutic comment. A promising option is the use of GABA-related compounds. γ-Aminobutyric acid (GABA) is also used as a basis for rational antiepileptic treatment in a new class of drugs such as γ-vinyl-GABA or vigabatrin,[43] and is sometimes considered as a basis for memory improvement.[40] Thus far the memory-enhancing effects of such drugs have not been established.

Putative memory modulators

The administration of putative memory modulators has been proposed, using several types of neuropeptides, such as vasopressin. Of the 20 or more potentially active peptides, ACTH, vasopressin and opioid peptides have been studied. Although results in experimental animal studies proved successful, effective treatment in humans is reported only in specific groups such as in people with diabetes insipidus.[44] In general the assumed effects of neuropeptides are now being seriously questioned.[45]

Drugs that increase CBF

Several types of drugs are available that claim to increase cerebral blood flow (CBF) or to enhance cellular metabolism in the brain. This may be a promising approach for the treatment of memory in epilepsy, because several trials with these drugs showed protective properties against amnesia in models that may allow for generalization of the results to epilepsy. Examples are the electroshock model and induced cerebral hypoxia.[46,47] Lagergren and Levander[48] induced artificial hypoxia by means of a controlled reduction of heart rate. Piracetam, the first drug to be developed in this class, had little effect on performance at normal heart rate, but significantly decreased the cognitive deterioration caused by the hypoxia when the heart beat was reduced. The same mode of operation may be assumed if, for reasons other than hypoxia, hypofunction of cerebral metabolism occurs, such as in epilepsy.[8] Drugs in this class also showed protection against amnesia caused by noxious stimuli that were induced by several amnesic agents.[37,47,49–51] In epilepsy these types of drugs may be used as add-on treatment against the sedative side effects of the antiepileptic drugs, which may be clinically relevant when changes in the antiepileptic drug regimens are not possible. Some positive results have been reported in normalizing diazepam-induced changes[52] and in recovery from drug intoxication.[37]

A sub-class of these drugs are the 'nootropic drugs', which not only act as vigilance-enhancing psychostimulants, but may also influence specific cognitive targets.[47,49,51] The mechanism of action of this class of drugs is assumed to be a selective effect on integrative mechanisms in the telencephalon, with no alteration in neuronal excitability or neurotransmitter activity.[49–51] Several specific cognitive targets for these drugs have been proposed. Some studies suggest that cognitive improvement of nootropic drugs may be the result of general psychostimulant effects on arousal and vigilance.[53]

The EEG profiles of this class of drugs are very similar to those in the class of non-specific CNS-stimulating drugs, e.g. an alpha-enhancing effect, an increase in the average EEG frequency and a decrease of delta activity.[51,52,54] In addition, an effect on verbal processing is suggested. Piracetam, for example, has been studied in children with dyslexia. This approach was based on the observation in early studies that substantial improvement of verbal-sequential processing occurs after administration of piracetam.[55–57] An extensive investigation brought up some neurophysiological support for this observation. This prompted Conners to postulate a specific 'left-hemisphere function' of the drug,[58,59] though this is questioned by others.[54] A multi-centre study showed that, on the whole, the results did not support this claim.[56,60] Improvement of the reading disability was found, but only in limited areas, and most effects had to be characterized as weak. More pronounced changes were shown in enhanced short-term memory, especially in the greater availability of verbal information, as indicated by word recall. Therefore, short-term memory might be a more promising target for this class of drug treatment. This is in line with other clinical studies on piracetam, such as the studies of Helfgott et al[61,62] and Levi and Sechi[63] or on studies of related drugs such as etiracetam[64] or aniracetam.[46]

We have evaluated the effect of the last class of drugs, i.e. nootropic-type drugs, on memory in patients with refractory, localization-related epilepsy and severe memory impairment. A first trial involved oxiracetam (4–hydroxy-2–oxo-pyrrolidine-acetamide), a pyrrolidinone derivative, structurally related to a cyclic form of γ-amino-β-hydroxybutyric acid (GABOB).[65] For oxiracetam, the same mode of action is proposed as found in piracetam, only with more distinctive effects on memory,[66] especially in elderly people with organic brain syndrome,[67] in patients with primary degenerative dementia[68] and in a heterogeneous group of dementia patients.[69] Our study used a double-blind, placebo-controlled, between-patient randomized study.[70] During a 12-week period either oxiracetam (800 mg three times daily) or placebo was given to 30 patients. The study showed significant improvements in patients, suggesting the involvement of speed factors as well as of language comprehension. If we also take the tests with a systematic trend into consideration, the greatest improvement is found again for tests in which speed factors are predominant and for language. No specific improvements in memory were found. These findings are in agreement with reports about piracetam-induced effects on verbal processing,[56,60] and with the studies that found primary effects on alertness and vigilance.[37,53] However, we must be extremely cautious when interpreting the results in our study as drug effects. In most of the tests, improvement for oxiracetam is only very weak.

A second trial involved sabeluzole (R 58 735 (4–[(2–benzothiazolyl)methylamonil-α-[(4-fluorophenoxy)-methyl]-1–piperidine ethanol)), a benzothiazol derivative that was shown to be an effective protector against several types of hypoxia in animal experiments.[71] The results in normal volunteers showed that sabeluzole ameliorated both learning and recall from memory in conditions of age-related mild hypofunction.[72] Consolidation of information appeared to be more efficient and recall of verbal information from long-term memory was improved even one week after withdrawal of the drug.[73] Further experiments consistently showed most of the positive effects in subjects with relatively poor performance, i.e. in the sub-group with the lowest scores on baseline memory tests.[74] This suggests that sabeluzole does not improve memory function itself, but reactivates or restores *impaired* function. Although the cerebral working mechanisms of sabeluzole are not completely understood, its improvement of fast axonal transport and its effect on voltage-dependent outward K^+ currents may be implicated in the effects on memory.[75] Our study used a randomized, double-blind, placebo-controlled, parallel-group design[75] with 38 patients, assigned to a 12-week treatment with either sabeluzole or placebo. The number of 'responders', i.e. patients with an improvement that was more than 1 SD on at least three of the memory tests in the sabeluzole group, was nearly twice the number of responders in the placebo group (64 per cent vs 36 per cent). This suggested a clinically relevant effect of sabeluzole. The analysis of the memory tests showed a statistically significant improvement with sabeluzole on the verbal long-term memory test. This could represent a specific drug effect and is in line with previous results of normal volunteer studies, which also found improvement to be mainly restricted to the area of verbal long-term memory. Unfortunately, the company hesitates about whether or not the drug will be marketed because the primary target was Alzheimer's disease.

Summary

The overall results of both approaches, behavioural and pharmacological, may seem somewhat disappointing, in that the expected gains in memory functioning are certainly not dramatic. However, an important point to be made is that, in some patients, small improvements can make the difference between long-term institutional care and living at home, and in such cases treatment would certainly be justified in terms of costs and benefits.

It may be possible, of course, to develop new forms of memory training that are more effective than those we have now. For example, most internal strategies are basically strategies for learning new information, but memory-impaired patients with epilepsy may also have difficulties with the complex active search processes that may be involved in retrieving old information,[3,76] which was stored away a long time ago, perhaps without any deliberate attempt to make the information somehow easier to remember at a later date. Conceivably, these active retrieval strategies can be systematically trained, but relatively little work has been done on the development of retrieval strategies that can be used by memory-impaired patients. Most research on retrieval strategies is concerned with the retrieval of long-past memories in normal subjects.[77,78]

An additional option is the use of training programmes designed for patients who have had a cerebrovascular accident (CVA) and in patients with a unilateral epileptic focus. The rationale of such an approach is that unilateral CVA damage may resemble the dysfunctions that occur in patients with a unilateral focus.[79]

The results of the pharmacotherapeutic approach may be improved when motivational factors are considered more carefully. Whereas most of the memory training programmes seem to meet the need for the patient and his or her family 'to do something', pharmacotherapy seems to produce a passive attitude. In our trial with oxiracetam, neither the subjective reports of well-being nor the responses on a standardized mood rating scale showed any improvement. The same finding was obtained for the placebo condition. Normally, placebo treatment results in subjective improvements. This suggests that drug treatment may be regarded by the patients as 'ego alien', possibly because their role during treatment was, essentially, passive. It may well be that a combination of cognitive training and pharmacological treatment is more effective than a trial that exclusively uses drug treatment, although such a combination introduces several additional methodological problems that have yet to be resolved.

References

1. Stores G. Memory impairment in children with epilepsy. *Acta Neur Scand* 1981;**89**:21–9.
2. Loiseau P, Strube E Signoret JL. Memory and epilepsy. In: Trimble MR, Reynolds EH, eds. *Epilepsy, behaviour and cognitive function.* New York: John Wiley & Sons, 1988:165–77.
3. Thompson PJ. Epilepsy and memory. In: Manelis J, Bental E, Loeber EN, Dreifuss FE, eds. *Advances in epileptology*, Vol. 17, Raven Press: New York, 1989.
4. Overweg J, Verhoeff NPLG, van Royen EA, et al. Memory disorders and focus localisation with ⁹⁹ᵐTC HMPAO SPECT, EEG and CT in patients with partial epilepsy. *Eur J Nucl Med* 1991;**16**:522–3.
5. Aldenkamp AP, Vermeulen J, Alpherts WCJ, et al. Validity of computerized testing: patient dysfunction and complaints versus measured changes. In: Dodson WE, Kinsbourne M, eds. *Assessment of cognitive function.* New York: Demos, 1992:51–68.
6. Hermann BP, Wyler AR, Richey ET, Rea JM. Memory function and learning ability in patients with complex partial seizures of temporal lobe origin. *Epilepsia* 1987; **28**:547–54.
7. Herrmann DJ. Know thy memory: the use of questionnaires to assess and study memory. *Psychol Bull* 1982;**92**:434–52.
8. Verhoeff NPLG, Aldenkamp AP, Overweg J, Van Royen EA, Verbeeten B Jr, Weinstein H. Memory complaints, memory disorders and focus localization in patients with partial epilepsy. *Seizure* 1992;**1**:149–56.
9. Guilford JP. *The nature of human intelligence.* London: McGraw Hill, 1971.

10. Squire LR, Slater P, Chase PM. Retrograde amnesia: temporal gradient in very long-term memory following electroconvulsive therapy. *Science* 1975;**187**:77–9.

11. Neisser U, Herrmann DJ. An inventory of every-day memory experiences. In: Gruneberg MM, Morris PE, Sykes RN, eds. *Practical aspects of memory*. London: Academic Press, 1978.

12. Dodrill CB. Correlates of generalized tonic-clonic seizures with intellectual, neuropsychological, emotional and social function in patients with epilepsy. *Epilepsia* 1986;**27**:399–411.

13. Trimble MR, Reynolds EH. *Epilepsy, Behaviour, and Cognitive Function*. Chichester: John Wiley & Sons, 1988.

14. Aldenkamp AP. Cognitive side-effects of antiepileptic drugs. In: Aldenkamp AP, Dreifuss FE, Renier WO, eds. *Epilepsy in children and adolescents*. New York: CRC Press Publishers, 1995:161–83.

15. Ladavas E, Umilta C, Provincialli L. Hemisphere dependent cognitive performance in epileptic patients. *Epilepsia* 1979;**20**:493–502.

16. Binnie CD. Seizures, EEG discharges and cognition. In: Trimble MR, Reynolds EH, eds. *Epilepsy, behaviour and cognitive function*. New York: John Wiley & Sons, 1987:45–51.

17. Ojemann GA, Dodrill CB. Verbal memory deficits after left temporal lobectomy for epilepsy: mechanisms and intraoperative prediction. *J Neurosurg* 1985;**62**:101–7.

18. Scoville WB, Milner B. Loss of recent memory after bilateral hippocampal lesions. *J Neurol Neurosurg Psychiatry* 1957;**20**:11–21.

19. Penfield W, Milner B. Memory deficit produced by bilateral lesions in the hippocampal zone. *Arch Neurol Psychiatry* 1958;**79**:475–9.

20. Deonna T, Ziegler AL, Despland PA, Van Melle G. Partial epilepsy in neurologically normal children: clinical syndromes and prognosis. *Epilepsia* 1986;**27**:241–7.

21. Lorayne H, Lucas J. *The Memory Book*. New York: Stein & Day, 1974.

22. Yates FA. *The Art of Memory*. Chicago: University of Chicago Press, 1966.

23. Young MN, Gibson WB. *How to develop an exceptional memory*. Radnor, PA: Chilton, 1962.

24. Powell EP. *Brain function therapy*. Aldershot: Gower, 1981.

25. Wilson BA. *Rehabilitation of memory*. New York: Guildford Press, 1987.

26. Sohlberg G, McKay Moore F, Mateer CA. *Introduction to Cognitive Rehabilitation*. New York: Guildford Press, 1989.

27. Harris JE, Sunderland A. A brief survey of the management of memory disorders in rehabilitation units in Britain. *Int Rehabil Med* 1981;**3**:206–9.

28. Prigatano G, Fordyce D, Zeiner H, Roueche J, Pepping M, Wood B. Neuropsychological rehabilitation after closed head injury in young adults. *J Neurol Neurosurg Psychiatry* 1984;**47**:505–13.

29. Schacter D, Rich S, Stampp A. Remediation of memory disorders. Experimental evaluation of the spaced retrieval technique. *J Clin Exp Neuropsychol* 1985;**7**:79–96.

30. Harris JE. Memory aids people use: two inter-view studies. *Mem Cog* 1980;**8**:31–8.

31. Harris J. Methods of improving memory. In: Wilson B, Moffat N, eds. *Clinical management of memory problems*. London: Croom Helm, 1984.

32. Prins RS, Schoonen R, Vermeulen J. Efficacy of two different types of speech therapy for aphasic stroke patients. *Appl Psycholing* 1989;**10**:85–123.

33. Schoonen R. The internal validity of efficacy studies: design and statistical power in studies of language therapy for aphasics. *Brain Lang* 1991;**41**:446–64.

34. Aldenkamp AP, Vermeulen J. Neuropsychological rehabilitation of memory function in epilepsy. *J Neuropsychol Rehab* 1992;**1**:199–214.

35. Smith WL, ed. *Drugs and cerebral function*. Springfield, IL: Charles C Thomas, 1970.

36. Dunn A. Neurochemistry of learning and memory: an evaluation of recent data. *Annu Rev Psychol* 1980;**31**:343–90.

37. Ashton H. *Brain Systems, disorders and psychotropic drugs*. Oxford University Press, 1987, Oxford/New York.

38. Bradley C. The behavior of children receiving benzedrine. *Am J Orthopsychiatry*. 1937;**94**:577–85.

39. Bender L, Cottington F. The use of amphetamine sulfate (benzedrine) in child psychiatry. *Am J Psychiatry* 1942;**99**:116–21.

40. Mondadori C. Pharmacological modulation of memory: trends and problems. *Acta Neurol Scand* 1981;**64**(Suppl 89):129–40.

41. Squire LR, Davis HP. The pharmacology of memory: a neurobiological perspective. *Annu Rev Pharmaco Toxicol* 1981;**21**:323–56.

42. Drachman DA. Central cholinergic system and memory. In: Lipton MA, DiMascio A, Killam KF, eds. *Psychopharmacology: a generation of progress*. New York: Raven Press, 1978: 651–62.

43. Dam M. Long-term evaluation of vigabatrin (Gamma Vinyl GABA) in epilepsy. *Epilepsia* 1989;**30**(Suppl 3):S26–31.

44. Kovacs GL, Bohus BE, Versteeg DHG, Telegdy G, De Wied D. Neurohypophyseal hormones and memory. In: H Yoshida, Hagihara Y, Ebashi S, eds. *Advances in phamacology and therapeutics II*. Vol. I, *CNS Parmacology-Neuropeptides*. Oxford: Pergamon Press, 1982:175–87.

45. De Wied D. The importance of vasopressin in memory. *Trends Neurosci* 1984;**7**:63–4.

46. Saletu B, Grünberger J. The hypoxia model in human psychopharmacology: neurophysiological and psychometric studies with aniracetam. *Human Neurobiol* 1984;**3**:171–81.

47. Saletu B, Grünberger J. Memory Dysfunction and vigilance: neurophysiological and psychopharmacological aspects. *Ann NY Acad Sci* 1985;**444**:406–27.

48. Lagergren K, Levander S. A double-blind study on the effects of piracetam (1–acetamide-2–pyrrolidine) upon perceptual and psychomotor performance at varied heart rates in patients treated with artificial pacemakers. *J Pharmacol* 1974;**5**:55–60.

49. Giurgea C. Piracetam: nootropic pharmacology of neurointegrative activity. In: Essman WB, Vazelli L, eds. *Current developments in psychopharmacology*. Vol. 3. New York: Spectrum Publications, 1976:223–73.

50. Giurgea C. Experimental animal models relevant to learning disabilities. *Child Health Dev* 1987;**5**:1–8.

51. Giurgea, Salama CM. Nootropic drugs. *Prog Neuro-Psychopharmacol* 1977;**1**:235–47.

52. Giaquinto S, Nolfe G, Vitali S. EEG-changes induced by oxiracetam on diazepam medicated volunteers. *Clin Neuropharmacol* 1986;**9**: (Suppl):79–84.

53. Wolkowitz OW, Tinklenberg JR, Weingartner H. A psychopharmacological perspective of cognitive functions. *Neuropsychobiology* 1985; **14**:88–96.

54. Volavka J, Simeon J, Simeon S, Cho D, Reker D. Effect of piracetam on EEG spectra of boys with learning disorders. *Psychopharmacology* 1981;**72**:185–8.

55. Dimond SJ, Brouwers EYM. Increase in the power of human memory in normal man through the use of drugs. *Psychopharmacology* 1976;**49**:307–9.

56. Wilsher C, Atkins G, Manfield P. Piracetam as an aid to learning in dyslexia. *Psychopharmacology* 1979;**65**:107–9.

57. Simeon J, Waters B, Resnick M. Effects of piracetam in children with learning disorders. *Psychopharmacol Bull* 1980;**16**:65–7.

58. Connors CK. The use of stimulant drugs in enhancing performance and learning. In: WL Smith, ed. *Drugs and cerebral function*. Springfield, IL: Charles C Thomas, 1970:85–98.

59. Conners CK, Blouin AG, Winglee BS, et al. Piracetam and event-related potentials in dyslexic children. *Psychopharmacol Bull* 1984; **20**:667–73.

60. Conners CK, Reader MJ. The effects of piracetam on reading achievement and visual event-related potentials in dyslexic children. *Child Health Dev* 1987;**5**:75–90.

61. Helfgott E, Rudel RG, Krieger J. Effect of piracetam on the single word and prose reading of dyslexic children. *Psychopharmacol Bull* 1984;**20**:688–90.

62. Helfgott E, Rudel RG, Koplewicz H, Krieger J. Effect of piracetam on reading test performance of dyslexic children. *Child Health Dev* 1987;**5**:110–22.

63. Levi G, Sechi E. A study of piracetam in the pharmacological treatment of learning disabilities. *Child Health Dev* 1987;**5**:129–39.

64. Sara SJ. Memory retrieval deficits: alleviation by etiracetam, a nootropic drug. *Psychopharmacology* 1980;**68**:235–41.

65. Guazelli M, Rocca R, Lattanzi L, et al. Effects of oxiracetam on electroencephalogram at rest in healthy young subjects. *Therap Res* 1987;**41**:234–43.

66. Banfi S, Dorigotti L. Experimental behavioral studies with oxiracetam on different types of

chronic cerebral impairment. *Clin Neuro-pharmacol* 1986;**9**(Suppl):519–26.

67. Villardita C, Parini J, Grioli S. Clinical and neuropsychological study with oxiracetam versus placebo in patients with mild to moderate dementia. *J Neurol Transm* 1987;**24** (Suppl):293–8.

68. Mangoni A, Perin C, Smirne S. A double-blind, placebo-controlled study with oxiracetam in demented patients administered the Luria–Nebraska Neuropsychological Battery. *Drug Dev Res* 1988;**14**:217–22.

69. Maina G, Fiori L, Torta R, et al. Oxiracetam in the treatment of primary degenerative and multi-infarct dementia: a double-blind, placebo-controlled study. *Neuropsychobiology* 1989;**21**:141–5.

70. Aldenkamp AP, van Wieringen A, Alpherts WCJ, et al. Double-blind placebo-controlled, neuropsychological and neurophysiological investigations with oxiracetam (CGP 21690e) in memory-impaired patients with epilepsy. *Neuropsychobiology* 1991;**46**:41–52.

71. Wauquier A, Clincke G, Ashton D, De Ryck M, Fransen J, van Clemen G. R 58 735: a new antihypoxic drug with anticonvulsant properties and possible effects on cognitive functions. *Drug Dev Res* 1986;**8**:373–80.

72. Clincke GHC, Tritsman L, Idzikowski C, Amery WK, Janssen PAJ. The effect of R 58 735 (Sabeluzole) on memory functions in healthy elderly volunteers. *Psychopharmacology* 1988;**94**:52–7.

73. Clincke GHC, Tritsman L. Sabeluzole (R 58 735) increases consistent retrieval during serial learning and relearning of nonsense syllables. *Psychopharmacology* 1988;**96**:309–10.

74. Tritsman L, Clincke G, Amery WK. The effect of sabeluzole (R 58 735) on memory retrieval functions. *Psychopharmacology* 1988;**94**:527–31.

75. Aldenkamp AP, Overweg J, Smakman J, et al. Effect of sabeluzole (R58 735) on memory functions in patients with epilepsy. *Neuropsychobiology* 1995;**32**:37–44.

76. Baddeley AD. Domains of recollection. *Psychol Rev* 1982;**6**:708–29.

77. Wagenaar WA. My memory. A study of autobiographical memory over six years. *Cogn Psychol* 1986;**18**:225–52.

78. Linton M. Memory for real world events. In: Norman DA, Rumelhart DE and the LNR Research Group. *Explorations in cognition*. San Francisco: Freeman, 1975.

79. Gasparrinini B, Satz P. A treatment of memory problems in left hemisphere CVA patients. *J Clin Neuropsychol* 1979;**2**:137–50.

23

The ten most common treatment errors in epilepsy

Dieter Schmidt

Introduction

Two recent surveys on epilepsy care in Europe indicated that as many as 51 per cent and 53 per cent of patients respectively, had uncontrolled seizures during the last year.[1,2] In addition, 20 per cent had more than one seizure per month.[1] However, only 7.3 per cent of patients were referred to specialized epilepsy units by neurologists.[2] Errors in the treatment of epilepsy could be responsible, at least in part, for the failure to achieve complete seizure control in more patients. It is difficult to be certain, however, since the incidence and the type of treatment errors in the case of patients with epilepsy are unknown. In an effort to identify the most common errors in the treatment of epilepsy, a panel of epilepsy experts was asked to rank the five most common errors they themselves had made and those they had observed in the cases of patients referred. The error deemed most common by each expert received 5 points, followed by 4 points for the second most common error; errors ranked 3, 4 and 5 received 3, 2 and 1 point, respectively. Eight of the nine German-speaking clinical epileptologists serving in commissions of the International League against Epilepsy in 1996 returned the questionnaire and one did not reply. The experts noted a total of 69 errors receiving a total of 221 points. The 10 most common consolidated errors (Figure 23.1) will be discussed briefly in this chapter.

All 69 answers from the eight experts were pooled and the number of points each error received is given in parentheses (see text).

1. Failure to ensure the maximum tolerated dose in uncontrolled epilepsy (26)
2. Adding a second drug before the original one has failed (21)
3. Delayed referral to specialized epilepsy units (9)
4. Misdiagnosis of frontal lobe seizures as non-epileptic psychogenic seizures (9)
5. Failure to diagnose the epilepsy syndrome (8)
6. Suboptimal use of new AEDs (8)
7. Unnecessarily high dosages of AEDs (8)
8. Failure to choose the optimum drug for seizure type (8)
9. Premature discontinuation of anticonvulsants in seizure-free patients (7)
10. Failure to persistently pursue treatment goals (7)

Figure 23.1
The top ten errors in the treatment of epilepsy.

Error no. 1: Failure to ensure the maximum tolerated dose in uncontrolled epilepsy

In the view of the experts, failure to use the maximum tolerated dose in patients still having disabling seizures is the most common error in the treatment of epilepsy. Controlled trials and clinical practice have demonstrated a dose–response relationship for standard antiepileptic drugs (AEDs), e.g. valproate,[3] and most new AEDs, e.g. oxcarbazepine, topiramate[4] and vigabatrin.[5] For some of the newer drugs, such as lamotrigine and gabapentin, the maximum tolerated dose needs to be determined in phase IV trials and in clinical practice. There is no doubt that failure to reach the maximum tolerated dose curbs the therapeutic potential of AED treatment. In one study, 11 of 35 patients referred for uncontrolled partial seizures became seizure-free by taking a higher dose of the anticonvulsant they had presented with at the clinic.[6] The patient's drug compliance should be reviewed as a possible cause for failure to reach the effective dose. However, if the maximum tolerated dose is shown not to provide complete control—and this is unfortunately not uncommon in patients with chronic refractory epilepsy—then the dosage should be slowly reduced to avoid unnecessary overtreatment (see Chapter 17).

Clinical guidelines

1. Ensure that the patient is treated with the appropriate first-line anticonvulsant for that patient's specific seizure type and epilepsy syndrome.
2. In patients still having seizures, review patient compliance.
3. Verify that the maximum tolerated dose has been prescribed and taken as prescribed. Do not rely on serum concentrations for the determination of maximum tolerated dose; instead, titrate stepwise until initial clinical adverse effects appear.
4. In case the patient does not respond satisfactorily to the maximum tolerated dose,

the dosage should be reduced to prevent chronic toxicity, and a second drug should then be introduced.

Error no. 2: Adding a second drug before the original one has failed

Earlier claims that adding a second drug at low dosage to a first drug would lead to higher efficacy and, at the same time, lower the toxicity, have not been confirmed.[7] In fact, failure to ensure the maximum tolerated dose of the first drug before adding another one makes it very difficult to disentangle the effects of either drug. Yet, a number of physicians insist that adding a drop of this or one tablet of that anticonvulsant will do the trick. However, in most cases, the same effect would probably have been possible if the first drug had been given at a higher dose. The evidence that two drugs are more effective than one drug in refractory epilepsy is surprisingly weak. The evidence is limited to a small series of patients with refractory absence seizures in whom the combination of valproate and ethosuximide was more effective than either drug alone.[8] In a larger series of 50 patients with refractory partial epilepsy treated with phenytoin and carbamazepine, the combination of both drugs was more effective than either drug alone.[9] This is of interest because conventional wisdom suggests combinations of drugs with different mechanisms of action, whereas phenytoin and carbamazepine both appear to work via voltage-dependent sodium channel blockade. In summary, the current experimental and clinical evidence supports the use of polytherapy only in failures of adequate monotherapy.[10]

Clinical guidelines

1. If the first drug is not effective at the maximum tolerated dose, an alternative drug should be added slowly. In patients with intolerable side effects from the original drug, the dose of the original drug can often be reduced without an unacceptable increase in seizure frequency.
2. If the patient's seizures have responded favorably to the addition of the second drug, withdrawal of the first drug is an option. The patient may benefit from the second drug alone (alternative monotherapy). However, if adding the second drug has not been effective, the first drug should be replaced by an alternative drug.

Error no. 3: Delayed referral to specialized epilepsy units

In a recent survey, < 10 per cent of patients with refractory epilepsy were referred to specialized epilepsy units.[2] Unfortunately, many patients referred to epilepsy units have a history of many years of uncontrolled seizures and the psychosocial problems associated with intractable epilepsy. About 20 per cent of those presenting in specialized units with a history of refractory epilepsy turn out to have non-epileptic seizures. Failure to supply the results of previous investigations may result in unnecessarily repeated laboratory tests and other examinations. Furthermore, the reverse flow of information back to the referring physician is often seen as unsatisfactory, and may disrupt continuous epilepsy care.

Clinical guidelines

1. Any patient with uncontrolled and disabling seizures or with intolerable adverse effects despite adequate drug treatment should be evaluated within 1 year in a specialized epilepsy unit.
2. Surgical options, including vagal nerve stimulation, should be assessed in any patient with refractory and disabling seizures.
3. Any patient with psychological, psychiatric, or social problems should be evaluated in due course by a multidisciplinary team in an epilepsy unit.

Error no. 4: Misdiagnosis of frontal lobe epilepsy as non-epileptic psychogenic seizures

In the past, a number of patients with frontal lobe seizures, specifically those with complex partial seizures, were mistakenly diagnosed as having non-epileptic psychogenic seizures and vice versa. Failure to diagnose psychogenic seizures may result in inappropriate anticonvulsant therapy and may deny patients the appropriate psychological care and antidepressant treatment. Conversely, patients with frontal lobe epilepsy mistaken for psychogenic disorders are denied adequate anticonvulsant and surgical care. The difficulties of distinguishing between frontal lobe seizures, psychogenic seizures, and other non-epileptic seizures have been well described.[11]

Clinical guidelines

1. When in doubt, refer any patient with an uncertain seizure type to a specialized epilepsy unit for diagnostic re-evaluation. Video-EEG monitoring may help in patients with sufficient seizure frequency.
2. Consider the diagnosis of psychogenic seizures if standard anticonvulsants fail to control the seizures.

3. Allow for the uncommon co-existence of both epileptic and non-epileptic seizures in the same patient.
4. Any patient diagnosed with psychogenic seizures should receive a full neurological examination, including magnetic resonance imaging (MRI).

Error no. 5: Failure to diagnose the epilepsy syndrome

An international classification of epileptic syndromes, approved by the International League Against Epilepsy, appeared in 1989.[12] An epileptic syndrome is defined as an epileptic disorder characterized by a cluster of signs and symptoms occurring together. The advantages of a syndromic diagnosis, as opposed to a mere seizure diagnosis, are that it provides much more information—e.g. about age of onset, etiology, seizure type(s), seizure-provoking factors, chronicity, prognosis and choice of treatment. As many of the epilepsy syndromes are age-related, the age at onset of seizures may provide a clue to the correct syndrome diagnosis. Finally, a syndromic diagnosis may offer guidance on the optimum medical treatment—the choice of the anticonvulsant may not only depend on the type of seizures, but also on the syndrome. In his review, Gram gave two examples.[13] In children with Rolandic epilepsy, the response to AEDs is good, quite in contrast to symptomatic frontal lobe seizures syndrome, and the seizures spontaneously remit by age 16. In addition, parents may defer starting drug treatment in cases with mild and infrequent seizures altogether. Furthermore, MRI is not necessary in this genetic syndrome, again in distinction to the syndromes of symptomatic frontal lobe epilepsy. Another example is juvenile myoclonic epilepsy (JME). This is an idiopathic generalized epilepsy with bilateral synchronous generalized spike–wave discharges and onset during adolescence. The common precipitation of seizures in this syndrome requires careful counselling in order to avoid specific and unspecific precipitating factors and to select the right choice of anticonvulsant, e.g. valproate. Failure to recognize the syndrome may result in the inappropriate choice of anticonvulsants such as phenytoin, carbamazepine, vigabatrin, tiagabine, or gabapentin—which will not only be ineffective against the myoclonic and absence seizures, but may even exacerbate them.[14]

Clinical guidelines

1. Identify not only the seizure type or types of patient, but also diagnose the epilepsy syndrome before ordering neuroimaging. In positively identified epilepsy syndromes of genetic (idiopathic) etiology, neuroimaging is not essential.
2. Be sure to identify the epilepsy syndrome before starting drug treatment. In some syndromes, such as Rolandic epilepsy or JME with mild and infrequent myoclonic seizures alone, drug treatment may not be necessary. Instead, counseling the patient with JME about the importance of avoiding seizure precipitants may be sufficient for seizure control. Make sure you know the syndrome diagnosis before discussing the prognosis of the epilepsy.

Error no. 6: Suboptimal use of new anticonvulsants

Considering that a host of new anticonvulsants has been introduced in recent years and that new drugs continue to be introduced into the market, it is not surprising that the optimal use of new anticonvulsants may be problematic. More specifically, failure to recognize the specific indication or, in other words, the limitations of the new drugs, may result in unsuccessful therapy. For example, the selective GABA-ergic compounds gabapentin, tiagabine, and vigabatrin are of no use for the treatment of generalized absence or myoclonic seizures. In fact, seizure exacerbation, or in the case of tiagabine, non-convulsive status epilepticus, has been reported in some patients.[15] In addition, the adverse effect profile differs and that will again limit the use of these drugs for some patients. Patients with a history of kidney stones would be well advised to avoid topiramate, which produces kidney stones in some patients. Patients with acute hematological disorders or acute liver disease should not receive felbamate, which may cause aplastic anemia and acute hepatic failure. Also, in those receiving valproate, lamotrigine should be titrated very slowly because valproate acutely inhibits the metabolism of lamotrigine. Likewise, the dosage of standard anticonvulsants should be reduced by 25 per cent when felbamate is added, because felbamate inhibits, in a dose-dependent fashion, the metabolism of valproate, phenytoin and carbamazepine-epoxide. Although controlled trials have shown that the new anticonvulsants (e.g. lamotrigine, oxcarbazepine and gabapentin) are effective for partial seizures, most experts advise against using them as first-line treatment at this time, simply because they are more costly, and advocate their use when the patient does not tolerate first-line drugs such as valproate and carbamazepine. However, some of the new drugs have advantages that would favor their use in early epilepsy, e.g. fewer sedative side effects—which is especially valuable in the treatment of the elderly (e.g. gabapentin and lamotrigine)—and lack of drug–drug interaction—which is very welcomed in the treatment of patients who need to take other drugs for medical disorders or contraception (e.g. gabapentin, lamotrigine).

Clinical guidelines

1. Any patient with uncontrolled seizures or adverse side effects from treatment with standard anticonvulsants should be assessed for possible use of newer anticonvulsants. More specifically, gabapentin and lamotrigine may have fewer sedative side effects, while vigabatrin or topiramate may be more effective for seizure control in patients with intractable epilepsy. Do not expect and promise too much in terms of added seizure control. No more than 10 per cent, at most, of the patients with intractable epilepsy will become seizure-free.[16] It should be noted that a similar percentage was seen when divalproex was tested as add-on therapy.[17]

2. Make sure that you select one or two new drugs of your choice, e.g. one for partial seizures and one broadly effective for partial, generalized absence and myoclonic seizures. Become familiar with the optimum use of these compounds, learn about their characteristic side effects, and common drug–drug interactions.

3. Make sure that you note anything unusual in patients receiving new drugs—new adverse reactions, although rare, may emerge with more widespread use.

Error no. 7: Unnecessarily high dosages of AEDs

Overtreatment with unnecessarily high dosages of AEDs may, in principle, occur at the start of treatment in previously untreated patients with early epilepsy, and perhaps more often, in partially responsive patients with chronic epilepsy receiving further dose increments (Chapter 17).

Ideally, each patient with early epilepsy should be treated with the lowest effective dose of an anticonvulsant at the onset of treatment; but there are two problems. The lowest effective dose (which is more effective than placebo) has not been determined for most AEDs, and physicians eager to suppress seizures as soon as possible may choose a higher-than-necessary dose rather than risk another seizure. In fact, many patients are overtreated because they would have responded to a lower dose. A recent study of 500 mg valproate for initial treatment of patients with newly diagnosed JME showed that this dose was sufficient for complete seizure control in patients,[18] suggesting that the usually recommended starting dose of anticonvulsants may be higher than is necessary for some patients. However, the impact and the incidence of overtreatment is unknown. In addition, it has been shown that patients with tonic–clonic seizures alone require lower serum concentrations (and lower effective doses) for treatment than patients with simple and partial seizures.[19]

In patients continuing to have seizures, increasing the dosage of the AED may be beneficial, as discussed before. In one report, 31 per cent of patients with previously uncontrolled partial seizures became seizure-free when the dosage of the drug they presented with in an epilepsy clinic was increased.[6] Unfortunately, as many as two thirds of the patients with uncontrolled partial seizures do not benefit from treatment with the maximum tolerated dose. In fact, seizure frequencies in some patients may even increase with the further dose increments, as discussed recently in a review on the exacerbation of seizures induced by AEDs.[20] The maximum tolerated dose should be maintained only in those who show a meaningful reduction in seizure frequency or intensity at the highest tolerated dose. In all other cases, the dose should be reduced to the previous lower dosage that provided a similar benefit. Leaving the patient on the maximum tolerated dose despite its failure to benefit the patient is a common cause of overtreatment and of chronic AED toxicity. In fact, some patients may even have fewer seizures when the dose is reduced.[21]

Clinical guidelines

1. Any patient who does not clearly benefit from the maximum tolerable dose should undergo a slow dose reduction. This may offer fewer side effects without compromising the level of seizure control.
2. Any patient with uncontrolled seizures on more than one anticonvulsant should be assessed for slow transfer to monotherapy.
3. Any patient who requires more than the maximum tolerated dose of an anticonvulsant for seizure control should be referred for therapeutic evaluation of surgical options, including vagal nerve stimulation.

Error no. 8: Failure to choose the correct drug for the seizure type

Errors in the choice of drugs due to misdiagnosis of seizure type are common. Failure to recognize generalized absence seizures and mistake them for short complex partial seizures and treat them (unsuccessfully) with phenytoin or carbamazepine is not rare. The second most common error is to treat patients with JME (unsuccessfully) with carbamazepine, phenytoin, or the newer selective GABA-ergic drugs—gabapentin, tiagabine and vigabatrin—because the seizures are mistaken for clonic seizures of partial origin. It is not always well appreciated that in some patients with JME the generalized myoclonic seizures may appear to occur on one side only. Bilateral frontal spike waves are not uncommon and may be mistaken for bilateral synchrony. Misdiagnosis of non-epileptic seizures and subsequent mistreatment with anticonvulsants has been discussed above. Treating patients with tonic–clonic seizures with ethosuximide is a thing of the past, given the infrequent use of ethosuximide today.

Clinical guidelines

1. Any patient whose seizures do not respond to an appropriate dose of a first-line anticonvulsant should be diagnostically re-evaluated for three reasons:
   (i) the seizure diagnosis may be incorrect and the wrong anticonvulsant may have been chosen;
   (ii) to review the diagnosis of the epilepsy syndrome;
   (iii) to determine whether the patient has epilepsy or a non-epileptic seizure syndrome.
2. If it is unclear whether the patient has partial seizures or generalized absence or myoclonic seizures, be sure to choose a broadly acting anticonvulsant such as valproate, clobazam, lamotrigine, or topiramate.
3. Some patients may have seizures that are difficult to classify as either partial or generalized; in these cases, use a broadly effective anticonvulsant such as valproate or lamotrigine.

Error no. 9: Premature discontinuation of anticonvulsants in patients thought to be in remission

Finding the optimum time to recommend discontinuation of anticonvulsants in patients who have been seizure-free for a while is a complex task that needs to reconcile two opposing principles of drug treatment. Some patients are very eager to withdraw their medication after a few months of entering remission, while others hang on to their treatment and diagnosis and would prefer to remain on the medication forever, if possible. Both scenarios are unsatisfactory. Premature

The global risk of relapse within 2 years following discontinuation is ~ 30 per cent. After assessing the risks and benefits of withdrawal to the patient and others, discontinuation may be considered by the physician and informed patient or parent/guardian if the patient meets the following profile. However, it should be emphasized that successful discontinuation may be possible in patients not meeting the complete profile, while a patient not showing any of the factors would be advised not to discontinue the medication.

- normal neurological examination and normal IQ
- normal EEG prior to withdrawal
- seizure-free for 2–5 years or longer
- single type of seizure
- juvenile myoclonic epilepsy with myoclonic seizures alone

Figure 23.2
Practical guide as to when to withdraw antiepileptic drugs.[7]

withdrawal is clearly more common, despite the evidence from a landmark study on withdrawal that the longer the duration of remission, the lower the rate of relapse.[22]

Clinical guidelines

1. Any patient entering remission should be counseled on the risk factors for relapse (Figure 23.2) and the safeguards to prevent a relapse, including a 1-year period of remission as a minimum.
2. Two-year remission is recommended for all patients who did not become seizure-free easily, i.e. with a low-to-medium dosage of the initial anticonvulsant. A remission of 3 years or longer is recommended for all patients with any risk factors for relapse.
3. Never urge an unwilling patient in remission to discontinue the medication. The relapse will be blamed on you. Inform the patient to specifically avoid seizure precipitation once the drug is discontinued, and to seek help in case of relapse.

Error no. 10: Failure to relentlessly pursue treatment goals

Understandably, patients and relatives of patients with chronic intractable epilepsy may lose confidence in the effectiveness of treatment and the physician to control seizures and the associated problems. After failures of past treatment efforts, physicians and patients may lose the motivation to control the seizures aggressively with the maximum tolerated dose and to pursue surgical options in failures of drug treatment. Patients and physicians may become complacent and resigned. This is unfortunate, because new drugs are continuously coming on the market and the patient may be one of the few that will respond miraculously to one of the drugs. In addition, surgical outcomes are improving because of better surgical and neuroimaging techniques. New non-pharmacological options have become available, such as vagal nerve stimulation, which is free of significant side effects and offers partial relief from frequent seizures.

Clinical guidelines

1. The outcome of treatment should be reviewed annually and the patient should be informed about new developments in the field.
2. Avoid complacency. Pursue treatment goals relentlessly.
3. A second opinion should be sought if the treatment is not considered to be successful by either the patient or the physician.

References

1. Hart YM, Shorvon SD. The nature of epilepsy in the general population. I. Characteristics of patients receiving medication for epilepsy. *Epilepsy Res* 1995;**21**:43–50.
2. Pfäfflin M, May TW, Stefan H, Adelmeier U. Prävalenz, Behandlung und soziale Aspekte von Epilepsien in Deutschland. Erste Ergebnisse einer epidemiologischem Querschnittstudie (EPIDEG-Studie). *Epilepsieblätter* 1997;**10**:15–20.
3. Beydoun A, Uthman BM, Sackellares JC. Gabapentin: pharmacokinetics, efficacy, and safety. *Clin Neuropharmacol* 1995;**18**:469–81.

4. Faught E, Wilder BJ, Ramsay RE, et al. Topiramate placebo-controlled dose ranging trial in refractory partial epilepsy using 200-, 400-, and 600-mg daily dosages. Topiramate YD Study Group. *Neurology* 1996;**46**:1684–90.

5. French JA, Mosier M, Walker S, et al. A double-blind, placebo-controlled study of vigabatrin three g/day in patients with uncontrolled complex partial seizures. *Neurology* 1996;**46**:54–61.

6. Schmidt D. Single drug therapy for intractable epilepsy. *J Neurol* 1983;**229**:221–6.

7. Schmidt D, Gram L. Monotherapy versus polytherapy in epilepsy: a reappraisal. *CNS Drug* 1995;**3**:194–208.

8. Rowan AJ, Meijer JWA, de Beer-Pawlikowski N, van der Geest P. Valproate–ethosuximide combination therapy for refractory absence seizures. *Arch Neurol* 1983;**40**:797–802.

9. Hakkarainen H. Carbamazepine vs diphenylhydantoin vs their combination in adult epilepsy. *Neurology* 1980;**30**:354.

10. Schmidt D. Modern management of epilepsy: rational polytherapy. *Baillière's Clin Neurol* 1996;**5**:757–63.

11. Schmidt D, Lempert Th. Differential diagnosis in adults. In: Dam M, Gram L, eds. *Comprehensive epileptology*. New York: Raven Press, 1991:449–72.

12. Commission on Classification and Terminology of the International League against Epilepsy. Proposal for revised classification of epilepsies and epileptic syndromes. *Epilepsia* 1989;**30**:389–99.

13. Gram L. Classification of seizures and syndromes. *Lancet* Review Epilepsy, 1990;**336**:161–3.

14. Schmidt D. Response to antiepileptic drugs, and the rate of relapse after discontinuation of drug treatment in patients with juvenile myoclonic epilepsy, 1999; in press.

15. Steinhoff BJ, Freudenthaler N, Paulus W. The influence of established and new antiepileptic drugs on visual perception. I. A placebo-controlled, double-blind, single-dose study in healthy volunteers. *Epilepsy Res* 1997;**29**:35–47.

16. Walker MC, Sander JWAS. The impact of new antiepileptic drugs on the prognosis of epilepsy. Seizure freedom should be the ultimate goal. *Neurology* 1996;**46**:912–14.

17. Willmore LJ, Shu V, Wallin B, the M88-194 Study Group. Efficacy and safety of add-on divalproex sodium in the treatment of complex partial seizures. *Neurology* 1996;**46**:49–53.

18. De Toffel B, Autret A. Traitement de l'epilepsie myoclonique juvenile par les faibles doses de valproate de sodium. *Rev Neurol (Paris)* 1996;**152**:708–10.

19. Schmidt D, Haenel D. Therapeutic plasma levels of phenytoin, phenobarbital and carbamazepine: individual variation in relation to seizure frequency and type. *Neurology* 1984;**34**:1252–5.

20. Perucca E, Gram L, Avanzini G, Dulac O. Antiepileptic drugs as a cause of worsening seizures. *Epilepsia* 1998;**39**:5–17.

21. Schmidt D. Reduction of two-drug therapy in intractable epilepsy. *Epilepsia* 1983;**24**:368–76.

22. Medical Research Council Antiepileptic Drug Withdrawal Study Group. Randomised study of antiepileptic drug withdrawal in patients in remission. *Lancet* 1991;**337**:1175–80.

VIII

CHILDHOOD EPILEPSY

24

The ketogenic diet revisited

*John M Freeman, Eileen PG Vining, Jane C Casey and
Jane R McGrogan*

Preface

Mrs Smith comes to your office with Robby, her 4-year-old son. You have been treating Robby's difficult-to-control seizures for >1 year. She says, 'This medicine is not working either, doctor. I saw something about a diet for epilepsy on the evening news last week and I checked it out on the Internet. There's lots of stuff out there about a ketogenic diet. I wanted to ask what you thought of it'.

You reply:

- 'I know a lot about the diet and it will be very difficult for you and even worse for Robby. Not even someone with Robby's problems should be made to give up cookies and ice-cream. What will he do in daycare when the others have a snack? I don't recommend it.'
- 'I know the diet has received a lot of publicity lately, but it is only used as a very last resort, and we haven't exhausted all of our options yet. There are three new anticonvulsants which have been approved in the last year or so. I think we should try them first. There are also two medications which can be obtained from outside the US. If they don't work, and nothing else has become available, then we can always try the diet.'
- 'The last time I tried the diet the child had terrible cramps and nausea from all the

MCT oil. I think that was 8 years ago. If it were any good we wouldn't be developing all these new medications. Don't believe all those claims you see on the Internet.'
- 'Yuck!! What normal child would eat that stuff? Can you really believe that a high-fat diet is good for you? You've read about avoiding fats; what can those "kooks" be thinking of? I don't know anyone who is using that diet with any success. Those doctors at Johns Hopkins are crazy.'

Hopefully, none of these replies will be your response. The purpose of this chapter is to acquaint you, or reacquaint you, with the ketogenic diet, with its current role in the treatment of children with difficult-to-control epilepsy, and to make you aware of the potential role of the diet for adults.

Introduction

The ketogenic diet is a high-fat diet that was successfully utilized during the 1920s and 1930s to control seizures. After the discovery of diphenylhydantoin (Dilantin) in 1938, the diet was not often used. However, there has been a recent resurgence of interest in the diet as a treatment for children with difficult-to-control seizures,[1,2] coupled with continued scepticism about both its efficacy and its tolerability. This chapter will attempt to place the

Table 24.1
Results of studies of the effectiveness of the ketogenic diet: 1925–92.

Study	Year	Number of patients	>90 per cent control	>50 per cent control	No control
Peterman	1925	37	60	35	5
Helmholz	1927	91	31	23	46
Livingston	1954	300	43	34	22
Hopkins	1970	34	29	12	...
Kinsman	1992	58	29	38	33
Huttenlocher MCT	1971	12	...	50	...

current use of the ketogenic diet in its proper perspective.

What is the ketogenic diet?

The 'classic' ketogenic diet is a high-fat, moderate protein, low-carbohydrate diet designed to mimic the biochemical changes associated with prolonged starvation, which had been reported to produce a dramatic decrease in uncontrollable seizures.[1,3] Starvation forces the body to burn stored fat for energy. When there are insufficient carbohydrates available, fat is incompletely metabolized, resulting in residual ketones. The ketogenic diet forces the body to first burn its own stored fats for energy, and then provides exogenous fat as the primary energy source. As the diet provides minimal carbohydrate, the fats are incompletely metabolized and ketone bodies result.[3] The diet provides adequate protein for growth.

Is the ketogenic diet effective in treating seizures?

Yes.[2] Table 24.1 shows the reported outcomes of studies of the ketogenic diet carried out over many decades.[3] The study by Huttenlocher is of the medium-chain triglyceride (MCT) diet. Although none of these studies were prospective, blinded or controlled, they reported that 41–95 per cent of children placed on the diet at different institutions, over multiple decades, achieved better than 50 per cent control of their seizures. A recent multi-centre study has demonstrated its efficacy in a wide range of settings.[4] A recent prospective study[5] of 150 consecutive children with difficult-to-control seizures confirms these results.

In the latter study,[5] the average age of the children at the time of initiating the diet was 5.3 years and the children averaged 410 seizures, of various types, per month prior to initiating the diet. The percentage of children remaining on the diet at each time period after initiating the diet, and their degree of seizure control are shown in Table 24.2.

In all, 83 per cent of the 150 children initiating the diet remained on the diet for 3 months and 71 per cent for 6 months; 55 per cent were still on the diet 1 year after starting. One year after initiating the diet, 11 of the original 150 children (7 per cent) were seizure-free and 30 additional children (20 per cent) had a 90 per cent or greater decrease in seizures. (These included children who suffered

Table 24.2

Outcomes of the ketogenic diet at varying times after the diet was initiated in 150 children.[5]

Seizure control and diet status	Number (%) after		
	3 months	*6 months*	*12 months*
Seizure free	4 (3)	5 (3)	11 (7)
>90 per cent	46 (31)	43 (29)	30 (20)
50–90 per cent	39 (26)	29 (19)	34 (23)
<50 per cent	36 (24)	29 (19)	8 (5)
Continued the diet	125 (83)	106 (71)	83 (55)

only one seizure with illness during the month prior to the assessment.) An additional 34 children (23 per cent) had a 50–90 per cent decrease in seizures. Thus, 75 of the original 150 children (50 per cent) had achieved a better than 50 per cent decrease in their seizures. Forty-one of the 150 children (27 per cent) had achieved better than a 90 per cent decrease in their seizure frequency at 12 months. Only eight children (5 per cent) , with less than a 50 per cent decrease in seizures remained on the diet. The remainder had discontinued the diet, most of them after a trial of 3 months or longer.

There were no statistically significant differences in seizure control based on age, sex, or seizure type. Even teenaged children tolerated the diet—if it was effective—but were somewhat more likely to discontinue the diet if it did not result in a substantial decrease in seizure frequency.

Efficacy and tolerability of the diet were closely inter-related in this study. If the diet was effective in decreasing the seizure frequency by at least 50 per cent, most children remained on the diet. Only a minority (10 per cent) of the children remaining on the diet at 1 year had less than a 50 per cent decrease in seizure frequency.

Who do you start on the diet, and at what point?

The diet has been used for children, usually >2 years of age and less than teen age. The reason for those old boundaries is unclear. We have successfully utilized the diet in children <6 months of age as well as in motivated older adolescents. The efficacy and tolerability of the diet in adults are not yet established.

We have restricted our use of the diet predominantly to children with refractory seizures who have failed to respond to multiple anticonvulsants. As the diet is more effective in controlling seizures than most of the newer anticonvulsants, it is unclear why children 'must have failed all anticonvulsants' prior to using the diet. Because the diet requires a substantial commitment from the child and the family, we would not use the diet as the initial therapy. Medication is far easier and is usually effective. As children whose seizures have failed to improve with two anticonvulsants have less than a 15 per cent chance of having their seizures controlled with other medications, we often recommend the use of the diet when two medications have been unsuccessful. While the proper role of the diet in the management of children with seizures

- For 1–2 days before fasting the family is instructed to decrease their child's intake of carbohydrates and starches. Fasting is begun after dinner, the evening before admission. Whenever possible, carbohydrate-free anticonvulsant medications should be used.
- Day 1: The child is admitted to the hospital. Fluids (caffeine-free and carbohydrate-free) are limited to 60–75 ml/kg of body weight with an upper limit of 1200 ml/day. Blood glucose is measured by Dextrostix every 6 h unless the level falls below 40 mg/100 ml in which case it is measured every 2 h. Symptoms simulating hypoglycemia warrant an immediate blood glucose test. Symptoms, or glucose levels below 25 mg/100 ml, warrant giving 30 ml of orange juice and measuring the blood glucose level again. Symptomatic hypoglycemia during this fasting is uncommon, even in small children.
- Day 2: Lack of energy and lethargy are common during the second 24 h of fasting. Hunger is uncommon. On the evening of the second day, after 48 h of fasting, one third of the calculated ketogenic diet is given as an 'egg-nog'. The diet is generally calculated on the basis of a given number of calories/kg to be provided in a given day, divided into three equal meals. Usually a 4:1 ratio is used. A 4:1 ratio egg-nog would contain 60 g of 36 per cent cream, 25 g of egg, vanilla and saccharine for flavor. This would yield 245 calories, approximately 4 g of protein, 2 g of carbohydrate and 24 g of fats (24:6 or 4:1 ratio). Therefore, if 120 ml of a 4:1 ratio egg-nog would usually serve as a meal for a given child, one third would be 60 ml of the egg-nog and two thirds would be 120 ml of the egg-nog. Although most children will have reached 4+ urinary ketosis (>160 mmol/100 ml on Ketostix) by this time, we begin feeding even if this degree of ketosis is not reached. Excess ketosis may be manifested by nausea or vomiting and may be relieved with small amounts of orange juice followed by continuation of the protocol.
- Day 3: One third of the calculated diet is given as egg-nog for breakfast and lunch. Two thirds is given beginning with dinner. As the body is shifting to the utilization of ketones as the primary energy source, general lack of energy and lethargy persist; they will be regained over the ensuing 2 weeks.
- Day 4: The child continues with two thirds of the calculated diet as egg-nog and dinner is the first full meal. Occasionally, the child becomes too ketotic or acidotic as evidenced by failure to drink, Kussmaul breathing, pallor or limpness. In such an event the child is rehydrated with carbohydrate-free fluids and the diet is continued.
- Day 5: The child receives a full ketogenic breakfast and is discharged.
- Every child should receive a sugar-free multivitamin supplement and additional calcium.

The Johns Hopkins protocol for initiating the ketogenic diet.

remains to be established, it has become clear that it does have a role.

How is the diet initiated?

We admit children to the hospital, fast them for 48 h, and usually start them on the 'classical' 4:1 diet (ratio of grams of fat to grams of protein plus carbohydrate) using the Johns Hopkins protocol (see Box).[6]

Each day while the child is in the hospital, the parents (and older children) are involved in classes to learn the rationale behind the diet, and how to calculate meals, weigh foods, labels and manage the diet during childhood illnesses.

After discharge, parents are instructed to measure urinary ketones daily, in the evening. The diet is then individually adjusted by telephone consultation, changing the calories or the ratio, to provide maximum seizure control, to maintain the child in 3–4+ ketosis, and to avoid both significant weight gain and weight loss. As many of our patients come from great distances we may only see them at 3–6 month intervals. Such visits are important to assess nutrition and to evaluate seizure control and medications. We do not routinely monitor blood glucose or electrolytes after discharge, nor do we follow serum lipids, except for research purposes. We do not alter or abandon the diet even if the serum lipids are elevated.

Calculating the diet

The caloric content of the ketogenic diet is generally based on 75 per cent of the recommended daily allowance (RDA) for the child's *ideal* weight. This requirement *must* be modified for the child's activity level.

Profoundly disabled, inactive children require fewer calories than their hyperactive counterparts. A child in a spica cast uses less calories than one running around the playground. Some children are so sedated by medications that they use few calories. When medication is reduced the child may then require more calories.

If the diet is to be effective, children who are overweight for their height must have diets that are calculated so that they lose weight. Those who are underweight may be allowed to gain weight until they reach their ideal weight. Calculating the ketogenic diet is three parts science and one part art. The art is a combination of common sense, empathy and intuition. Each child's individual needs and preferences must be taken into account. If the initial estimate is too high or too low it can be corrected by 'fine-tuning' the diet.

The calculated number of calories/kg varies with the child's age, weight and activity.	
Under age 1	75–80 Kcal/kg
Ages 1–3	70–75 Kcal/kg
Ages 4–6	65–68 Kcal/kg
Ages 7–10	55–60 Kcal/kg
11 and over	30–40 Kcal/kg

Our most common error is beginning with too many calories and thereby not producing sufficient ketosis. It is better to underestimate the child's caloric requirements than to overestimate them. It is psychologically far harder to remove calories than to add them.

Caloric requirements

Multiply the child's weight by the child's caloric requirement (as in the Box above, adjusted for weight and activity) to obtain the child's caloric allotment per day. *For example*: A 4-year-old child weighing 15 kg needs 68 Kcal $\times$15 kg = 1020 calories/day.

Dietary units

- A 4:1 diet has 4 g of fat for each 1 g of protein + carbohydrate.
- A 3:1 diet has 3 g of fat for each 1 g of protein + carbohydrate.

Fat has 9 calories/g, and protein and carbohydrate each have 4 calories/g. Therefore, a 4:1 diet has 36 calories as fat (9 calories/g $\times$ 4 g) and 4 calories from protein and carbohydrate combined (4 calories/g $\times$ 1) = 4. Thus a dietary unit on a 4:1 diet ratio contains 36 + 4 = 40 calories.

Dividing the caloric requirements by the number of calories in a dietary unit gives the number of dietary units the child receives each day. *Example continued*: If the child illustrated above requires 1020 calories/day then:

1020 (calories)/40 (units)
= 25.5 dietary units/day.

Multiply the number of dietary units by the units of fat to determine the number of grams of fat permitted daily. *Example continued*: On a 4:1 diet the child requires:

fat: 25.5 (dietary units) $\times$ 4
=102 g of fat/day.
protein + carbohydrate 25.5 (dietary units) $\times$ 1 = 25.5 grams of carbohydrate and protein per day.

As most growing children require 1 g/kg of protein for growth, that child requires 15 $\times$ 1 = 15 g of protein. Subtracting the protein requirement from the total protein + carbohydrate allotment results in: 25.5 (the number of

	Grams/day	Grams/meal
Fat	102	34.0
Protein	15.0	5.0
Carbohydrate	10.5	3.5
Calories	1020	340

Table 24.3
Example of a child's dietary meal plan.

units) minus 15 (the number of grams of protein required per day) leaving 10.5 g as the total amount of carbohydrate allotted per day. The child's dietary meal plan therefore comes to the allocation shown in Table 24.3.

These total allotments can also be divided into more meals per day for smaller children or into three meals and a snack by subtracting the number of calories in the snack and then re-dividing the calories per meal.

Liquids are restricted to 1 ml/calorie or a maximum of 1200 ml per day. This is a fluid restriction which may need to be liberalized in hot weather, or if the child develops kidney stones or crystals in the urine. Liquids must be caffeine-free and carbohydrate-free. The rational behind fluid restriction is lost in antiquity and has not been retested. Liquids are spread throughout the day.

Once the diet order is calculated, meal plans are calculated by hand using a system of exchange lists and average food values.[6] A computer program that performs the calculations discussed above and which will calculate the portions of each component of each meal is available from: Epilepsy Foundation of the Chesapeake Region, 300 E Joppa Road, Suite 1103, Towson, MD 21204–3018, USA (tel. 001-410–828–7700).

The ketogenic diet is deficient in vitamins, iron and in calcium. All children must be supplemented with sugar-free multivitamins, iron and calcium. The diet is possibly also deficient in trace minerals, but we know of no evidence of trace mineral deficiency. Occasional zinc deficiency is manifested by hair loss and can be rectified by the administration of two macadamia nuts per day or zinc supplements.

Note: All medications, supplements such as vitamins, even toothpaste, must be free of carbohydrates. Carbohydrates include all sugars, polysaccharides and starches (anything that ends in -ose or -ol). When intravenous fluids are required they must also be sugar-free.

Fine-tuning the diet

Calculating and initiating the diet in the hospital are but the first steps towards achieving success. The initial estimates of caloric requirements are educated guesses. After hospital discharge the child is weighed weekly at home and the calories are adjusted up or down to maintain a constant weight. Except in small, rapidly growing infants, the child's weight should remain proportional to the height over the first year. Children who are gaining weight out of proportion to their increase in height, or who are losing weight must have their diet adjusted.

Ketones suppress appetite. If ketosis is sufficient, children should rarely be excessively hungry, despite the small portions. Hunger usually indicates insufficient ketosis and further caloric restriction, or a change in diet ratio may be needed.

Many children who are at their ideal body weight on the diet have insufficient stores of fat to continue providing ketosis throughout the night. We find this most often in young children who have supper at 5.30 pm, are put to bed at 7.30 pm and do not get breakfast until 7.00 am. Such children may have low morning ketones, and early morning seizures.

Moving dinner to 7.00 pm, or giving a snack as late as possible in the evening, will often provide sufficient ketones to last until morning and prevent the seizures.

In case of illness

Children on the ketogenic diet, like most children, will develop intercurrent illnesses. Children who are seizure-prone, as are all children on the diet, often have an increase in seizures during such illnesses. Children on the ketogenic diet should be treated just as other children, with fluids and with antibiotics when appropriate. However, it is crucial that *all medications and all fluids must be carbohydrate-free.*

Occasionally during illnesses associated with vomiting and diarrhoea, children on the diet become excessively ketotic or acidotic. Symptoms of these states include nausea, vomiting, pallor and occasionally Kussmaul breathing. Physicians, emergency rooms, and most of all parents, should be alert to such symptoms. A bolus of saline (without dextrose) or occasionally one containing bicarbonate is usually sufficient to reverse the excess keto-acidosis. On rare occasions when a child is very sick it may be necessary to break the diet with intravenous glucose or with orange juice with sugar. As the diet is rarely the cause of the problem, it can be reinstituted when the illness is passed by fasting for 1 day and then restarting the previous diet.

Medications

All medications given to the child on the diet must be carbohydrate-free. Many medications for children are formulated in carbohydrate-containing syrups or sugar-containing pills.

Many medications labelled 'sugar-free' use sucrose or other carbohydrates as sweeteners. Pills and capsules often have starch as a filler. Whenever possible utilize the form of medication that is carbohydrate-free so that the small amounts of allotted carbohydrate are not wasted on medicine.

Some newer anticonvulsants and some other medications come only in formulations containing carbohydrate. If the carbohydrate content of the daily amount of such medications is >1 g, that amount should be calculated into the child's total carbohydrate allotment.

Cholesterol and other lipids

Everyone 'knows' that a high-fat diet is bad for your health. How then can we justify feeding children a diet which is 90 per cent fat?

- Even if the diet were atherogenic (and we do not know for certain whether it is or is not), a patient would have to remain on the diet for many years to develop atherosclerosis. Few of our patients remain on the diet for this duration of time. When they terminate the diet they essentially go on a (relatively) low-fat diet and atheromata should then resorb.

- The significance of cholesterol and triglyceride levels and of the concomitant changes in the high- and low-density lipoproteins is currently under study. Preliminary data indicate that cholesterol levels increase to the low 200s in many children while on the diet. A small percentage of children have levels in the 400–500 range. Even these levels would have to be sustained for many years to be atherogenic, therefore we do not alter or discontinue the diet just because the lipid levels are high. Indeed, we would not even monitor them if we were not doing a study.

Even if the diet is atherogenic, and even if it were to shorten the child's life span by some finite amount, would that be better or worse than the continuing seizures that led to the start of the diet in the first place, or than the medications that were being used in an unsuccessful attempt to stop the seizures?

Growth

Most children seem to grow well on the diet. A few, particularly those who are severely impaired and undersized when starting the diet, may even have a growth spurt. A small percentage of children seem to stop growing while on the diet. It is said that they will have a spurt when they discontinue the diet, but that has not been clearly established. While on the diet, weight should increase (or decrease) to the ideal weight for the child's height. With growth, weight gain should then parallel the increase in height. A child who is gaining significant weight on the diet should have the calories reduced.

Prepubertal females may have a delay in menstruation while on the diet and adolescent females may cease menstruating until the diet is discontinued and the normal body fat is replenished.

Beta-hydroxybutyrate and urinary ketosis

The classic standard of adequate ketosis in children who are on the ketogenic diet has been and currently remains 3–4+ ketones in the urine, in the evening, as measured by the nitroprusside dipstick. It has been observed that when the urine consistently shows <3+ ketones the child's seizures are less likely to be controlled and the child is more likely to be hungry. Similarly it has been observed that while 4+ ketones are necessary for seizure control they are not necessarily sufficient. A child who has 4+ ketones in the urine and who continues to have seizures may still benefit by further caloric restriction or by a higher dietary ratio.

The reason for this old observation is becoming apparent. The ketostick is insensitive to higher levels of beta-hydroxybutyrate (BOHB) or acetone in the blood. Therefore once the serum level of BOHB reaches 2–3 mmol, the urine registers 4+. It is beginning to appear that seizure control may improve with serum BOHB levels >6 mmol. The correlation of seizure control to serum BOHB is currently under study, and the coming availability of the ability to measure BOHB on blood from a finger stick may facilitate the optimization of serum ketones.

The diet in other countries

We have rarely attempted to instigate the diet in children from countries other than the US. The differences in local foods and their contents, the differences in food habits and customs, and the need for frequent telephone support for the families make this a daunting task. We are aware of centers in many countries where the diet is being adapted successfully to the local conditions and preferences.

How long do we continue the diet?

It is unclear how long to continue the diet. Classically, children who have been seizure-free on the diet for 2 years are tapered off the diet by decreasing the ratio every 3 months. This has not been adequately studied. The families of children whose seizures have not been completely controlled face a choice. They may either continue on the diet or attempt to discontinue it. We tell them that either option is reasonable. If the diet is tapered, and the seizures increase, then the child can be re-fasted and replaced on the previous diet. If the child's seizures remain unchanged off the diet, medications remain an option. Some of our more impaired children have remained on the diet for more than a decade.

Summary

There has been a recent resurgence of interest in the ketogenic diet as an alternative therapy for children with difficult-to-control seizures. Even with the many newer medications now available for seizure control, many children continue to be substantially impaired by seizures and their treatment. Fifty per cent of such children appear to benefit from the diet and achieve better than a 50 per cent decrease in their seizures. The role of the diet in adult epilepsy remains to be established.

Now that it has been established that there is still a role for the diet in seizure management in children,[2,7] it is hoped that further studies will refine answers to questions about when and for whom the diet should be used. Since the diet, unlike many medications, appears to work equally well in patients with various seizure types and of varied ages, perhaps future studies will establish the mechanisms by which the diet works. Hopefully, these investigations will also lead to new understanding of some of the mechanisms underlying epilepsy.

References

1. Wheless J. The ketogenic diet: fa(c)t or fiction. *J Child Neurol* 1995;**10**:419–23.

2. Nordli DR, DeVivo DC. The ketogenic diet revisited: back to the future. *Epilepsia* 1997;**38**: 743–9.

3. Swink TD, Vining EPG, Freeman JM. The ketogenic diet: 1997. *Adv Pediatr* 1997;**44**: 297–329.

4. Vining EPG, Freeman JM, Ballaban-Gil K, et al. A multi-center study of the efficacy of the ketogenic diet. *Arch Neurol* 1998;**55**:1433–7.

5. Freeman JM, Vining EPG, Pillas DJ, et al. The efficacy of the ketogenic diet-1998: a prospective evaluation of intervention in 150 children. *Pediatrics* 1998;**162**:1358–63.

6. Freeman JM, Kelly MT, Freeman JB. *The epilepsy diet treatment: an introduction to the ketogenic diet*, 2nd edn. New York: Demos, 1994.

7. Freeman JM, Vining EPG. The ketogenic diet: a reprise. *Epilepsia* 1998;**39**:450–1.

25

Therapeutic challenges in infantile epileptic encephalopathies

Richard E Appleton

Introduction

The neonatal period and subsequent first 12 months of life ('infancy') comprise the time of life when the incidence of seizures—and the onset of epilepsy—is at its highest.[1] In addition, seizures presenting during this period are generally frequent, refractory to treatment, accompanied by additional and often severe neurological dysfunction, and are often symptomatic (of an underlying cerebral, metabolic, infectious or other aetiology).

The term 'epileptic encephalopathy' is commonly defined by frequent, multiple and usually drug-resistant seizures, and severe, often persistent, generalized or multifocal electro-encephalographic (EEG) abnormalities, which are generally considered to result in impaired neurological and cognitive development. The 1989 ILAE Classification of epilepsies and epilepsy syndromes[2,3] recognizes two 'epileptic encephalopathies': early myoclonic encephalopathy (frequently with a neonatal onset) and early infantile epileptic encephalopathy with suppression burst (sometimes termed 'Ohtahara's syndrome'). Severe myoclonic epilepsy, infantile spasms (West's syndrome – which is discussed in Chapter 27), early onset Lennox-Gastaut syndrome and myoclonic–astatic epilepsy, which also appear in the 1989 ILAE Classification,[2] should be regarded as lying within the spectrum of the infantile epilep-

tic encephalopathies; a number of others remain unclassified, including the 'hemiconvulsion–hemiplegia–epilepsy (HHE) syndrome'. These syndromes may be both symptomatic and cryptogenic in terms of aetiology. It is important to realize that a transient epileptic encephalopathy may also occur in many other children who do not have any of the recognized epilepsy syndromes described above, including infants with a clearly identified aetiology, and that any detrimental or adverse effect on intellectual development in these children may arise as a direct result of the transient encephalopathy and independent of the natural history of the underlying condition. A wide range of conditions may give rise to an epileptic encephalopathy:

- Cerebral dysgeneses (e.g. abnormalities of neuronal migration, heterotopias and dysplasias).
- Neurocutaneous syndromes (e.g. tuberous sclerosis, Sturge–Weber syndrome, linear sebaceous naevus syndrome).
- Metabolic or biochemical disorders:
  - pyridoxine (vitamin B_6) dependency;
  - biotinidase deficiency;
  - sulphite oxidase and molybdenum co-factor deficiency;
  - non-ketotic hyperglycinaemia;
  - mitochondrial and peroxisomal disorders;

- Tay–Sachs and Sandhoff's diseases;
- biopterin deficiency ('malignant phenyl-ketonuria variant');
- early infantile neuronal ceroid lipo-fuscinosis (Santavuori–Haltia–Hagberg disease).

All epileptic encephalopathies, whether cryptogenic or symptomatic, are characterized by the following:

- Frequent and intractable seizures that are predominantly generalized (myoclonic, tonic, clonic, tonic–clonic and atypical absence) or, less commonly, partial but often with secondary generalization.
- Episodes of status epilepticus (usually myo-clonic) or epilepsia partialis continuans.
- A persistently abnormal EEG, showing patterns of slow spike and wave, poly-spikes (and slow waves) or burst suppression.

A further and universally frustrating characteristic of the epileptic encephalopathies is their invariable drug resistance, the inevitability of multiple drug treatments (polytherapy) and the use of alternative therapies. Not infrequently, the clinical seizures may be temporarily controlled but the EEG abnormalities persist. Finally, there is the difficult but obvious question: 'do frequent seizures (and possibly continuous 'subclinical' spike activity on the EEG) damage the developing brain?[4,5] The answer to this question is clearly important because it would dictate the general principles and specific methods of treating infants with severe epilepsy.

General therapeutic approach

The overall therapeutic approach in these infants tends to be relatively aggressive in trying to control the seizures and suppress the abnormal epileptiform activity on the EEG, with the primary objective of maximizing their neurological and cognitive development. However, it is important to realize that there is limited information about the natural history of the epileptic encephalopathies and whether such aggressive treatment, which may have to be continued for many weeks or even months, has any significant effect on improving the long-term developmental and cognitive outcome. In addition, and unfortunately, an aggressive approach is not without its problems; the use of multiple drugs, often in very high doses, may result in sedation, stupor, irritability and other central nervous system-related side effects, which may themselves impair cognitive development, as well as producing systemic complications including hypotension and immune dysfunction. In this situation, a 'therapeutic compromise' may be a not unreasonable objective, whereby the 'major' (e.g. tonic, tonic–clonic or spasms) seizures are controlled, although more 'minor' (e.g. atypical absence and some myoclonic) seizures remain largely uncontrolled without the child being oversedated or intoxicated by the treatment. This therapeutic compromise would also appear to be a more realistic goal because the seizures that characterize the epileptic encephalopathies are, by definition, never fully controlled.[6]

Finally, any degree of seizure control is often temporary and unsustained; seizure recurrence is common and should even be anticipated. In these situations, the usual 'automatic' response is to add or change treatment. Although this is likely to be necessary in many cases, it is not always effective and may not always be justified; the apparent deterioration may be only transient and could be related to some other event, including an intercurrent infection. A radical change of treatment at this time may therefore not only be unnecessary but could potentially exacerbate the overall situation—by increasing seizure frequency or by causing side effects, or both. Conversely, however, there may be situations in which electively rotating or changing therapies may be of value, particularly if there appears to be a clear cyclical pattern to relapses or periods of acute seizure deterioration. Finally, there is the 'no treatment' option if all treatments have proved to be ineffective and/or accompanied by adverse side-effects.

Aetiology

As for any child who presents with seizures or develops epilepsy, one of the first steps in management is the identification of an underlying cause; this is particularly relevant for children aged under one year, because a relatively high proportion will be symptomatic, with an obvious aetiology. This has implications for prognosis and genetic counselling, but particularly for treatment. Two conditions in particular should be considered in any infant who presents with an 'epileptic encephalopathy': pyridoxine dependency and biotinidase deficiency.

Pyridoxine (vitamin B₆) dependency[7,8]

Infants with this autosomal recessive disorder commonly present within the first few hours of birth with frequent and multiple seizures; rarely they may have an onset either *in utero* or up to the age of 18 months. Other common features include the following: status epilepticus (partial/unilateral as well as generalized); reflex (e.g. light- or startle-induced) myoclonic seizures; 'infantile spasms' and non-specific features, including irritability, disturbed sleep and vomiting, which may precede the seizures; and minimal developmental progress. The EEG shows a poorly organized and often chaotic background with frequent ictal and interictal irregular spike/spike-and-wave discharges; a burst-suppression pattern may also occur. Although a common presentation is with an onset of 'cryptogenic' seizures in a previously normal infant, it is not uncommon for some infants with pyridoxine dependency also to have structural cerebral abnormalities (e.g. dysgenesis or dysplasias).

Whenever pyridoxine dependency is considered, a therapeutic trial of pyridoxine is indicated:

- Intravenous pyridoxine (20–50 mg/kg) should be given during an EEG. In many infants this will result in a dramatic improvement in the EEG and cessation of the seizures. However, this immediate response is not always seen and both the clinical and the EEG improvement may be delayed for some days.

- As a result of this possibly delayed response, oral (or intravenous if enteral administration is not possible) pyridoxine (50 or 100 mg twice daily, or higher depending on the age of the child) should be given for at least 3 or 4 weeks, irrespective of the response to the initial high-dose intravenous 'diagnostic' pyridoxine challenge that is given under EEG control.

- A repeat EEG should be recorded before withdrawal of the pyridoxine at the end of this 3- or 4-week period; if seizures recur, pyridoxine should be restarted and continued indefinitely, and all other antiepileptic drugs should be withdrawn gradually. Finally, it is important to realize that seizure recurrence in pyridoxine dependency may occur from 2–3 days to many weeks after the withdrawal of pyridoxine.

Pyridoxine is also reported to be effective in treating other 'intractable' seizures, including infantile spasms, and other types of seizures and epilepsy syndromes in older children.

Biotinidase deficiency[9]

Children with this very rare, autosomal, recessively inherited, metabolic disorder may present with frequent and prolonged seizures in the neonatal period or, more commonly, in later infancy/childhood, when they may be accompanied by developmental delay. The seizures are resistant to both conventional antiepileptic drugs and pyridoxine. The skin rash and hair abnormalities (including alopecia) develop only in a minority; the accompanying biochemical disturbances of metabolic acidosis, hyperammonaemia and ketosis occur late and are clearly not pathognomic for biotinidase deficiency. The treatment is with oral biotin 5–10 mg/day, although occasionally higher doses are used. Multivitamin preparations may contain enough biotin to suppress the seizures and correct the other features of the disorder.

Antiepileptic drugs

Most if not all antiepileptic drugs will, at some point, have been used to treat the infantile epileptic encephalopathies, irrespective of the specific syndrome or aetiology. It is important to emphasize that the literature describing the use of these drugs in this specific population is based almost exclusively on open and anecdotal data, often reflecting clinicians' personal experiences and prejudices (including my own). The antiepileptic drugs that tend to be most commonly used include the following:

- phenobarbitone
- phenytoin
- benzodiazepines (clonazepam and nitrazepam)
- sodium valproate.

(Lamotrigine, vigabatrin, topiramate and felbamate are used less frequently, primarily because of less 'infant-friendly' formulations, but also because of limited data on their use in infancy, in addition to concerns over toxicity.)

Phenobarbitone is frequently prescribed for neonatal seizures, including early myoclonic encephalopathy. Although it is clearly a potent anticonvulsant and is particularly effective in treating generalized seizures, high doses are often required, with resulting sedative and possibly hypotensive and respiratory complications. Phenytoin is an alternative and commonly used antiepileptic drug in the treatment of neonatal seizures, but it may exacerbate myoclonic seizures and is therefore of limited value in the early myoclonic and early infantile epileptic encephalopathies. In addition, phenytoin's pharmacokinetics make the drug relatively difficult to use and there is the additional concern that potentially irreversible cerebellar damage may be associated with high doses of the drug;[10] this complication could also theoretically be more likely to occur in young infants.

The benzodiazepines,[11] principally clonazepam[12] and nitrazepam[13] (1,4-benzodiazepines), but also clobazam[13] (a 1,5-benzodiazepine), are the most commonly prescribed—and arguably the most effective—drugs in the epileptic encephalopathies. Lorazepam and diazepam are also effective but tend to be used more intermittently, particularly for episodes of status epilepticus, rather than on a regular and long-term basis. A clear advantage of using clonazepam is that it can be given intravenously as well as orally, and is therefore of particular value when rapid seizure control is required, including status epilepticus (both convulsive and non-convulsive or electrical). However, when treating myoclonic or non-convulsive status epilepticus in the Lennox–Gastaut syndrome, clonazepam (and the other benzodiazepines) may occasionally induce tonic[14] or tonic–clonic status epilepticus. Clonazepam is effective in treating myoclonic and typical/atypical absence seizures and appears to be particularly useful in early myoclonic encephalopathy. In combination with sodium valproate, the drug is arguably the most commonly prescribed (and effective) combination 'polytherapy' in early Lennox–Gastaut syndrome and severe myoclonic epilepsy of infancy (although it is possible that valproate and lamotrigine may have already become the 'new' combination of choice). The main disadvantages of the benzodiazepines (as a group) are their adverse effects of sedation, irritability and excessive salivation and tolerance (or tachyphylaxis), which may develop over a few weeks. Clobazam is perhaps the best tolerated but is not easy to use because of its usual, and relatively non-infant-friendly, formulation. Nitrazepam seems to have a different antiepileptic spectrum to clonazepam; its main and almost its only use is in treating infantile spasms, for which clonazepam is largely ineffective.

In contrast, sodium valproate is arguably the drug of choice in treating myoclonic seizures although, not uncommonly, very high doses (≥ 60 mg/kg per day) have to be used, particularly in early myoclonic encephalopathy and severe myoclonic epilepsy of infancy. It also has a broad spectrum of anticonvulsant activity, including being at least partly effective in tonic and atonic seizures. However, the drug should be used cautiously (particularly if there is an underlying metabolic disorder) in view of the reported hepatotoxic effects, which appear to complicate its use in a particular 'at risk' population[15] (i.e. age under 2 years, severe epilepsy including myoclonic seizures, and marked, global, developmental delay). It remains unclear whether the drug has a direct hepatotoxic effect, but it may 'unmask' or exacerbate an underlying metabolic disorder, particularly those involving fatty acid oxidation.[16] Unfortunately, assessments of liver function undertaken before, and during, the use of valproate are unreliable in predicting which children are likely to develop subsequent hepatotoxicity.

Lamotrigine seems to have a similar antiepileptic profile to valproate, although it may not be as effective in controlling myoclonic seizures,[17] and there is some evidence that the drug may even exacerbate the frequent myoclonic seizures in severe myoclonic epilepsy of infancy.[18] Liver toxicity is rarer than with valproate, but the drug may cause a severe morbilliform rash (including Stevens–Johnson syndrome) which, although primarily idiosyncratic, is also related both to the starting dose and its rate of increase and to whether the child is also receiving sodium valproate. As a result, the drug has to be introduced gradually and therefore the initial target maintenance dose, and resulting seizure control, may be reached only after 5–8 weeks, which could obviously limit its usefulness. There is, however some evidence that, in infants, lamotrigine can be introduced safely and more rapidly over 2–3 weeks. Lamotrigine may also have a direct and beneficial effect on the EEG in suppressing interictal (i.e. subclinical) spike or spike and slow-wave activity, that could contribute to the developmental stagnation and intellectual impairment which so frequently characterizes the epileptic encephalopathies. Lamotrigine also appears to be better tolerated than sodium valproate, in the long term. As a result of all these features, many clinicians now regard lamotrigine, rather than sodium valproate, as the drug of choice in treating one of the epileptic encephalopathies—early onset Lennox–Gastaut syndrome. Finally, there is a clear synergistic effect between sodium valproate and lamotrigine, in terms of both efficacy and adverse effects.

Vigabatrin is clearly effective in one of the infantile epileptic encephalopathies (West's syndrome; infantile spasms), but its role in the other epileptic encephalopathies is far less clear.[19,20] Anecdotal evidence suggests that myoclonic seizures in the non-progressive epilepsies (e.g. juvenile myoclonic epilepsy) may be exacerbated by vigabatrin, although it may be effective in early myoclonic encephalopathy or severe myoclonic epilepsy of infancy.[21] There are conflicting reports of its value in the Lennox–Gastaut syndrome, but the overall impression is that it is not effective and should not be regarded as a first-line drug; however, this observation derives from older children with established Lennox–Gastaut syndrome and it is possible, although unlikely, that a different response may be seen if the drug were used earlier. One of the main benefits of vigabatrin is its relative ease of use; it is available in a powder preparation, can usually be introduced and, unlike in older children and adults, increased rapidly (over 7–10 days without causing unacceptable drowsiness or irritability), and does not have a clear dose–response relationship. The reports of peripheral visual field constriction that have occurred in adults have yet to be demonstrated in children and may be extremely difficult to detect in infants, particularly in this population because of the frequent accompanying visual and neurological problems.

Topiramate appears to have a broad spectrum in its antiepileptic action; early data in older children indicate that it may be particularly effective in treating 'drop' (atonic and tonic) seizures, partial seizures and intractable infantile spasms.[22] There are no reports of its use in infants with either early myoclonic/early infantile encephalopathy or severe myoclonic epilepsy. Anorexia and consequent weight loss in adults may pose a significant theoretical risk to infants and young children because of their rapid growth and development, thereby limit-ing its potential usefulness and role in this age group.

Felbamate was shown to be effective in older children[23] (and adults) with largely intractable Lennox–Gastaut syndrome; there is no information about its use in early-onset Lennox–Gastaut syndrome or other epileptic encephalopathies, primarily because the drug was withdrawn before any experience could be gained from using it in these other malignant epilepsies. A potentially fatal aplastic anaemia and hepatic failure have led to a marked restriction of its prescription in most countries apart from the US.

Ethosuximide has a relatively narrow spectrum of antiepileptic action, but it may be useful in myoclonic and typical/atypical absences, more frequently as polytherapy (with a benzodiazepine, sodium valproate or lamotrigine), rather than as monotherapy.[24]

Although carbamazepine may be effective in tonic seizures, it does not have a particularly broad spectrum of antiepileptic activity, and myoclonic seizures that are common in many of the encephalopathies may be exacerbated by this drug, including inducing myoclonic status. This is particularly relevant for severe myoclonic epilepsy of infancy in which unilateral or partial motor seizures may be the presenting seizure type, occurring many weeks before the development of myoclonic and absence seizures.

Corticosteroids

Short courses of steroids (adrenocorticotrophic hormone [ACTH], hydrocortisone and prednisolone)[25] are commonly prescribed in the epileptic encephalopathies, often in the belief that the 'encephalopathy' (in its broadest definition) may be inflammatory in origin and is therefore best treated with an anti-inflammatory drug. Although the mechanism of action of steroids in seizure suppression is unclear, it may modulate the function of the GABA-A receptor;[26] the antiepileptic effects of steroids are not thought to be the results of their anti-inflammatory action. In a few infants, acceptable seizure control may be achieved, but quite often at a price in terms of adverse effects, including immunosuppression, hypertension and electrolyte disturbances. An additional and not infrequent problem is that, as the steroid is being withdrawn, seizure relapse is frustratingly common. Occasionally some degree of seizure control may be regained by reintroducing the drug and continuing to give it in a very low dose for a number of weeks or even months, although this will necessitate close supervision of the child for the development of side effects.

Unlike in West's syndrome and infantile spasms, there is very little information about the comparative response rates between the different steroid preparations in the other infantile epileptic encephalopathies. In some countries, including the UK, ACTH is only available on a 'named patient basis'. In addition many clinicians are reluctant to use ACTH in view of its mandatory intramuscular route of administration, and the greater risk and incidence of adverse effects compared with prednisolone. Finally, as with infantile spasms, a wide range of doses of both ACTH and prednisolone is used in treating these epilepsies.

Ganaxolone, one of a group of neuroactive (and theoretically neurospecific) steroids called epalons (epiallopregnanolone), may offer a similar antiepileptic effect to ACTH/prednisolone, but without the side effects. The drug has a high specificity for GABA-A receptor sites and preliminary data suggest that it may be effective in some of the refractory childhood epilepsies, including infantile spasms.[27] As yet there is no information about its use (or effect) in the other infantile epileptic encephalopathies.

Immunoglobulins

Pooled immunoglobulins contain antibodies directed against a variety of autoantibodies, and might theoretically be capable of 'switching off' production of putative neuronal antibodies. Alternatively, like steroids, immunoglobulins may have an unspecified immune effect that reduces seizure frequency. However, currently their mechanism of action is unknown and they are an unproven therapy. Immunoglobulin infusions have been used in the Lennox-Gastaut syndrome and other intractable epilepsies, usually in older children but also in infants.[28] Different doses have been used ranging from 10 to 1000 mg/kg per dose, given either as a 'once only' dose or repeated every 2–4 weeks for a number of months, even indefinitely. Limited evidence suggests that, if there has been no response after two or three doses, then it is unlikely to be effective. Immunoglobulin therapy is relatively safe. Anaphylaxis is a potential risk in patients with total immunoglobulin subclass deficiency, and there is a remote but theoretical risk of the transmission of blood-borne infections including new variant Creutzfeldt–Jakob disease.

Ketogenic diet

Although the ketogenic diet is recognized to be of benefit in the management of older children with medically intractable epilepsies for whom the surgical option is not possible,[29,30] its role in infants[31] is perhaps less clear. This is primarily because of conflicting concerns over the nutritional and metabolic requirements of this particular population, and the effects that this might have on subsequent growth and development, as well as its efficacy. Theoretically, the diet could be regarded as being potentially more effective in younger children, first because they tend to produce and utilize ketone bodies more readily, and second because the diet and their overall food intake should be easier to supervise. A successful response to the diet could also provide the opportunity of reducing or withdrawing one or more antiepileptic drugs with a consequent improvement in alertness and behaviour. Further efficacy and safety data about the use of the ketogenic diet are clearly required in this specific population.

Surgery

Surgery has now become recognized, if not established, as a realistic therapeutic option for many children with 'medically intractable' epilepsies. However, the types of surgery available for infants are relatively limited and largely restricted to major procedures, including functional or anatomical hemispherectomy[32-34] (e.g. hemimegalencephaly, and Sturge–Weber, Rasmussen's and HHE syndromes), lesionectomy (e.g. focal cortical dysplasia) or hippocampectomy and, rarely, corpus callosotomy (e.g. cryptogenic Lennox-Gastaut syndrome). Corpus callosotomy is the least effective surgical procedure and should probably be undertaken only for very frequent 'drop attacks'. Vagal nerve stimulation remains an evolving and largely empirical surgical procedure with as yet ill-defined criteria and is currently of limited use in treating the infantile epileptic encephalopathies; further scientific evaluation and clinical experience with this technique may clarify its role in this specific population.

The most important aspect of surgery is that, as soon as it is considered to be a viable therapeutic option (based on the overall clinical situation and results of detailed evaluation/ investigation) it should be undertaken sooner rather than later, even in young infants.[33,34] This is important to reduce the risk of prolonged status and potentially life-threatening seizures, and to minimize the deleterious effect on cognitive and motor function of the unaffected hemisphere by the epileptogenic hemisphere. In addition, there is the theoretical risk that the frequently, although not continually, spiking abnormal hemisphere may 'kindle' the contralateral hemisphere, which could result in other additional epileptogenic foci, thereby precluding surgery. However, for an individual child it may still be unclear whether surgery should be performed early, to prevent adverse development of the 'normal' hemisphere, or delayed, to ensure that the only source of the seizures is the abnormal hemisphere.[35]

Holism (management of the whole child within the family)

It is important to realize and understand that the psychological impact of frequent seizures on families and siblings of these children can be considerable, and is always stressful and frequently devastating; there is often accompanying minimal, or absent, developmental progress and frequent hospitalization. Support for these families is crucial, but it is usually inadequate and relies on scarce resources, including nurse specialists in paediatric epilepsy[36] and the relevant voluntary epilepsy associations (e.g. the British Epilepsy Association, 'Brainwave' [The Irish Epilepsy Association], the International Bureau for Epilepsy [the Netherlands] and the Epilepsy Foundation of America). Unfortunately, despite the immense value of both these associations and the nurse specialists, neither are ubiquitous or particularly experienced in dealing with the severe infantile epileptic encephalopathies—

primarily because of the relatively low incidence of these epilepsies compared with the epilepsies starting in mid and late childhood.

Additional important treatment issues that must be considered in these children include the prescription of helmets or other forms of protective headwear (for mobile and ambulant children), the provision of regular respite care for these children (specifically so that their parents may have time for themselves or their other children) and appropriate use of genetic counselling. Finally, despite the inevitable difficulties—and despair—the clinician, and all involved healthcare personnel, should attempt to adopt an approach that is positive, as well as realistic, to the management of these children and their families.

All of these issues represent and reflect total or holistic medicine; failure to address them is a failure of medical treatment.

References

1. Anderson VE, Hauser WA, Rich SS. Genetic heterogeneity in the epilepsies. In: Delgado-Escueta AV, Ward AA Jr, Woodbury DM, Porter RJ, eds. *Advances in Neurology*. New York, Raven Press, 1986.

2. Commission on Classification and Terminology of the International League Against Epilepsy. Proposal for classification of epilepsies and epileptic syndromes. *Epilepsia* 1989;**30**:389–99.

3. Roger J, Bureau M, Dravet Ch, et al. *Epileptic syndromes in infancy, childhood and adolescence*, 2nd edn. London: John Libbey, 1992.

4. Wasterlain CG. Recurrent seizures in the developing brain are harmful. *Epilepsia* 1997;**38**:728–34.

5. Camfield PR. Recurrent seizures in the developing brain are not harmful. *Epilepsia* 1997;**38**:735–7.

6. Guerrini R, Dravet Ch. Severe epileptic encephalopathies of infancy, other than West syndrome. In: Engel J Jr, Pedley TA, eds. *Epilepsy: a comprehensive textbook*. Philadelphia: Lippincott-Raven, 1998:2285–302.

7. Bankier A, Turner M, Hopkins IJ. Pyridoxine-dependent seizures – a wider clinical spectrum. *Arch Dis Child* 1983;**58**:415–18.

8. Baxter P, Griffiths P, Kelly T, Gardner-Medwin D. Pyridoxine-dependent seizures: demographic, clinical, MRI and psychometric features, and effect of dose on intelligence quotient. *Dev Med Child Neurol* 1996;**38**:998–1006.

9. Salbert BA, Pellock JM, Wolf B. Characterisation of seizures associated with biotinidase deficiency. *Neurology* 1993;**43**:1351–5.

10. Kuruvilla T, Bharucha NE. Cerebellar atrophy after acute phenytoin intoxication. *Epilepsia* 1997;**38**:500–2.

11. Henriksen O. An overview of benzodiazepines in seizure management. *Epilepsia* 1998;**39** (Suppl 1):S2–6.

12. Tassinari CA, Michelucci R. The use of diazepam and clonazepam in epilepsy. *Epilepsia* 1998;**39**(Suppl 1):S7–14.

13. Shorvon S. The use of clobazam, midazolam, and nitrazepam in epilepsy. *Epilepsia* 1998;**39**(Suppl 1):S15–23.

14. Bittencourt PR, Richens A. Anticonvulsant-induced status epilepticus in Lennox–Gastaut syndrome. *Epilepsia* 1981;**22**:129–34.

15. Konig SA, Siemes H, Blaker F, et al. Severe hepatotoxicity during valproate therapy: an update and report of eight new fatalities. *Epilepsia* 1994;**35**:1005–15.

16. Appleton RE, Farrell K, Applegarth DA, et al. The high incidence of valproate hepatotoxicity in infants may relate to familial metabolic defects. *Can J Neurol Sci* 1989;**17**:145–8.

17. Besag FMC, Wallace SJ, Dulac O, et al. Lamotrigine for the treatment of epilepsy in childhood. *J Pediatr* 1995;**127**:991–7.

18. Guerrini R, Dravet C, Genton P, et al. Lamotrigine and seizure aggravation in severe myoclonic epilepsy. *Epilepsia* 1998;**39**:508–12.

19. Chiron C, Dulac O, Luna D, et al. Vigabatrin in childhood epilepsy. *J Child Neurol* 1991; 6(Suppl 2):S30–7.

20. Appleton RE. Vigabatrin in the management of generalised seizures in children. *Seizure* 1995; 4:45–8.

21. Baxter PS, Gardner-Medwin D, Barwick DD, et al. Vigabatrin monotherapy in resistant neonatal seizures. *Seizure* 1995;4:57–9.

22. Glauser TA. Preliminary observations on topiramate in pediatric epilepsies. *Epilepsia* 1997;38(Suppl 1):S37–41.

23. Felbamate Study Group in Lennox–Gastaut syndrome. Efficacy of felbamate in childhood epileptic encephalopathy (Lennox–Gastaut syndrome). *N Engl J Med* 1993;328:29–33.

24. Aicardi J. *Epilepsy in children*, 2nd edn. Raven Press: New York, 1994.

25. Prasad AN, Stafstrom CF, Holmes GL. Alternative epilepsy therapies: the ketogenic diet, immunoglobulins, and steroids. *Epilepsia* 1996;37(Suppl 1):S81–95.

26. O'Regan ME, Brown JK. Is ACTH a key to understanding anticonvulsant action? *Dev Med Child Neurol* 1998;40:82–9.

27. Lechtenberg R, Villeneuve N, Monaghan EP, et al. An open-label dose-escalation study to evaluate the safety and tolerability of ganaxolone in the treatment of refractory epilepsy in pediatric patients. *Epilepsia* 1996;37(Suppl 5):204 (abstract).

28. Etzioni A, Jaffe M, Pollack S, et al. High dose intravenous gamma-globulin in intractable epilepsy of childhood. *Eur J Pediatr* 1991; 150:681–3.

29. Schwartz RH, Eaton J, Aynsley-Green A. Ketogenic diets in the treatment of epilepsy: short-term clinical effects. *Dev Med Child Neurol* 1989;31:145–51.

30. Swink TD, Vining EPG, Freeman JM. The ketogenic diet: 1997. *Adv Pediatr* 1997;44: 297–329.

31. Nordli DR, Koenigsberger D, Carroll J, De Vivo DC. Successful treatment of infants with the ketogenic diet. *Ann Neurol* 1995;38:523 (abstract).

32. King M, Stephenson JBP, Ziervogel M, et al. Hemimegalencephaly – a case for hemispherectomy? *Neuropediatrics* 1985;16:46–55.

33. Appleton RE, Gardner-Medwin D, Mendelow D. Hemispherectomy for intractable seizures. *Dev Med Child Neurol* 1991;33:273–4.

34. Wyllie E, Comair YG, Kotagal P, et al. Epilepsy surgery in infants. *Epilepsia* 1996;37:625–37.

35. Jahan R, Mischal PS, Curran JG, et al. Bilateral neuropathological changes in a child with hemimegalencephaly. *Pediatr Neurol* 1997;17:344–9.

36. Appleton RE, Sweeney A. The management of epilepsy in children: the role of the clinical nurse specialist. *Seizure* 1995;4:287–91.

26

Epilepsy surgery in children: when and how to operate
Christian E Elger and Martin Kurthen

Introduction

The question of when and how to operate on children with chronic epilepsy is even more intricate than the question of surgical therapy in adults with epilepsy. In adults, there are quite well-defined epileptic syndromes—paradigmatically, the syndrome of mesial temporal lobe epilepsy (MTLE)[1]—which are known to be successfully treated by standard surgical procedures such as anterior temporal lobectomy or, more recently, selective amygdalohippocampectomy. Surgery can be considered as soon as the disease is identified as medically intractable, or at least as soon as the development of medical intractability can be expected with a high probability in an individual patient. The diagnostic procedures required for presurgical decision-making are also fixed and standardized to a considerable degree. The aim of epilepsy surgery is defined in a straightforward fashion as seizure freedom (or reduction) without postoperative impairments of any kind. All of this does not hold equally for epilepsy surgery in children.

Childhood epilepsies are often difficult to classify and, at an early stage of the disease, it may even be difficult to identify the 'benign' epileptic syndromes with their high rate of spontaneous remission. Standardized surgical procedures such as anterior temporal lobectomy are the exception rather than the rule; in children, surgical procedures such as cortical resections are often tailored to the individual patient, and more radical surgical procedures such as (functional) hemispherectomy and corpus callosotomy play a major role. The question of timing is perhaps the most difficult one in childhood epilepsies, because it depends not only on the intractability criterion, but also on a variety of criteria, some of which are not easy to evaluate. In fact, there are good reasons to prefer early surgery for epilepsy in children, which means that presurgical assessment has to be performed at an early stage with all the methodical diagnostic problems found in very young patients. Two of these problems—cerebral plasticity and development—are mentioned here. First, there is evidence that both seizures and antiepileptic drugs can interfere with brain maturation; second, recovery from postoperative deficits will often be more complete in children than in adults as a result of the greater plasticity of the young brain. When making decisions about diagnostic procedures, the pathway is less fixed in children than in adults, because the specific value of, for example, functional imaging techniques and seizure semiology is still controversial. Finally, the possible aims of epilepsy surgery in children are more complex than those in adults: in addition to freedom from seizures and no postoperative impairments, more specific aims have to be considered, such as acceleration of cognitive development, reduction of behavioral abnormalities and even interictal EEG improvement.

In what follows, these specific aspects of decision-making about epilepsy surgery in children are discussed with a special emphasis on timing of and selection for presurgical evaluation; this selection is based on the prevalent literature and our own experience with presurgical assessment of epilepsy in children. Although, in the literature, reports on epilepsy surgery in children often refer to patients up to the age of 18, this tends to obscure the specific pediatric aspects of surgery, because older children and adolescents, who often form the major parts of the reported samples, resemble adults: they have intractable seizures much more often than do younger children. These constraints must be taken into account in any review of previous reports on epilepsy surgery in 'children'. The following three sections address the questions of timing, selection and choice of surgical procedure; these seem to be the crucial points of decision-making in epilepsy surgery in children. The following are three questions that need answers:

1. What is the optimal time of presurgical assessment and surgery with respect to patient's age and development of the disease?
2. What are the best criteria for patient selection for presurgical evaluation and surgery?
3. How can the optimal surgical procedure be determined as a result of a conclusive presurgical assessment?

It must be borne in mind that any actual review of epilepsy surgery in children will be preliminary in character, because currently, the published experience with children is limited in many respects when compared with the literature on surgical procedures and their outcome in adults. Accordingly, the answers to the three questions listed above should be the subject of constant reconsideration and revision.

Timing

Postoperative studies on adults can give indirect clues to the question of timing of surgery, because in most patients, presurgical evaluation and surgery are not performed directly after the diagnosis of intractability. Wyllie[2] gave an average delay of 11 years from onset of intractability to surgery. This means that, in postoperative studies, there is a large number of young adults who could (or should) have been operated on as children. However, there are no decisive studies comparing long-term outcome from childhood surgery with outcome from late surgery in patients with presumed childhood intractability. It has at least been argued that a favorable surgical outcome correlates with a shorter duration of epilepsy presurgically.[3] This is partially reflected by the opinions of patients and families about timing of surgery; in a recent Japanese study,[4] most of the patients and relatives would have liked surgery to have been carried out earlier than it actually had, although few patients, in retrospect, wanted an operation before they were 15. Although many aspects of timing of surgery are inseparable from questions of patient selection (see below), some general points can be made.

First, in addition to the well-known metabolic aberrations that are associated with status epilepticus, there may be brain injury caused by prolonged and/or recurrent seizures, perhaps as a result of an excessive release of excitatory amino acids.[5] Clinically, recurrent seizures in children may be associated with cognitive impairment.[6] In a recent review of studies on medically and surgically treated children with infantile spasms,[7] it was shown that seizure control leads to a significant improvement in non-verbal communication, which was taken to be an established developmental measure. Duration of illness and the underlying pathology (in surgically treated children) were identified as the factors with major impact on early development. In both infantile spasms and the Lennox-Gastaut syndromes—and, in general, in catastrophic childhood epilepsies—one may ask whether early surgery can prevent the severe mental deterioration that is often prominent in the course of these diseases. At present, there are no conclusive data to answer this question. At least for seizure outcome, age at surgery and duration of epilepsy seem to have some relevance to prediction.[8] As well as the literature on the effects of seizures on cerebral development, there is also evidence that antiepileptic drugs may have negative effects on the developing brain: in rats, phenobarbitone (phenobarbital) and sodium valproate (valproic acid) have been shown to induce brain growth retardation[9,10] and, at least for phenobarbitone, negative effects on IQ have been reported in children.[11] Negative effects of anticonvulsants on fetal growth have been noted in human fetuses who were exposed to antiepileptic drugs *in utero* from the treatment of their mothers with antiepileptic drugs.[12] The consequences of these adverse effects of seizures and antiepileptic drugs on brain function are much more severe in children than in adults, because negative effects on the developing brain may result in a delay of developmental stages or even an irreversible failure to acquire socially relevant cognitive skills. Therefore, one of the specific aims of epilepsy surgery in children must be the prevention of these potentially life-long impairments.

The second point is that a complementary aspect of timing of surgery is represented by the fact that, as a result of decreasing cerebral plasticity, functional recovery after late surgery is worse or more incomplete than after early surgery. This is illustrated best by drastic examples such as left-sided hemispherectomy:

performed at a very early age, this surgical procedure leads to a favorable long-term outcome in respect of higher cognitive functions of the left and right hemispheres,[13–15] whereas in adult patients who have a dominant left hemisphere, the sequelae would be disastrous. Vargha-Khadem and Mishkin[16] also report evidence that the earlier the hemispherectomy for treatment of drug-resistant seizures is carried out, the more favorable the cognitive developmental outcome. The effect of a better functional reorganization after early surgery is, however, also found in patients with less radical resections. In patients with left temporal lobe epilepsy, there is a relationship between increased risk of pre- to postoperative verbal memory decline after anterior temporal lobectomy and increasing age at onset of epilepsy.[17] In a recent study from our clinic on 20 children with temporal lobe epilepsy aged under 16 who underwent surgery, it was found that they showed a lower risk of postoperative memory deterioration than the equivalent adult patients.[18] As for infantile spasms, a series of 24 children operated on at UCLA (University of California at Los Angeles) also confirmed the relevance of early surgery,[19] because the variable 'age at surgery' turned out to be the main predictor of developmental outcome. Another study on corpus callosotomy in 25 children revealed greater neuropsychological gains in the 'younger' (age at surgery < 13 years) subgroup.[20] Finally, in patients with the Landau–Kleffner syndrome, who were treated surgically by multiple subpial transections,[21] it seemed that language recovery after early performance of the surgery was far better than recovery after spontaneous resolution of epileptic activity in teenagers.

The final point is that social disadvantages and behavioral impairments are among the most serious unwanted sequelae of epilepsies in children, because without an effective therapy, the lost 'social ground' is hard to recover. It has been pointed out that the psychosocial costs of uncontrolled seizures in children differ from those in adults.[2] These costs include poor peer relations, poor school performance, poor self-esteem, parental overprotection, and early psychiatric problems, which together can potentially lead to permanent disability and unemployment in adulthood. When the negative behavioral features of the disease that are often directly related to the social problems respond to surgical treatment, the children may be enabled to return to a normal social life. Impairments in social behavior can be found in many epilepsy syndromes in children. Symptomatic temporal lobe epilepsy and atypical Landau–Kleffner syndrome have been reported to be accompanied by autistic features, which can respond to surgical treatment.[22]

As a more common example, temporal lobe epilepsy in children is known to be frequently accompanied by behavioral disturbances. In a recent study on 37 children with temporal lobe epilepsy from our clinic aged between 3 and 17,[23] it was demonstrated that about one third of the children had severe behavioral impairments, mainly aggressiveness and outbursts of rage, followed by social maladjustment. The behavioral features were associated with an early onset of the epilepsy, a high focal interictal spike frequency, and the occurrence of neoplastic lesions as depicted on magnetic resonance imaging (MRI) scans. Seven of twelve children with severe behavioral disturbances dramatically improved in social behavior immediately after temporal lobe surgery. This improvement was not strongly associated with the degree of postoperative seizure relief, but with a moderate focal spike activity in the presurgical EEG recordings. For the patients and their families, postoperative improvement in social behavior is often considered to be a major aspect of the perceived success of epilepsy surgery, on a par with seizure relief.

These points together indicate that there are some good independent reasons for early surgery in childhood epilepsy. The seizures themselves, the antiepileptic drug, and the psychological and social sequelae of the disease all have a negative influence on the development of the young person, leading to potentially irreversible disadvantages in adulthood. The earlier that this negative influence is eliminated by successful treatment, the better for the development of the child. As an epileptologist, one is, however, forced into a dilemma. On the one hand, surgical treatment of epilepsy should be considered as early as possible: the younger the child, the more critical the undesired sequelae of the disease will be. On the other hand, epilepsy surgery should not be performed too early: the earlier presurgical evaluation is done, the greater the risk of error with respect to candidacy and surgical indication. The second horn of the dilemma calls for a thorough consideration of selection criteria and, in a second step, a well-advised choice of a specific surgical procedure. These problems are discussed in the next two sections. The preliminary conclusion of this section is: presurgical evaluation and surgery in childhood epilepsy should be performed as early as possible, but not before the history of the disease allows a comprehensive assessment of the individual epileptic syndrome and its prognosis under non-surgical therapy.

Selection

An adequate selection of surgical candidates requires a prior clarification of the aims of epilepsy surgery. Although one can argue that improvement of the quality of life is the one general aim of epilepsy surgery, it may be helpful to formulate some concrete subordinate aims, the achievement of which may contribute to an improvement in quality of life in general. It is often said that in adults, the two major concrete aims of epilepsy surgery are seizure control and the avoidance of additional deficits of any kind. The second point holds equally for children. In fact, the general and specific risks of postoperative deficits are the main source of argument for the well-established selection criterion of medical intractability: if surgery were without risk, one could even operate on children who could also be successfully treated with antiepileptic drugs, thus avoiding undesired side effects of these drugs. The first point will, however, have to be slightly modified in epilepsy surgery in children.

Adult patients are usually excluded from surgical therapy when there is no realistic perspective of achieving freedom from seizures (adult callosotomy candidates will form an exception to this rule). In children, partial seizure control may be considered a sufficient success for surgery, if it can be expected to have a positive effect on development. Relief from secondary generalized seizures or reduction of seizure frequency may be advantageous for mental development, and elimination of seizures with sudden falls helps to avoid disabling injuries and is therefore socially advantageous. Thus, in addition to seizure control and avoidance of additional deficits, a major aim of epilepsy surgery in children is the prevention of secondary consequences—particularly in the cognitive domain—of the disease specifically related to the patient's development. Another aspect, which will rarely have to be considered in adults, is the improvement of the above-mentioned, often socially disabling, behavioral disturbances that accompany many childhood epileptic syndromes.

As our own study on children with temporal lobe epilepsy has shown,[23] behavioral improvement is not necessarily paralleled by adequate seizure control. If prevention of cognitive deficits and disabling behavioral patterns are dependent on a postsurgical improvement of interictal EEG patterns, then EEG improvement may itself be considered a goal of surgical therapy in certain cases; this is particularly the case in syndromes where continuous interictal epileptiform discharges are predominant or even represent the only manifestation of the epileptic disturbance. For example, in the Landau–Kleffner syndrome treated with multiple subpial transections, EEG normalization seems to be one of the main determining factors of language improvement after surgery.[21]

In individual patients, the specific aims of surgery will have to be formulated according to the patient's overall presurgical status and a complete set of data from presurgical evaluation. Future research could systematize this sort of assessment and categorize patients presurgically in terms of their expected benefits from surgery (see Taylor et al[24] for a preliminary proposal).

According to these major aims of epilepsy surgery in children, some selection criteria can be discussed. The focus here is on the selection of patients for presurgical evaluation, not for therapeutic surgery itself. The choice of a specific surgical procedure is considered in the next section. The main aspects of patient selection are: medical intractability; exclusion of a symptomatic cause; exclusion of epileptic syndromes that do not need surgical treatment; identification of syndromes with favorable outcome; and evidence of acute or subacute worsening of patient status.

Medical intractability

This term can be defined as 'inadequate seizure control in spite of appropriate medical therapy with AED or adequate seizure control but with unacceptable side effects from the AEDs'.[25] Obviously, this general definition does not yield an all-or-none criterion in individual patients, because it is left open to interpretation or individual judgement as to what will count as adequate, appropriate and acceptable. As mentioned above, the adequacy of seizure control in children is difficult to estimate, because low-frequency (and at first sight tolerable) seizures may still have disadvantageous developmental consequences. The appropriateness of medical therapy is even harder to establish, and even more so for childhood epilepsies. With the availability of a selection of new antiepileptic drugs with proven or presumed effectiveness in seizure control in children, it would now take an enormous amount of time to demonstrate that a patient fails with all drugs that are presumed to be effective. If patients are not meant to spend their whole childhood on drug trials, for each distinct epileptic syndrome or class of syndromes a limited set of mono- and polytherapies would have to be defined, failure of which would render a patient's epilepsy 'medically intractable' in a wide, but pragmatically reasonable, sense.

In children in whom time is particularly limited, this set of appropriate therapies would have to be kept as short as possible (but, yet, as long as necessary—this is the well-known dilemma). With regard to the acceptability of side effects, we again face the problem that the negative consequences of long-term antiepileptic drug treatment on the physical, cognitive and social development of epileptic children are not well known. At the very least, the concept of momentary acceptability of side effects, which is often pragmatically applied in adults, cannot easily be transferred to children. Furthermore, in children we have to consider, to a much higher degree than in adults, not only medical intractability of seizures, but also

'intractability' of interictal epileptiform EEG patterns, particularly in epileptic syndromes with rare or absent seizures (see above).

Exclusion of a symptomatic cause of the seizures

Seizures that have a symptomatic cause and could be treated successfully otherwise should be excluded. This may seem a matter of course, but it should at least be mentioned that before surgery (in fact, before any anticonvulsive treatment, except in very acute cases) seizures that are just the symptoms of an underlying disease of metabolic, inflammatory, etc. origin should be excluded, as these could be treated successfully by a specific non-surgical therapy. When children are considered for presurgical evaluation, a symptomatic origin of this kind will be the exception rather than the rule. On the other hand, one may well find a symptomatic origin that does not allow for a causal therapy, e.g. tuberous sclerosis or the Sturge–Weber syndrome. Some of these patients can be treated successfully by surgery, even in the presence of multiple cerebral lesions. Although adult patients with progressive diseases of the central nervous system (CNS) are usually excluded from surgery, there is at least one exception to that rule in children, namely Rasmussen's encephalitis, which can often be treated successfully by hemispherectomy, when non-surgical therapies such as immunosuppression have failed.[26]

Exclusion of epileptic syndromes not to be treated surgically

This includes syndromes that need not or cannot be treated surgically and may sound trivial even in our age of sophisticated diagnostics, however, epileptologists must take care not to operate on a normal brain for a spontaneously remitting condition such as benign rolandic epilepsy or benign focal epilepsy with occipital spikes. Mostly, these conditions are easily recognized by their clinical course and characteristic EEG patterns.

The same holds true for most of the idiopathic syndromes, such as idiopathic epilepsies with generalized tonic–clonic seizures, absences or myoclonic seizures. These syndromes need not and cannot be treated surgically, because they become manifest with seizures that are primarily generalized and usually respond well to treatment with an antiepileptic drug such as valproate or ethosuximide. There is, however, a gray area of syndromes that may be treated surgically, although they have long been looked upon as 'benign' and indeed have a high rate of spontaneous remissions. The most well known of these conditions is the Landau–Kleffner syndrome,[27] which is, however, only 'benign' in a weak sense—when symptoms persist for less than a year, there is a good chance of at least partial spontaneous recovery. The main problem with the Landau–Kleffner syndrome is that patients tend to remain severely compromised with respect to linguistic capacities, even when the EEG returns to normal.[28]

In this gray area of controversial surgical indications, one should be cautious not to rush to conclusions about the in-principle 'inoperability' of certain epileptic syndromes, because this would preclude some surgical candidates from evaluation. For example, infantile spasms and other 'catastrophic' epilepsy syndromes have long been thought to be the result of diffuse cerebral damage, but recent research has shown that a subgroup of patients has circumscribed epileptogenic lesions and may profit from resective surgery.[29,30]

Identification of epileptic syndromes with a known favorable surgical outcome

This is the first of two positive criteria, the fulfilment of which is not mandatory, but desirable. In some cases, an epileptic syndrome with known good surgical outcome can be assumed in outpatients on the basis of medical history, seizure semiology, interictal EEG patterns and MRI scans. This holds particularly for patients with mesial temporal lobe epilepsy, a syndrome that is, however, rarely diagnosed in younger children with their variable seizure semiology and lack of MRI changes.[29] In older children with mesial temporal lobe epilepsy, it may suffice to perform additional video-EEG seizure recordings and neuropsychological assessment to submit a patient to temporal lobe surgery. Another example of a syndrome with good surgical outcome is focal epilepsy in a patient with a history of drug-resistant seizures of monohemispheric origin; this is based on severe early damage of one hemisphere and a normally developed contralateral hemisphere. If patients who display this syndrome show a severe spastic hemiparesis with loss of independent finger movements, they may be good candidates for hemispherectomy with a low risk of additional motor deficits postoperatively.[31,32]

Even if it cannot be assumed that a distinct epileptic syndrome with a well-known good surgical outcome is a good candidate based on outpatient data, there may still be diagnostic markers or indicators of possible candidacy for surgery. These are mainly focal features such as partial seizures, focal neurological signs and focal radiological signs.[33,34] Focal interictal epileptiform discharges on surface-EEG recordings made on outpatients also represent an important diagnostic marker, although, in epileptic children, such focal EEG changes are not found as regularly as, for example, in adults with temporal lobe epilepsy. On the other hand, bilateral EEG changes will not preclude children from evaluation for unilateral resections, because the impression of bilaterality may be the result of secondary bilateral synchrony.

In our own experience,[35] the unilateral origin of these secondary bilateral discharges in children can be demonstrated by selective Wada tests of the artery that supplies the presumed epileptogenic area. Ideally, these tests will demonstrate a bilateral suppression of epileptiform discharges with an injection on the side of the seizure origin.

Evidence of an acute or subacute worsening of the patient's status

This can be a result of an aggravation of the disease: priority should be given to the evaluation of children with a recent history of either developmental stagnation or impairment, or the occurrence of disturbances in social behavior, or of any other acute or subacute undesired effects of the disease on development. In such patients, there is evidence of a 'dynamic' negative development of the epilepsy, which may lead to irreversible deficits in later life. Taking this subacute worsening or developmental stagnation as a warning sign may contribute to early presurgical evaluation in those patients who, otherwise, would be at risk of undergoing an irreversibly disadvantageous development. The value of this early evaluation and operation is not, however, easily substantiated in clinical studies, because one would have to compare the development of two groups of children with similar syndromes after either surgical or non-surgical therapy. This is difficult to do, because surgically treated children will always differ from those who are non-surgically treated in some important clini-

cal features. In any case, in view of the frequent disastrous sequelae of drug-resistant epileptic syndromes in early childhood, presurgical evaluation should be performed before the development of an epileptic syndrome with poor prognosis.

Choice of surgical procedure

Surgical procedures can be subdivided according to their 'where', 'what' and 'how', i.e. which area of the brain is operated on, what is the assumed underlying pathology and what sort of surgical strategy is chosen. In terms of the 'where' question in children, distinction into temporal lobe surgery, extratemporal surgery, hemispherectomy and callosotomy is usually made. With regard to the underlying pathology, pediatric epileptologists are mainly concerned with neuronal migration disorders, tumors, phakomatoses, inflammatory processes, vascular or hypoxic lesions and less frequently, traumatic lesions and hippocampal scleroses. Surgical strategies are either resective (cortical resection, hemispherectomy, amygdalohippocampectomy), non-resective (callosotomy, multiple subpial transections), or mixed resective and non-resective (cortical resection plus multiple subpial transections, or functional hemispherectomy as a combination of resection and disconnection). The choice of a surgical procedure depends on the totality of information gathered before and during presurgical evaluation. The details of the diagnostic procedures (imaging, electrophysiology, neuropsychology) and their relative importance for surgical decision-making are not comprehensively discussed in this chapter. As space is limited, the same restriction holds for the consideration of outcome and prognosis of the various surgical procedures. In what follows, we just go through the various surgical procedures under the 'where' aspect and point to the procedures of choice for the respective syndromes or pathologies.

Temporal lobe surgery

In some centers (such as ours), selective amygdalohippocampectomy is favored as the most selective procedure for the treatment of mesial temporal lobe epilepsy,[36] but, as the fully fledged syndrome is rather infrequent in children, there are as yet no published series for comparison of selective amygdalohippocampectomy and anterior temporal lobectomy in younger patients. In our view, as for in adults, the former can be seen as the therapy of choice in older children with mesial temporal lobe epilepsy. Surgical strategies that focus on maximal resection of mesial structures and only limited resection of the temporal neocortex have also been proposed.[37,38] Traditional anterior temporal lobectomy can also be performed in temporal lobe epilepsy, but there is evidence that sparing of the lateral temporal neocortex results in a better neuropsychological outcome.[39] In patients with circumscribed extrahippocampal lesions, such as cortical dysplasias or benign tumors, an extended lesionectomy will be the resective strategy of choice, unless there is evidence of involvement of the hippocampus or the whole temporal lobe in seizure generation.

Generally, temporal lobe surgery can be performed when interictal and ictal EEG recordings, MRI scans and recordings of seizure semiology yield concordant results in terms of unilateral temporal lobe epilepsy. On the other hand, evidence of bitemporal disease or additional extratemporal disease, normal MRI or dual pathology increases the risk of poor outcome from temporal lobe surgery. Non-invasive EEG recordings may suffice in patients with positive MRI findings and unequivocal epileptiform discharges;[40] invasive recordings[41] with subdural strip and/or grid electrodes or intrahippocampal depth electrodes will often be necessary in the absence of morphological lesions, in patients with dual pathology or in patients with insufficient correspondence of data from different diagnostic procedures. Functional imaging with positron emission tomography (PET) is helpful for localization of the epileptic focus in the absence of abnormalities on MRI scans.[42] Seizure outcome is generally favorable in childhood temporal lobe surgery, but reliable predictors of outcome have not yet been established.[43]

Extratemporal surgery

The outcome from extratemporal surgery is generally poorer than the outcome from temporal lobe surgery.[44] As seizure semiology and surface EEG recordings are often inconclusive in childhood seizures of extratemporal origin, there is an emphasis on imaging techniques and invasive EEG recordings (including intraoperative electrocorticography for the determination of the borders of resection or multiple subpial transections) in these syndromes. In the absence of MRI pathologies, ictal single photon emission computed tomography (SPECT) seems to be more helpful for the localization of the focus than PET,[45] although conclusive data are only available in adults.[46] High-quality MRI for detection of small and subtle lesions is crucial in extratemporal epilepsy, to guide planning of electrode implantation and the final resective strategy. Even in non-lesional patients, however, favorable outcome is achieved when the zones of ictal onset and interictal abnormalities are completely resected.[47] If this is not possible as a result of involvement of eloquent brain areas (especially motor or language cortex, but also visual cortex, somatosensory cortex and supplementary motor area), cortical resections can be combined with multiple subpial transections, but, even then, complete seizure freedom is rare.[48] If the epileptogenic area is completely located within eloquent brain areas, pure multiple subpial transections may lead to sufficient reduction of seizure frequency. This new approach extends the indications of epilepsy surgery to patients who would otherwise be inoperable. Specific data from childhood epilepsies treated with pure multiple subpial transections are available for the Landau–Kleffner syndrome, in which 11 of 14 patients significantly improved neuropsychologically.[21]

Hemispherectomy

The term 'hemispherectomy' is used to describe a number of resective strategies,[49] namely: anatomical hemispherectomy (total excision of one hemisphere), modified hemispherectomy (anatomical hemispherectomy with subsequent reduction of the subdural hemispherectomy cavity), hemidecortication (removal of the cortex of one hemisphere), functional hemispherectomy (temporal and frontocentroparietal resection plus disconnection of all residual frontal and parieto-occipital fibers) and hemispherotomy (versions of functional hemispherectomy with minor excision and major disconnection). Many centers currently prefer some sort of functional hemispherectomy, with its smaller access and exposure and its lower risks of hydrocephalus and infection.

The typical hemispherectomy candidate is a young patient with a history of drug-resistant seizures of monohemispheric origin, based on severe early damage of one hemisphere and, ideally, a normally developed contralateral hemisphere. Etiologically, Rasmussen's encephalitis, severe cortical dysplasia, early vascular lesions, hemiatrophy and the Sturge–Weber syndrome are the most common.

If such a patient shows a severe spastic hemiparesis with loss of independent finger movements, he or she runs only a low risk of additional postoperative motor deficits.[31,32] Before surgery, a high risk of postoperative hemianopsia and/or language deficits has to be excluded by the Wada tests, transcranial magnetic stimulation, ophthalmological examinations and, if necessary, functional imaging of the visual cortex. If cases are carefully selected, the percentage of seizure-free patients comes close to 70 per cent, but there is still a perioperative mortality rate of up to 10 per cent.

Callosotomy

Corpus callosotomy can be incomplete (mostly anterior) or complete; the modern techniques usually spare the anterior commissure, fornix and intermediate mass.[50] The typical callosotomy candidate is a young patient with a history of medically intractable, bilateral motor seizures, especially seizures with sudden falling and a high risk of injury, and in whom presurgical assessment reveals no resectable epileptic focus. Drop seizures associated with bilateral (synchronous) epileptiform discharges are known to respond best to callosotomy, but generalized tonic–clonic seizures may also be reduced. Postoperatively, many patients suffer from a transitory disconnection syndrome with mutism and left-sided apraxia,[51] but permanent neuropsychological deficits are rare, at least after incomplete callosotomy.[52] To prevent postoperative dysphasia, interhemispheric antagonism and limb apraxia, preoperative Wada tests are recommended to exclude mixed language dominance and/or dissociation of language and motor dominance.[53] It is still a matter of discussion whether complete callosotomy is superior to anterior section with regard to seizure control; in some centers, callosotomy is completed in a second step if incomplete section turns out to be insufficient.[54] Generalized seizures may convert into partial ones after callosotomy;[52,54] in rare cases, the resulting partial seizures can again be evaluated with respect to focal resectability.

Summary

Epilepsy surgery in children has evolved rapidly over the last decades, as a result mainly of increasing knowledge about the natural course of the various epileptic syndromes in childhood and the major advances in morphological (cranial computed tomography, MRI) and functional (PET, SPECT) imaging techniques, which have improved the detection of focal abnormalities as causes or correlates of epileptic diseases. Unlike in adults, epilepsy surgery in children aims not only at seizure control with no additional postoperative impairments, but also at acceleration of cognitive development, reduction of behavioral abnormalities and even improvement in interictal EEG in some cases. As a result of the vulnerability of the developing brain to damage and/or functional deterioration caused by recurrent or prolonged seizures and unwanted antiepileptic drug effects, presurgical evaluation should be performed as early as possible, i.e. as soon as a poor spontaneous prognosis and medical intractability have been established pragmatically. Some well-defined surgical procedures have been demonstrated to result in a good outcome in a high proportion of patients, although for some techniques (e.g. multiple subpial transections) and some syndromes (e.g. infantile spasms) the available data are not yet conclusive. In this chapter, we have pointed to some specific aspects of timing and patient selection in childhood epilepsies. Generally, early surgery is recommended to prevent further mental deterioration and unfavorable psychosocial development.

References

1. Engel J Jr, Williamson PD, Wieser HF. Mesial temporal lobe epilepsy. In: Engel J Jr, Pedley J, eds. *Epilepsy: a comprehensive textbook*, Vol. 3. New York: Lippincott-Raven, 1998:231.

2. Wyllie E. Candidacy for epilepsy surgery special considerations in children. In: Lüders HO, ed. *Epilepsy surgery*. New York: Raven Press, 1992:127–30.

3. Vaernet K. Temporal lobectomy in children and young adults. In: Parsonnage M et al, eds. *Advances in epileptology: XIVth Epilepsy International Symposium*. New York: Raven Press, 1983:255–61.

4. Inoue Y, Mihara T, Seino M. Timing of epilepsy surgery: its relevance for psychosocial rehabilitation. In: Tuxhorn I, Holthausen H, Boenigk H, eds. *Paediatric epilepsy syndromes and their surgical treatment*. London: John Libbey, 1997:76–84.

5. Olney JW, Collins RC, Sloviter RS. Excitotoxic mechanisms of epileptic brain damage. *Adv Neurol* 1986; **44**:857–77.

6. Bourgeois BFD, Prensky AL, Palkes HS, et al. Intelligence in epilepsy: a prospective study in children. *Ann Neurol* 1983;**14**:438–44.

7. Caplan R. Epilepsy in early development: the lesson from surgery for early intractable seizures. *Semin Pediatr Neurol* 1995;2:238–45.

8. Shewmon DA, Shields WD, Sankar R, et al. Follow-up on infants with surgery for catastrophic epilepsy. In: Tuxhorn I, Holthausen H, Boenigk H, eds. *Paediatric epilepsy syndromes and their surgical treatment*. London: John Libbey, 1997:513–25.

9. Diaz J, Schain R, Bailey B. Phenobarbital induced brain growth retardation in artificially reared rat pups. *Biol Neonate* 1977;**32**:77–82.

10. Diaz J, Shields WD. Effects of dipropylacetate on brain development. *Ann Neurol* 1981;**10**: 465–8.

11. Farwell JR, Lee YJ, Hirtz DB, et al. Phenobarbital for febrile seizures: effects on intelligence and on seizure recurrence. *N Engl J Med* 1990;**322**:364–9.

12. Hiilesma VK, Teramo K, Granstrom ML, Bardy AH. Fetal growth and antiepileptic drugs: preliminary results of the prospective Helsinki study. In: Janz D et al, eds. *Epilepsy, pregnancy, and the child.* New York: Raven Press, 1982:203–5.

13. Ogden JA. Language and memory functions after long recovery periods in left-hemispherectomized subjects. *Neuropsychologia* 1988;**26**:645–59.

14. Ogden JA. Visuospatial and other 'right-hemispheric' functions after long recovery periods in left-hemispherectomized subjects. *Neuropsychologia* 1989;**27**:765–76.

15. Fusco L, Vigevano F. Reversible operculum syndrome caused by progressive epilepsia partialis continua in a child with left hemimegalencephaly. *J Neurol Neurosurg Psychiatry* 1991;**54**:556–8.

16. Vargha-Khadem F, Mishkin M. Speech and language outcome after hemispherectomy in childhood. In: Tuxhorn I, Holthausen H, Boenigk H, eds. *Paediatric epilepsy syndromes and their surgical treatment.* London: John Libbey, 1997:774–84.

17. Hermann BP, Seidenberg M, Haltiner A, Wyler AR. The relationship of age at onset, chronological age, and adequacy of preoperative performance to verbal memory change following anterior temporal lobectomy. *Epilepsia* 1995;**36**:137–45.

18. Lendt M, Helmstaedter C, Elger CE. Pre- and postoperative neuropsychological profiles in children and adolescents with temporal lobe epilepsy. Submitted.

19. Asarnow RF, Lopresti C. Adaptive functioning in children receiving resective surgery for medically intractable infantile spasms. In: Tuxhorn I, Holthausen H, Boenigk H, eds. *Epilepsy syndromes and their surgical treatment.* London: John Libbey, 1997:526–536.

20. Lassonde M, Sauerwein C. Neuropsychological outcome of corpus callosotomy in children and adolescents. *J Neurosurg Sci* 1997;**41**:67–73.

21. Morrell F, Whisler WW, Smith MC, et al. Landau–Kleffner syndrome: treatment with subpial intracortical transection. *Brain* 1995; **118**:1529–46.

22. Neville BG, Harkness WF, Cross JH, et al. Surgical treatment of severe autistic regression in childhood epilepsy. *Pediatr Neurol* 1997; **16**:137–40.

23. Elger CE, Brockhaus A, Lendt M, et al. Behavior and cognition in children with temporal lobe epilepsy. In: Tuxhorn I, Holthausen H, Boenigk H, eds. *Paediatric epilepsy syndromes and their surgical treatment.* London: John Libbey, 1997:311–25.

24. Taylor DC, Cross JH, Harkness W, Neville BGR. Defining new aims and providing new categories for measuring outcome of epilepsy surgery in children. In: Tuxhorn I, Holthausen H, Boenigk H, eds. *Paediatric epilepsy syndromes and their surgical treatment.* London: John Libbey, 1997:17–25.

25. Bourgeois BFD. General concepts of medical intractability. In: Lüders HO, ed. *Epilepsy surgery.* New York: Raven Press, 1992:77–82.

26. Andermann F, ed. *Chronic encephalitis and epilepsy: Rasmussen's syndrome.* Boston: Butterworth–Heinemann, 1991.

27. Landau W, Kleffner F. Syndrome of acquired aphasia with convulsive disorder in children. *Neurology* 1957;**7**:523–30.

28. Deonna T, Peter CL, Ziegler AL. Adult follow-up of the acquired aphasia-epilepsy syndrome in children. *Neuropediatrics* 1989;**20**:132–8.

29. Brockhaus A, Elger CE. Complex partial seizures of temporal lobe origin in children of different age groups. *Epilepsia* 1995;**36**: 1137–81.

30. Chugani HT, Shewmon DA, Shields WD, et al. Surgery for intractable infantile spasms: neuroimaging perspectives. *Epilepsia* 1993;**34**: 764–71.

31. Vining EP, Freeman JM, Pillas DJ, et al. Why would you remove half a brain? The outcome of 58 children after hemispherectomy—the Johns Hopkins experience: 1968 to 1996. *Pediatrics* 1997;**100**:163–71.

32. Peacock WJ, Wehby-Grant MC, Shields WD, et

al. Hemispherectomy for intractable seizures in children: a report on 58 cases. *Childs Nerv Syst* 1996;**12**:376–84.

33. Kramer U, Sue WC, Mikati MA. Focal features in West syndrome indicating candidacy for surgery. *Pediatr Neurol* 1997;**16**:213–17.

34. Dietrich RB, El-Saden S, Chugani HT, et al. Resective surgery for intractable epilepsy in children: radiologic evaluation. *AJNR* 1991;**12**:1149.

35. Brundert S, Elger CE, Solymosi L, et al. Selective amobarbital test in epilepsy surgery [German]. *Radiologe* 1993;**33**:213–18.

36. Helmstaedter C, Elger CE, Hufnagel A, et al. Different effects of left anterior temporal lobectomy, selective amygdalohippocampectomy, and temporal cortical lesionectomy on verbal learning, memory, and recognition. *J Epilepsy* 1996;**9**:399–405.

37. Crandall PH. Cortical resections. In: Engel J Jr, ed. *Surgical treatment of the epilepsies.* New York: Raven Press, 1987:377–404.

38. Peacock WJ, Comair Y, Chugani HT, et al. Epilepsy surgery in childhood. In: Lüders HO, ed. *Epilepsy surgery.* New York: Raven Press, 1992:589–98.

39. Wieser HG. Behavioral consequences of temporal lobe resections. In: Trimble MR, Bolwig RG, eds. *The temporal lobes and the limbic system.* Petersfield: Wrightson Biomed, 1992: 169–88.

40. Blume WT, Girvin JP, McLachlan RS, Gilmore BE. Effective temporal lobectomy in childhood without invasive EEG. *Epilepsia* 1997;**38**:164–7.

41. Wyllie E, Lüders H, Morris HH, et al. Subdural electrode in the evaluation for epilepsy surgery in children and adults. *Neuropediatrics* 1988;**19**:80–6.

42. Adelson PD, Peacock WJ, Chugani HT, et al. Temporal and extended temporal resections for the treatment of intractable seizures in early childhood. *Pediatr Neurosurg* 1992;**18**:169–78.

43. Goldstein R, Harvey AS, Duchowny M, et al. Preoperative clinical, EEG, and imaging findings do not predict seizure outcome following temporal lobectomy in childhood. *J Child Neurol* 1996;**11**:445–50.

44. Bizzi JW, Bruce DA, North R, et al. Surgical treatment of focal epilepsy in children: results in 37 patients. *Pediatr Neurosurg* 1997;**26**:83–92.

45. Menzel C, Steidele S, Grünwald F, et al. Evaluation of technetium-99m-ECD in childhood epilepsy. *J Nucl Med* 1996;**37**:1106–12.

46. Newton MR, Berkovic SF. Ictal SPECT. In: Pedley TA, Meldrum BS, eds. *Recent advances in epilepsy*, vol. 6. Edinburgh: Churchill Livingstone, 1995:41–55.

47. Jayakar P, Harvey S, Duchowny M, et al. Epilepsy surgery in children with normal or non-specific imaging studies. *Epilepsia* 1995;**36**(Suppl):139.

48. Polkey CE. Experiences with multiple subpial transection. In: Tuxhorn I, Holthausen H, Boenigk H, eds. *Paediatric epilepsy syndromes and their surgical treatment.* London: John Libbey, 1997:876–9.

49. Villemure JG. Hemispherectomy: techniques and complications. In: Wyllie E, ed. *The treatment of epilepsy: principles and practice.* Philadelphia: Lea & Febiger, 1993:116–19.

50. Zentner J. Surgical aspects of corpus callosum section. In: Tuxhorn I, Holthausen H, Boenigk H, eds. *Paediatric epilepsy syndromes and their surgical treatment.* London: John Libbey, 1997:830–49.

51. Ross MK, Reeves AG, Roberts DW. Post-commissurotomy mutism. *Ann Neurol* 1984;**16**:114.

52. Cendes F, Ragazzo PC, daCosta V, Martins LF. Corpus callosotomy in treatment of medically resistant epilepsy: preliminary results in a pediatric population. *Epilepsia* 1993;**34**:910–17.

53. Sass KJ, Spencer DD, Spencer SS, et al. Corpus callosotomy for epilepsy. II. Neurological and neuropsychological outcome. *Neurology* 1988;**38**:24–8.

54. Nordgren RE, Reeves AG, Viguera AC, Roberts DW. Corpus callosotomy for intractable seizures in the pediatric age group. *Arch Neurol* 1991;**48**:364–72.

27

West's syndrome: the role of new antiepileptic drugs

Catherine Chiron

Introduction

West's syndrome or so-called infantile spasms is the most frequent type of epilepsy in the first year of life. Diagnosis is based on particular seizures (epileptic spasms), particular EEG patterns between seizures (hypsarrhythmia) and psychomotor regression. This syndrome has a special place among types of childhood epilepsy as a result of the severe epileptic and mental prognosis, the usual resistance to conventional antiepileptic drugs, and a non-satisfactory and poorly tolerated standard treatment, consisting of steroid therapy, although there is some efficacy of new compounds emerging.

Both the aetiology and epilepsy itself contribute to the prognosis of infantile spasms. A large number of cerebral lesions can induce infantile spasms (symptomatic infantile spasms), including cortical malformations, sequelae of pre-, per- or postnatal hypoxic ischaemia, infection of the central nervous system (CNS), neuro-cutaneous syndromes and inherited metabolic disorders; all of these are associated with a certain degree of neurological and mental impairment. Epilepsy adds its own severity to this status. The mental prognosis is often unfavourable in cases that have no detectable cerebral lesion (cryptogenic infantile spasms). The severity of the infantile spasms results not only from the seizures, but also from the diffuse and subcontinuous interictal paroxysmal activity recorded on the EEG—the hypsarrhythmia; this interferes with normal brain activity and produces an epileptic encephalopathy.[1] This activity impairs cognitive development, thus contributing to the poor prognosis. The treatment of infantile spasms should therefore have two goals: control of both the seizures and the hypsarrhythmia. Complete cessation of spasms is a necessary treatment goal.

Infantile spasms are known to be one of the most drug resistant of the epilepsy syndromes. Conventional antiepileptic drugs are usually inefficient, except the benzodiazepines and valproate in a limited number of cases. Deterioration has even been observed using carbamazepine.[2] Since the first reports in 1958 of a remarkable effect of adrenocorticotrophic hormone (ACTH),[3] steroids have been considered the main treatment for infantile spasms around the world. However, their tolerance by patients is widely recognized as poor and their long-term effects as controversial. Moreover, there is no consensus about the dose, duration or type of steroid compound to be used to provide the best benefit–risk profile. In some countries, steroids are prescribed only secondary to vitamin B_6 or valproate at high doses.[4,5] Some authors are even reluctant to administer steroids to patients who have a clear cerebral lesion, because they consider that the disadvantageous side effects outweigh any reasonably favourable mental outcome, in those cases where spasms are controlled.[6]

Finally, the efficacy of steroids is difficult to assess retrospectively, being based on so many different treatment schedules. The response seems to differ according to the aetiology, but the various causes of infantile spasms are rarely individualized in the various studies. The level of relapse seems to be relatively high, although long-term surveys are few and the mental benefit from the control of spasms during the initial phase of the disease remains uncertain. Fortunately, favourable results have been obtained over recent years with new antiepileptic drugs that are tolerated much better than steroids, mainly vigabatrin; this encourages the inclusion of trials of infantile spasms in the development of further new compounds. As a small proportion of patients (1–2 per cent) can recover spontaneously,[7,8] trials with new drugs need to be controlled. Specific problems indicate that most trials are open: rapid mental deterioration usually accompanies the onset of spasms, so using placebo is difficult; the high frequency of adverse events with reference drugs used in studies prevents blinding of any comparative trial; seizure quantification requires precise methodology; and endpoints for favourable response must include not only the disappearance of spasms but also some EEG criteria. Some successful studies have demonstrated the interest in use of vigabatrin for infantile spasms. Finally, such a need for particular controlled designs, which are specifically dedicated to a given type of epilepsy occurring at a given age, has increased interest in development of trials for childhood epilepsy in general.

Conventional treatments in West's syndrome[9]

Conventional treatments, mainly steroid therapy, still have a large role to play in the treatment of infantile spasms, even though vigabatrin tends to be used more and more as the first-line drug in most of the countries that have given it approval. However, as of 1998, the experience with vigabatrin might be not extensive enough to consider this drug as an alternative to steroids for all types of infantile spasms. It is still therefore useful to bear in mind the most significant results obtained with more conventional therapeutic approaches to infantile spasms.

Steroids

ACTH has been the first and the most extensively studied steroid used. A dose of 40 IU is usually advised, which controls seizures initially in about 75 per cent of patients. A lower dose (20 IU) is less efficient and a higher dose (150 IU) more efficient, but the long-term response rate does not disclose a significant difference between 150 IU and 40 IU. More than 5 months of treatment at 40 IU induced an initial response rate of 87 per cent compared with only 32 per cent for less than 1 month's treatment. Although the relapse rate is not reported according to treatment duration, the lowest rate was observed in patients who had been treated with prolonged high doses, with the relapse rate ranging from 33–56 per cent. After a first relapse, a second course of therapy may produce a response in 74 per cent of patients. The incidence of adverse events is dramatically high, reaching almost 100 per cent if one considers the Cushing effect. The other most common problems include infections, increased arterial blood pressure, gastritis and hyperexcitability. These problems are often reported as severe with a mortality rate of between 2 and 5 per cent. Tetracosactrin (a synthetic ACTH) seems to be even less tolerated than ACTH.

Oral steroids are not now prescribed so extensively, although they seem to be better tolerated than ACTH, with only 17 per cent of adverse events occurring with hydrocortisone. In a prospective, randomized, blind study, the efficacy of prednisone (at 2 mg/kg per day) was inferior to that of ACTH given for 2 weeks at 150 IU,[10] although it was the same when ACTH was given at lower doses.[11] No control data are available that compare hydrocortisone with ACTH, although a prospective study, including 94 patients treated for 2 weeks with hydrocortisone 15 mg/kg per day who received tetracosactrin for another 2 weeks if spasms persisted, showed that 74 per cent of them had benefited from low doses of oral steroids, with only minor side effects and a relapse rate of 18 per cent.[12] Among the ten treated with tetracosactrin, nine ceased to have any spasms.

A favourable outcome in terms of intelligence ranges from 14 to 58 per cent, being more frequent in cryptogenic than in symptomatic cases. Perhaps surprisingly, 64 per cent of the surviving patients who had had symptomatic infantile spasms, from a series of 214 children followed for 20–35 years, had normal intelligence and socioeconomic status.[13] All had received steroid therapy. This gives an important argument in favour of steroid prescription, even in symptomatic cases, when spasms persist, which is against the advice of some authors who deny any contribution by this treatment to improvement in mental outcome.

The mechanisms of steroid action remain unclear and include non-specific effects, such as: a decrease in cerebral blood flow; an increase in permeability of the blood–brain barrier; an acceleration of enzymatic activity and maturation of the brain; an increase in the level of nerve growth factor in cerebrospinal fluid, with a decrease in NAA synthesis in mitochondria, which produces cellular hyper-polarization; or an increase in γ-aminobutyric acid (GABA) receptor affinity.[14,15]

Benzodiazepines

Nitrazepam has been reported to achieve complete control of infantile spasms at a dose of between 0.6 and 1 mg/kg per day in about 50 per cent of cases; clonazepam achieves this at a daily dose of 0.1 mg/kg in about 33 per cent. Open studies concluded that benzodiazepines are less effective than steroids, but a single, randomized, prospective comparison between ACTH and nitrazepam showed no difference between the two.[16]

Tolerance by patients is no better than that achieved with steroids because more than half of the patients experienced severe side effects, mainly increased secretion of saliva, difficulty in swallowing and mucus obstruction of the bronchi. A mortality rate of 25 per cent has been reported with nitrazepam for doses higher than 0.8 mg/kg per day.

Valproate

Valproate was used as initial monotherapy in infantile spasms at doses of between 20 and 60 mg/kg per day; complete seizure control was achieved in 27 per cent of cases, and partial control in more than 27 per cent, with no side effects except transient hypotonia and lethargy. A prospective escalation dose study showed that 50 per cent of the patients were controlled within 4 weeks, at a mean dose of 74 mg/kg per day and a mean plasma level of 114 mg/l, with good tolerance and no cases of hepatitis, although 64 per cent relapsed.[9]

Pyridoxine

A recovery rate of up to 37.5 per cent has been claimed using vitamin B_6 (pyridoxine) either at the usual doses of between 100 and 400 mg/day or at high doses ranging from 1 to 2.4 g/day. Others did not confirm monotherapy as efficacious, but reported seizure control in 84 per cent of cases when ACTH was added at a low dose.[17] Relapse was observed in 29 per cent of this group, although half of the patients experienced normal development and none developed serious side effects.

Immunoglobulins

Since the first study, which reported six of six patients with cryptogenic infantile spasms controlled by intravenous administration of immunoglobulin 100–200 mg/kg at intervals of 2–3 weeks (one to eight administrations), further results have been rather disappointing. No more than 21 per cent of patients experienced a lasting cessation of seizures in a study using Veinoglobulin 1 g/kg per day for 2 days, repeated every 3 weeks for 6 months.

Miscellaneous

Various treatment attempts have been made, based on pathophysiological hypotheses; treatments include thyrotrophin-releasing hormone, naloxone, and antiserotoninergic or anticatecholaminergic agents. All have had disappointing results.

Finally, among the classic treatments for infantile spasms, steroids remain the drug of choice, more by practice than from control data. As steroid therapy is unanimously recognized as poorly tolerated and often dangerous, other drugs are now preferred as the first-line treatment, such as vitamin B_6 or high-dose valproate. As a result, therapeutic approaches to infantile spasms may be totally different in different countries.[4]

New antiepileptic drugs in West's syndrome

The development of new drugs, particularly vigabatrin, has totally changed the therapeutic approach to infantile spasms in the last few years. As vigabatrin provided evident improvement when compared with steroids (similar or even superior efficacy, good tolerance by patients and rapid effect), it rapidly became the drug of first choice for infantile spasms in Europe and in most countries that have given it approval. Control data have now justified this attitude for some aetiologies such as tuberous sclerosis. However, the superiority of vigabatrin over steroids has not, to date, been completely established for other aetiologies in which steroids could bring some benefit. Long-term data are still scarce, especially with monotherapy, about efficacy as well as tolerance by patients.

Vigabatrin

Vigabatrin (γ-vinyl-GABA) is an irreversible inhibitor of GABA transaminase, the main enzyme involved in GABA catabolism. It therefore increases the level of GABA in the brain, which is the basis for its antiepileptogenic activity. Vigabatrin has been shown to reduce seizure frequency significantly in partial epilepsy in both adults[18] and children.[19] The latter, together with a multicentre open study of children,[20] have suggested that vigabatrin could also be useful in epilepsies with generalized seizures, such as the Lennox-Gastaut or West's syndromes.

The first study specifically dedicated to infantile spasms was published in 1991,[21] preliminary short-term data were reported in 1990.[22] The study involved 70 children aged from 2 months to 13 years, who had infantile spasms refractory to other treatments, which were classified as cryptogenic in 37 cases and symptomatic in 33, including 14 with tuberous sclerosis. Children received vigabatrin up to 200 mg/kg per day, as open and add-on treatment; they were evaluated after a mean 3-month duration of treatment. Spasms had disappeared in 43 per cent of patients, from the first week of treatment, and efficacy was maintained in 55 per cent of them after 8–33 months of follow-up. The best response was obtained in patients with tuberous sclerosis; 71 per cent of them were seizure-free short term and 100 per cent long term (13 of the 13 who continued vigabatrin), whereas the other symptomatic and cryptogenic patients experienced cessation of seizures in 30 per cent of cases, although 26 per cent of the cryptogenic cases had a recurrence of spasms long term. Tolerance by patients was excellent compared with steroids, because only two patients had to stop vigabatrin, one for hypertonia and the other for hypotonia; only 13 per cent of the patients experienced side effects, mainly sedation or excitation, which were moderate and transient.

Further open trials dedicated to vigabatrin as add-on therapy included patients with refractory infantile spasms and pointed out cessation of spasms in 25–100 per cent, depending on the relative proportion of different aetiologies included, especially tuberous sclerosis.[23-27]

Based on the evidence of safety and efficacy of vigabatrin used for intractable spasms, vigabatrin monotherapy has been advocated as a first-line drug in newly diagnosed infantile spasms.[28] Since 1992, a significant number of newly diagnosed patients should have received vigabatrin as a first-line treatment for infantile spasms, but there have been reports on only a small proportion.[29-36] Spasms initially disappeared respectively in 4 of 11, 3 of 6, 4 of 7, 8 of 12, 9 of 18, 4 of 7, 13 of 26 and 8 of 19 of cases, respectively, although the aetiology was not given.

A retrospective European survey collected together as many of these observations as possible, in order to assess the efficacy of vigabatrin as the initial treatment of infantile spasms.[37] Among 192 infants confirmed as having infantile spasms and treated with vigabatrin as first-line therapy, 68 per cent experienced initial suppression of spasms. The best response was observed in tuberous sclerosis at 96 per cent (27 of 28 had complete cessation of spasms), compared with 60 per cent in the other symptomatic patients and 69 per cent in cryptogenic patients. Vigabatrin was initiated at a median dose of 50 mg/kg per day and maintained at 100 mg/kg per day; 59 per cent of the patients needed a modification of the vigabatrin dose to control spasms. A high rate of suppression of spasms (90 per cent) was also obtained in the 20 patients aged under 3 months at the onset of spasms. Response was obtained at a median time of 4 days, with 82 per cent of the patients responding within 7 days. Twenty-one per cent of all responders (28 of 131) relapsed for spasms, 77 per cent within 3 months. Tolerance by patients was good with only 13 per cent of infants exhibiting adverse events; of these the most common were somnolence and hyperkinesia. In only two cases was vigabatrin withdrawn.

These retrospective data were followed by three randomized trials that compared vigabatrin either with steroids, the reference treatment, or with placebo.

The first trial compared vigabatrin (at 150 mg/kg per day) with hydrocortisone (oral steroid at 15 mg/kg per day), randomly assigned as first-line monotherapy in 22 infants with infantile spasms resulting from tuberous sclerosis.[38] All 11 who received vigabatrin as the first-line drug experienced cessation of spasms, compared with 5 of the 11 who received hydrocortisone ($p < 0.01$). The six non-responders were switched to vigabatrin at

1 month and all became spasm-free. The mean time to the disappearance of spasms was 3.5 days on vigabatrin against 13 days on hydrocortisone ($p < 0.01$). Five patients exhibited side effects on vigabatrin and nine patients on hydrocortisone ($p = 0.006$). The conclusion was that vigabatrin was superior in efficacy, more rapidly effective and better tolerated than the reference treatment, and it should therefore be considered as the first choice for the treatment of infantile spasms caused by tuberous sclerosis.

The second trial compared vigabatrin (at 100–150 mg/kg per day) with ACTH (10 IU/day), randomly assigned as the first-line drug in 42 infants with untreated infantile spasms.[39] Of the 23 receiving vigabatrin as the first-line drug, 11 (48 per cent) experienced cessation of spasms: 4 of 7 (57 per cent) cryptogenic and 7 of 16 (44 per cent) symptomatic patients, and all three with tuberous sclerosis. Of the 19 receiving ACTH as the first-line drug, 14 (74 per cent) became spasm-free: 7 of 8 (87 per cent) of the cryptogenic and 7 of 11 (64 per cent) of the symptomatic patients. Eleven of twelve who did not respond to vigabatrin and two of the five who did not respond to ACTH had a better response when switched to the second drug after 20 days. However, six cases of relapse were observed in patients treated with ACTH, compared with only one with vigabatrin, and 37 per cent of the patients exhibited side effects on ACTH compared with only 13 per cent on vigabatrin. Therefore, despite initial efficacy in favour of ACTH, particularly in cryptogenic cases, we recommend vigabatrin as the first choice of treatment for infantile spasms, before initiation of ACTH, for both safety and long-lasting response.

The third study was a blind, placebo-controlled study that compared vigabatrin (50–150 mg/kg per day) with placebo as the first-line drug in 39 untreated infants with infantile spasms; treatment was for a 5-day period, after which all the continuing infants were treated openly with vigabatrin for 6 months.[40] Vigabatrin significantly reduced the number of spasms compared with placebo and there were no more side effects on vigabatrin than there were on placebo, thus justifying the use of vigabatrin as the first choice in infantile spasms.

Several authors have pointed out the appearance of partial seizures on vigabatrin therapy, used as an add-on or monotherapy for infantile spasms.[21,37,41] However, focal features are now well known to be a major component of infantile spasms of most aetiologies[1,42] and partial seizures are often associated with spasms whatever the therapy.[43,44] Therefore, partial seizures are more likely to be the result of the cerebral lesion from which the infantile spasms originated than to be induced by vigabatrin. Moreover, vigabatrin has proved to have relatively good efficacy in partial seizures in infants.[45]

At this stage in the development of vigabatrin—a drug now approved in most countries around the world—we need to collect more information about the efficacy of the drug according to the different causes of infantile spasms, both initially and on follow-up. There are a number of ongoing studies in these fields, the preliminary results of which are too limited to draw definite conclusions.

In a prospective multicentre French study, 59 infants received vigabatrin as first-line monotherapy, 100–150 mg/kg per day, for previously untreated infantile spasms (22 cryptogenic, 37 symptomatic).[46] Cryptogenic patients experienced cessation of spasms in 82 per cent of cases compared with 27 per cent in symptomatic cases. This is contrary to what has been reported in the literature with regard to the response of infantile spasms to vigabatrin.

However, patients with tuberous sclerosis were not included in the study nor were patients with mental disability, but normal MRI scans, were classified as symptomatic, whereas such patients would have been considered as having cryptogenic infantile spasms in previous studies. Both contributed to diminish the proportion of symptomatic responders in this work. Indeed, the lower response rate was observed in patients with mental disability but normal MRI (one in 14 was spasm-free) and authors discouraged the use of vigabatrin in such patients.

Moreover, this series provided major information for the practical use of vigabatrin. All responder patients who remained with spikes on their EEG after 15 days on vigabatrin later experienced a relapse of their spasms. Thus, considering that these EEG features indicated the incomplete efficacy of vigabatrin, the authors added steroids (hydrocortisone) at this stage. Definite control of spasms was thus obtained in all cryptogenic patients, and in half of the symptomatic patients with cerebral malformation.

Others proposed initially to combine vigabatrin with ACTH in infantile spasms complicating cerebral palsy, and to discontinue the latter after 4–6 weeks in order to maintain vigabatrin alone.[47] All patients but one experienced complete cessation of spasms with a mean follow-up of 19 months.

Long-term results were more disappointing in the population of choice for the use of vigabatrin as first-line therapy—patients with tuberous sclerosis. In a series of 21 children, all initially controlled by vigabatrin monotherapy (11 as the first-line drug, 10 after hydrocortisone failure), five relapsed for spasms (four having received vigabatrin as the first-line drug), at a time interval ranging from 2.5 to 12 months, and only three could be recontrolled secondarily using prolonged cortitherapy.[48] This contrasts with the excellent long-lasting effect of vigabatrin in tuberous sclerosis patients initially treated with vigabatrin as an add-on.[21,26] Of 16, only one relapsed for spasms: he was the only one in whom vigabatrin had been stopped after less than 2 years of treatment.

Tolerance by patients can be assessed from data about more than 700 infants who received vigabatrin as add-on or monotherapy before the age of 2 years. Severe side effects have been noted in no more than 3 per cent, and all patients recovered. Most of the side effects were moderate and transient, the most common being drowsiness, hypotonia or hyperexcitability. Reduction in the vigabatrin dose was often sufficient to stop them.

There is no case of a myelin disorder attributed to vigabatrin in humans, although there were cases in dogs and rats treated with doses higher than those recommended for humans.[49] In a personal series of 16 epileptic children with normal MRI scans who were treated with vigabatrin, there was no evidence of an abnormal signal in the white matter, and no abnormality was observed in maturation of the myelin after 11 months of treatment at the usual doses. In our personal experience of 10 years using vigabatrin in young children, we have never had any suspicion of white matter abnormality induced by this drug, including neuropathological specimens.

Some rare cases of constriction of the visual field have recently been reported in adults treated with vigabatrin.[50] The relationship to vigabatrin needs to be clarified. The GABAergic hypothesis could be one to consider. To date, there is no report in children, although cases might go unrecognized because the problems may remain asymptomatic. Further information is needed in adults and older children able to undergo examination of the visual field before any conclusion can be drawn regarding the population of infants, in terms of benefit–risk ratio.

The benefit of vigabatrin in infantile spasms to mental development after the control of spasms should be evaluated. Unfortunately, studies are almost non-existent in this population. Measurement of the developmental quotient, in 11 previously untreated patients with infantile spasms from tuberous sclerosis, both before the initiation of vigabatrin and after 2 months of monotherapy,[38] meant that we could assume that the drug did not induce any deleterious effect on cognitive functions (unpublished personal data). The neuropsychological follow-up of a series of seven children with tuberous sclerosis who received vigabatrin as an add-on treatment for infantile spasms gave us more convincing evidence.[51] Mental outcome was evaluated after over 30 months of treatment. The control of spasms was associated with a significant improvement in cognition and behaviour in six cases, although partial seizures persisted or appeared in four. Cognitive development, mainly involving verbal abilities and social interaction, was particularly dramatic because the early signs of autism had disappeared in all cases.

Lamotrigine

Some interesting results were reported in 1994 from a study using lamotrigine in infantile spasms.[52] Thirty patients with refractory infantile spasms were entered in a single-blind, placebo-controlled, add-on study; their ages ranged from 1 month to 11 years. At 3 months, nine patients were responders, five with complete cessation of spasms. Among the responders, the proportion of symptomatic cases (eight of nine) and of valproate co-medication was significantly higher than in the group of non-responders. At a mean follow-up of 2 years, the response was maintained and

the five seizure-free patients were receiving the combination of lamotrigine and valproate. Three patients showed adverse side effects, including one cutaneous rash. However, the potential usefulness of lamotrigine in infantile spasms still needs to be confirmed.

Felbamate

Based on the demonstrated efficacy of felbamate in the Lennox-Gastaut syndrome, a type of epilepsy that frequently follows infantile spasms, this drug was used as an add-on for four infants with spasms refractory to conventional therapies.[53] Three showed complete resolution of spasms within 1 week of starting felbamate. Safety and long-lasting response were not reported. None of these patients had received vigabatrin before felbamate was tested.

Another preliminary report mentioned a decrease in seizure frequency of more than 75 per cent in four of six patients with symptomatic infantile spasms that were refractory to steroids, vigabatrin and lamotrigine, and treated with felbamate.[54]

Ganaxolone

In an ongoing trial, ganaxolone was given as add-on, in an open titration study, to 21 children with infantile spasms refractory to steroids and other conventional therapies, including vigabatrin and lamotrigine.[55] Spasms disappeared in only one of these children, but decreased by more than 50 per cent in 50 per cent of them, with dramatic improvement in behaviour. In two, hyperkinesia required withdrawal of ganaxolone.

Ketogenic diet

Whether there is any effect of this diet on infantile spasms is impossible to determine from the literature, because the epilepsy syndromes of responders are not specified.[56] In a population of 18 infants aged less than 2 years, four were seizure-free at 3 months, six at 6 months and three at 1 year.[57]

Of a personal series of 32 patients, who received a ketogenic diet in addition to their antiepileptic treatment for at least 1 month, 14 had infantile spasms that were refractory to therapies, including vigabatrin.[58] Seven of them experienced a decrease of more than 50 per cent in the frequency of spasms but none had complete disappearance.

Summary: role of new antiepileptic drugs in infantile spasms

Until recently, infantile spasms were one of the epilepsy syndromes with the most controversial treatment. Steroids were not unanimously considered to be first-line treatment because of their high toxicity. There were no convincing data about the type, dose and duration of therapy that should be used. Controlled studies were too few to draw definite conclusions, and even the control of spasms was subject to discussion, in terms of long-term mental outcome. Finally, treatment of infantile spasms was based on local protocols rather than scientifically-based schedules. There was a great need for novel innovative approaches.

It took a long time until childhood epilepsy was included in the strategy of development of new antiepileptic drugs. Guidelines specifically dedicated to this population were established in 1994.[59] However, controlled trials were especially difficult to initiate in infantile spasms. Interestingly, surgery appeared as a treatment for infantile spasms before new drugs. Focal cortical resection can control spasms caused by focal lesion,[42] as well as

hemipsherectomy for hemimegalencephaly.[60] Complete callosotomy may improve patients with multifocal lesions, provided that they have been operated on before the age of 10 years.[61]

Among the first 'new generation' drugs, vigabatrin provided a 'standard' development. In 1998, vigabatrin is close to being the consensus choice of first-line drug in the treatment of infantile spasms; this is based on excellent tolerance by patients and demonstrated efficacy, which are at least similar to those of steroids, although much more rapid. However, it must be borne in mind that experience is still limited (< 10 years, < 500 cases reported) and incomplete, making it difficult to answer the following questions:

- What is the specific vigabatrin efficacy according to the different aetiologies of infantile spasms apart from tuberous sclerosis?
- What are the right criteria for initial efficacy?
- What is the long-term efficacy in terms of epilepsy and mental outcome?
- Is prolonged monotherapy an advantage compared with add-on?
- How long should vigabatrin be continued if found to be either effective or ineffective?
- What about long-term tolerance?

On the other hand, infantile spasms that are refractory to vigabatrin and steroids do exist, thus justifying the development of other new drugs for this indication. Indeed, this population represents one of the most severe forms of childhood epilepsy with the most disappointing outcome. Therapeutics based on physiopathological hypothesis have not succeeded up to now, but they remain the only logical method for research. A surgical approach relies on such a strategy.

As a result of previous considerations, it is premature to establish any definite rules for current treatment of infantile spasms. Based on our own experience, the numerous discussions with colleagues and the review of literature, the following is proposed:

- Use vigabatrin as the first-line drug, at 50, 75, then 100 mg/kg per day if necessary, as monotherapy, for 2 weeks, whatever the aetiology of the infantile spasms.
- Conclude the initial efficacy at 15 days if the spasms have completely disappeared, as well as the spikes on an EEG. If this is the case, continue vigabatrin as monotherapy for at least 2 years. A benzodiazepine may need to be added to patients with tuberous sclerosis.
- If vigabatrin is ineffective, add steroids— oral steroids and then ACTH if necessary. Most aetiologies seem to benefit from this combination.

- For pharmacoresistant cases, use focal resection if possible, or other conventional treatments (valproate, benzodiazepines, vitamin B_6, etc.); then new drugs (lamotrigine, felbamate, ganaxolone, etc.) or ketogenic diet should be considered.

Vigabatrin represents a dramatic improvement in the therapy for infantile spasms and can now be advised as the first-line drug in this epilepsy syndrome. However, further data still need to be collected for rational optimization of the use of this new compound.

Acknowledgement

I am grateful to Professor O Dulac and Dr C Dumas for their advice.

References

1. Dulac O, Chugani HT, Dalla Bernardina B. *Infantile spasms and West syndrome.* London: WB Saunders, 1994.
2. Talwar D, Amora MS, Sher PK. EEG changes and seizure exacerbation in young children treated with carbamazepine. *Epilepsia* 1994;**35**: 1154–9.
3. Sorel L, Dusaucy-Bauloye A. A propos de 21 cas d'hypsarythmie de Gibbs. Son traitement spectaculaire par l'ACTH. *Acta Neurol Belg* 1985;**58**:130–41.
4. Watanabe K, Medical treatment of West syndrome in Japan. *J Child Neurol* 1995;**10**: 143–7.
5. Siemes H, Spohr HL, Michael T, Nau H. Therapy of infantile spasms with valproate: results of a prospective study. *Epilepsia* 1988;**29**:553–60.
6. Aicardi J. *Epilepsy in children.* New York: Raven Press, 1986:17–38.
7. Bachman D. Spontaneous remission of infantile spasms with hypsarrhythmia. *Arch Neurol* 1981;**38**:785 (letter).
8. Hrachovy RA, Glaze DG, Frost JP. A retrospective study of spontaneous remission and long-term outcome in patients with infantile spasms. *Epilepsia* 1991;**32**:212–14.
9. Dulac O, Schlumberger E. Treatment of West syndrome. In: Wyllie, E, ed. *The treatment of epilepsy: principles and practice.* Philadelphia: Lea & Feibiger, 1993:595–604.
10. Baram TZ, Mitchell WG, Tournay A, Snead OC, Hanson RA, Horton EJ. High dose corticotropin (ACTH) versus prednisone for infantile spasms: a prospective, randomized, blinded study. *Pediatrics* 1996;**97**:375–9.
11. Hrachovy RA, Frost JD, Kellaway P, Zion TE. Double-blind study of ACTH vs prednisone therapy in infantile spasms. *J Pediatr* 1983;641–5.
12. Schlumberger E, Dulac O. A simple, effective and well-tolerated regime for West syndrome. *Dev Med Child Neurol* 1994;**36**:863–72.

13. Riikonen R. Long-term outcome of West syndrome: a study of adults with a history of infantile spasms. *Epilepsia* 1996;**37**:367–72.

14. Riikonen R, Soderstrom S, Vanhala R, Ebendal T, Lindholm DB. West syndrome: cerebrospinal fluid, nerve growth factor and effect of ACTH. *Pediatr Neurol* 1997;**17**:224–9.

15. Maeda H, Furune S, Nomura K, et al. Decrease of *N*-acetylaspartate after ACTH therapy in patients with infantile spasms. *Neuropediatrics* 1997;**28**:262–7.

16. Dreifuss F, Farwell J, Holmes G, et al. Infantile spasms: comparative trial of nitrazepam and corticotropin. *Arch Neurol* 1986;**43**:1107–10.

17. Takuma Y, Seti T. Combination therapy of infantile spasms with high-dose pyridoxal phosphate and low-dose corticotropin. *J Child Neurol* 1996;**11**:35–40.

18. Gram L, Klosterskov P, Dam M. Gamma-vinyl-GABA: a double-blind placebo-controlled trial in partial epilepsy. *Ann Neurol* 1985;**17**:262–6.

19. Luna D, Dulac O, Pajot N, Beaumont D. Vigabatrin in the treatment of childhood epilepsies: a single-blind placebo-controlled study. *Epilepsia* 1989;**30**:430–7.

20. Livingston JH, Beaumont D, Arzimanoglou A, Aicardi J. Vigabatrin in the treatment of epilepsy in children. *Br J Clin Pharmacol* 1989;**27**:S109–12.

21. Chiron C, Dulac O, Beaumont D, Palacios L, Pajot N, Mumford J. Therapeutic trial of Vigabatrin in refractory infantile spasms. *J Child Neurol* 1991;**6**:S52–9.

22. Chiron C, Dulac O, Luna D, et al. Vigabatrin in infantile spasms. *Lancet* 1990;**335**:363–4 (letter).

23. Lopez-Valdes E, Hernandez-Lain A, Simon R, Porta J, Mateos F. Treatment of refractory infantile epilepsy with vigabatrin in a series of 55 patients. *Rev Neurol* 1996;**24**:1255–7.

24. Coppola G, Terraciano AM, Pascotto A. Vigabatrin as add-on therapy in children and adolescents with refractory epilepsy: an open trial. *Brain Dev* 1997;**19**:459–63.

25. Herranz JL, Sellers J, Viteri C, the spanish collaborative group (GABA 2000). Efficacy and tolerability of vigabatrin add-on therapy in 434 children with epilepsy. *Epilepsia* 1977;**38**:54 (abstract).

26. Hadac J, Siskova D, Slapal R, Misurcova H. The effect of vigabatrin therapy in epilepsy caused by tuberous sclerosis. *Epilepsia* 1997;**38**:101 (abstract).

27. Slapal R, Zouhar A, Misurkova H. Vigabatrin in the treatment of epileptic syndromes in children. *Epilepsia* 1997;**38**:99 (abstract).

28. Appleton RE, Monteil-Viecca F. Vigabatrin in infantile spasms. Why add-on? *Lancet* 1992;**341**:962 (letter).

29. Appleton RE. The role of vigabatrin in the management of infantile epileptic syndromes. *Neurology* 1993; S21–3.

30. Vles BI, Van Der Heyden AM, Ghijs A, Troost J. Vigabatrin in the treatment of infantile spasms. *Neuropediatrics* 1993;**24**:230–1.

31. Schmitt B, Wohlrab G, Bolthauser E. Vigabatrin in newly diagnosed infantile spasms. *Neuropediatrics* 1994;**25**:54 (letter).

32. Buti D, Rota M, Lini M, et al. First-line monotherapy with vigabatrin in infantile spasms: long term clinical and EEG evolution in 12 patients. *Epilepsia* 1995;**36**:S102 (abstract).

33. Granström ML, Gaily E, Lindhl E, et al. Vigabatrin as first drug in infantile spasms. *Epilepsia* 1995;**36**:S102 (abstract).

34. Kwong L. Vigabatrin as first line therapy in infantile spasms: review of seven patients. *J Pediatr Child Health* 1997;**33**:121–4.

35. Rufo M, Santiago C, Castro E, Ocana O. Monotherapy with vigabatrin in the treatment of West's syndrome. *Rev Neurol* 1997;**25**:1365–8.

36. Djuric M, Marjanovic B, Zamurovic D. Vigabatrin monotherapy in infantile spasms. *Epilepsia* 1997;**38**:129 (abstract).

37. Aicardi J, Sabril IS. Investigator and peer review groups, Mumford J, Dumas C, Wood S. Vigabatrin as initial therapy for infantile spasms: a European retrospective survey. *Epilepsia* 1996;**37**:638–42.

38. Chiron C, Dumas C, Jambaqué I, et al. Randomized trial comparing vigabatrin and hydrocortisone in infantile spasms due to tuberous sclerosis. *Epilepsy Res* 1997;**26**:389–95.

39. Vigevano F, Cilio MR. Vigabatrin versus ACTH as first-line treatment for infantile spasms: a randomized, prospective study. *Epilepsia* 1997;**38**:1270–4.

40. Peters AC, Appleton RE, Roi L, Thornton JL. Vigabatrin as first line monotherapy in newly

diagnosed infantile spasms: a placebo-controlled double-blind study. *Epilepsia* 1996;37:118 (abstract).

41. Lortie A, Chiron C, Dumas C, Mumford J, Dulac O. Optimizing the indication of vigabatrin in children with refractory epilepsy. *J Child Neurol* 1997;**12**:253–9.

42. Chugani HT, Shields WD, Shewmon DA, et al. Infantile spasms: PET identifies focal cortical dysgenesis in cryptogenic cases for surgical treatment. *Ann Neurol* 1990;**27**:406–13.

43. Donat JF, Wright FS. Simultaneous infantile spasms and partial seizures. *J Child Neurol* 1991;**6**:246–50.

44. Plouin P, Dulac O, Jalin C, Chiron C. Twenty-four-hour ambulatory EEG monitoring in infantile spasms. *Epilepsia* 1993;**34**:686–91.

45. Nabbout R, Chiron C, Mumford J, Dumas C, Dulac O. Vigabatrin in partial seizures in children. *J Child Neurol* 1997;**12**:172–7.

46. Villeneuve N, Soufflet C, Plouin P, et al. Treatment of infantile spasms with vigabatrin as first-line therapy and in monotherapy: apropos of 70 infants. *Arch Pediatr* 1998;**5**:731–8.

47. Zafeiriou DI, Kontopoulos EE, Tsikoulas IG. Adrenocorticotropic hormone and vigabatrin treatment of children with infantile spasms underlying cerebral palsy. *Brain Dev* 1996;**18**:450–2.

48. Villeneuve N, Dulac O, Chiron C, Dumas C. Vigabatrin in infantile spasms due to tuberous sclerosis. *Epilepsia* 1996;**37**:S4, 118 (abstract).

49. Hauw JJ, Trottier S, Boutry JM, Sun P, Sazdovitch V, Duyckaerts C. The neuropathology of vigabatrin. *Br J Clin Pract* 1988;**61**:S10–13.

50. Eke T, Talbot JF, Lawden MD. Severe persistent visual field constriction associated with vigabatrin. *BMJ* 1997;**314**:180–1.

51. Jambaqué I, Chiron C, Dumas C, Mumford J, Dulac O. Mental improvement following control of infantile spasms by vigabatrin in tuberous sclerosis patients.

52. Veggiotti P, Cieuta C, Rey E, Dulac O. Lamotrigine in infantile spasms. *Lancet* 1994;**44**:1375–6 (letter).

53. Hurst DL, Rolan TD. The use of felbamate to treat infantile spasms. *J Child Neurol* 1995;**10**:134–6.

54. Coppola G, Pascotto A. Felbamate in refractory infantile spasms. *Epilepsia* 1997;**38**:37 (abstract).

55. Soufflet C, Villeneuve N, Monaghan E, Dulac O. Etude préliminaire de l'action du ganaxolone sur 23 enfants. *Arch Fr Pediatr* (abstract) (in press).

56. Freeman JM, Vining EP. Ketogenic diet: a time-tested, effective, and safe method for treatment of intractable childhood epilepsy. *Epilepsia* 1998;**39**:450–1.

57. Swink T, Vining E, Casey, et al. Efficacy of the ketogenic diet in children under 2 years of age. *Epilepsia* 1997;**38**:26 (abstract).

58. Villeneuve N, Pinton F, Heron B, et al. Régime cétogène dans les épilepsies rebelles: à propos de 32 patients. *Arch Fr Pediatr* (abstract) (in press).

59. Commission on Antiepileptic Drugs of the International League against Epilepsy. Guidelines for antiepileptic drug trials in children. *Epilepsia* 1994;**35**:94–100.

60. Vigevano F, Bertini E, Boldrini, et al. Hemimegalencephaly and intractable epilepsy: benefits of hemispherectomy. *Epilepsia* 1989;**30**:833–43.

61. Pinard JM, Delalande O, Plouin P, Dulac O. Callosotomy in West syndrome suggests a cortical origin of hypsarrhythmia. *Epilepsia* 1993;**34**:780–7.

28

Intractable myoclonic absences

Olivier Dulac and Anna Kaminska

Introduction

Myoclonic absences are one type of absence seizure in which loss of contact is combined with bilateral rhythmic jerks of the limbs.[1,2] Intractability to common anti-absence drugs is usual, because it affects approximately 50 per cent of cases, and has severe consequences as it is combined with mental disability. In intractable cases, proper identification of the epilepsy syndrome is the first step, preceding optimization of drug treatment.

Definition of myoclonic absences

As a seizure type

Myoclonic absences consist of rhythmic jerks of the limbs, predominantly in the upper limbs, which involve mainly the shoulders and arms, and less frequently the lower limbs, with hypertonia and which last from 10–60 s.[3] Perioral jerks are frequent but eyelid myoclonus is very unusual. Impairment of consciousness is variable and the patient remains aware of the limb movements. He or she often tries to control the jerks with voluntary movements, which could appear as automatisms, such as lacing up the shoes. Jerks may be asymmetrical or unilateral, and are often precipitated by hyperventilation, although photosensitivity is rare.

Polygraphic recording shows bilateral and symmetrical spike and slow-wave discharges, which, at first sight, look like pyknoleptic absence. However, the recording most often comprises a series of polyspikes, each followed by a slow wave. The myographic recording shows that the jerk is linked to the first, negative component of the polyspike, whereas the second component of the polyspike is linked to an inhibitory motor phenomenon that produces negative myoclonus. Thus, each myoclonic jerk comprises a brief jerk followed by a drop of the affected limb.[4]

As a specific epilepsy syndrome (myoclonic absence epilepsy)

Myoclonic absences are the predominant seizure type of myoclonic absence epilepsy, although two thirds of the patients exhibit other kinds of generalized seizures, including typical absences, tonic–clonic seizures and drop attacks. Neurological examination is normal, but 45 per cent of the patients are mentally disabled at onset and another 25 per cent develop mental disability during the course of the disease; most of these are patients with intractable myoclonic absence epilepsy. Onset ranges from 1–12 years (mean 7), and myoclonic absence epilepsy is more frequent than childhood absence epilepsy during the second year of life.[5] There is male predominance (69 per cent) and the family history of epilepsy (19 per cent) is clearly less frequent than in childhood absence epilepsy. The disorder remits in half the cases, after a mean course of 5.5 years, but in the remaining cases it persists for over two decades.[3] Thus, some patients meet the characteristics of idiopathic generalized epilepsy, whereas others have cryptogenic or symptomatic characteristics.

Differential diagnosis of myoclonic absence epilepsy

Absences with rhythmic jerks of the limbs may occur in a number of generalized epilepsies of childhood.

Childhood or juvenile absence epilepsies

The confusion with myoclonic absences is possible only when there is an important myoclonic component. The occurrence of jerks in the eyes and upper eyelids is a common event, affecting over 80 per cent of patients studied with video-EEG, but it does rarely affect the upper limbs.[6] Stefan et al[6] have shown that, in this case, the latency to involvement of the eyelids is the shortest, followed by the face and then the limbs; this is not the case with myoclonic absences, in which involvement of the limbs starts at the onset of the seizure, and the intensity of the jerks is more prominent.

Perioral myoclonus with absences

This syndrome, with onset in childhood or adolescence, comprises jerks of the mouth and jaws.[7] There is a higher risk of developing absence status and generalized tonic–clonic seizures.

Continuous spike waves in slow sleep

The absences comprise jerks of the upper limbs, but these jerks are the result of atonia, and therefore negative myoclonus, not of classic myoclonus. In addition to absences, there are one or several foci of slow-spike waves. As soon as the patient falls asleep, in slow-wave sleep, the tracing shows continuous spikes and slow-wave activity.[8] It has been shown that, when the focus affects the rolandic area, there is negative myoclonus as a result of intermittent loss of tone, which looks like clusters of jerks.[9] This requires benzodiazepine, monotherapy or combination with steroid treatment, which produces a high incidence of positive response.

Lennox–Gastaut syndrome

The onset is also between the ages of 2 and 8 years, and atonic absences comprise eventual raising of the upper limbs, because of the tonic axial component, which may predominate in the upper limbs.[10] However, tonic axial seizures occur when falling asleep, and an interictal EEG shows slow spike–wave activity when awake and bursts of polyspike waves in sleep. Nevertheless, almost 10 per cent of myoclonic absence epilepsy may evolve to Lennox–Gastaut syndrome.[3]

Myoclonic–astatic epilepsy

This may be particularly difficult to distinguish from myoclonic absence epilepsy because of the age of onset—between 2 and 5 years—and the combination of absences with myoclonus. However, mental development is normal before the first seizures in myoclonic–astatic epilepsy and there are tonic–clonic seizures over a few weeks or months before the occurrence of absences.[11] In addition, there are drop attacks, caused by massive myoclonus, by the time the patient exhibits absences.

Juvenile myoclonic epilepsy

Here, also, the jerks are rhythmic and occur in clusters, although the clusters are brief, lasting 1–2 s without loss of consciousness; the EEG shows variable amplitude of spike activity within a burst, and frequent photosensitivity.[12] In addition, although cases with onset in childhood have been reported,[9] this is a rare event.

Late-onset infantile spasms

Jerks and intermittent loss of consciousness are characteristic of this condition, which may start after the end of the first year of life, up to 4 years of age.[13] Drop attacks are often caused by the spasms. The interictal EEG shows long runs of irregular spikes and slow-wave activity, which are increased and more synchronous during sleep. Polygraphic recording of ictal events is necessary to identify the seizures as being epileptic spasms. Although a small proportion of patients responds to vigabatrin or lamotrigine, most of them require steroid therapy and half the patients remain intractable to conventional treatment. Cognitive impairment mainly affects speech and interpersonal contact, which improves when seizures are controlled.

Treatment of myoclonic absence epilepsy

Many antiepileptic drugs should not be administered to patients with myoclonic absences because they may increase the frequency and severity of the seizures: carbamazepine, phenytoin, phenobarbitone, vigabatrin and gabapentin.[14] About half the patients respond to valproate, ethosuximide or lamotrigine, as monotherapy or in combination.[3,15,16]

In the other cases for which it is not possible to obtain complete seizure freedom, optimization of the effect of drugs must be the aim. Too high a dose of medication may produce a paradoxical effect, with an increase in seizure frequency that is probably related to drug-induced alteration of vigilance.[14] From this perspective, the interaction of drugs must be kept in mind. The interaction may be pharmacokinetic, as with the combination of valproate and ethosuximide in which the blood levels of the latter are increased by valproate.[17] Therefore, the ethosuximide dose should be reduced by half when combined with valproate. The interaction may be both pharmacokinetic and pharmacodynamic, as with the combination of lamotrigine and valproate.[18] In the latter, lamotrigine should be introduced particularly slowly in order to prevent skin rash and the pharmacodynamic interaction that increases the incidence and severity of side effects, particularly tremor, which is increased by this combination.[18]

In case of pharmacoresistance, mildly effective drugs, such as epidione and benzodiazepines, may be tried although the response rate is very low. No clinically relevant effect has been obtained with steroids. The potential effect or ketogenic diet, vagal nerve stimulation or other surgical procedures, or new antiepileptic drugs such as topiramate or remacemide, has not been evaluated to date. Keeping the patient in a mentally active condition contributes to a reduction in the frequency of seizures.

Summary

Myoclonic absences are clearly distinct from typical absences because they often occur in the context of pharmacoresistant epilepsy. Although the limited number of patients who respond to drug treatment do so with the very drugs that are most effective in typical absences, this does not indicate that the mechanisms and neurophysiological pathways involved are the same as in typical absences. In fact, the mechanism that determines intractability remains unclear, but the neurophysiological background appears to be distinct because polygraphic recordings show a distinct pattern. There is a clear need for further research in this field, particularly with regard to the areas of the brain that are most affected by the discharge. In addition, it still needs to be determined whether the syndrome is single or a combination of different conditions that respond differently to treatment.

References

1. Roger J, Bureau M, Dravet C, Dreifuss FE, Perret A, Wolf P. *Epileptic syndromes in infancy, childhood and adolescence*, 2nd edn. London: John Libbey, 1992.

2. Commission on Classification and Terminology of the International League Against Epilepsy. Proposal for revised classification of epilepsies and epileptic syndromes. *Epilepsia* 1989; 30:389–99.

3. Tassinari CA, Bureau M, Thomas P. Epilepsy with myoclonic absences. In: Roger J et al, ed. *Epileptic syndromes in infancy, childhood and adolescence*. London: J Libbey, 1992:151-60.

4. Tassinari CA. Myoclonus and epilepsy in childhood. 1996 Royaumont meeting. *Epilepsy Res* 1998;30:91–106.

5. Aicardi J. Typical absences in the first two years of life. In: Duncan JS, Panayiotopoulos CP, eds. *Typical absences and related epileptic syndromes*. London: Churchill Livingstone, 1995:338–43.

6. Stefan H, Burr W, Hildenbrand K, Penin H. Basic temporal structure of absence symptoms. In: Akimoto H, Kazamatsuri H, Seino MD, Ward A, eds. *Advances in epileptology: the XIIIth Epilepsy International Symposium*. New York: Raven Press, 1982:55–60.

7. Panayiotopoulos CP, Obeid T, Waheed G. Differentiation of typical absences in epileptic syndromes: a video-EEG study of 224 seizures in 20 patients. *Brain* 1989;112:1039–56.

8. Patry G, Lyagoubi S, Tassinari CA. Subclinical 'electric status epilepticus' induced by sleep in children. *Arch Neurol* 4:242–52.

9. Guerrini R, Dravet C, Genton P, et al. Epileptic negative myoclonus. *Neurology* 1993;43:1078–83.

10. Niedermeyer E, Degen R, eds. *The Lennox–Gastaut syndrome*. New York: Alan R Liss Inc, 1988.

11. Doose H, Gerken H, Leonhardt R, Voltzke E, Colz C. Centrencephalic myoclonic–astatic petit mal. *Neuropediatrics* 1970;2:59–78.

12. Janz D. Epilepsy with impulsive petit mal (juvenile myoclonic epilepsy). *Act Neurol Scand* 1985;72:439–59.

13. Bednarek N, Motte J, Plouin P, Soufflet C, Dulac O. Evidence for late onset infantile spasms. *Epilepsia* 1988;39:55–60.

14. Perucca E, Gram L, Avanzini G, Dulac O. Antiepileptic drugs as a cause of worsening of seizures. *Epilepsia* 1998;39:5–17.

15. Manonmain V, Wallace SJ. Epilepsy with myoclonic absences. *Arch Dis Child* 1994;70: 288–90.

16. Schlumberger E, Chavez F, Palacios L, Rey E, Pajot N, Dulac O. Lamotrigine in treatment of 120 children with epilepsy. *Epilepsia* 1994; 35:359–67.

17. Sato S, White BG, Penry JK et al. Valproic acid versus ethosuximide in the treatment of absence seizures. *Neurology* 1982;32:157–63.

18. Panayiotopoulos CP, Ferrie CD, Knott C, Robinson RO. Interaction of lamotrigine and sodium valproate. *Lancet* 1993;i:445.

IX
PROGNOSIS OF EPILEPSY

29

Long-term prognosis of epilepsy

Josemir WAS Sander and Deb K Pal

Introduction

The epilepsies are a heterogeneous group of disorders, often grouped under the single rubric of 'epilepsy'. Epilepsy is now regarded as a condition in which the majority of patients will achieve long-term remission with treatment. This view contrasts with the pessimism with which epilepsy was described for much of the 19th and 20th centuries,[1,2] and which is still expressed by many patients and families at the mention of the diagnosis. Physicians treating epilepsy are often asked to predict prognosis and make decisions about commencing and withdrawing treatment. Practice can be guided by epidemiological studies of prognosis and the recent advances in syndrome classification. Our understanding now is that prognosis depends largely on the aetiology of the seizures and the clinical background of the patient rather than on the seizures themselves or the treatment prescribed.[3] Psychosocial aspects of the disorder frequently have the most far-reaching implications for the patient and family, and these should be borne in mind when planning comprehensive management.

This chapter considers the prognosis of epilepsy in terms of seizure remission, psychosocial adjustment and mortality, and the influence of antiepileptic drug (AED) treatment. Causes of death, status epilepticus and prognosis after epilepsy surgery are dealt with in separate chapters.

Syndromic approach

The separation of benign epilepsy syndromes with good outcome, and malignant syndromes in which there is strong evidence of cognitive deterioration, coincident with a severe phase of the epilepsy, has arisen from paediatric studies.[4] Syndromes are generally based on age and clinical phenomenology; therefore prognosis can largely be inferred from syndrome classification. Epilepsy is also a common concomitant of acute and chronic brain syndromes, in which the underlying pathology may be static or progressive. Indications for surgical treatment are increasing the options available for intractable epilepsy and thereby alter the prognosis for patients in this group.

Benign syndromes

The benign syndromes are usually age-limited, stereotyped, often provoked or provokable and occur in otherwise normal children. Genetic predisposition is common. Many seizure disorders do not fit a syndrome classification, but the prognostic features in Table 29.1 may be used to predict outcome.[5]

Rolandic epilepsy

Rolandic epilepsy is the most common benign epileptic syndrome. Benign epilepsy with Rolandic (centrotemporal) interictal foci has an onset between 2 and 12 years, most commonly

Good outcome	Adverse outcome
Single seizure type	Multiple seizure types
No additional impairment	Additional neurological impairment (especially cognitive)
Late age at onset (for the syndrome)	Early age at onset (for the syndrome)
Provoked	Unprovoked
Short seizures	Status epilepticus
Low frequency of seizures	High frequency of seizures
Good initial response to AEDs	Poor initial response to AEDs; polytherapy required

From Neville (1997)[5]

Table 29.1
Prognostic factors for epilepsy outcome.

between 7 and 10 years, and remits by 14 years.[6] About 30 per cent of patients have a family history of epilepsy. The children are free of major impairments, but may have neuropsychological deficits.[7] Further investigation is indicated if there are features predictive of poor outcome (Table 29.1). Only 2 per cent of patients with benign partial epilepsies (Rolandic or occipital) develop chronic epilepsy.

Occipital epilepsy

Some children with typical partial seizures with visual phenomena, post-ictal headache and migrainous characteristics have a benign prognosis, but others have a poorer cognitive and seizure outcome, and some have lesions.[8,9] The features in Table 29.1 should be used as a guide to prognosis.

Absence epilepsy

The absence epilepsies are uncommon in the general population, representing only 1–2 per cent of all epilepsies. The prognosis of childhood absence epilepsy is ~80 per cent for seizure remission with treatment, and most favourable with a late age of onset and in the absence of generalized tonic–clonic seizures (GTCS).[10,11] Phenytoin, carbamazepine and vigabatrin are unhelpful or may aggravate the condition, particularly myoclonic absence seizures. The risk of tonic–clonic seizures in adult life can be predicted from past history of tonic–clonic seizures, an IQ of <90, and a family history of seizures. Ten per cent of those with none or one adverse factor continue to have absence seizures, with all of those having three adverse features going on to have GTCS.[10] Absence seizures can be a benign self-limiting condition or form part of a malignant syndrome of multiple seizure types, e.g. the Lennox-Gastaut syndrome.

Febrile convulsions

Febrile convulsions are often considered to be a special group, separate from the benign syndromes, although sharing many characteristics. Febrile convulsions are epileptic seizures provoked by fever of extracranial origin and occur in at least 3 per cent of children, mainly between the ages of 6 months and 5 years. The seizures are usually brief, bilateral clonic, or tonic–clonic attacks. The risk of a second febrile seizure is ~34 per cent.[12] The risk of a third febrile convulsion after a second is ~50 per cent.[13] Risk factors for a second or subsequent febrile convulsion include young age at the first febrile convulsion and a family history of febrile convulsions. About 10 per cent of children with febrile seizures have complex, focal, or prolonged seizures requiring emergency treatment for status epilepticus. Severe sequelae of febrile status, such as hemiplegia, are now uncommon because of modern medical treatment. Overall, 2–7 per cent of children with febrile convulsions go on to have an unprovoked seizure in childhood or early adult life; their risk is therefore at least four times that of the rest of the population.[14–17] A family history of epilepsy, complex febrile convulsions and prior neurological abnormality are associated with an increased risk of subsequent epilepsy.

Prophylaxis of febrile convulsions has been a controversial topic over the past 20 years. Both phenobarbitone and sodium valproate have been shown to have preventive effects in a meta-analysis of available studies, but side effects outweigh the benefits in this generally benign condition.[18] Other drugs have been used, but the most popular treatment in many countries is rectal diazepam given at the time of a recurrence. Many convulsions herald the onset of a febrile illness and so cannot be prevented by antipyretic measures. Investigation into causes of recurrent infection may be indicated, and alternative diagnoses such as severe polymorphic epilepsy of infancy should also be considered if development is abnormal and there are many seizures. Febrile convulsions and epilepsy are epidemiologically distinct syndromes and there is no evidence to suggest that treating febrile convulsions with AEDs prevents the onset of subsequent epilepsy.[19]

Malignant syndromes

Although developmental arrest and regression as a consequence of malignant syndromes of epilepsy are common, it is essential to consider metabolic, degenerative and structural brain diseases. Cerebral malformations (including migrational disorders and neurocutaneous syndromes) are particularly associated with a poor prognosis for seizure control, except in cases where surgical options are available. Metabolic causes of epilepsy are often fatal, and seizures may be intractable. Progressive myoclonic epilepsies include Lafora's disease, Unverricht-Lundeborg disease and mitochondrial disorders, which have a uniformly poor prognosis for seizure control, and a variable pace of degeneration.

Infantile spasms

West's syndrome is symptomatic of many static cortical diseases, with only 10 per cent being truly idiopathic or cryptogenic. Traditionally, treatment has been with steroids—adrenocorticotrophic hormone (ACTH) or prednisolone—but recent studies have shown vigabatrin to be effective, with about 50 per cent of infants becoming seizure-free, the best response occurring in those patients younger than 3 months at onset or with tuberous sclerosis.[20] Twenty-two per cent went on to have other types of seizures and 21 per cent of responders had recurrence of infantile spasms. Comparison with conventional steroid treatment is favourable in terms of both efficacy and side effects.[21] The overall mortality of treated West's syndrome is 20 per cent, with 30–50 per cent developing cerebral palsy, and cognitive impairment in up to 85 per cent.[22] Outcome varies according to pathology: cognitive and social disorders (frequently autism) are more common in children with tuberous sclerosis. Hypoxic-ischaemic damage and metabolic disorders are aetiologies that are also associated with a poor developmental and seizure prognosis. Type I neurofibromatosis is one of the few symptomatic forms with a favourable prognosis. In contrast, 50 per cent of patients with cryptogenic West's syndrome may go on to have normal development. Most infants with unprovoked seizure disorders in the first year of life, whether they have West's syndrome or not, have a poor developmental outcome.[23]

Lennox-Gastaut syndrome

It is likely that Lennox-Gastaut syndrome (LGS) represents a final common pathway for several diverse pathologies. Prognosis for seizure control (80 per cent continue to have seizures) and development (80–90 per cent with developmental delay) are overall poor, although slightly better in idiopathic cases.[24] Half of all affected children have primary developmental delay, and all have learning difficulties after 5 or more years of the condition. The short-term mortality is estimated as 4–7 per cent, partly as a result of tonic status.[25] Only about 10 per cent have a reasonable chance of independent living. Preceding infantile spasms or abnormalities on neuroimaging are associated with poorer prognosis.[26] Seizures are often refractory to AEDs, and benzodiazepines, corticosteroids and a ketogenic diet are often used. Drug intoxication may contribute to the disability. Episodes of non-convulsive status complicate the clinical course. Occasionally, palliative callosotomy may reduce the frequency of severe drop attacks that cause sudden falls and head injury.

Severe myoclonic epilepsy of childhood

This syndrome often begins at 4–10 months, often with a prolonged partial clonic seizure associated with moderate fever. Later attacks, in the second or third year of life, are of multiple seizure types, including complex absences, myoclonias, complex partial seizures and apnoeic attacks, and developmental regression accompanies this phase.[27] Most children eventually are severely or moderately retarded, often with attention deficit and hyperactivity.[28] Most patients develop mild motor problems of myoclonus, ataxia, and pyramidal signs. Myoclonic attacks disappear in 4–7 years, but generalized tonic–clonic, alternating clonic, or complex partial seizures persist. At least 16 per cent of patients die in the first decade, and the ability to live independently is rare.[29]

Partial seizures of lesional origin

Partial seizures of lesional origin may be static or progressive. Static disorders include vascular and traumatic pathologies and some benign tumours. Cavernous angiomas and arteriovenous malformations respond well to surgical removal, but less discrete, early onset lesions may be associated with motor impairment and intractable partial seizures. The long-term prognosis for patients with temporal lobe epilepsy due to lesions is of one third achieving remission, one third with continuing functional impairments and one third being completely dependent.[30] A mortality of 0.5 per cent per annum occurs.[31] Adverse prognostic features can be identified early and justify surgery in childhood. Young children with developmental tumours of the temporal lobe may present with cognitive and autistic regression, which may respond to surgery.[32] Rasmussen's syndrome is a progressive intractable partial epilepsy syndrome with cognitive deterioration, aphasia, and hemiplegia, for which medical treatment with immunoglobulins or steroids is disappointing[33] and early surgery is the only treatment modality leading to a chance of long-term freedom from seizures.[34]

Landau–Kleffner syndrome (LKS)

LKS is uncommon. Typically, partial or generalized seizures (including atypical absences) begin and language comprehension and speech are lost after 2 or more years of normal development. The range of impairments includes behavioural disorders and global cognitive, motor and social regression with many autistic features, sometimes without clinical seizures.[35] Although AEDs may reduce seizures and electro-encephalogram (EEG) abnormalities, the prognosis for aphasia and cognitive deficit is more pessimistic, often with little response to AEDs. High doses of sodium valproate, often in combination with lamotrigine, are sometimes helpful. A clinically significant, sometimes dramatic, response to steroids can occur, but problems with side effects and long-term dependency may arise. The preliminary results of multiple subpial transections suggest that about half of those patients with clear evidence of a driving hemisphere can be helped.[36]

Recurrence after first seizure

Most people experiencing an initial seizure will go on to develop epilepsy. A large population-based study showed that 60 per cent of patients had a recurrence within 6 months, 67 per cent within 12 months and 78 per cent within 36 months.[37] Most recurrences occur within the first 3 months and the risk of a second seizure declines as time passes.[3,38] In both adults and children, first seizures in sleep are more likely to recur than first seizures during the daytime.[39,40] Recurrence also depends on the type of seizure, the presence of underlying pathology and the age of the patient. For example, absence seizures are not usually isolated and complex partial seizures usually have a chronic course.[41–43] Risk factors for recurrence are summarized below.

Risk factors

Aetiology

The underlying cause of a seizure is probably the most important determinant of recurrence risk, but this has not been formally tested for most of the epilepsy syndromes. Seizures associated with a postnatally acquired central nervous system (CNS) lesion are more likely to recur compared with idiopathic seizures.[43,44] Recurrence is more likely to occur (100 per cent) in children with neurological deficit presumed present at birth (e.g. cerebral palsy or severe mental retardation), 75 per cent for remote symptomatic seizures and 40 per cent for acute symptomatic seizures.[37] Seizures of idiopathic origin have a 69 per cent recurrence risk after 12 months.

Head injury

Recurrent seizures after head injury depend on the severity of the trauma and the presence of complications, including prolonged loss of consciousness, post-traumatic amnesia, intracranial haemorrhage and dural tear or skull fracture.[45] Seizures following mild head injury (amnesia or loss of consciousness for <30 min, and no skull fracture) carry a 2 per cent risk of recurrence. Risk for recurrence following moderate head injury (non-depressed skull fracture, or loss of consciousness or amnesia lasting from 30 min to 24 h) is 2–5 per cent. Severe head injury (intracranial haemorrhage, brain contusion, dural tear, unconsciousness or amnesia lasting <24 h) increases the risk to 12–15 per cent. The highest risk occurs for patients with penetrating head injury (50 per cent).[46] Seizures immediately following the injury or in the first week do not necessarily lead to chronic epilepsy.[47]

Intracranial infection

Postnatal meningitis, encephalitis or brain abscess all increase the risk of chronic seizures by three-to-ten-fold, depending on the severity of infection, extent of damage and age at which infection occurs.[48]

Family history

Family history is often assumed to increase the risk of seizure recurrence, but the evidence is conflicting, probably because ascertainment of family history can be difficult or unreliable.[39,41–43,49]

Usefulness of EEG

The EEG does not reliably predict relapse after a first seizure, although some studies suggest that the risk of recurrence is higher in those with clear-cut EEG abnormalities.[41,50,51]

Treatment and chronicity

AED treatment

There are few placebo-controlled trials to justify much of the use of AEDs in epilepsy. Thus arguments about whether to start treatment after the first, second or third seizure are based on convention rather than evidence. Two studies have shown an increased risk of recurrence in patients not treated after the first seizure compared with those treated.[37,52] In one trial, the risk was 2.5 times that in the untreated group (95 per cent CI: 1.9–4.2), in the other, respective recurrence rates were 57 per cent versus 78 per cent at 36 months. However, there is no evidence that early treatment leads to earlier remission.[53,54] AEDs can prevent seizures in acute encephalopathies, prevent the recurrence of febrile convulsions and can control seizures, but there is no evidence that they prevent the development of chronic epilepsy. They may, however, improve cognitive function in certain epilepsy syndromes, and change the quality of life of people with epilepsy.[55]

Natural history of treated epilepsy

Most studies of the treatment of newly diagnosed epilepsy have reported 1-year remission rates of 65–80 per cent.[38,56–59] The prognosis for seizure remission is not as good for pure partial seizures (16–43 per cent at 1 year) as it is for secondarily generalized seizures (48–53 per cent).[60] Similarly, seizure remission is less probable in patients with multiple seizure types or associated neurological impairments.[3,38] The most important predictors of remission are aetiology and syndrome type, although many studies of remission have not used syndromic classification. Large population-based studies have shown that the likelihood of remission is greatest in the first 2 years, thereafter the probability diminishes.[58,61] A further large-scale study has shown that age and seizure type have little effect on the chance of 5-year remission, although patients with acute and remote symptomatic epilepsies were more likely to die prematurely.[62] There is no evidence that any one particular first-line AED in monotherapy is associated with a superior seizure outcome.[3,63] In a Canadian population-based study, about 17 per cent of children treated with a first-line AED in monotherapy had inadequate seizure control, and 42 per cent of them achieved control with a second AED.[64] Complex partial seizures and neurological impairments were associated with less favourable response to the first AED. It would seem logical therefore to use the natural history of the epilepsy syndrome, or the presence of adverse clinical features, to guide the decision to commence and finally withdraw treatment.

Risk of relapse after AED withdrawal

Most patients with epilepsy treated with AEDs eventually become seizure-free, and it is common clinical practice to consider discontinuing drugs after a substantial remission period. Withdrawal in itself carries a risk of relapse, reportedly lower in children than in adults.[65] Large studies of AED withdrawal indicate that the risk for relapse is greatest in the first 2 years after discontinuing medication, but is actually greater in those continuing medication in the period after that, although this may be due to voluntary withdrawal of medication.[66] Risk factors for seizure recurrence after discontinuing therapy include a long history of seizures before remission, occurrence of more than one seizure type, presence of cerebral impairment, past history of remission or relapse and diagnosis of juvenile myoclonic epilepsy (JME). Patients with remote symptomatic seizures or an abnormal EEG pattern are more likely to relapse.[65] Relapse is usually easily controlled by reinstituting previously effective treatment.[67]

Predictors of intractability

Intractability is not an absolute phenomenon, and some patients are inadequately treated.[68] Some patients labelled as having chronic epilepsy do not in fact have epilepsy (e.g. pseudoseizures). However, when these reasons are discounted, about 20–30 per cent of patients with epilepsy do not enter remission, and still others are resistant to surgical treatment.[58,62] The inherently poor prognosis for remission in Lennox-Gastaut syndrome and polymorphic epilepsy of infancy is well recognized. Only a small fraction of patients with intractable epilepsy will be rendered seizure-free by adjunctive treatment with vigabatrin, lamotrigine, gabapentin or felbamate.[69] Risk factors for intractability in childhood include infantile spasms, age at onset (a decreasing risk with increasing age), remote symptomatic epilepsy and a history of status epilepticus

either before or after a diagnosis of epilepsy has been made.[70]

Co-morbidity

People with epilepsy are less physically fit than healthy counterparts, participate less often in regular sports and have higher body fat ratios.[71] Overprotective attitudes, as well as insufficient knowledge on the part of sports instructors and health professionals were believed to be contributory in a German study. Somatic diseases are no more common in young adult survivors of childhood onset epilepsy alone than in the general population, but the risk of psychiatric and psychosomatic disorders (e.g. neck and back pains, insomnia) is three-to-four times higher in young adults with childhood onset epilepsy and no other impairments.[72] Heart diseases, diabetes mellitus and asthma were recorded more often in these cohort members dying prematurely than in the general population.

Mortality

People with epilepsy have a higher mortality than the rest of the population, in contrast to the common perception of epilepsy as a condition with a relatively low mortality rate. The standardized mortality rate (SMR) can be between two and three times higher than the general population, and in a retrospective community study was maximum in the year after diagnosis,[73] suggesting an effect of the underlying pathology (e.g. brain tumours, head injury, strokes). However, the SMR was raised (overall 2.4, in the first year after diagnosis 3.5) even in people with cryptogenic epilepsy, as confirmed in a large British population-based cohort.[74] Mortality seems to be greatest in the period around diagnosis, declining thereafter, and consistently higher in males.

Symptomatic epilepsy carries a higher mortality, as do myoclonic and other severe or chronic epilepsies.[73,75] Chapter 30 discusses the causes and mechanisms of death in patients with epilepsy.

Psychosocial outcome

Social adjustment

Children with epilepsy seem to have more difficulty in social adjustment and more behavioural problems than children with other chronic disorders.[76–78] As they grow to become adults, even children with epilepsy but without additional impairments face disadvantages in education, employability and marriage. They more often feel a loss of control over, and dissatisfaction with their lives—more commonly if their epilepsy continues to be active or they are on polytherapy.[79] Cognitive limitations and behavioural problems have a major effect on social and educational success, but family and socio-cultural factors are increasingly recognized as dominant influences.[80,81] The relationship between behavioural and emotional problems, seizure control and family factors can be complex.[82,83] Parent–child relationships are important predictors of behavioural problems and social adjustment in children with epilepsy, even when biological factors have been taken into account.[84,85] For example, parental overprotection, low expectations and inconsistent behavioural management are common.[86] Maternal ratings of family stress and feelings of parental mastery independently predict behavioural problems in children with epilepsy.[83] Parental overprotection and lowered expectations from parents and teachers may have a negative impact on behaviour, performance and self-perception.[87,88] In turn, poor self-esteem may lead to educational underachievement. Parental perceptions of their child's health, their expectations for them and their positive handling have been shown to be important predictors of social adjustment.[89] Self-perceived seizure severity is important in predicting psychosocial functioning in adults with epilepsy.[90] The implications of these studies are therefore that parental adjustment reactions at the time of diagnosis are predictive of adverse psychosocial consequences for their child with epilepsy.

Education

Children with epilepsy as a group have lower academic achievements and qualifications than their peers because of learning difficulties and behavioural problems,[91] and this undoubtedly contributes to employment disadvantage. About 30 per cent of children with epilepsy are in special schools.[92,93] Epilepsy may be associated with specific neuropsychological problems in information processing and occasional cognitive decline,[94] and temporal lobe epilepsy with hippocampal damage has often been associated with specific cognitive problems involving memory. Such deficits may be exacerbated by AED treatment, especially polytherapy.[95] Stasis in learning has been associated with phenobarbital in febrile convulsions, but is not convincingly demonstrated for other AEDs.[96] Reading skills and attention may be impaired by phenytoin.[97] Few newer AEDs have been systematically studied for their effects on cognition in children.

Employment

Most people with active epilepsy are able to work, but employment chances are affected by a lower overall level of qualifications, negative self-perceptions, discrimination among employers and public prejudice. Of all patients with epilepsy, a higher rate than the general population are unemployed or receiving state benefits.[98,99] However, a high proportion of people with well-controlled epilepsy are employed. In a British study, of those who were not employed, few attributed this to their epilepsy, although a third of the whole sample felt that their epilepsy affected their ability to gain employment.[100] Good seizure control, good experiences with work colleagues and management and the perception that epilepsy has little effect on job prospects are all related to good employability.[101] Only 11 per cent of people with severe uncontrolled epilepsy, some with associated neurological impairment, were employed in the open labour market, and only 47 per cent reported past employment.[102] In general, however, people with epilepsy are probably employed below their potential, with resultant low socio-economic status. A Finnish study showed that only 1 per cent of people with epilepsy in work were employers, 7 per cent were self-employed, 27 per cent were employees and 65 per cent were manual workers.[103] Fear of stigma in employment was reported by 69 per cent of people with newly diagnosed epilepsy, and this was related to the severity of the seizure disorder.[104] Prospective employers may be unaware of the employment problems faced by people with epilepsy, or through the absence of defined policy, allow individual line managers to actively discriminate against them.[105,106] In Denmark, for example, 7 per cent of the general public had objections to equal employment for people with epilepsy, and half of the full-time employees with epilepsy in the UK reported discrimination in the workplace.[107] In fact, it is a common fallacy that people having epileptic seizures are more prone to cause accidents in the workplace.[108] Principles for good employment practice are available in many countries,[109] and there is some support for the positive effect of changing attitudes on employment patterns.[110] Legislative protection has been put into place in the US (the Americans with Disabilities Act) to provide clear guidance for employers and workers regarding rights and responsibilities in the workplace.[111] In summary, mild or no impairments, good seizure control, strong qualifications, appropriate employment training, and a combination of public awareness, positive employer attitudes and supportive legislation offer the best chances for the person with epilepsy seeking a job.

Summary

Modern population-based epidemiological studies have contributed significantly to our knowledge of prognosis of the epilepsies. Most people with epilepsy will enter long-term remission. The delineation of epilepsy syndromes allows a more specific prediction of outcome, associated problems and need for treatment. Adverse prognostic factors are known for epilepsies that cannot be classified into syndromes. Associated cognitive impairments usually signify poor outcome for seizure, developmental and social outcomes. The indications for early surgery are increasing quickly, and this will undoubtedly alter the prognosis for many patients in intractable groups for whom historically the outlook has been grave. Early life predictors of social adjustment and educational success have also been identified and, with appropriate intervention, should lead to timely assessment and intervention to prevent psychosocial complications which could otherwise have pervasive damaging effects on personality and livelihood. Premature mortality in epilepsy has recently been recognized, but is not yet adequately understood. AEDs probably do not alter the natural history of epilepsies, but can control seizures and in certain syndromes they can improve cognitive, motor and social function. Future developments in identifying aetiological mechanisms in the epilepsies, and of models of psychosocial adjustment in disability, will increase understanding of prognosis and permit the development of preventive and health-promoting measures.

References

1. Gowers WR. *Epilepsy and other chronic convulsive diseases: their causes, symptoms and treatment*. London: J & A Churchill, 1901.
2. Rodin EA. *The prognosis of patients with epilepsy*. Springfield, IL: Charles C Thomas, 1968.
3. Sander JWAS. Some aspects of prognosis in the epilepsies: a review. *Epilepsia* 1992;**34**:1007–16.
4. Aicardi J. Syndromic classification in the management of childhood epilepsy. *J Child Neurol* 1994;**9**:15–17.
5. Neville BGR. Epilepsy in childhood. *BMJ* 1997;**315**:924–30.
6. Beaussart M. Benign epilepsy of children with Rolandic (centro-temporal) paroxysmal foci: a clinical entity. Study of 221 cases. *Epilepsia* 1972;**13**:795–811.
7. Weglage J, Demsky A, Pietsch M, Kurlemann G. Neuropsychological, intellectual, and behavioral findings in patients with centrotemporal spikes with and without seizures. *Dev Med Child Neurol* 1997;**39**:646–51.
8. Gastaut H. Benign epilepsy of childhood with occipital paroxysms. In: Roger J, Bureau M, Dravet C, Dreifuss FE, Perret APW, eds. *Epileptic syndromes in infancy, childhood and adolescence*. 2nd edn. London: Libbey, 1992:201–17.
9. Panayiotopoupos CP. Vomiting as an ictal manifestation of epileptic seizures and syndromes. *J Neurol Neurosurg Psychiatry* 1988;**51**:1448–51.
10. Sato S, Dreifuss FE, Penry JK. Prognostic factors in absence seizures. *Neurology* 1976;**26**:788–96.
11. Sander JWAS. The epidemiology and prognosis of typical absence seizures. In: Duncan JS, Panayiotopoulos CP, eds. *Typical absences and related epileptic syndromes*. Edinburgh: Churchill Livingstone, 1995:135–45.
12. Berg AT. Febrile seizures and epilepsy: the contributions of epidemiology. *Paediatr Perinatal Epidemiol* 1992;**6**:145–52.
13. Berg AT, Shinnar S, Hauser WA, Leventhal JM. Predictors of recurrent febrile seizures: a meta-analytic review. *J Pediatr* 1990;**116**:329–37.
14. Nelson KB, Ellenberg JH. Predictors of epilepsy in children who have experienced febrile seizures. *N Engl J Med* 1976;**295**:1029–33.
15. Nelson KB, Ellenberg JH. Prognosis of children with febrile seizures. *Pediatrics* 1978;**61**:720–7.
16. Annegers JF, Hauser WA, Elveback LR, Kurland LT. The risk of epilepsy following febrile convulsions. *Neurology* 1979;**29**:297–303.
17. Annegers JF, Hauser WA, Shirts SB. Factors prognostic of unprovoked seizures after febrile convulsions. *N Engl J Med* 1987;**316**:493–8.
18. Rantala H, Tarkka R, Uhari M. A meta-analytic review of the preventive treatment of recurrences of febrile seizures. *J Pediatr* 1997;**131**:922–5.
19. Berg AT, Shinnar S. The contributions of epidemiology to the understanding of childhood seizures and epilepsy. *J Child Neurol* 1994;**9** (Suppl 2):S19–S26.
20. Aicardi J, Mumford JP, Dumas C, Wood S. Vigabatrin as initial therapy for infantile spasms: a European retrospective survey.

Sabril IS Investigator and Peer Review Groups. *Epilepsia* 1996;**37**:638–42.

21. Chiron C, Dumas C, Jambaque I, et al. Randomized trial comparing vigabatrin and hydrocortisone in infantile spasms due to tuberous sclerosis. *Epilepsy Res* 1997;**26**: 389–95.

22. Aicardi J. *Epilepsy in children*. 2nd edn. New York: Raven Press, 1994.

23. Chevrie JJ, Aicardi J. Convulsive disorders in the first year of life: neurological and mental outcome and mortality. *Epilepsia* 1978;**19**: 67–74.

24. Gastaut H, Dravet C, Loubier D, et al. Evolution clinique et prognostic du syndrome de Lennox–Gastaut. In: Lugaresi E, Pazzaglia P, Tassinari CA, eds. *Evolution and prognosis of epilepsy*. Bologna: A. Gaggi, 1973:133–54.

25. Erba G, Browne TR. Atypical absence, myoclonic, atonic and tonic seizures, and the Lennox–Gastaut syndrome. In: Browne TR, Feldman RG, eds. *Epilepsy: diagnosis and management*. Boston: Little, Brown, 1983: 75–94.

26. Aicardi J, Gomes AL. The Lennox–Gastaut syndrome: clinical and electroencephalographic features. In: Niedermeyer E, Degen R, eds. *The Lennox–Gastaut syndrome*. New York: Alan R. Liss, 1988:25–46.

27. Cavazutti GB, Ferrari P, Lalla P. Follow-up of 482 cases with convulsive disorders in the first year of life. *Dev Med Child Neurol* 1984; **26**:425–37.

28. Aicardi J. Myoclonic epilepsies in childhood. *Int Pediatrics* 1991;**6**:195–200.

29. Dravet C, Bureau M, Guerrini R, et al. Severe myoclonic epilepsy in infants. In: Roger J, Bureau M, Dravet C, et al. eds. *Epileptic syndromes in infancy, childhood and adolescence*. London: John Libbey, 1992:75–88.

30. Harrison RM, Taylor DC. Childhood seizures: a 25 year follow-up. *Lancet* 1976;**327**:948–51.

31. Nashef L, Sander JWAS, Shorvon SD. Mortality in epilepsy. In: Pedley TA, Meldrum BS, eds. *Recent advances in epilepsy*. Vol. 6. Edinburgh: Churchill Livingstone, 1995: 271–87.

32. Neville BGR, Harkness WFJ, Cross JH, et al. Surgical treatment of autistic regression. *Pediatr Neurol* 1997;**16**:137–40.

33. Hart YM, Cortez M, Andermann F, et al. Medical treatment of Rasmussen's syndrome (chronic encephalitis and epilepsy): effect of high-dose steroids or immunoglobulins in 19 patients. *Neurology* 1994;**44**:1030–6.

34. Dulac O. Rasmussen's syndrome. *Curr Opin Neurol* 1996;**9**:75–7.

35. Beaumanoir A. The Landau–Kleffner syndrome. In: Roger J, Dravet C, Bureau M, et al. eds. *Epileptic syndromes in infancy, childhood and adolescence*. London: Libbey, 1993:231–43.

36. Morrell F, Whisler WW, Smith MC, et al. Landau–Kleffner syndrome: treatment with subpial intracortical transection. *Brain* 1995; **118**:1529–46.

37. Hart YM, Sander JWAS, Johnson AL, Shorvon SD. National General Practice Study of Epilepsy: recurrence after a first seizure. *Lancet* 1990;**336**:1271–4.

38. Hauser WA, Hesdorffer DC. *Epilepsy: frequency, causes and consequences*. Maryland: Demos Publications, 1990.

39. Hopkins A, Garman A, Clark C. The first seizure in adult life: value of clinical features, electroencephalography, and computerised tomographic scanning in prediction of seizure recurrence. *Lancet* 1988;**18**:721–6.

40. Shinnar S, Berg AT, Ptachewicz Y, Alemany M. Sleep state and the risk of seizure recurrence following a first unprovoked seizure in childhood. *Neurology* 1993;**43**:701–6.

41. Annegers JF, Shirts SB, Hauser WA, Kurland LT. Risk of recurrence after an initial unprovoked seizure. *Epilepsia* 1986;**27**:43–50.

42. Camfield PR, Camfield CS. Epilepsy after a first unprovoked seizure in childhood. *Neurology* 1985;**35**:1657–60.

43. Shinnar S, Berg AT, Moshe SL. Risk of seizure recurrence following a first unprovoked seizure in childhood: a prospective study. *Pediatrics* 1990;**85**:1076–85.

44. Hauser WA, Anderson VE, Loewenson RB, McRoberts S. Seizure recurrence after a first unprovoked seizure. *N Engl J Med* 1982; **307**:522–8.

45. Annegers JF, Grabow JD, Groover RV. Seizures after head trauma: a population study. *Neurology* 1980;**30**:638–9.

46. Salazar AN, Jabbari B, Vance SC. Epilepsy

after penetrating head injury. Clinical correlates: a report of the Vietnam Head Injury Study. *Neurology* 1985;**35**:1406–15.

47. Sander JWAS. The prognosis, prevention, morbidity and mortality of epilepsy. In: Duncan JS, Fish DR, Shorvon SD, eds. *Clinical epilepsy.* Edinburgh: Churchill Livingstone, 1995:299–320.

48. Annegers JF, Hauser WA, Beghi E, et al. The risk of unprovoked seizures after encephalitis and meningitis. *Neurology* 1988;**38**:1407–10.

49. Hirtz DG, Ellenberg JH, Nelson KB. The risk of recurrence of non-febrile seizures in children. *Neurology* 1984;**34**:637–41.

50. Dean JC, Penry JK. Discontinuation of antiepileptic drugs. In: Levy R, Mattson R, Meldrum B, et al eds. *Antiepileptic drugs.* New York: Raven Press, 1989:133–42.

51. Shinnar S, Kang H, Berg AT, et al. EEG abnormalities in children with a first unprovoked seizure. *Epilepsia* 1994;**35**:471–6.

52. First Seizure Trial Group. Randomised clinical trial on the efficacy of antiepileptic drugs in reducing the risk of relapse after a first unprovoked tonic–clonic seizure. *Neurology* 1993;**43**:478–83.

53. Musicco M, Beghi E, Solari A. Effects of antiepileptic treatment initiated after the first unprovoked seizure in the long term prognosis of epilepsy. *Neurology* 1994;**44**:A337–8.

54. O'Donoghue MF, Sander JWAS. Does early antiepileptic drug treatment alter the prognosis for remission in the epilepsies? *J Ro Soc Med* 1996;**89**:245–6.

55. Shinnar S, Berg AT. Does antiepileptic drug therapy alter the prognosis of childhood seizures and prevent the development of chronic epilepsy? *Semin Pediatr Neurol* 1994;**1**:111–17.

56. Sander JWAS, Shorvon SD. Remission periods in epilepsy and their relation to long-term prognosis. *Adv Epileptology* 1987;**16**:353–60.

57. Brorson LO, Wranne L. Long-term prognosis of childhood epilepsy: survival and seizure prognosis. *Epilepsia* 1987;**28**:324–30.

58. Annegers JF, Hauser WA, Beghi E. Remission of seizures and relapse in patients with epilepsy. *Epilepsia* 1979;**27**:43–50.

59. Camfield C, Camfield P, Gordon K, et al. Outcome of childhood epilepsy: a population-based study with a simple predictive scoring system for those treated with medication. *J Pediatr* 1993;**122**:861–8.

60. Mattson RH, Cramer JA, Collins JF. Comparison of carbamazepine, phenobarbital, phenytoin and primidone in partial and secondarily generalized tonic–clonic seizures. *N Engl J Med* 1985;**313**:145–51.

61. Goodridge DMG, Shorvon SD. Epileptic seizures in a population of 6000. *BMJ* 1983;**287**:641–7.

62. Cockerell OC, Johnson AL, Goodridge DMG, et al. The remission of epilepsy: results from the National General Practice Study of Epilepsy. *Lancet* 1995;**346**:140–4.

63. De Silva M, Macardle B, McGowan M, et al. Randomised comparative monotherapy trial of phenobarbitone, phenytoin, carbamazepine, or sodium valproate for newly diagnosed childhood epilepsy. *Lancet* 1996;**347**:709–13.

64. Camfield PR, Camfield CS, Gordon K, Dooley JM. If a first antiepileptic drug fails to control a child's epilepsy, what are the chances of success with the next drug? *J Pediatr* 1997;**131**:821–4.

65. Berg AT, Shinnar S. Relapse following discontinuation of antiepileptic drugs: a meta-analysis. *Neurology* 1991;**44**:601–8.

66. MRC Antiepileptic Drug Withdrawal Group. Randomised study of antiepileptic drug withdrawal in patients in remission. *Lancet* 1991;**337**:1175–80.

67. Todt H. The late prognosis of epilepsy in childhood. *Epilepsia* 1984;**25**:137–44.

68. Aicardi J. Clinical approach to the management of intractable epilepsy. *Dev Med Child Neurol* 1988;**30**:429–40.

69. Walker MC, Sander JWAS. The impact of new antiepileptic drugs on the prognosis of epilepsy: seizure freedom should be the ultimate goal. *Neurology* 1996;**46**:912–14.

70. Berg A, Levy SR, Novotny EJ, Shinnar S. Predictors of intractable epilepsy in childhood: a case-control study. *Epilepsia* 1996;**37**:24–30.

71. Steinhoff BJ, Neususs K, Thegeder H, Reimers CD. Leisure time activity and physical fitness in patients with epilepsy. *Epilepsia* 1996;**37**:1221–7.

72. Jalava M, Sillanpaa M. Concurrent illnesses in

adults with childhood-onset epilepsy: a population-based 35-year follow-up study. *Epilepsia* 1996;37:1155–63.

73. Hauser WA, Annegers JF, Elveback LR. Mortality in patients with epilepsy. *Epilepsia* 1980;21:339–412.

74. Cockerell OC, Johnson AL, Sander JWAS, et al. Mortality from epilepsy: results from a prospective population-based study. *Lancet* 1994;344:918–21.

75. Henriksen B, Juul-Jensen P, Lund M. The mortality of epileptics. In: Brackenridge RD, ed. *Proceedings of the 10th International Congress of Life Assurance Medicine.* London: Pilomen, 1970:55–8.

76. Sillanpaa M. Social adjustment and functioning of chronically ill and impaired children and adolescents. *Acta Paediatr Scand* 1987;76:1–70.

77. Hoare P, Mann H. Self-esteem and behavioural adjustment in children with epilepsy and children with diabetes. *J Psychosom Res* 1994;38:859–69.

78. Austin JK, Smith MS, Risinger MW, McNelis AM. Childhood epilepsy and asthma: comparison of quality of life. *Epilepsia* 1994;35:608–15.

79. Jalava M, Sillanpaa M, Camfield C, Camfield C. Social adjustment and competence 35 years after onset of childhood epilepsy: a prospective controlled study. *Epilepsia* 1997;38:708–15.

80. Mitchell WG, Chavez JM, Lee H, Guzman BL. Academic underachievement in children with epilepsy. *J Child Neurol* 1991;6:65–72.

81. Mitchell WG, Sheier LM, Baker SA. Psychosocial, behavioural and medical outcomes in children with epilepsy: a developmental risk factor model using longitudinal data. *Pediatrics* 1994;94:471–7.

82. Hoare R, Kerley S. Psychosocial adjustment of children with chronic epilepsy and their families. *Dev Med Child Neurol* 1991;33:201–15.

83. Austin JK, Risinger MW, Beckett LA. Correlates of behaviour problems in children with epilepsy. *Epilepsia* 1992;33:1115–22.

84. Pianta RC, Lothman DJ. Predicting behaviour problems in children with epilepsy: child factors, disease factors, family stress, and child–mother interaction. *Child Dev* 1994;65:1415–28.

85. Lothman DJ, Pianta RC. Role of child–mother interaction in predicting competence of children with epilepsy. *Epilepsia* 1993;34:658–69.

86. Austin JK, McDermott N. Parental attitude and coping behaviours in families of children with epilepsy. *J Neurosci Nurs* 1988;20:174–9.

87. Holdsworth L, Whitmore K. A study of children with epilepsy attending ordinary schools. 1. Their seizure patterns, progress and behaviour in school. *Dev Med Child Neurol* 1974;16:746–58.

88. Hartlage LC, Green JB. The relation of parental attitudes to academic and social achievement in epileptic children. *Epilepsia* 1972;13:21–6.

89. Carlton-Ford S, Miller R, Brown M, et al. Epilepsy and children's social and psychological adjustment. *J Health Soc Behav* 1995;36:285–301.

90. Baker GA, Jacoby A, Chadwick DW. The associations of psychopathology in epilepsy: a community study. *Epilepsy Res* 1996;25:29–39.

91. Kokkonen J, Kokkonen ER, Saukonnen AL, Pennanen P. Psychosocial outcome of young adults with epilepsy in childhood. *J Neurol Neurosurg Psychiatry* 1997;62:265–8.

92. Sillanpaa M. Social functioning and seizure status of young adults with onset of epilepsy in childhood. *Acta Neurol Scand* 1983;68:1–81.

93. Seidenberg M. Academic achievement and school performance of children with epilepsy. In: Hermann BP, Seidenberg M, eds. *Childhood epilepsies: neuropsychological, psychosocial and intervention aspects.* Chichester: John Wiley, 1989:105–18.

94. Holmes GL. The long-term effects of seizures on the developing brain: clinical and laboratory issues. *Brain Dev* 1991;13:393–409.

95. Hirtz DG, Nelson KB. Cognitive effects of antiepileptic drugs. In: Pedley TA, Meldrum BS, eds. *Recent advances in epilepsy.* Vol. 2. Edinburgh: Churchill Livingstone, 1985:161–81.

96. Farwell JR, Lee YJ, Hirtz DG, et al.

Phenobarbital for febrile seizures: effects on intelligence and on seizure recurrence. *N Engl J Med* 1990;322:364–9.

97. Stores G. School children with epilepsy at risk for learning and behaviour problems. *Dev Med Child Neurol* 1978;20:502–8.

98. Elwes RD, Marshall J, Beattie A, Newman PK. Epilepsy and employment. A community based survey in an area of high unemployment. *J Neurol Neurosurg Psychiatry* 1991;54:200–3.

99. Hart YM, Shorvon SD. The nature of epilepsy in the general population. I. Characteristics of patients receiving medication for epilepsy. *Epilepsy Res* 1995;21:43–9.

100. Jacoby A. Impact of epilepsy on employment status: findings from a UK study of people with well-controlled epilepsy. *Epilepsy Res* 1995;21:125–32.

101. Collings JA, Chappell B. Correlates of employment history and employability in a British epilepsy sample. *Seizure* 1994;3:255–62.

102. Thompson PJ, Oxley J. Socioeconomic accompaniments of severe epilepsy. *Epilepsia* 1988;29:9–18.

103. Sillanpaa M. Children with epilepsy as adults. *Acta Paediatr Scand* 1990;79:1–78.

104. Chaplin JE, Yepez Lasso R, Shorvon SD, Floyd M. National General Practice study of epilepsy: the social and psychological effects of a recent diagnosis of epilepsy. *BMJ* 1992;304:1416–18.

105. Cooper M. Epilepsy and employment: employers' attitudes. *Seizure* 1995;4:193–9.

106. Moody GA, Probert CS, Jayanthi V, Mayberry JF. The attitude of employers to people with inflammatory bowel disease. *Soc Sci Med* 1992;34:459–60.

107. Scambler G, Hopkins A. Social class, epileptic activity, and disadvantage at work. *J Epidemiol Community Health* 1980;34:129–33.

108. US Department of Labor. The performance of psychically impaired workers in manufacturing industries. Washington, DC: US Government Printing Office, 1972.

109. The Employment Commission of the International Bureau for Epilepsy. Employing people with epilepsy: principles for good practice. *Epilepsia* 1989;30:411–12.

110. Hicks RA, Hicks MJ. Attitudes of major employers toward the employment of people with epilepsy: a 30-year study. *Epilepsia* 1991;32:86–8.

111. Troxell J. Epilepsy and employment: the Americans with Disabilities Act and its protections against employment discrimination. *Med Law* 1997;16:375–84.

30

Excess mortality in epilepsy: impact on clinical management

Lina Nashef

Introduction

There is an observed excess mortality in patients with epilepsy that is about two-to-three times that of the general population.[1-7] This overall figure conceals large differences among different patient groups. The excess mortality is related partly to the underlying disease associated with or causing the epilepsy and partly to the epilepsy itself. This chapter focuses on mortality caused by epilepsy, particularly that which is potentially preventable.

Do you tell newly diagnosed patients with epilepsy about the risk of dying from their condition? I am asked this question most often and indeed patient information is at the heart of this subject. It is one of two important issues that will be addressed,[8] the other being the impact of the observed excess mortality on clinical management in the care of the individual patient.[9] The latter may be approached at two interdependent levels: the first is the scope for prevention of premature death; the second is the extent to which the knowledge of this excess mortality directly impinges on treatment decisions, whether they are medical or surgical. Another important area is that of service provision,[10] which is outside the scope of this chapter.

Much has been learnt in this field in the past few years, particularly in epidemiology, but we still lack some of the information needed to give categorical advice about prevention. The clinical guidelines in this chapter are therefore based on my evaluation of current evidence, with the knowledge that some of the advice given may later have to be revised.

Patient information

With regard to patient information, our role has perhaps recently eased. For much of the last 25–50 years, the emphasis on management has been on the encouragement of independence in those with epilepsy, consequently, inadvertently or otherwise, minimizing the extent of some of the associated risks. Although excess mortality and risk of injury in epilepsy have been recognized and documented for more than a century,[11-13] the experience and writings of our predecessors appear to have been, for a period at least, largely ignored. Until recently, the message most often given to patients and carers was that seizures, although very disturbing to witness, pose very little risk, except in the event of an unfortunate (and rare) accident. Only a few years ago, at least in the UK, it was quite commonly stated that, alarming though generalized seizures may be, they 'appear worse than they are'.

Although each seizure carries a low risk, there is no doubt of the significantly increased risk of premature death in uncontrolled severe epilepsy. Over the past few years, however, with parallel publications in both the medical and the lay press, the latter sometimes alarmist in tone, the general public has become increasingly aware of this issue. The risk to life in other common conditions is already generally appreciated. It is widely known, for example, that the diagnosis of asthma carries with it a small excess risk to life, depending on the severity of the condition; the same applies to epilepsy, and both, to some extent, are potentially preventable.

The revival of interest in this field, particularly in the syndrome of sudden unexpected death in epilepsy (SUDEP), can be attributed to three factors.[14] The first relates to the laudable and dedicated efforts of the UK-based self-help group 'Epilepsy Bereaved?'.[15] The second is the direct support, and indeed sometimes the instigation, by the pharmaceutical and allied industries of related research and education in the field.[16,17] Large trials of new antiepileptic drugs in patients with intractable epilepsy inevitably meant that unexpected deaths were observed during those trials. Thus, it became important that such deaths were documented to occur in intractable epilepsy, irrespective of the drug or treatment under study. Finally, litigation issues have begun to surface, at least in the US, and in Leestma's words 'precisely when SUDEP entered the consciousness of the greater public cannot be known, but it has arrived so far as the courts are concerned'.[18]

Undoubtedly, with increased general awareness of the risks associated with epilepsy, the clinician will find it easier to discuss the subject with an individual patient. The overall message to be conveyed, and one that needs to be included in general information booklets, is that there is a small overall excess risk of premature death in association with epilepsy; it should also be conveyed that this risk varies depending on individual circumstances, medical and social, and that it is minimal or negligible in those whose epilepsy is fully controlled. The role of the physician becomes that of broadly estimating the risk for individual patients under their care, advising about preventive measures that they may wish to take, and helping them to make choices about treatment options and lifestyle. The question is therefore not one of inappropriately confronting a newly diagnosed patient with the spectre of premature death.

Before proceeding with a brief review of causes of death from epilepsy, let me address the understandable reservations of the clinician who is wary of approaching this subject. There are, as yet, no studies that look at the potential harm that discussion of mortality may cause an individual patient for use in guidance of clinical practice. Such studies are no doubt needed. Those who favour withholding information may use the argument of potential harm or distress to support their stand—an argument that has been abandoned in many other areas of medicine. They will need to be able to justify their position to relatives of patients with epilepsy who die unexpectedly. Such relatives have argued that the deceased person had a right to know the risks attached to his or her condition, that they may have acted differently and perhaps, although this is difficult to prove, they may have avoided a premature death.[8,19]

In my view, any discussion must be tailored to the individual patient and recorded in the medical notes. On the one hand, unwanted information, except where specific social or treatment decisions need to be made, should not be forced on the patient. Conversely, all patients should be given the opportunity of asking relevant questions and receiving truthful and accurate answers to the detail that they require. There may be specific situations in which the clinician may consider such discussions to be harmful and choose to withhold information. Such situations, except in the case of children and those with learning disability, must be considered the exception. For the hesitant clinician, let me add that it is my impression that most patients, carers and relatives are already concerned about safety issues. Addressing these issues allows them to place these concerns in perspective. Avoiding discussion of risk does not necessarily mean peace of mind, because that peace of mind is often not there in the first place.

Safety issues are also usefully discussed with relatives or carers. This should be encouraged with the permission of the individual with epilepsy, without eroding the independence acquired in recent years by those with epilepsy. In any activity or situation that carries no risk to others, it is up to individuals to decide about the level of risk or curtailment of freedom that they are willing to accept.

Prevention of avoidable mortality: a treatment aim in epilepsy

For the clinician who treats people with epilepsy, prevention of avoidable injury and mortality should now be one of three overlapping aims of treatment, along with freedom from seizures and improved quality of life.[20] This chapter reviews causes of death from epilepsy within the context of overall mortality, including the category of SUDEP, as well as the potential for prevention of premature death.

Overall mortality in epilepsy

Methodological problems relating to definitions, case identification, selection bias, incomplete follow-up and difficulties in ascertaining causes of death bedevil mortality studies in epilepsy. The prevalence of epilepsy (approximately 0.5 per cent) depends on incidence (approximately 0.05 per cent annually), remission and mortality. Remission is an important factor, accounting for the difference between prevalence and cumulative incidence.[21] The relative contribution of mortality has not, however, been emphasized. In unselected population-based series,[3,5] excess mortality is highest in the first few years after diagnosis and is mainly *but not exclusively* the result of the underlying disease associated with or causing the epilepsy. In the UK National General Practice Study of Epilepsy, 114 of 564 definite incident cases died during the follow-up period (mean 6.9 years), instead of an estimated 37 with a standardized mortality ratio of 3.[5] (Standardized mortality ratio (SMR) is the ratio of deaths observed in the group under study to those expected during the follow-up period if the group in question had experienced the same age- and sex-specific death rates as in the control population. The overall SMR in epilepsy is 2–3.) These figures indicate an effect of mortality on prevalence. As expected in such a cohort, some 60 per cent of cases achieved remission. Thus, only a subgroup of those identified in studies of newly diagnosed cases contributes to the pool of chronic epilepsy, and mortality findings in such studies cannot be extrapolated to cohorts with active epilepsy. Underlying or associated disease is a main cause of death in the first years after diagnosis in population-based studies.[1,3,5] Even in these studies, mortality is also increased, though to a lesser extent, when patients with idiopathic/cryptogenic epilepsy are considered separately (Table 30.1).

Wannamaker[22] quotes different, largely selected studies with deaths attributed to epilepsy that account for between 25.9 and 62.2 per cent of the total. Excess mortality from the epilepsy itself is most evident in institution-based

	SMR	95 % CI
Rochester, USA[1,3]		
Overall	2.3	1.9–2.6
Idiopathic/cryptogenic	1.8	1.4–2.3
National General Practice		
Study of Epilepsy, UK[2,5]		
Overall	2.5	2.1–2.9
Idiopathic	1.6	1.0–2.4

95% CI, 95% confidence limits.

Table 30.1
Standardized mortality ratios (SMRs) in two population-based studies of epilepsy.

series. In two recent studies of patients with chronic, largely uncontrolled epilepsy, age- and sex-matched SMRs of 5.1[23] and 15.9[24] were observed, with 58 per cent and 71 per cent of deaths, respectively, classified as caused by epilepsy. Epilepsy-related deaths are also likely to be more frequent in untreated populations, although studies are few.[25,26]

Variables affecting overall excess mortality in epilepsy

Within the two-to-three times overall increase in mortality, there is a wide range from no increased risk (for example, in childhood absence epilepsy) to much higher risks with SMRs of 8 and above. The impact of the excess mortality, which is a little higher in males, decreases with increasing age, with deaths resulting from epilepsy 'lost' within higher overall death rates from all causes. It is possible, however, that the risk of dying from a given disease is compounded by the presence of secondary epilepsy, for example, in the elderly

population or other subgroups with multiple pathology.[27] Information on mortality in children and older age groups is generally limited.[28–32] Seizure type is important, and tonic–clonic seizures in particular are associated with a higher mortality. Patients with more severe epilepsy in terms of seizure frequency are at higher risk, as are patients with remote symptomatic epilepsy, compared with patients with cryptogenic/idiopathic epilepsy. Mortality is also higher in association with mental handicap, although, co-existing neurological disease and abnormalities in other systems make this difficult to assess.[33,34]

Causes of death in epilepsy

Death in epilepsy may be apparently unrelated, related to underlying or associated disease or related to epilepsy and its treatment. Some of the epilepsy-related and epilepsy-associated deaths are:

- Seizure-related:
  - status epilepticus
  - trauma, burns or drowning consequent to a seizure
  - the majority of sudden unexpected deaths in epilepsy
  - deaths in a seizure with severe aspiration and/or airway obstruction by food, etc.
  - deaths provoked by habitual seizures resulting from co-existing cardiorespiratory disease.
- Deaths as a consequence of medical or surgical treatment of epilepsy.
- Suicides.

There is overlap between the categories and classification may be difficult.

Drowning, trauma and burns

Advice to patients in this context overlaps with advice given to prevent injury. Two main risk factors for injury are seizure frequency and seizure type, namely generalized tonic–clonic seizures.[35] Drug-related ataxia and drug-induced osteoporosis also need to be considered. In a recent study, treatment with antiepileptic drugs was found to be one of the risk factors for hip fractures in white women.[36] It is self-evident that epilepsy should be treated aggressively. The best way to prevent seizure-associated injury is by controlling seizures, and patients need to be informed of potentially hazardous situations. The extent of the precautionary measures needed depends on the control of their epilepsy. There are, in addition, legal requirements that they need to be informed of, particularly in relation to driving.

There is an increased risk of drowning in epilepsy,[37–42] which is dependent on exposure and is highly amenable to prevention. It is greater in the absence of supervision and in association with other disability. Deaths from non-intentional drowning constitute 1.8–10 per cent of deaths in epilepsy.[2] All patients with epilepsy should be given appropriate advice. Baths, except where there is direct *constant* supervision, should be avoided. Pulling the plug while maintaining the head above water in the event of a seizure is likely to be easier in the first instance than pulling an adult out of a bath. Sit-down showers with thermostat-controlled water temperatures are considered to be the safest option. Swimming should be supervised by someone who is capable of giving assistance and has been informed of the epilepsy. Waterfronts need to be avoided as do heights, and flotation devices need to be worn during accompanied water sports.

The magnitude of other accidental mortality is difficult to assess because epilepsy may not be recorded when death certificates are issued, and it is not always possible to know if an accident was secondary to a seizure. Nevertheless, accidental deaths are known to be increased in cohorts with epilepsy. The Rochester and Warsaw population-based studies reported that 5–6 per cent of deaths in people with epilepsy were caused by accidents.[3] In proportional mortality studies, non-drowning accidental deaths constitute up to 18 per cent of total deaths.[2] Driving restrictions aim to limit driver-related vehicle accidents as a result of epilepsy, although such restrictions are not in force in all countries.[43-46] According to Taylor,[47] in police-reported road traffic accidents resulting from driver collapse in Britain in 1984, 39 per cent had suffered tonic–clonic seizures confirmed by witnesses. Seizures themselves may result in potentially fatal head injuries, cervical trauma or limb fractures. In one study, the incidence of seizures resulting in injury presenting to an emergency department was 29.5 in 100 000 of the population (32 : 100 000 of injury and death).[48] Another study, of a cohort of patients with more severe epilepsy, who were living in a sheltered environment, showed that the risk of serious head injury *per seizure* was relatively low.[49] However, non-drowning accidents in a mortality study at the same centre constituted only 0.8 per cent of total deaths.[50] This emphasizes the preventable nature of these accidental deaths.

It is not possible to caution against every eventuality, but to advise that potentially dangerous situations are best avoided in the event of a seizure. These would include avoiding heights and waterfronts, proximity to fires or dangerous machinery, and taking care as a pedestrian. Helmet or wheelchair use is appropriate only in very severe epilepsy with frequent drop attacks. With regard to avoidance of burns, mention has already been made of thermostat-controlled water sources. Similarly, good insulation of hot pipes and storage tanks, care with cooking and heating water, and care with home appliances are advised.[51,52]

Status epilepticus

There have been some conflicting reports about the mortality risk from status epilepticus in those with known epilepsy. Nevertheless, convulsive status epilepticus remains a life-threatening medical emergency where prompt treatment is essential. Although status epilepticus is more common in children, mortality is higher in adults. In 12 series, the mortality rate was 18 per cent of all cases: 7 per cent of children and 28 per cent of adults.[53] Status epilepticus is listed as the cause in some 10 per cent or fewer of epilepsy deaths in various series of treated cohorts with epilepsy.[2] The accuracy of the figures is uncertain because, in the past, in the UK at least, unwitnessed deaths, which would currently be classified as SUDEP, were often certified as having died of status epilepticus. Death from convulsive status, was however, reported as higher in historical series of untreated groups[54] and in a recent study from Kenya.[25] Death from status epilepticus in idiopathic/cryptogenic epilepsy has declined in recent reported hospital series. Deaths are considered to result mainly from underlying disease with only 2 per cent of deaths directly attributable to the status epilepticus itself.[52] These reports are from tertiary centres and should not give rise to complacency in the acute management and prevention of this life-threatening state. Recent data from Hauser and colleagues[55] suggest that the overall mortality from status has not altered in recent years. However, the inclusion of proportionally more cases with acute neurological insults in older age groups is one probable explanation for this apparent discrepancy. Interestingly,

however, Hauser's data suggest that those with epilepsy, who present with or who are susceptible to status epilepticus, have a greater medium-term and overall mortality and are a group at special risk.[55,56]

Sudden unexpected death in epilepsy

Otherwise well patients with epilepsy may die unexpectedly, with post-mortem examination showing pulmonary or other organ congestion, but not the cause of death.[16,24,25,57–78] The definition of SUDEP, the acronym most commonly used to denote this category, has been subject to debate, as indeed have potential underlying mechanisms:

> Sudden, unexpected, witnessed or unwitnessed, non-traumatic and non-drowning death in epilepsy, with or without evidence for a seizure and excluding documented status epilepticus, where post-morten examination does not reveal a cause for death.

These deaths have been difficult to investigate because, for the most part, they are unwitnessed. Many investigators believe, myself among them, that most of these deaths occur during or soon after convulsive seizures,[79] when potentially life-threatening cardiorespiratory changes are known to occur. Different possible mechanisms are not mutually exclusive and indeed may contribute in a given case. The previous emphasis on possible cardiac arrhythmias has been supplemented by evidence in favour of hypoventilation as a common occurrence in seizures, likely to be a significant mechanism in SUDEP. Cardiac mechanisms are likely to be more important in older people with ischaemic heart disease who die suddenly of their cardiac disease during habitual seizures. They are also important in cases of misdiagnosis of cardiac syncope as epilepsy.[80]

In the younger, otherwise previously well SUDEP case, the frequent presence of pulmonary oedema (almost a sine qua non) argues against an instantaneous primary cardiac arrhythmia.[77] Pulmonary oedema is well documented after seizures.[81–84] Systematic studies of ambulatory ECG, both ictally and interictally, have generally shown malignant tachyarrhythmias to be rare,[85] although, as reviewed by Jallon,[86,87] there are a number of case reports of severe bradyarrhythmias with secondary syncope in complex partial seizures of temporal lobe origin. Such cases probably constitute a special subgroup at risk, but are not likely to account for most SUDEP deaths.

Animal studies support an important role for apnoea/hypoventilation, which has been known for many years to occur commonly during seizures.[88] Ictal fatal central apnoea, amenable to simple resuscitation, is observed to occur in the DBA2 mouse.[14] In Simon's sheep model of ictal sudden death, animals that died were those with a greater rise in pulmonary vascular pressure and hypoventilation, thought to be central rather than obstructive.[89] A further study of tracheotomized sheep observed central apnoea and hypoventilation in all the animals studied (eight). This caused or contributed to death in two; a third also developed heart failure with significant pathological cardiac ischaemic changes.[90] Systematic ictal recordings in humans, with techniques used in polysomnography,[91,92] show that central apnoea is observed commonly during seizures and is infrequently accompanied by transient bradycardia.

Obstructive apnoea is also observed but less commonly. Studies in telemetry units are likely to underestimate intrinsic/positional and extrinsic obstructive apnoea because of intervention from attending staff. In an interview study looking at detailed circumstances in SUDEP, in 11 of 26 cases, the position of the head was such that obstructive apnoea may well have occurred.[80] The tragic EEG/video-recorded case of death in a seizure is also in keeping with apnoea. In this case, respiratory parameters were not recorded, but the persistence of pulse artefact, seen on one of the intracranial depth EEG electrode channels for 120 s after complete EEG flattening, indicated adequate perfusion until the late stages of the terminal event. Death in this case occurred after the ictal discharge and appeared to be the result of cessation of all brain activity.[93]

In summary, obstructive and central apnoea, which may be amenable to intervention by an observer, occurs not only as part of an ictal discharge but also post-ictally. Emphasis on the role of apnoea in SUDEP does not exclude an important role for cardiac autonomic changes.[94,95] These may occur in association with apnoea caused by the same ictal discharge; it may also occur as a secondary event, as part of a cardiorespiratory reflex, or indeed independently of apnoea, as is likely in the cases of severe bradycardia/sinus arrest in temporal lobe epilepsy cited above. Mameli's animal data, recording cardiac autonomic changes with activation of brain-stem arrhythmogenic trigger zones, showed that cardiac changes were transient and not life threatening, unless accompanied by alteration in metabolic parameters.[96] Studies of heart rate variability comparing nocturnal and daytime recordings, the influence of the epilepsy syndrome, left and right temporal discharges, and antiepileptic drugs are being carried out and may throw light on the risk factors identified in descriptive studies.[97]

The incidence of SUDEP depends on the cohort under study and has been reviewed.[75,98] Data from patients in remission suggest that controlled patients, whether as a result of either treatment or inherently less severe disease, as judged by seizure control, have an extremely low risk of sudden death.[99]

O'Donaghue and Sander[98] estimate that those in the general population with epilepsy carry a risk of approximately 1:500–1000 per year. Those with more severe epilepsy seen at specialized units have a risk of about 1:250 per year, whereas those being considered for epilepsy surgery have a risk of 1 : 100 per year or more. Those rejected for epilepsy surgery and those with failed surgery are at particularly high risk. Background rates of sudden unexpected death in the general population are age related and range from 5–10 per 100 000 per year in young adults (<45) to 300 per 100 000 per year in elderly people.[100]

The following risk factors for SUDEP have been suggested, although these, for the most part, have yet to be confirmed by ongoing case–control studies. They include youth (those aged 20–40 appear to be at higher risk), uncontrolled epilepsy, a history of generalized tonic–clonic seizures, unwitnessed seizures, nocturnal seizures, remote symptomatic epilepsy, male sex, a history of psychotropic drug prescriptions and non-compliance or abrupt drug withdrawal.[101] Neuropathological studies indicate a higher incidence of macroscopic abnormalities in SUDEP cases.[58,102,103] Specialized cardiac pathology has only been performed in a small series of SUDEP cases with a higher incidence of pathological findings compared with a control group without epilepsy.[104]

Suicides

Whether there is a higher incidence of suicide among patients with epilepsy has been subject to debate. The topic has been reviewed by Barraclough[105] and Mathews and Barabas,[106] with both self-poisoning and suicides apparently increased in patients with epilepsy. Although increased suicide was not reported in the population-based Rochester study, with only three suicides reported in 8233 person-

years,[3] it is generally considered that suicide rates are increased four to five times in cohorts with epilepsy, compared with the general population. In other more selected series, suicides constitute 2–10 per cent of total deaths. It is likely that selected subgroups, particularly those with temporal lobe epilepsy, are at greater risk.[2] In the Warsaw series a higher incidence was observed among those in the community, compared with institutionalized patients with epilepsy.[6]

An increased number of suicides was also reported in older series of post-temporal lobectomy, particularly in the first few years.[107,108] A younger age at suicide than in the general population and an association with more severe epilepsy has also been reported.[109] Mendez and Doss[110] suggest a greater association with psychotic behaviours and psychic symptoms than with major depression or the psychosocial burden of having epilepsy. This would appear to be supported by the observation of a much higher risk in those with a diagnosis of temporal lobe epilepsy, estimated at 25 times that of the general population.[103] Also of interest is the observation that depression is more common in left temporal lobe epilepsy, whereas postoperative depression appears to be more common after right temporal lobe resections. Another potentially important issue is the effect of different antiepileptic drugs on mood, some being beneficial and others detrimental.[111] Suicides are potentially preventable and joint care with psychiatric services is needed where appropriate.

Deaths secondary to medical and surgical treatment of epilepsy

In addition to specific points outlined below, an important issue relevant to treatment interventions, which is not often emphasized, is the potential for antiepileptic drugs to make epilepsy worse,[111] in particular the potential for a medication (or surgery) to alter seizure severity including the post-ictal phase, thus altering the risks associated with an individual seizure. Surprisingly, scales of seizure severity do not address cardiorespiratory distress occurring during seizures (e.g. cyanosis or severe changes in respiratory pattern), although the potential for injury has been included.[113,114] The potential risk of injury from drug-related ataxia and osteoporosis has already been mentioned, as have risks resulting from non-compliance and abrupt drug changes.

On more specific issues, an association between antiepileptic drugs and an increased long-term risk of secondary neoplasia has been suggested.[2,115-120] In a study of over 2000 residents with epilepsy, White et al[115] defined the limits of an overall increase in risk for cancer (excluding CNS) at between 1.1 and 1.8 times the average. Clemmesen et al[116] and Shirts et al[120] found no such overall increase. A more recent study of 7864 Danish patients with epilepsy showed no overall increased risk when brain cancers were excluded.[116] The available evidence suggests that, once CNS neoplasms are excluded, any excess reported is small or borderline, although doubt remains regarding neoplasms of the lung and non-Hodgkin's lymphomas.

Idiosyncratic reactions to antiepileptic drugs, generally viewed as rare, may be life threatening, and include blood dyscrasias, hepatic failure and sinus arrest.[2,121-123] The exact magnitude of risk in established antiepileptic drugs is uncertain, but is considered very low compared with the risk inherent in uncontrolled epilepsy. However, the risk is unknown in any newly introduced drug. At the time of licensing, the total number of people exposed to a new treatment is usually only a few thousand. Thus, the risk of a potentially life-threatening idiosyncratic reaction occurring, even relatively commonly, would not have been excluded.

Post-marketing surveillance and caution on the part of the prescribing clinician are essential.

The recent experience of liver failure and aplastic anaemia occurring with relative frequency with felbamate, a highly effective new antiepileptic drug (though with many drug interactions), is salutary.[124] Thus, the clinician needs to take the severity of the epilepsy into account, including the risk of injury and death, before recommending a relatively untried antiepileptic drug. The same applies to other techniques, such as vagal nerve stimulation. The raised SMR observed in patients treated using the Neurocybernetic Prosthesis (Cyberonics, Inc) system were comparable with those observed in studies of young adults with intractable epilepsy, as was the rate of definite/probable SUDEP of 4.5 per 1000 person-years.[17] Continued monitoring, as with any newly introduced treatment, is essential. Vigilance is also required when any antiepileptic drug, new or old, is first prescribed, particularly in the first few weeks or months.

In surgical candidates, relatively low mortality from presurgical assessment and from epilepsy surgery needs to be balanced against the risks associated with intractable epilepsy. It may be expected that mortality after surgery for epilepsy would decline. Two older series, however, report elevated long-term mortality after surgery, with some half to two thirds of deaths related to seizures or suicides.[107] In a recent cohort of 248 people who underwent diagnostic evaluation for epilepsy surgery,[125] those not operated on had a significantly higher mortality than the surgical group. Furthermore, a significantly higher proportion of those who died were noted to have ongoing seizures at last recorded follow-up compared with survivors. Unfortunately, the number of person-years is not provided.

In a 5-year follow-up study of temporal lobectomy for refractory epilepsy, a seizure-free state was found to be associated with reduced mortality and increased employment.[126] In the Maudsley series, overall postoperative mortality was elevated, compared with the general population, particularly in the right temporal lobectomy group, but to a lesser extent than would be expected in an intractable cohort. Most deaths were epilepsy related and included one suicide, accidents, deaths from status epilepticus and sudden unexpected deaths. The last constituted the largest category, who for the most part were still experiencing seizures or undergoing medication withdrawal. It was of note, however, that in certain cases, despite a decrease in overall seizure frequency, a change in seizure type to more severe generalized or more prolonged attacks may have altered their risk.[127]

The potential for prevention

Apart from seizure prevention, and in addition to avoiding seizure-related injury, the potential for prevention of excess mortality related to epilepsy lies in the response to an individual seizure and in the prevention of seizures, particularly generalized convulsions, although complex partial seizures are not totally without risk. This emphasizes the need to treat epilepsy aggressively, and the importance of compliance with medical treatment and avoiding precipitated seizures such as those associated with sleep deprivation, alcohol or photosensitivity. The issue of response to seizures is often only cursorily addressed in the clinical setting and in patient literature. Advice is usually given with regard to cushioning the fall if possible, protection from sharp objects, and placing the individual in the recovery position after the event. There is little discussion about the need for supervision or more specific resuscitative measures. The former, with its potential for curtailing independence, should be based on

informed choice. For some with severe epilepsy, knowledge of the excess mortality and the possible benefit of supervision needs to be taken into account in deciding on optimum residence. The drive for complete independence at all costs, particularly if there is associated handicap, may not always be wise. In my view, timely assistance when a seizure occurs is likely to reduce the risk of death or injury, and there is direct and indirect evidence in support of this statement. Supervision has been shown to be helpful in preventing fatal drowning[52] and it is reasonable to assume that other accidental deaths would be reduced by appropriate assistance.

With regard to sudden unexpected deaths, it is worth emphasizing that most of these are unwitnessed, ranging from 3 to 43 per cent of cases. In my experience less than 20 per cent are witnessed.[23,24,80] In an ongoing case–control study, only 10 per cent of more than 100 cases identified so far were witnessed (Y Langan, personal communication). A probable explanation for this is that unwitnessed seizures carry a higher risk of death. A significant proportion of SUDEPs, are however, nocturnal, and there may be physiological reasons why a nocturnal seizure may lead to death, such as a higher likelihood of respiratory compromise or increased vagal tone. Others have suggested an influence of sudden intense increases in geomagnetic activity.[128]

The observations in a cohort of pupils with epilepsy and learning difficulty at a special residential school are of interest.[24] During the period under study, no SUDEP cases occurred while the pupils were under the supervision of the school (866 person-years), with 14 SUDEP cases occurring either after the pupils had left the school or during holidays or weekend leave (3269 person-years). Although the difference did not reach statistical significance, there was certainly a strong trend supporting the premise that supervision at the school was providing some protection, despite the pupils having severe epilepsy and very frequent seizures. The pupils were supervised constantly, including at night when four night staff, an on-call resident nurse and a sound-monitoring system ensured prompt response to seizures. Compliance in that environment was also assured. Similar experience has been noted at Lingfield School in the UK (F. Besag, personal communication).

Response to seizures/advice to carers

Ictal or post-ictal apnoea occurs commonly in seizures. Both the central and obstructive components of apnoea are amenable to intervention. Central apnoea may respond to stimulation and obstructive apnoea to positioning. The post-ictal state is a period of risk and the individual should not be left unsupervised even if in the recovery position. A carer of someone with severe epilepsy needs to be taught (where possible) not only to assess respiration, but also to feel the pulse and start cardiopulmonary resuscitation if appropriate. Failed attempts at resuscitation in witnessed events undoubtedly occur, although the timing of the resuscitation in relation to the collapse is not always clear. There are also anecdotal reports of witnessed 'near-miss' events, where intervention by an observer appeared to influence the outcome. Finally, early intervention, as already stated, to prevent established status epilepticus is strongly advised.

Risk per individual seizure

Attempts at quantifying the risk of death per generalized tonic–clonic seizure are meaningless because seizures vary greatly in severity. A description from a reliable observer of an individual's seizures is, however, likely to be important in assessing, qualitatively if not quantitatively, the risk in an individual case. Of particular interest is severity of respiratory involvement both during the seizure and post-ictally, and the occurrence of near-miss events. Treatment interventions may alter the seizure severity/type, both in a beneficial and in an adverse direction that needs to be monitored. This is not currently routinely assessed in trials of new medication. The risk in an individual case will depend on the habitual seizures experienced, as well as the presence of the risk factors for injury and SUDEP referred to.

Treatment after a first seizure

The current position in the UK is that treatment is not usually advised for someone with an unprovoked first seizure. Discussions on the validity of this approach have centred on whether seizures beget seizures, and whether the occurrence of more than one seizure before treatment affects outcome.[129] Mortality has not been deemed an issue. There would be a strong case for earlier treatment were evidence to emerge that a significant number of epilepsy-related deaths occur in a second or third seizure. At present, available limited data do not suggest that many deaths occur at that stage, although some undoubtedly do. Furthermore, diagnostic issues often arise following a first event. A large prospective study of SUDEP cases would provide the necessary information in this regard. This will also be addressed in a National Sentinel Audit supported by the Department of Health in the UK.

With current knowledge, the decision regarding when treatment should be started is made following discussions with the individual concerned, depending on the exact circumstances of the case. The likelihood of compliance also needs to be assessed, because it is often the case that a young otherwise fit young adult has doubts about the diagnosis and the need for long-term treatment. In certain situations, there may be more risk from non-compliance than from an untreated second seizure. Assuming that there is no diagnostic doubt and unless there are specific circumstances that favour early treatment such as patient wishes and circumstances, a very high likelihood of early recurrence or the presence of progressive disease, or seizure descriptions that appeared particularly life threatening, my own practice is not to recommend treatment routinely after a first seizure.

Antiepileptic drug withdrawal

Withdrawal of antiepileptic drugs is contemplated by those in remission, as well as by young women before conception. Many patients and indeed physicians underestimate the risk of recurrence even after years of complete freedom from seizures. An estimate of the likelihood of recurrence can be based on the Liverpool MRC Antiepileptic Drug Withdrawal Study.[99] Many individuals chose at that point not to withdraw treatment to avoid potential consequences of seizure recurrence, be they social, employment related or because of driving regulations. For those who choose to withdraw, despite knowing the 'odds', they need to be informed that, in addition to potential social consequences, safety issues also need to be considered because seizures are not always benign and carry some risk. Further discussion is tailored to the individual. Where such planned withdrawal is undertaken, I always advise very gradual withdrawal because abrupt changes may carry an increased risk.

Treatment options

Patients contemplating presurgical work-up with a view to epilepsy surgery need to be informed, not only of the risks involved in the procedures and surgery proposed, but also of the risks inherent in uncontrolled epilepsy. Long-term overall postoperative mortality remains elevated, but to a lesser extent than

would be expected in an intractable cohort, with deaths occurring particularly in relation to unsuccessful surgery. Furthermore, a change in seizure type, which may alter risk if surgery is unsuccessful, needs to be considered.

In considering treatment options, patients and physicians need to weigh up the risk of the epilepsy against the risk of new or old antiepileptic drugs and of other therapeutic interventions, such as vagal nerve stimulation.

Summary

Every effort must be made to prevent avoidable deaths in epilepsy. All patients should be given general advice on safety. Dangers from heights, unprotected waterfronts, fires, unsupervised bathing or swimming, dangerous machinery and driving need to be highlighted. Epilepsy should be treated aggressively. Patients need to be cautioned of the dangers of non-compliance. Abrupt changes in prescribed medication should be avoided where possible, as should circumstances or drugs (including alcohol and sleep deprivation) known to precipitate seizures in specific cases. Vigilance is required when any antiepileptic drug is prescribed, particularly in the early stages. Depression associated with epilepsy needs to be actively managed. Relatives need to be advised on how to respond to seizures, and individuals given the opportunity to make informed choices about the level of supervision that they require depending on the severity of their epilepsy. Those involved in making treatment decisions need to be aware of the background risk of the epilepsy itself.

Since this chapter was written, a case-control study of SUDEP has been published showing an increased relative risk of SUDEP with number of seizures per year, increased number of AEDs and frequent changes of medication.[130]

References

1. Hauser WA, Hesdorffer DC Mortality. In: *Epilepsy: frequency, causes and conse-quences*. Maryland: Epilepsy Foundation of USA, 1990.
2. Nashef L, Sander JWAS, Shorvon SD. Mortality in epilepsy. In: Pedley TA, Meldrum BS, eds. *Recent advances in epilepsy 6*. Edin-burgh: Churchill Livingstone, 1995: 271–87.
3. Hauser WA, Annegers JF, Elveback LR. Mortality in patients with epilepsy. *Epilepsia* 1980;**21**:399–412.
4. Nashef L, Shorvon SD. Mortality in epilepsy (editorial commentary). *Epilepsia* 1997;**38**: 1059–61.
5. Cockerell OC, Johnson AL, Sander JWAS, et al. Mortality from epilepsy: results from a prospective population-based study. *Lancet* 1994;**344**:918–21.
6. Zielinski JJ. Epilepsy and mortality rate and cause of death. *Epilepsia* 1974;**15**:191–201.
7. Henriksen B, Juul-Jensen P, Lund M. The mortality of epileptics. In: Brackenridge RDC, ed. *Proceedings of the 10th International Congress of Life Assurance Medicine*. London: Putman, 1970:139–48.
8. Preston J. Information on sudden deaths from epilepsy. *Epilepsia* 1997;**38**(Suppl 11): S72–74.
9. Fish DR. Sudden unexpected death in epilepsy: impact on clinical practice. *Epilepsia* 1997;**38**(Suppl 11):S60–2.
10. Brown SW. Impact on priority setting. *Epilepsia* 1997;**38**(Suppl 11):S70–1.
11. Bacon GM. On the modes of death in epilepsy. *Lancet* 1868;**1**:555–6.
12. Munson JF. Death in epilepsy. *Medical Rec* 1910 Jan 8;**58**:62.
13. Spratling WP. Prognosis. In: *Epilepsy and its treatment*. Philadelphia: WB Saunders, 1904: 304.
14. Nashef L, Annegers JF, Brown SW. Introduction and overview. Proceedings of the international workshop on sudden death in epilepsy, London 28/10/96. *Epilepsia* 1997; **38**(Suppl 11):S1–2.
15. Epilepsy Bereaved? PO Box 1777, Bournemouth BH5 1YR, UK.
16. Leestma JE, Annegers AF, Brodie MJ, et al. Incidence of sudden unexplained death in the Lamictal (Lamotrigine) clinical development program. *Epilepsia* 1994;**35**:12.
17. Annegers JF, Coan SP, Hauser WA, et al. Epilepsy, vagal nerve stimulation by the NCP system, mortality and sudden unexpected unexplained death. *Epilepsia* 1998;**39**:206–12.
18. Leestma JE. Forensic considerations in sudden unexpected death in epilepsy. *Epilepsia* 1997;**38**(Suppl 11):S63–6.
19. Hanna J. Epilepsy and sudden death: a personal view. *Epilepsia* 1997;**38**(Suppl 11): S3–5.
20. Baker GA, Nashef L, van Hout BA. The impact of frequent seizures on cost of illness, quality of life and mortality. Current issues in the management of epilepsy. *Epilepsia* 1997;**38**(Suppl 11):S1–S8.
21. Sander JWAS. Some aspects of prognosis in the epilepsies: a review. *Epilepsia* 1993; **34**: 1007–16.
22. Wannamaker BB. A perspective on death of persons with epilepsy. In: Lathers CM, Schraeder PL, eds. *Epilepsy and sudden death*. New York: Marcel Dekker, 1990:27–37.
23. Nashef L, Sander JWAS, Fish DR, Shorvon SD. Incidence of sudden unexpected death in an outpatient cohort with epilepsy at a tertiary referral centre. *J Neurol Neurosurg Psychiatry* 1995;**58**:462–4.
24. Nashef L, Fish DR, Garner S, et al. Sudden death in epilepsy – a study of incidence in a young cohort with epilepsy and learning diffi-culty. *Epilepsia* 1995;**36**:1187–94.
25. Snow RW, Williams REM, Rogers JE, et al. The prevalence of epilepsy among a rural Kenyan population: its association with premature mortality. *Trop Geogr Med* 1994;**46**:175–9.
26. Senanayake N, Peiris H. Mortality related to convulsive disorders in a developing country in Asia: trends over 20 years. *Seizure* 1995;**4**:273–7.
27. Nilsson L. Tomson T. Farahmand BY, et al. Cause specific mortality in epilepsy: a cohort

study of more than 9,000 patients once hospitalized for epilepsy. *Epilepsia* 1997;**38**: 1062–8.

28. Chevrie JJ, Aicardi J. Convulsive disorders in the first year of life. Neurological and mental outcome and mortality. *Epilepsia* 1978;**19**: 67–74.

29. Brorson LO, Wranne L. Long-term prognosis in childhood epilepsy: survival and seizure prognosis. *Epilepsia* 1987;**28**:324–30.

30. Harvey AS, Hopkins IJ, Nolan TM, Carlin JB. Mortality in children with epilepsy: an epidemiological study. AES proceedings. *Epilepsia* 1991;**32**(Suppl 3):54.

31. Luhdorf K, Jensen LK, Plesner AM. Epilepsy in the elderly: life expectancy and causes of death. *Acta Neurol Scand* 1987;**76**:183–90.

32. Appleton RE. Sudden unexpected death in epilepsy in children. *Seizure* 1997;**6**:175–7.

33. Williams CE. Accidents in mentally retarded children. *Dev Med Child Neurol* 1973;**15**: 660–2.

34. Forsgren L, Edvison SO, Nystrom K, Blomquisk HK. Influence of epilepsy on mortality in mental retardation: an epidemiologic study. *Epilepsia* 1996;**37**:956–63.

35. Buck D, Baker G, Jacoby A, et al. Patients' experience of injury as a result of epilepsy. *Epilepsia* 1997;**38**:439–44.

36. Cummings SR, Nevitt MC, Browner WS, et al. Risk factors for hip fracture in white women. *N Engl J Med* 1995;**332**:767–73.

37. Kemp AM, Sibert JR. Epilepsy in children and the risk of drowning. *Arch Dis Child* 1993;**68**:684–5.

38. Ryan CA, Dowling G. Drowning deaths in people with epilepsy. *Can Med Assoc J* 1993; **148**:781–84.

39. Diekema DS, Quan L, Holt VL. Epilepsy as a risk factor for submersion injury in children. *Paediatrics* 1993;**91**:612–6.

40. Orlowski JP, Rothner DA, Lueders H. Submersion accidents in children with epilepsy. *Am J Dis Child* 1982;**136**:777–80.

41. Smith NM, Byard RW, Bourne AJ. Death during immersion in water in childhood. *Am J Forensic Med Pathol* 1991;**12**:219–21.

42. Sonnen AEH. *Epilepsy and swimming.* Monograph of Neural Science Vol. 5. Basel: Karger, 1980:256–70.

43. Brown SW. Sudden death and epilepsy: clinical review. *Seizure* 1992;**1**:71–3.

44. Bener A, Murdoch JC, Achan NV, et al. The effect of epilepsy on road traffic accidents and casualties. *Seizure* 1996;**5**:215–9.

45. Hansotia P, Broste SK. The effect of epilepsy or diabetes mellitus on the risk of automobile accidents. *N Engl J Med* 1991;**324**:22–6.

46. Hansotia P, Broste SK. Epilepsy or diabetes and auto accidents. *N Engl J Med* 1991;**324**:1511 (letter).

47. Taylor J. Epilepsy and driving. In: Duncan JS, Gill JQ, eds. *Lecture Notes: 4th Epilepsy Teaching Weekend, International League Against Epilepsy* (British Branch)1993: 275–8.

48. Kirby S, Sadler RM. Injury and death as a result of seizures. *Epilepsia* 1995;**36**:25–8.

49. Russell-Jones DL, Shorvon SD. The frequency and consequences of head injury in epileptic seizures. *J Neurol Neurosurg Psychiatry* 1989; **52**:659–62.

50. Klenerman P, Sander JWAS, Shorvon SD. Mortality in patients with epilepsy: a study of patients in long-term residential care. *J Neurol Neurosurg Psychiatry* 1993;**56**:149–52.

51. Spitz MC, Towbin JA, Shantz D, Adler LE. Risk factors for burns as a consequence of seizures in patients with epilepsy. *Epilepsia* 1994;**35**:764–7.

52. Spitz MC. Injury and death as consequences of epilepsy. *Sudden Death and Epilepsy* (Syllabus). American Epilepsy Society, Dec 1997:18–20.

53. Shorvon SD. Prognosis and outcome of status epilepticus. In: *Status Epilepticus.* Cambridge: Cambridge University Press, 1994:293–301.

54. Nashef L. Sudden unexpected death in epilepsy: incidence, circumstances and mechanisms. University of Bristol, 1995 (thesis).

55. Hesdorffer DC, Logroscino G, Cascino G, et al. Incidence of status epilepticus in Rochester, Minnesota 1965–84 *Neurology* 1998;**50**: 735–41.

56. Waller M. The epidemiology and management of status epilepticus. *Curr Opin Neurol* 1998;**11**:149–54.

57. Dasheiff RM. Sudden unexpected death in epilepsy: a series from an epilepsy surgery programme and speculation on the relation-

ship to sudden cardiac death. *J Clin Neurophysiol* 1991;**8**:216–22.

58. Earnest MP, Thomas GE, Randall AE, Kenneth FH. The sudden unexplained death syndrome in epilepsy. *Epilepsia* 1992;**33**:310–16.

59. Freytag E, Lindenberg R. Medicolegal autopsies on epileptics. *Arch Pathol* 1994;**78**:274–86.

60. Hashimoto K, Fukushima Y, Saito F, Wada K. Mortality and causes of death in patients with epilepsy over 16 years of age. *Jpn J Psychiatry Neurol* 1989;**43**:546–7.

61. Hirsch CS, Martin DL. Unexpected death in young epileptics. *Neurology* 1971;**21**:682–90.

62. Iivanainen M, Lehtinen J. Causes of death in institutionalized epileptics. *Epilepsia* 1979;**20**:485–92.

63. Jallon P, Haton F, Maguin P. Death among epileptics. *Adv in Epileptol* 1989;**17**:351–5.

64. Jay GW, Leetsma JE. Sudden death in epilepsy. A comprehensive review of the literature and proposed mechanisms. *Acta Neurol Scand* 1981;**63**(Suppl B2):5–66.

65. Jick SS, Cole TB, Mesher RA, et al. Sudden unexplained death in young persons with primary epilepsy. *Pharmcoepidemiol and Drug Safety* 1992;**1**:59–64.

66. Keeling JW, Knowles SAS. Sudden death in childhood and adolescence. *J Pathol* 1989;**159**:221–4.

67. Krohn W. Causes of death among epileptics. *Epilepsia* 1963;**4**:315–21.

68. Lathers CM, Schraeder PL, eds. *Epilepsy and sudden death*. New York: Marcel Dekker, 1990.

69. Leestma JE, Hughes JR, Teas SS, Kalelkar MB. Sudden epilepsy deaths and the forensic pathologist. *Am J Forensic Med Pathol* 1985;**16**:215–18.

70. Leestma JE, Annegers AF, Brodie MJ, et al. Incidence of sudden unexplained death in persons with seizure disorder treated with antiepileptic drugs in Saskatchewan, Canada. *Epilepsia* 1995;**36**:29–36.

71. Leetsma JE. A pathological review. In: Lathers CM, Schraeder PL, eds. *Epilepsy and sudden death*. New York: Marcel Dekker, 1990:61–88.

72. Leetsma JE, Walczak T, Hughes JR, et al. Prospective study on sudden unexpected death in epilepsy. *Ann Neurol* 1989;**26**:195–203.

73. Lip GYH, Brodie MJ. Sudden death in epilepsy: an avoidable outcome? *J R Soc Med* 1992;**85**:609–11.

74. Nashef L, Brown S. Epilepsy and sudden death (commentary). *Lancet* 1996;**348**:1324–5.

75. Nashef L, Sander JWAS. Sudden death in epilepsy – where are we now? *Seizure* 1996;**5**:235–8.

76. Schwender LA, Troncoso JC. Evaluation of sudden death in epilepsy. *Am J Forensic Mec Pathol* 1986;**7**:283–7.

77. Wilson JB. Hazards of epilepsy. *BMJ* 1978;**2**:200.

78. Brown SW. Sudden death and epilepsy: clinical review. *Seizure* 1992;**1**:71–3.

79. Nashef L, Garner S, Sander JWAS, et al. Circumstances of death in sudden death in epilepsy: interviews of bereaved relatives. *J Neurol Neurosurg Psychiatry* 1998;**64**:349–52.

80. Hordt M, Haverkamp W, Oberwittler C, et al. The idiopathic QT syndrome as a cause of epileptic and nonepileptic seizures. *Nervenartzt* 1995;**66**:282–7.

81. Archibald RB Armstrong JD. Recurrent post-ictal pulmonary oedema. *Postgrad Med* 1978;**63**:210–13.

82. Bloom S. Pulmonary edema following a grand mal epileptic seizure. *Am Rev Respir Dis* 1968;**97**:292–4.

83. Bonbrest HC. Pulmonary edema following an epileptic seizure. *Am Rev Respir Dis* 1965;**91**:97–100.

84. Ohlmacher AP. Acute pulmonary oedema as a terminal event in certain forms of epilepsy. *Am J Med Sc* 1910;**139**:417–22.

85. Blumhardt LD, Smith PEM, Owen L. Electrographic accompaniments of temporal lobe epileptic seizures. *Lancet* 1986;**1**:1051–5.

86. Jallon P. Epilepsie et coeur. Rev Neurol 1997;**153**:173–84.

87. Jallon P. Arrhythmogenic seizures. *Epilepsia* 1997;**38**:S43–7.

88. Singh B, Al Shahwan SA, Al Deeb S. Partial seizures presenting as life threatening apnea. *Epilepsia* 1993;**34**:901–3.

89. Simon RP. Epileptic sudden death: animal models. *Epilepsia* 1997;**38**(Suppl 11):S35–6.

90. Johnston SC, Siedenberg R, Min JK, et al. Central apnea and acute cardiac ischemia in a sheep model of epileptic sudden death. *Ann Neurol* 1997;**42**:588–94.

91. Nashef L, Walker F, Allen P, et al. Apnoea and bradycardia during epileptic seizures: relation to sudden death in epilepsy. *J Neurol Neurosurg Psychiatry* 1996;**60**:297–300.

92. Walker F, Fish DR. Recording respiratory parameters in patients with epilepsy. *Epilepsia* 1997;**38**(Suppl 11):S41–2.

93. Bird JM, Dembny KAT, Sandeman D, Butler S. Sudden unexplained death in epilepsy: an intracranially monitored case. *Epilepsia* 1997;**38**(Suppl 11):S52–6.

94. Annegers JF, Hauser WA, Shirts SB. Heart disease mortality and morbidity in patients with epilepsy. *Epilepsia* 1984;**25**:699–704.

95. Schraeder PL, Lathers CM, eds. The relation of paroxysmal autonomic dysfunction and epileptogenic activity. In: *Epilepsy and sudden death*. New York: Marcel Dekker, 1990:21–197.

96. Mameli O. Discussion. *Epilepsia* 1997;**38**: S58.

97. Tomson T, Kenneback G. Arrhythmia, heart rate variability and anti-epileptic drugs. *Epilepsia* 1997;**38**(Suppl 11):S48–51.

98. O'Donaghue MF, Sander JWAS. The mortality associated with epilepsy, with particular reference to sudden unexpected death: a review. *Epilepsia* 1997;**38**(Suppl 11):S15–9.

99. Medical Research Council Antiepileptic Drug Withdrawal Study Group. Randomized study of antiepileptic drug withdrawal in patients in remission. *Lancet* 1991;**337**:1175–80.

100. Annegers JF. United States perspective on definitions and classifications *Epilepsia* 1997;**38**(Suppl 11):S9–12.

101. Bowerman DL, Levinsky JA, Urich RW, Wittenberg PH. Premature deaths in persons with seizure disorders: subtherapeutic levels of anticonvulsant drugs in postmortem blood specimens. *J Forensic Sci* 1978;**23**:522–6.

102. Thom M. Neuropathologic findings in postmortem studies of sudden death in epilepsy *Epilepsia* 1997;**38**(Suppl 11):S32–4.

103. Leestma JE. Sudden unexpected death associated with seizures: a pathological review. In: Lathers CM, Schraeder PL, eds. *Epilepsy and sudden death*. New York: Marcel Dekker, 1990:61–8.

104. Natelson BH, Suarez RV, Terence CF, Turizo R. Patients with epilepsy who die suddenly have cardiac disease. *Arch Neurol* 1998;**55**:857–60.

105. Barraclough BM. The suicide rate of epilepsy. *Acta Psychiatr Scand* 1987;**76**:339–45.

106. Mathews WS, Barabas G. Suicide and epilepsy: a review of the literature. *Psychosomatics* 1981;**22**:515–24.

107. Jensen I. Temporal lobe epilepsy. Late mortality in patients treated with unilateral temporal lobe resections. *Acta Neurol Scand* 1975;**52**: 374–80.

108. Taylor DC, Marsh SM. Implications of long-term follow-up studies in epilepsy: with a note on the cause of death. In: Penry JK, ed. *Epilepsy: the Eighth International Symposium*, New York: Raven Press, 1977:27–34.

109. Force L, Jallon P, Hoffman JJ. Suicide and epilepsy. *Adv Epileptol* 1989;**17**:356–8.

110. Mendez MF, Doss RC. Ictal and psychiatric aspects of suicide in epileptic patients. *Int J Psychiatr Med* 1992;**22**:231–7.

111. Robertson M. Mood disorders associated with epilepsy. In: McConnel HW, Snyder PJ, eds. *Psychiatric comorbidity in epilepsy*. Washington: American Psychiatric Press, 1998:133–67.

112. Perucca E, Gram L, Avanzini G, Dulac O. *Epilepsia* 1998;**39**:5–17.

113. O'Donoghue MJ, Duncan JS, Sander JWAS. The National Hospital Seizure Severity Scale: a further development of the Chalfont Seizure Scale. *Epilepsia* 1996;**37**:563–71.

114. Baker GA, Smith DF, Dewey M, et al. The development of a seizure severity scale as an outcome measure in epilepsy. *Epilepsy Res* 1991;**8**:245–51.

115. White SJ, McLean AEM, Howland C. Anticonvulsant drugs and cancer. A cohort study in patients with severe epilepsy. *Lancet* 1979;**ii**:458–60.

116. Clemmesen J, Fuglsang-Frederiksen V, Plum C. Are anticonvulsants oncogenic? *Lancet* 1974;**i**:705–7.

117. Olsen JH, Boice JD, Jensen JPA, Fraumeni JF. Cancer among epileptic patients exposed to antiepileptic drugs. *J Natl Cancer Inst* 1989;**81**:803–9.

118. Anthony JJ. Malignant lymphoma associated with hydantoin drugs. *Arch Neurol* 1970;**22**:450–4.

119. Friedman GD. Barbiturates and lung cancer in humans. *J Natl Cancer Instit* 1981;**67**:291–5.

120. Shirts SB, Naaegers JF, Hauser AW, Kurland LT. Cancer incidence in a cohort of patients with seizure disorders. *J Natl Cancer Instit* 1986;**77**:83–7.

121. Dreifuss FE, Santilli N, Langer DH, et al. Valproic acid hepatic fatalities: a retrospective review. *Neurology* 1987;**37**:379–85.

122. Jacome DE. Syncope and sudden death attributed to carbamazepine. *J Neurol Neurosurg Psychiatry* 1987;**50**:1245.

123. Stone S, Lange LS. Syncope and sudden unexpected death attributed to carbamazepine in a 20-year-old epileptic. *J Neurol Neurosurg Psychiatry* 1986;**49**:1460–1.

124. Kaufman DW, Kelly JP, Anderson T, et al. Evaluation of case reports of aplastic anaemia among patients treated with felbamate. *Epilepsy* 1997;**38**:1265–69.

125. Vickrey BG. Mortality in a consecutive cohort of 248 adolescents and adults who underwent diagnostic evaluation for epilepsy surgery. *Epilepsia* 1997;**38**:S70–1.

126. Sperling MR, O'Connor MJ, Saykin AJ, Plummer C. Temporal lobectomy for refractory epilepsy. *JAMA* 1996;**276**:470–5.

127. Hennessy M, Langan Y, Elwes RDC, et al. A study of mortality following temporal lobe epilepsy surgery. *Neurology* 1999; in press.

128. Persinger MA, Psych C. Sudden unexpected death in epileptics following sudden, intense increases in geomagnetic activity: prevalence of effect and potential mechanisms. *Int J Biometeorol* 1995;**38**:180–7.

129. Berg AT, Shinnar S. Do seizures beget seizures? An assesment of the clinical evidence in humans. *J Clin Neurophysiol* 1997;**14**: 102–10.

130. Nilsson L, Farahmand BY, Persson PG, et al. Risk factors for sudden unexpected death in epilepsy: a case-control study. *Lancet* 1999;**353**:888–93.

31

Predicting surgical outcome in epilepsy: how good are we?

Thomas Grunwald, Martin Kurthen and Christian E Elger

Introduction

The presurgical evaluation of patients with intractable epilepsy has three primary goals: to localize the primary epileptogenic area; to determine individual risks of potential surgical therapy; and to evaluate chances of postoperative seizure control. Eventually, the aim is to counsel patients adequately about surgery, with regard to their individual prospects and risks, so that they can decide for or against this elective treatment. Thus, prognosis is essential for the preoperative work-up, not only to identify candidates who may profit from epilepsy surgery but also to counsel the individual patient. Postoperative quality of life is, of course, influenced by numerous factors such as neurological and neuropsychological outcome or vocational rehabilitation. Seizure control is, however, one of the most important of these factors and, within the bounds of the present chapter we concentrate on prognosis of seizure outcome.

How can an adequate prognosis be made? Obviously, prognosis depends on the results that epilepsy surgery can achieve on the whole. Therefore, to evaluate the chances of postoperative seizure control in individual patients it is first necessary to identify characteristic syndromes of patients who have been operated on previously. If it is possible to subsume an individual patient under one of these syndromes, the outcome of surgery within this

subgroup can then be used to assess individual chances of seizure control. Essentially, the concepts of 'prognosis' and 'outcome' are closely related, even mutually dependent. A better outcome for a certain patient group improves the prognosis of individual patients within this group. Conversely, more accurate classification of individual patients under specific syndromes may influence surgical outcome if it leads to a more restrictive choice of patients for surgery. However, if efforts to improve the accuracy of prognosis led to the clinical practice of offering surgery only to *ideal* candidates, a considerable number of patients would be denied surgery in spite of its possible success. Accordingly, improvement in the accuracy of prognosis may also mean better identification of candidates who are not *ideal*, but may still benefit from surgery.

That prognosis is best for candidates who are ideal and worse for those who are not may appear as a truism. Yet, different centers will draw different conclusions from this fact. It is conceivable that some centers may decide to operate only on ideal candidates and deny surgery to all others, which would result in a high percentage of postoperative seizure freedom. Alternatively, other centers may be less restrictive, which would worsen outcome statistics but make it possible that certain (ideal) candidates have a better prognosis than the overall outcome statistics at these specific centers. In any case, both to identify ideal candidates and to offer surgery to patients who are not ideal, but still have the chance to become seizure-free, calls for the reliable assessment of the potential surgical outcome.

Over the past few years, it has become evident that to predict surgical outcome, it is advisable to distinguish between patients with temporal lobe epilepsy and those with seizures of extratemporal origin. For both groups, it has been shown that prospects are significantly better if there is evidence of a morphological correlate of the primary epileptogenic area, as detected by magnetic resonance imaging (MRI).[1,2] In the following, we address prognosis in temporal lobe epilepsy and extratemporal epilepsy separately. Moreover, we give special consideration to the question of whether imaging studies may suffice for evaluation of the prospects of epilepsy surgery.

Prognosis in temporal lobe epilepsy

The outcome of epilepsy surgery for temporal lobe epilepsy has improved over the last few decades. A comparison between two surveys presented at the Palm Desert conferences of 1986 and 1992 shows that, while in the first survey 1296 temporal lobe resections led to seizure cessation in 55.5 per cent of the patients, the second survey could report on a seizure-free rate of 67.9 per cent after 2429 anterior temporal lobectomies and of 68.8 per cent after selective amygdalohippocampectomies.[3] A good outcome has been shown to persist over the longer term.[4-6]

Medical history

The medical history of patients with temporal lobe epilepsy who are eligible for resective surgery may be of predictive value. In particu-

lar, the age at seizure onset and a history of febrile convulsions have been shown to indicate good prognosis for postoperative seizure cessation, most probably because both factors are associated with the development of Ammon's horn sclerosis.[7] As earlier studies of brain pathology in epilepsy patients have directed attention to mesial temporal lobe structures,[8-10] an increasing number of investigations has underlined the importance of 'Ammon's horn sclerosis', 'hippocampal' or 'mesial temporal sclerosis' for temporal lobe epilepsy.[11-13] Today, it is widely accepted that mesial temporal lobe epilepsy with Ammon's horn sclerosis represents a well-defined syndrome.[13] It is characterized by hippocampal atrophy and sclerosis, onset of unilateral or bilateral anterotemporal interictal epileptiform abnormalities, mesial temporal seizures, and, in many cases, a history of febrile convulsions or another initial precipitating injury. Histopathology demonstrates sprouting of mossy fibers and a decline in densities of Ammon's horn neurons, typically sparing the CA-2 subfield.[14,15]

A second group of patients with temporal lobe epilepsy includes those in whom MRI shows signs of structural temporal lobe abnormalities other than Ammon's horn sclerosis; postsurgical histopathological analyses demonstrate either neoplastic or non-neoplastic focal lesions. Seizure control in these patients has been found to compare favorably with that of patients with mesial temporal lobe epilepsy, while the outcome is significantly worse in patients without Ammon's horn sclerosis and without any temporal lobe lesions. In a study of 178 patients who received temporal lobe surgery in Bonn, the rate of seizure-free outcome was 68.5 per cent for patients with neoplastic lesions, 66.7 per cent for those with Ammon's horn sclerosis, and 54 per cent for those with non-neoplastic focal lesions.[16] By contrast, none of the patients in whom histopathological findings were normal became seizure-free postoperatively. In a study by O'Brien et al, of 46 patients, 87 per cent of the patients with Ammon's horn sclerosis became seizure-free, compared with 60 per cent of the patients with temporal neocortical lesions.[17] Even patients with dual pathology, i.e. Ammon's horn sclerosis in addition to an extrahippocampal lesion, can become seizure-free if surgery includes resection of both the lesion and the atrophic hippocampus.[18]

Magnetic resonance imaging

As the presence of a morphological correlate of the primary epileptogenic area influences surgical prognosis decisively, evidence of Ammon's horn sclerosis or other temporal lobe pathology in MRI studies is one of the most important diagnostic findings in the presurgical work-up. Kuzniecky et al examined the predictive value of MRI findings in 34 patients with temporal lobe epilepsy selected for surgical treatment.[19] MRI abnormalities were found in 25 of their patients, whereas in nine patients, the MRI scan was normal. In this study, the predictive value of abnormal MRI scans for surgical success was 82 per cent compared with 56 per cent of normal MRI scans. Garcia et al prospectively evaluated the prognostic value of MRI findings in 51 temporal lobe epilepsy patients; in 25 the MRI scan showed evidence of Ammon's horn sclerosis on the side that was eventually operated on.[20] Of these patients 24 (96 per cent) became seizure-free postoperatively. Arruda et al found complete seizure cessation in 85.1 per cent of their patients with unilateral hippocampal atrophy.[21] By contrast, only about half of the patients with either bilateral or no significant atrophy of the mesial temporal lobe became seizure-free. Thadani et al reported on 22 patients with temporal lobe epilepsy who

had MRI signs of a localized abnormality and concordant clinical seizure pattern, interictal and ictal scalp EEG, neuropsychological testing, and results of the intracarotid amobarbitone (amobarbital) procedure.[22] Of these patients, 18 (82 per cent) became seizure-free. In 60 patients with temporal lobe lesions, Eliashiv et al found a seizure-free rate of 80 per cent after standard *en bloc* anterior temporal lobe resection, including mesiotemporal structures.[23] Berkovic et al studied the outcome after temporal lobectomy in 135 patients classified into subgroups according to preoperative MRI findings.[24] After a follow-up of at least 2 years, 80 per cent of patients with foreign tissue lesions, 62 per cent with Ammon's horn sclerosis and 36 per cent with normal MRI scans were completely seizure-free.

In summary, MRI findings that indicate the presence of Ammon's horn sclerosis or a foreign tissue lesion in temporal lobe epilepsy are of indisputable importance for the presurgical work-up and have a high positive predictive value. On the other hand, there are MRI findings in temporal lobe epilepsy that may worsen the prognosis of temporal lobe surgery, including widespread extrahippocampal structural abnormalities,[25] periventricular nodular heterotopia[26] and, possibly, cerebellar atrophy.[27]

Electrophysiological studies

In spite of the importance of MRI studies, it still remains necessary to demonstrate the epileptogenicity of structural abnormalities. Fish and Spencer communicated their results from intracranial EEG recordings in 51 patients with unilateral Ammon's horn sclerosis[28] and stated that, although 29 were localized to the atrophic hippocampus, 12 remained unlocalized and 9 were localized elsewhere. These authors emphasize the need to search for more dual pathology that has remained undetected on MRI scan, because the removal of the EEG focus led to complete seizure control in half of the patients who had EEG localization other than in Ammon's horn sclerosis. Consistent with the view that electrophysiological studies are necessary, King et al described 5 patients in a series of 53 who had bilateral hippocampal atrophy and in whom surgery was performed on the side of ictal onset. Four of these patients became seizure-free.[29] The same group also reported that, in a larger group of 101 patients with Ammon's horn sclerosis, they found three with discordant EEG and Ammon's horn sclerosis.[30] While, in these patients, resection of the non-atrophic hippocampus yielded excellent results, 4 patients with seizure onset on the side of Ammon's horn sclerosis failed to achieve seizure control by hippocampectomy. It can be concluded that the presence of hippocampal atrophy is not an independent predictor of the site of epileptogenesis.

Thus, in spite of the sensitivity of MRI for Ammon's horn sclerosis, electrophysiological studies remain indispensable for the presurgical work-up. If only non-invasive monitoring is performed, unequivocal recordings of one or several, more or less circumscribed, electrophysiological seizures are required by most centers before surgery, and patients without localized seizure onset or with multifocal seizures will not usually be operated on. Therefore, it is not possible to test the prognostic value of non-invasively recorded seizures statistically, and the prognosis of surgical outcome, based on electrophysiology, draws on interictal findings. Well-localized unilateral temporal spikes on the interictal scalp EEG, as opposed to an extratemporal spread of interictal spikes, have been shown to be indicative of a favorable outcome.[31] By contrast, Holmes et al found a postoperative cessation of seizures in only 50 per cent of their 44 patients with bitemporal interictal epileptiform patterns.[32] This is consistent with the fact that onset of bilateral independent seizures correlates strongly with bitemporal excitability, as shown by scalp EEG recordings.[33] However, there are patients with bilateral epileptiform EEG potentials who do profit from temporal lobe surgery.[34] In these patients, invasive recordings from hippocampal depth and subdural strip electrodes often are necessary to lateralize and localize the primary epileptogenic focus.

For data derived from invasive long-term monitoring, the following have been found to be favorable prognostic parameters:[35] the unilateral onset of seizures, fast spike trains as electrical pattern of onset, the absence of frontal lobe background desynchronization at the onset, and an interhemispheric propagation time of more than 8 s. Compatible with this, Hufnagel et al found that 89 per cent of patients (n = 59) investigated with subdural electrodes who had unilateral seizure onset and ipsilateral interictal epileptiform discharges became seizure-free after surgery.[36] By contrast, only half of those patients who showed unilateral seizure onset but bitemporal spikes or sharp waves were seizure-free. Furthermore, Spencer and Spencer argue that not only the site of seizure origin but also the site of seizure termination has prognostic value.[37] They found that localizing the site of seizure termination to cortical regions that differ from those of the focal onset is associated with a poorer surgical prognosis; this possibly indicates additional epileptogenic cortical regions. A more recent study could not, however, replicate these results.[38] The fact that patients with residual spikes in postoperative EEG studies have a higher risk of recurrent seizures,[39,40] may argue for more widespread epileptogenicity being a cause of a less favorable outcome.

Other imaging methods

Functional imaging methods have also been used to predict seizure outcome with variable success. While ictal[41] and interictal single photon emission computed tomography (SPECT)[42,43] may be of limited value, positron emission tomography (PET) studies that indicate anterolateral[44] or lateral[45] (rather than mesial) areas of hypometabolism, may be more promising. In a study by Theodore et al, 18 of 23 patients (78 per cent) with unilateral temporal fluorodeoxyglucose (FDG)-PET hypometabolism became seizure-free after temporal lobectomy; 14 patients had no lateralized PET abnormalities; seven were operated on but only four became seizure-free.

Other tests

Functional disturbances are also evaluated by the intracarotid amobarbital test (Wada test), which has been shown to contribute to the prediction of postoperative seizure control.[46,47] Perrine et al found that this test correlated with the side of surgery in 98 per cent of 70 patients with left-sided speech dominance, and correctly predicted 80 per cent of those patients who became seizure-free.[48] Lancman et al demonstrated that the Wada test has a high specificity but a low sensitivity for seizure-free outcome, with a positive predictive value of 87 per cent and a negative predictive value of 38 per cent.[49] However, they underscored the drawback that this test is not standardized in its application at different centers.

Sawrie et al used the performance in neuropsychological tests to predict the surgical outcome in 79 patients with left and 62 with right temporal lobe epilepsy.[50] The comparison of the predictive accuracy of these data in 'optimal' (55 per cent) and 'suboptimal' patients (72 per cent) with temporal lobe epilepsy showed that the results of neuropsychological tests may contribute to predictive accuracy in the latter group, although it may even reduce the prognostic exactness in patients who fit standard criteria for anterior temporal lobectomy perfectly. Presurgical IQ scores are also related to seizure outcome in temporal lobe epilepsy. In a recent study, Chelune et al[51] found that the odds of becoming seizure-free were 2:1 for patients with baseline IQ scores of under 75, 3:1 among patients with IQ scores of 76–109, and 4:1 among patients with higher scores.

Finally, the extent of the surgical procedure influences the eventual outcome, as has been shown for the extent of mesiobasal resection (regardless of the extent of lateral resection) in mesial temporal lobe epilepsy[52] and the completeness of lesion resection in lesional temporal lobe epilepsy.[53,54] However, such data obviously become available only after a decision in favor of temporal lobe surgery has been made; they cannot be used to counsel patients preoperatively. Counseling has to draw on the presurgical findings of imaging, electrophysiological and neuropsychological studies.

In summary, the prognostic accuracy of the diagnostic methods discussed above can reach 80 per cent, as has also been shown for the combination of methods.[55,56] Although this percentage seems high, we have to remember that it includes a 20 per cent probability of error, which highlights the necessity of further studies of epileptogenicity in temporal lobe epilepsy and its presurgical evaluation.

Prognosis in extratemporal epilepsy

Prognosis of surgery of extratemporal epilepsy is difficult to evaluate because patients with this type of epilepsy form a very heterogeneous sample, which is, moreover, much smaller in size than the temporal lobe epilepsy sample in most epilepsy centers. Furthermore, there is some evidence that surgery for extratemporal epilepsy is generally more problematic than temporal lobe epilepsy surgery.[57] Surface EEG recordings may suffer from a paucity of inter-ictal epileptiform discharges and from poor localization of ictal onset. Moreover, different paths of seizure propagation may result in heterogeneous semiological features, even in individual patients. As for outcome and prognosis, some valid information is available for frontal lobe epilepsy surgery (see below), although reports on parietal and occipital lobe surgery are clearly underrepresented. Even more than in patients with temporal lobe epilepsy, the presence of a monofocal morphological lesion represents a very important prognostic factor in surgery for extratemporal epilepsy. Studies of outcome from extratemporal resections agree that most—if not all—patients who become seizure-free post-operatively had structural lesions on preoperative MRI and/or cranial computed tomography (CCT) (see Tran et al[58] for a review). This is mainly due to the difficulty in localizing the epileptic focus in the absence of structural abnormalities or in the presence of multifocal lesions.[59] Diagnostic procedures with a high localizing value in temporal lobe epilepsy are often insufficient in extratemporal epilepsy: in addition to the problems of surface EEG recordings mentioned above, functional imaging is often inconsistent with respect to focus localization in extratemporal epilepsy.[60] Furthermore, the localizing value of neuropsychological testing is also limited in these patients: although the neuropsychological profile may help to identify patients with extratemporal functional impairment, it is often non-specific with regard to lateralization and the differentiation of frontal and parietal

(and occipital) deficits. Only ictal SPECT recordings seem to have some clinical value in non-invasively localizing the epileptic focus in patients with non-lesional extratemporal epilepsy.[61,62]

As a consequence of these limiting factors, intracranial EEG recordings are required in most patients with extratemporal epilepsy. In lesional patients, planning of electrode placement will be guided mostly by the localization of the lesion, in accordance with supplementary information about the EEG, semiology, etc. In non-lesional patients, however, it may even be impossible to achieve a plausible hypothesis for electrode implantation, if the basic localization information is contradictory or discordant. In the worst case, patients will be implanted with various multilobar electrodes, and yet recording of the seizure onset will not be achieved. In a recent study on outcome from extratemporal resections,[63] the relevance of structural lesions was again demonstrated: although 61 per cent of the lesional patients became seizure-free during a mean follow-up of 4 years, only 20 per cent of the non-lesional patients were completely free of seizures. In the whole group, 54 per cent of the patients were completely seizure-free, and an additional 32 per cent showed a seizure reduction of at least 75 per cent. These results indicate that seizure outcome for surgery for extratemporal epilepsy is generally favorable, but still slightly worse than the outcome for surgery for temporal lobe epilepsy (see also Rougier et al[64]).

For frontal lobe epilepsy surgery, some additional prognostic data are available. Although some authors again emphasize the prognostic relevance of pathological monofocal MRI findings,[59] others find that the immediate disappearance of epileptiform discharges after resection, demonstrated by intraoperative electrocorticography, is also a good predictor of favorable outcome.[65] In some subgroups, even surface EEG recordings may be predictive: in a sample of 17 patients with frontal encephalomalacias, Kazemi et al found that the presence of a focal ictal beta pattern was the best predictor of seizure-free outcome, an EEG pattern that was observed in 12 (70 per cent) of the patients.[66] At the present time, the data and literature do not allow consideration of the prognostic relevance of different sites of foci within the frontal lobe.

In parietal and occipital lobe surgery, prognostic factors are even harder to evaluate as a result of comparably small sample sizes. Studies carried out by Cascino et al[67] and Salanova et al[68,69] suggest that seizure outcome is generally favorable in these patients. Particularly in non-tumoral patients, lack of immediate post-resection epileptiform discharges in intraoperative electrocorticography can serve as a predictor of good seizure outcome,[68,70] in addition to the presence of MRI-detectable lesions[70,71] which also seems to be the most important factor in these patients.

When the epileptogenic area is located in or adjacent to eloquent brain areas, such as the motor or language cortex, a complete resection often cannot be achieved. Consequently, seizure outcome is comparably less favorable in such patients. This also holds for recent studies with application of the multiple subpial transection technique as an exclusive surgical procedure. Patients treated with multiple subpial transection alone characteristically show a significant reduction of seizure frequency, but complete seizure relief is rare.[72,73] However, when multiple subpial transections are performed in addition to resective surgery, seizure freedom can be achieved in 50–100 per cent of the patients.[71,74,75] In most patients, postoperative neurological deficits are transient, but the exact rate of persistent deficits remains to be determined by further studies.

In extratemporal epilepsy, in contrast to temporal lobe epilepsy, the prognostic relevance of functional imaging techniques, neuropsychological testing, and interictal and ictal EEG patterns, with respect to postoperative seizure outcome, has not yet been proved. Ictal SPECT, neuropsychological evaluation and surface-EEG recordings are essential for the planning of invasive testing, especially in non-lesional patients. Of course, a high localizing value is attributed to ictal electrocorticography patterns, but the predictive power of these patterns, with regard to seizure outcome from surgery in extratemporal epilepsy, remains to be demonstrated in studies with larger patient groups. As, in many epilepsy centers, patients with inconclusive ictal electrocorticography recordings or lack of concordance between MRI and ictal electrocorticography are not submitted for therapeutic surgery, it will be difficult to separate 'ictal onset' and 'MRI lesion' as predictive factors in retrospective analyses.

Independent of the location of a structural brain lesion, the completeness of its resection influences seizure outcome decisively.[2] Thus, one reason for the lower percentage of seizure-free outcomes from surgery in epilepsy patients with extratemporal lesions is the fact that there are patients in whom the lesion cannot be resected completely because of its proximity to eloquent cortical areas. Conversely, prognosis is better if the lesion is located far from these regions.

In summary, a seizure-free outcome from surgery for extratemporal epilepsy can be expected in *at least* 60 per cent of all patients with MRI signs of a cerebral lesion, and prognostic accuracy depends on the concordance of MRI and EEG/electrocorticography studies. In patients in whom the extratemporal lesion is far from eloquent areas, the percentage of patients free from seizures postoperatively can approach that of patients with lesional temporal lobe epilepsy.

Summary

During the last several decades, outcome studies have contributed to the refinement of diagnostic tools for the presurgical evaluation of epilepsy patients and to the improvement of the prognostic accuracy of these methods. Moreover, the experience that has been gained by relating non-invasive studies to ictal and interictal recordings from subdural and depth electrodes, has made it possible to do without invasive monitoring in a growing number of patients. Thus, the percentage of patients with temporal lobe epilepsy who are postoperatively free of seizures now can reach up to 70–80 per cent, depending on the composition of patient groups in different centers.

As for seizure outcome, invasive recordings are not necessarily indicated in patients with temporal lobe epilepsy who have MRI signs of unilateral Ammon's horn sclerosis, unilateral temporal interictal spike- or sharp-wave activity and concordant ictal onset, supported by concordant PET and neuropsychological findings. In these patients, a seizure-free outcome can be predicted with an accuracy of about 80 per cent; in some patients, it may even be possible to do without ictal recordings at all. However, it should be noted that seizure outcome, although important, is not the only factor determining postoperative quality of life. If, for example, there are data indicating possible functional disturbances of the contralateral temporal lobe, more invasive methods, such as the Wada test[76] or depth recordings of event-related potentials,[77] may be helpful in predicting postoperative memory performance.

In patients with discordant findings on non-invasive studies, invasive recordings will still be necessary. For those patients, as for those 20–30 per cent of the seemingly 'perfect' patients with temporal lobe epilepsy who do not become seizure-free, new methods are required to improve the predictive accuracy of presurgical studies. Although contralateral spike activity has been found to reduce the chance of postoperative seizure cessation possibly down to 50 per cent, it is still far from clear which, if any, spikes point to possible contralateral epileptogenesis. Proton MR spectroscopic imaging may possibly contribute to the detection of mesial temporal functional disturbances.[78] Similarly, limbic event-related potentials have been found to indicate such disturbances.[79,80] Thus, evaluation of the effect of word repetitions on limbic N400 potentials, on the side contralateral to the primary epileptogenic area, can contribute significantly to the accurate prediction of seizure outcome in patients with temporal lobe epilepsy.[81,82]

In surgery for extratemporal epilepsy, the only unquestionable predictor of favorable seizure outcome is the presence of an MRI-detectable, monofocal, structural abnormality in agreement with the findings from other diagnostic procedures such as ictal EEG recordings. Further studies are urgently needed to establish additional—currently hypothetical—predictors such as ictal electrocorticography patterns and 'clean' postresectional electrocorticography recordings.

In clinical practice, the presurgical evaluation of extratemporal epilepsy patients may remain non-invasive if MRI shows an extratemporal mass lesion not located in the immediate vicinity of eloquent areas, and electrophysiological, neuropsychological and PET studies together indicate a well-defined perilesional epileptogenic area. In these patients, intraoperative electrocorticography may suffice to plan strategies of resective surgery. Otherwise, chronic invasive monitoring will often be necessary for functional electrostimulation mapping and to delineate the epileptogenic zone. Surgery can fail to result in postoperative freedom of seizures as a result of a widespread extension of the seizure-onset zone and/or additional mesial temporal epileptogenicity that was not detected by chronic subdural and depth recordings. New methods of signal analysis derived from the theory of non-linear dynamics may offer new possibilities for detecting such changes, and can contribute to outcome prediction, as has been shown for patients who underwent extended neocortical lesionectomies.[83]

In conclusion, how good are we at predicting surgical outcome in epilepsy? We could say that we are improving: many studies have contributed to the identification of those patients who can expect to benefit from epilepsy surgery, and there are groups of patients for whom we can give an 80 per cent chance of postoperative freedom from seizures. However, we have to admit that we are not good enough. We still have to learn how to exclude those patients from surgery who only *seem* to be perfect candidates, but have no benefit after all. We also have to improve our skills in identifying those patients with non-lesional imaging studies who *will* be helped by surgery. We hope that the pace at which diagnostic methods are being improved at present will make it necessary to rewrite this chapter in the near future.

References

1. Spencer DD, Spencer SS, Mattson RH, Williamson PD. Intracerebral mass lesions in patients with intractable partial epilepsy. *Neurology* 1984;34:432–6.
2. Awad IA, Rosenfeld J, Ahl H, et al. Intractable epilepsy and structural lesions of the brain: mapping, resection strategies, and seizure outcome. *Epilepsia* 1991;32:179–86.
3. Engel J Jr, Van Ness PC, Rasmussen TB, Ojemann LM. Outcome with respect to epileptic seizures. In: Engel J Jr, ed. *Surgical treatment of the epilepsies*. New York: Raven Press, 1993:609–21.
4. Walczak TS, Radtke RA, McNamara JO, et al. Anterior temporal lobectomy for complex partial seizures: evaluation, results, and long-term follow-up in 100 cases. *Neurology* 1990;40:413–18.
5. Sperling MR, O'Connor MJ, Saykin AJ, Plummer C. Temporal lobectomy for refractory epilepsy. *JAMA* 1996;276:470–5.
6. Wass CT, Rajala MM, Hughes JM, et al. Long-term follow-up of patients treated surgically for medically intractable epilepsy: results in 291 patients treated at Mayo Clinic Rochester between July 1972 and March 1985. *Mayo Clin Proc* 1996;71:1105–13.
7. Wieser H-G, Engel J Jr, Williamson PD, et al. Surgically remediable temporal lobe syndromes. In: Engel J Jr, ed. *Surgical treatment of the epilepsies*. New York: Raven Press, 1993:49–64.
8. Sommer W. Erkrankungen des Ammonshorns als ätiologisches Moment der Epilepsie. *Arch Psychiatr Nervenkr* 1880;10:631–75.
9. Bratz E. Ammonshornbefunde bei Epileptikern. *Arch Psychiatr Nervenkr* 1899;32:820–35.
10. Margerison JH, Corsellis JAN. Epilepsy and the temporal lobes: a clinical encephalographic and neuropathological study of the brain in epilepsy, with particular reference to the temporal lobes. *Brain* 1966;9:499–530.
11. Faconer MA, Taylor DC. Surgical treatment of drug resistant epilepsy due to mesial temporal sclerosis. *Arch Neurol* 1968;19:353–61.
12. Bruton CJ. *The neuropathology of temporal lobe epilepsy*. New York: Oxford University Press, 1988.

13. Gloor P. Mesial temporal sclerosis: historical background and an overview from a modern perspective. In: Lüders H, ed. *Epilepsy surgery.* New York: Raven Press, 1991:689–703.

14. Wolf HK, Campos MG, Zentner J, et al. Surgical pathology of temporal lobe epilepsy. Experience with 216 cases. *J Neuropathol Exp Neurol* 1993;**52**:499–506.

15. Mathern GW, Babb TL, Leite JP, et al. The pathogenic and progressive features of chronic human hippocampal epilepsy. *Epilepsy Res* 1996;**26**:151–61.

16. Zentner J, Hufnagel A, Wolf HK, et al. Surgical treatment of temporal lobe epilepsy: clinical, radiological, and histopathological findings in 178 patients. *J Neurol Neurosurg Psychiatry* 1995;**58**:666–73.

17. O'Brien TJ, Kilpatrick C, Murrie V, et al. Temporal lobe epilepsy caused by mesial temporal sclerosis and temporal neocortical lesions. A clinical and electroencephalographic study of 46 pathologically proven cases. *Brain* 1996;**119**:2133–41.

18. Li LM, Cendes F, Watson C, et al. Surgical treatment of patients with single and dual pathology: relevance of lesion and of hippocampal atrophy to seizure outcome. *Neurology* 1997;**48**:437–44.

19. Kuzniecky R, Burgard S, Faught E, et al. Predictive value of magnetic resonance imaging in temporal lobe epilepsy surgery. *Arch Neurol* 1993;**50**:65–9.

20. Garcia PA, Laxer KD, Barbaro NM, Dillon WP. Prognostic value of qualitative magnetic resonance imaging hippocampal abnormalities in patients undergoing temporal lobectomy for medically refractory seizures. *Epilepsia* 1994;**35**:520–4.

21. Arruda F, Cendes F, Andermann F, et al. Mesial atrophy and outcome after amygdalohippocampectomy or temporal lobe removal. *Ann Neurol* 1996;**40**:446–50.

22. Thadani VM, Williamson PD, Berger R, et al. Successful epilepsy surgery without intracranial EEG recording: criteria for patient selection. *Epilepsia* 1995;**36**:7–15.

23. Eliashiv SD, Dewar S, Wainwright I, et al. Long-term follow-up after temporal lobe resection for lesions associated with chronic seizures. *Neurology* 1997;**48**:621–6.

24. Berkovic SF, McIntosh AM, Kalnins RM et al. Preoperative MRI predicts outcome of temporal lobectomy: an actuarial analysis. *Neurology* 1995;**45**:1358–63.

25. Sisodiya SM, Moran N, Free SL, et al. Correlation of widespread preoperative magnetic resonance imaging changes with unsuccessful surgery for hippocampal sclerosis. *Ann Neurol* 1997;**41**:490–6.

26. Li LM, Dubeau F, Andermann F, et al. Periventricular nodular heterotopia and intractable temporal lobe epilepsy: poor outcome after temporal lobe resection. *Ann Neurol* 1997;**41**:662–8.

27. Specht U, May T, Schulz R, et al. Cerebellar atrophy and prognosis after temporal lobe resection. *J Neurol Neurosurg Psychiatry* 1997;**62**:501–6.

28. Fish DR, Spencer SS. Clinical correlations: MRI and EEG. *Magn Reson Imaging* 1995;**13**:1113–7.

29. King D, Spencer SS, McCarthy G, et al. Bilateral hippocampal atrophy in medial temporal lobe epilepsy. *Epilepsia* 1995;**36**:905–10.

30. King D, Spencer SS, McCarthy G, Spencer DD. Surface and depth EEG findings in patients with hippocampal atrophy. *Neurology* 1997;**48**:1363–7.

31. Barry E, Sussman NM, O'Connor MJ, Harner RN. Presurgical electroencephalographic patterns and outcome from anterior temporal lobectomy. *Arch Neurol* 1992;**49**:21–7.

32. Holmes MD, Dodrill CB, Ojemann GA, et al. Outcome following surgery in patients with bitemporal interictal epileptiform patterns. *Neurology* 1997;**48**:1037–40.

33. Steinhoff BJ, So NK, Lim S, Lüders HO. Ictal scalp EEG in temporal lobe epilepsy with unitemporal versus bitemporal interictal epileptiform discharges. *Neurology* 1995;**45**:889–96.

34. So N, Olivier A, Andermann F, et al. Results of surgical treatment in patients with bitemporal epileptiform abnormalities. *Ann Neurol* 1989;**25**:432–9.

35. Weinand ME, Wyler AR, Richey ET, et al. Long-term ictal monitoring with subdural strip electrodes: prognostic factors for selecting temporal lobectomy candidates. *J Neurosurg* 1992;**77**:20–8.

36. Hufnagel A, Elger CE, Pels H, et al. Prognostic

significance of ictal and interictal epileptiform activity in temporal lobe epilepsy. *Epilepsia* 1994;35:1146–53.

37. Spencer SS, Spencer DD. Implications of seizure termination location in temporal lobe epilepsy. *Epilepsia* 1996;37:455–8.

38. Brekelmans GJF, Velis DN, van Veelen CWM, et al. Intracranial EEG seizure-offset termination pattern: relation to outcome of epilepsy surgery in temporal lobe epilepsy. *Epilepsia* 1998;39:259–66.

39. Fiol ME, Gates JR, Torres F, Maxwell RE. The prognostic value of residual spikes in the postexcision electrocorticogram after temporal lobectomy. *Neurology* 1991;41:512–16.

40. Tuunainen A, Nousiainen U, Mervaala E, et al. Postoperative EEG and electrocorticography: relation to clinical outcome in patients with temporal lobe surgery. *Epilepsia* 1994;35:1165–73.

41. Lee BI, Lee JD, Kim JY, et al. Single photon emission computed tomography-EEG relations in temporal lobe epilepsy. *Neurology* 1997;49:981–91.

42. Grünwald F, Durwen HF, Bockisch A, et al. Technetium 99m HMPAO brain SPECT in medically intractable temporal lobe epilepsy: a postoperative evaluation. *J Nucl Med* 1991;32:388–94.

43. Tatum WO 4th, Sperling MR, O'Connor MJ, Jacobstein JG. Interictal single photon emission computed tomography in partial epilepsy. Accuracy in localization and prediction of outcome. *J Neuroimaging* 1995;5:142–4.

44. Wong CY, Geller EB, Chen EQ, et al. Outcome of temporal lobe epilepsy surgery predicted by statistical parametric PET imaging. *J Nucl Med* 1996;37:1094–110.

45. Theodore WH, Sato S, Kufta CV, et al. FDG positron emission tomography and invasive EEG: seizure focus detection and surgical outcome. *Epilepsia* 1997;38:81–6.

46. Loring DW, Meador KJ, Lee GP, et al. Wada memory performance predicts seizure outcome following anterior temporal lobectomy. *Neurology* 1994;44:2322–4.

47. Sperling MR, Saykin AJ, Glosser G, et al. Predictors of outcome after anterior temporal lobectomy: the intracarotid amobarbital test. *Neurology* 1994;44:2325–30.

48. Perrine K, Westerveld M, Sass KJ, et al. Wada memory disparities predict seizure laterality and postoperative seizure control. *Epilepsia* 1995;36:851–6.

49. Lancman ME, Benbadis S, Geller E, Morris HH. Sensitivity and specificity of asymmetric recall on Wada test to predict outcome after temporal lobectomy. *Neurology* 1998;50:455–9.

50. Sawrie SM, Martin RC, Gilliam FG, et al. Contribution of neuropsychological data to the prediction of temporal lobe epilepsy surgery outcome. *Epilepsia* 1998;39:319–25.

51. Chelune GJ, Naugle RI, Hermann BH, et al. Does presurgical IQ predict seizure outcome after temporal lobectomy? Evidence from the Bozeman Epilepsy Consortium. *Epilepsia* 1998;39:314–8.

52. Nayel MH, Awad IA, Luders H. Extent of mesiobasal resection determines outcome after temporal lobectomy for intractable complex partial seizures. *Neurosurgery* 1991;29:55–60.

53. Clarke DB, Olivier A, Andermann F, Fish D. Surgical treatment of epilepsy: the problem of lesion/focus incongruence. *Surg Neurol* 1996;46:579–85.

54. Li LM, Cendes F, Watson C, et al. Surgical treatment of patients with single and dual pathology: relevance of lesion and of hippocampal atrophy to seizure outcome. *Neurology* 1997;48:437–44.

55. Dodrill CB, Wilkus RJ, Ojemann GA, et al. Multidisciplinary prediction of seizure relief from cortical resection surgery. *Ann Neurol* 1986;20:2–12.

56. Guldvog B, Loyning Y, Hauglie-Hanssen E, et al. Predictive factors for success in surgical treatment for partial epilepsy: a multivariate analysis. *Epilepsia* 1994;35:566–78.

57. Quesney LF. Extratemporal epilepsy: clinical presentation, pre-operative EEG localization, and surgical outcome. *Acta Neurol Scand Suppl* 1992;140:81–94.

58. Tran TA, Spencer SS, Spencer DD. Epilepsy: medical and surgical outcome. In: Swash M, ed. *Outcomes in neurological and neurosurgical disorders*. New York: Cambridge University Press, 1998:407–40.

59. Lorenzo NY, Parisi JE, Cascino GD, et al. Intractable frontal lobe epilepsy: pathological and MRI features. *Epilepsy Res* 1995;20:171–8.

60. Salanova V, Morris HH, van Ness PC, et al. Comparison of scalp electroencephalogram with subdural electrocorticogram recordings and functional mapping in frontal lobe epilepsy. *Arch Neurol* 1993;**50**:294–9.

61. Newton MR, Berkovic SF. Ictal SPECT. In: Pedley TA, Meldrum BS, eds. *Recent Advances in epilepsy*, Vol. 6. Edinburgh: Churchill Livingstone, 1995:41–55.

62. Tiemeier H, Grunwald T, Menzel C, et al. Value of functional imaging in extratemporal epilepsy in relation to post-operative seizure control. *Epilepsia* 1997;**38**(Suppl 3):171 (abst).

63. Zentner J, Hufnagel A, Ostertun B, et al. Surgical treatment of extratemporal epilepsy: clinical, radiologic, and histopathologic findings in 60 patients. *Epilepsia* 1996;**37**:1072–80.

64. Rougier A, Dartigues JF, Commenges D, et al. A longitudinal assessment of seizure outcome and overall benefit from 100 corticectomies for epilepsy. *J Neurol Neurosurg Psychiatry* 1992;**55**:762–7.

65. Davies KG, Weeks RD. Cortical resections for intractable epilepsy of extratemporal origin: experience with seventeen cases over eleven years. *Br J Neurosurg* 1993;**7**:343–53.

66. Kazemi NJ, So EL, Mosewich RK, et al. Resection of frontal encephalomalacias for intractable epilepsy: outcome and prognostic factors. *Epilepsia* 1997;**38**:670–7.

67. Cascino GD, Hulihan JF, Sharbrough FW, Kelly PJ. Parietal lobe lesional epilepsy: electroclinical correlation and operative outcome. *Epilepsia* 1993;**34**:522–7.

68. Salanova V, Andermann F, Rasmussen T, et al. Parietal lobe epilepsy. Clinical manifestations and outcome in 82 patients treated surgically between 1929 and 1988. *Brain* 1995;**118**:607–27.

69. Salanova V, Andermann F, Rasmussen T, et al. Tumoural parietal lobe epilepsy. Clinical manifestations and outcome in 34 patients treated between 1934 and 1988. *Brain* 1995;**118**:1289–304.

70. Salanova V, Andermann F, Olivier A, et al. Occipital lobe epilepsy: electroclinical manifestations, electrocorticography, cortical stimulation and outcome in 42 patients treated between 1930 and 1991. *Brain* 1992;**115**:1655–80.

71. Williamson PD, Thadani VM, Darcey TM, et al. Occipital lobe epilepsy: clinical characteristics, seizure spread patterns, and results of surgery. *Ann Neurol* 1992;**31**:3–13.

72. Hufnagel A, Zentner J, Fernandez G, et al. Multiple subpial transection for control of epileptic seizures: effectiveness and safety. *Epilepsia* 1997;**38**:678–88.

73. Dogali M, Devinsky O, Luciano D, et al. Multiple subpial cortical transections for the control of intractable epilepsy in exquisite cortex. *Acta Neurochir Suppl* 1993;**58**:198–200.

74. Devinsky O, Perrine K, Vazquez B, et al. Multiple subpial transections in the language cortex. *Brain* 1994;**117**:255–65.

75. Sawhney IM, Robertson IJ, Polkey CE, et al. Multiple subpial transection: a review of 21 cases. *J Neurol Neurosurg Psychiatry* 1995;**58**:344–9.

76. Jokeit H, Ebner A, Holthausen H, et al. Individual prediction of change in delayed recall of prose passages after left-sided anterior temporal lobectomy. *Neurology* 1997;**49**:481–7.

77. Grunwald T, Elger CE, Lehnertz K, et al. Prediction of postoperative verbal memory performance by intrahippocampal cognitive potentials in temporal lobe epilepsy. *Epilepsia* 1994;**35**(Suppl 8):83 (abst).

78. Ende GR, Laxer KD, Knowlton RC, et al. Temporal lobe epilepsy: bilateral hippocampal metabolite changes revealed at proton MR spectroscopic imaging. *Radiology* 1997;**202**:809–17.

79. Grunwald T, Elger CE., Lehnertz K, et al. Alterations of intrahippocampal cognitive potentials in temporal lobe epilepsy. *Electroenceph Clin Neurophysiol* 1995;**95**:53–62.

80. Grunwald T, Lehnertz K, Heinze HJ, et al. Verbal novelty detection within the human hippocampus proper. *Proc Natl Acad Sci USA* 1998;**95**:3193–7.

81. Elger CE, Grunwald T, Lehnertz K, Heinze HJ. Prediction of postoperative seizure control by hippocampal event-related potentials. *Epilepsia* 1995;**36**(Suppl 4):85 (abst).

82. Grunwald T, Lehnertz K, Helmstaedter C, et al. Limbic ERPs predict verbal memory after left-sided hippocampectomy. *Neuroreport* 1998;**9**:3375–8.

83. Widman G, Lehnertz K, Elger CE. Neuronal complexity loss in lesional neocortical epilepsy: estimating the temporomesial involvement in the epileptogenic process. *Epilepsia* 1997;**38**(Suppl 8):71 (abst).

X

SUPPLEMENTAL NON-ANTIEPILEPTIC DRUG THERAPY

32

Hormones and epilepsy

Pavel Klein and Andrew G Herzog

Introduction

Hormones affect seizures and seizures, in turn, affect hormonal regulation and secretion. In women with epilepsy, the most commonly encountered endocrine problems relate to the effects of gonadal steroids on seizures, as in the case of catamenial epilepsy; to the change of seizure expression during changes of endocrine status such as menarche, pregnancy and menopause; and to the effect of seizures on reproductive endocrine function such as ovulation and sexuality. In men with epilepsy, the most commonly encountered endocrine problem is altered sexuality, usually hyposexuality. In both men and women, seizures cause acute as well as chronic alteration in hormonal secretion, for instance acute transient post-ictal hyperprolactinemia. In both men and women with epilepsy, antiepileptic drugs (AEDs) may affect endocrine function with clinically important consequences. Finally, in both men and women, hormonal treatment may in certain settings be successfully used as adjunctive anticonvulsant therapy. In this chapter, we shall address these issues.

Case 1: a 37-year-old woman with epilepsy

A 37-year-old woman had suffered head trauma at the age of 3 years. At the age of 13, 6 months after her menarche, she developed seizures with speech perseveration and facial automatisms followed by post-ictal drowsiness. EEG showed left temporal spikes. Her seizures occurred most frequently during a period from two days before to four days after the onset of her menses. Less frequently, they occurred at ovulation time, although they could occur at any other time of her menstrual cycle also.

In her early twenties, her menses became irregular, occurring every 6–8 weeks and she noted increased acne and hair on her chin, abdomen and breasts. She still had the feeling that her seizures occurred before her period, but she could no longer tell the exact temporal relationship between them and her menses. Seizures persisted in spite of treatment with phenytoin (DPH) and, subsequently, sodium valproate (VPA), and carbamazepine (CBZ). She was diagnosed as having polycystic ovarian syndrome. Natural progesterone 200 mg three times per day (t.i.d.) was added to her CBZ on days 15–26 of her menstrual cycle, with a tapering dose on days 26–28. Her seizures improved, from 1–3 per month to one every 2–3 months. At the age of 36, she developed perimenopausal symptoms (sweating, vaginal dryness). Her gynecologist started her on estrogen hormone replacement therapy (HRT) (premarin), and medroxyprogesterone was substituted for natural progesterone. Her sweating improved, but her seizures increased again, and for the first time in years, the seizures became secondarily generalized. Reinstitution of natural progesterone instead of medroxyprogesterone led to improvement of her seizures back to ~1 every 3 months.

This patient's history contains several points that illustrate the reciprocal interaction between reproductive hormones and seizures.

- Although she had suffered the cerebral insult (head trauma) during early childhood, she did not develop seizures until after menarche. Subsequently, her seizures were affected by her menstrual cycle—she had catamenial epilepsy. Did the hormonal changes associated with menarche activate her dormant seizure focus? Did hormonal fluctuations associated with the menstrual cycle alter her seizure threshold so as to facilitate seizure occurrence perimenstrually and at the time of ovulation?
- The patient then developed reproductive endocrine disturbances—polycystic ovarian syndrome and, eventually, premature perimenopause. Did her temporolimbic seizures predispose her to these gynecological abnormalities? Concomitantly with the alteration in her reproductive cycles, her seizure pattern changed also. Was there a relationship that could be explained, or was this a random change?
- Her seizures improved with adjunctive hormonal therapy with natural progesterone.
- Her seizures worsened at the time of perimenopause concomitantly with institution of estrogen HRT and substitution of the synthetic progestin for natural progesterone.

Catamenial epilepsy: what is it and how should it be evaluated and treated?

Catamenial (from Greek *katamenia: kata* by, *men* month) epilepsy refers to seizure exacerbation in relation to the menstrual cycle. Traditionally, the term has been used to refer to seizure exacerbation at the time of menstruation. In its purest form, catamenial epilepsy may occasion a woman to have seizures only at the time of menstruation. This form is uncommon. More commonly, a woman may tend to have seizures at particular times during her menstrual cycle, usually just before or during the onset of her menstruation or at the time of ovulation.[1-3] In this case, the best way of establishing whether or not seizures tend to worsen at certain points of the menstrual cycle is to have the patient keep a careful seizure diary in relation to the menstrual cycle (using the first day of menstrual bleeding as the first day of the cycle). The menstrual cycle is then divided into four phases: menstrual, counting days (−3) to (+3); follicular, days (+4) to (+9); ovulatory, days (+10) to (+16, equivalent to day −13 of the next menstrual cycle); and luteal, days (+17, equivalent to day −12) to (−4). The number of seizures in each phase is counted. The average daily number of seizures for each menstrual phase is then compared with average daily number of seizures for the whole month to see whether a pattern of exacerbation or remission at certain phases of the menstrual cycle is present. We define seizure exacerbation as a twofold or greater average daily seizure frequency during the affected part of the menstrual cycle compared with the remainder of the cycle.[2,4]

Three patterns of catamenial seizure exacerbation may be observed[3] (Figure 32.1): perimenstrually (C1), at the time of ovulation (C2), or throughout the whole second half of the menstrual cycle (C3). The former two patterns are seen in women with normal menstrual cycles. The latter pattern, which is the most difficult one to distinguish because the time of seizure exacerbation is prolonged rather than focused, is seen in women with

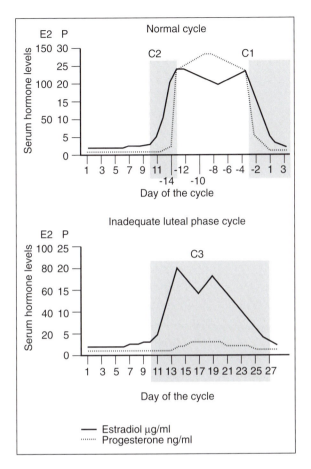

Figure 32.1
The three patterns of catamenial exacerbation of epilepsy—C1, C2, C3—in relation to serum estradiol (E2) and progesterone (P) levels.

abnormal menstrual cycles. Such women have anovulatory cycles and inadequate luteal phase syndrome.[5] Because they do not ovulate, no corpus luteum is formed during the second (luteal) half of the menstrual cycle and no progesterone is secreted. When catamenial epilepsy is defined as a twofold increase in seizure frequency during a particular phase of the menstrual cycle relative to the rest of the

menstrual cycle, it can be shown to affect about one third of women with intractable partial epilepsy.[2,4]

Menstrually related hormonal fluctuations of estrogen and progesterone underlie these different patterns of catamenial seizure exacerbation. Estrogens, in particular estradiol (E2), the most important of the different estrogen forms, have potent proconvulsant properties. They exert an excitatory effect on neurons by potentiating postsynaptic excitatory currents mediated by the glutamate receptor.[6] Estrogens also increase neuronal excitability by modulating structural connectivity. E2 increases the density of dendritic spines and of excitatory N-methyl-D-aspartate (NMDA)-receptor-containing synapses on hippocampal CA1 pyramidal neurons,[7] the neurons critical in generating ictal events from interictal spikes in temporolimbic epilepsy.[8] These effects may predispose hippocampal neuronal circuits to hyperexcitability associated with seizure generation. When administered intraperitoneally, intravenously, or topically to brain surface, estrogens cause seizures, including fatal status epilepticus, in various animal seizure models.[9–12] In female rats, temporolimbic seizures are most easily elicited at the time of ovulation, when serum estrogen levels are at their highest.[13] In women with epilepsy, intravenous administration of conjugated estrogens activates epileptiform discharges and may result in seizures.[14]

Progesterone has the opposite effect. It hyperpolarizes neurons, acting via one of its natural endogenous metabolites, allopregnanolone, as an agonist at the γ-aminobutyric acid (GABA)-A receptor with a potency almost a thousandfold greater than that of pentobarbital and greater than the most potent benzodiazepine, nitroflurazepam.[15,16] In animal seizure models, progesterone lessens epileptiform discharges, inhibits pre-existing seizures,[12,17] and protects against development of seizures.[11] In women with partial seizures, intravenous infusion of progesterone, resulting in luteal phase plasma levels, suppresses interictal epileptiform discharges.[18]

Thus, estrogens facilitate seizures whereas progesterone protects against seizures. During the menstrual cycle, serum levels of estradiol and progesterone fluctuate (Figure 32.1). In a normally menstruating woman, the surge of serum estrogen levels at the time of ovulation may be associated with increased seizure tendency, as may the fall in serum progesterone levels premenstrually to perimenstrually. In a woman with anovulatory cycles, estrogen levels rise at the end of the follicular phase and stay elevated throughout the luteal phase until premenstrually, as in normally menstruating women; but there is little or no progesterone secretion (hence the term *inadequate luteal phase syndrome*). Thus, there is estrogen–progesterone (E–P) imbalance with relative excess of estrogen (or deficiency of progesterone) throughout the whole second (luteal) half of the menstrual cycle, with associated seizure exacerbation.[19] A number of studies have suggested that it is both progesterone deficiency and estrogen excess relative to progesterone that contribute to the catamenial pattern of seizure exacerbation in both normal women and in women with menstrual irregularities, and that the E–P ratio is the determining factor of overall reproductive hormonal effect upon seizure frequency.[1,2,19] In addition, withdrawal of progesterone premenstrually also may potentiate seizures in a manner analogous to alcohol, benzodiazepine or barbiturate withdrawal seizures. Rapid withdrawal of progesterone leads to altered expression of the α-4 subunit of the GABA-A receptor. This decreases the GABA-A receptor sensitivity to GABA, benzodiazepines and barbiturates, and is associated with an eight-fold increase in seizure activity in animals.[20]

In addition, premenstrual exacerbation of seizures may also be related to a decline in anticonvulsant medication levels.[21,22] In women with catamenial epilepsy, DPH levels decline premenstrually, by up to one third.[21,22] This may be due to increased rate of clearance, with an associated reduction of half-life of DPH from 19 to 13 h.[21] Hepatic microsomal enzymes metabolize both gonadal steroids and anticonvulsants such as DPH, with competition between the two. The premenstrual decline in gonadal steroid secretion may therefore permit increased metabolism of antiepileptic drugs, resulting in lower serum levels.[21] However, it is not certain whether all AEDs are thus affected; phenobarbital is not, and catamenial fluctuation in serum levels of other AEDs has not been studied.

How should catamenial epilepsy be evaluated?

We suggest the following steps in evaluating catamenial epilepsy:[2]

1. Establish the presence of a catamenial pattern of seizure exacerbation using a careful seizure and menstrual diary as previously outlined.
2. Establish the menstrual pattern: normal or abnormal menstrual cycles.
3. Check mid-luteal serum progesterone levels (e.g. on day 22 of a 28-day menstrual cycle) to see whether an inadequate luteal phase is present.
4. If C1 (perimenstrual) catamenial seizure exacerbation is present, check trough AED levels on day 22 (when estradiol and progesterone are high and AED level should be 'normal'), and day 1 (menstrual, when estradiol and progesterone levels are low) to see whether the level is low at this time and could be the cause of perimenstrual seizure exacerbation.

For a discussion of the treatment of catamenial seizures, see the section on hormonal treatment in epilepsy at the end of this chapter.

Menarche, pregnancy, menopause: do they affect seizures?

Changes in reproductive hormonal status associated with menarche,[23] pregnancy[24,25] and menopause[26] may all affect clinical manifestation of seizures.

Menarche

Menarche may be associated with the resolution of some forms of partial seizures and the exacerbation of others. The former group includes the 'primary' partial seizures, such as benign Rolandic epilepsy of childhood and benign occipital epilepsy of childhood, which resolve spontaneously in both sexes in mid-teens.[27,28] The explanation for this is not clear and has not been investigated. Changes in both reproductive hormones and in adrenal steroid hormones associated with puberty and adrenarche could be involved.

Secondary partial seizures (idiopathic or lesional) may show exacerbation in relationship to menarche. A number of investigators have observed that late childhood and adolescence were peak periods for the first manifestation of epilepsy.[23,29] About 20 per cent of women report seizure onset in menarche.[23] This tendency is particularly strong among women with catamenial epilepsy, up to two thirds of whom may experience the onset of seizures within 3 years of menarche.[14,29] Pre-existing complex partial seizures in women may increase in frequency at the time of menarche.[23,30] The explanation for this may lie with the pattern of ovarian gonadal

hormonal secretion at the time of menarche. At the time of menarche, estrogen secretion by the ovary begins several months to a couple of years before the ovarian luteal secretion of progesterone. As we have seen, estrogen has proconvulsant properties while progesterone has anticonvulsant properties. Thus, the unopposed effect of estrogen on the brain may trigger or exacerbate seizures at this time, as happened in our patient. The finding in rats that oophorectomy prior to sexual maturation decreases susceptibility to seizures in subsequent adulthood supports the suggestion that increased neuronal excitability associated with elevation of estrogens at the time of menarche may explain this observation.[12]

Pregnancy

Pregnancy may have variable effects on epilepsy. A small number of women experience seizures for the first time during pregnancy and have seizures only during pregnancy.[24] In about one third of women, seizures worsen during pregnancy, probably because of decreased levels of AEDs, related to a greater volume of distribution and a higher rate of clearance.[24,25] In about one sixth of women, seizure frequency decreases, possibly because of increased medication compliance.[24,25]

Menopause

In some patients seizures may cease at the time of menopause, while other patients may experience seizure exacerbation.[26,31] The term *menopause* refers to a complex process and a variable end point that may differ significantly from person to person. Although estrogen levels decline as ovarian function diminishes, progesterone declines before estrogen, with resulting elevation of E–P serum ratios. Early during menopause, for example, anovulatory cycles may develop and lead to increased E–P ratios that would be expected to promote the occurrence of seizures. At the end of the process, estrogen production by the ovary may become essentially undetectable and potentially lead to a beneficial effect. Recently, 47 per cent of women with presumed partial seizures who responded to mailed questionnaires reported a decrease in seizure frequency at menopause, while 29 per cent reported no change and 24 per cent reported an increase in seizure frequency.[31] Patients with temporolimbic epilepsy (TLE) without hormone replacement were significantly more likely to have a reduction rather than increase in seizure frequency at the time of menopause.

Seizures may also be affected by HRT. In the study just mentioned, estrogen replacement therapy was associated with an increase in seizure frequency.[31] Seizure exacerbation with estrogen replacement therapy may occur even if progesterone replacement therapy is used concomitantly, because the progesterone commonly used is a synthetic progestin with little or no anticonvulsant activity. Synthetic progestins are much less effective anticonvulsants than natural progesterone. If a menopausal woman with epilepsy needs to be treated with estrogen HRT (e.g. for osteoporosis or to prevent ischemic heart disease), we suggest simultaneous use of natural progesterone to mimic normal luteal phase serum levels; for example, 100–200 mg t.i.d. cyclically 2 weeks per month[32] (see section on hormonal treatment).

In what other ways may hormones affect seizures?

Hormone-containing medication

Isolated reports exist of estrogenic oral contraceptives exacerbating and progestin-containing oral contraceptives ameliorating seizures, particularly in women with catamenial epilepsy.[26,29] For the most part, however, oral contraceptives have not been shown to have a significant direct effect upon seizures, other than affecting the levels of certain AEDs.

Pathological hormonal states

Reproductive endocrine disorders may favor the development of temporal lobe epilepsy in women. Conditions in which serum estrogen levels and E–P ratios are chronically elevated may be associated with an increased incidence of seizures by causing constant exposure of temporal lobe structures to estrogen without the normal luteal elevation of progesterone, thus heightening interictal epileptiform activity and the possibility of 'kindling'. In this regard, more than 50 per cent of women with anovulatory cycles or amenorrhea may have EEG abnormalities that may normalize after treatment with the antiestrogen, clomiphene citrate, and restoration of ovulation.[33] It is possible that partial seizures of temporal lobe origin may themselves promote the development of polycystic ovarian syndrome (PCOS) and hypothalamic hypogonadism (HH), two of the conditions associated with inadequate luteal phase syndrome.[34] Thus, epilepsy may alter the hormonal environment in such a way as to further facilitate seizures, as discussed below.

How does partial epilepsy affect endocrine reproductive function in women?

Reproductive dysfunction and endocrine disorders are unusually common among women with epilepsy.[34] Fertility is reduced by 20–30 per cent of the expected number of offspring among married epileptic women, although the reduction may only affect women whose seizures begin before the age of 10.[35] Thirty-five per cent of women with partial seizures of temporal lobe origin have anovulatory cycles.[36] About 60 per cent of women with TLE have menstrual cycle abnormalities, such as amenorrhea, oligomenorrhea, or abnormally long (>32 days) or short (<26 days) menstrual cycle intervals.[34] These abnormalities are often associated with distinct reproductive endocrine disorders. PCOS and HH are present in 20 per cent and 12 per cent, respectively, of women with TLE, as compared with 5 per cent and 1.5 per cent of women in the general population. Premature menopause and functional hyperprolactinemia occur in 4 per cent and 2 per cent of women with TLE, compared with less than 1 per cent for either condition in the general population.[34]

How do these disorders arise? The pathogenic mechanism has not been established. It may relate to the effect of temporal lobe seizures or interictal epileptiform discharges upon the functioning of the hypothalamo–pituitary–gonadal hormonal axis.

Ovulation is controlled by luteinizing hormone (LH) and follicular stimulating hormone (FSH), which are regulated by luteinizing hormone releasing hormone (LHRH) secreted by hypothalamic LHRH-containing neurons.[37] The LHRH neurons release LHRH into the portal hypophyseal circulation, which carries it to the anterior pituitary. There, LHRH stimulates LH and FSH into the systemic circulation. FSH acts on the ovary to stimulate the maturation of the follicle. This process is associated with ovarian estrogen production during the follicular phase of the menstrual cycle. When the follicle is mature, a surge of estrogen production stimulates a surge in LH secretion from the pituitary by a positive feedback. This is followed by ovulation—the release of the ovum from the follicle. The remaining follicle now becomes transformed into corpus luteum, which secretes progesterone and estrogen during the luteal half of the menstrual cycle. At the end of this phase, production of both estrogen and progesterone falls, leading to menstruation.[38]

LHRH, LH and FSH are secreted in a pulsatile manner (see[38] for a review). LH pulses in the peripheral blood are controlled by LHRH pulses. Alteration in the normal pulsatile pattern of LHRH and LH secretion may be important in the pathophysiology of reproductive disorders with abnormal ovulation, including PCOS and HH. Both diminished and excessive LH pulsatile secretion can lead to loss of ovulation. Women with PCOS may have increased LH pulse frequency.[38] Women with hypothalamic hypogonadism have decreased LH pulse frequency.[39]

The control of the pulsatile release of LHRH by LHRH cells is subject to modulatory influences from different parts of the brain,[40] including the amygdala.[41–43] LH pulsatile secretion is altered in women with epilepsy. Untreated women with epilepsy have higher LH pulse frequency than normal controls.[44] Women with TLE and PCOS tend to have left-sided epileptiform discharges and increased LH pulse frequency, whereas women with TLE and HH usually have right-sided epileptiform discharges and diminished LH pulse frequency.[39,45] Thus, involvement of temporal lobe structures, namely the amygdala, by ictal or interictal epileptiform discharges may disrupt normal limbic modulation of the LHRH pulse generator, thereby altering the frequency of LH pulse secretion and promoting the development of reproductive endocrine disorders. More particularly, discharges involving the left amygdala may lead to increased secretory activity of the hypothalamic LHRH neurons and their terminals, resulting in increased LH pulse frequency and PCOS.

In contrast, discharges involving the right amygdala may lead to reduced activity of the LHRH neurons, reduced LH pulse frequency, and subsequent hypothalamic hypogonadism.[39]

Reproductive endocrine disorders may, in turn, affect TLE. They may promote its development *de novo* in women with anovulatory cycles, and lead to its exacerbation in women with TLE in whom reproductive endocrine disorders develop as a consequence of TLE. Estrogen receptors are present in the amygdala and in the hippocampus.[46] As noted earlier, estrogen enhances excitatory neuronal activity[6] and facilitates seizure development,[9,11,14] while progesterone potentiates inhibitory synaptic transmission[15] and acts as an anticonvulsant.[11,18] PCOS and HH are characterized by anovulatory cycles, with failure of progesterone secretion during the luteal phase. Such cycles may, therefore, expose the amygdala and the hippocampus to continuous estrogen without the normal cyclical progesterone effects, and thereby promote interictal epileptiform activity and seizures. In fact, anovulatory cycles are associated with more frequent seizures.[19] Thus, the hormonal changes associated with anovulatory cycles may exacerbate seizures. A positive feedback cycle may be envisaged, whereby TLE leads to endocrine reproductive disorders with failure of ovulation which, in turn, further exacerbates the seizure disorder (Figure 32.2).

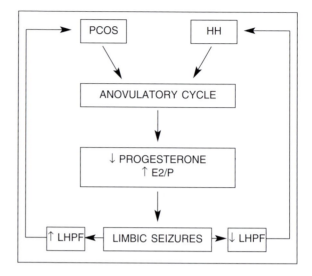

Figure 32.2

This figure illustrates the reciprocal relationship between reproductive endocrine disorders and temporolimbic epilepsy (TLE). By altering luteinizing hormone pulse frequency (LHPF), TLE may lead to the development of reproductive endocrine disorders such as polycystic ovarian syndrome (PCOS) or hypothalamic hypogonadism (HH), characterized by anovulatory cycles. Anovulatory cycles are associated with ovarian failure of progesterone (P) secretion, reduced serum progesterone levels and elevated serum estradiol (E2)-P ratio. This, in turn, may further facilitate seizures.

How should women with epilepsy and reproductive dysfunction be evaluated?

The most common reproductive complaint of women with partial epilepsy that may be related to epilepsy is an irregular menstrual cycle—usually prolonged, but sometimes shortened (or both). The two most common epilepsy-related causes of this irregularity are PCOS and HH. Other possible causes are functional hyperprolactinemia and premature menopause. Of course, if a woman complains of secondary amenorrhea, pregnancy should not be forgotten as a possible cause. We suggest the following approach:

1. History and examination to:
   a. Rule out pregnancy and menopause.

b. Evaluate for PCOS, HH, and hyperprolactinemia: hirsutism, acne (for PCOS-associated hyperandrogenism) and galactorrhea (for hyperprolactinemia).

2. Endocrine evaluation:
   a. During follicular phase, e.g. menstrual cycle day 4: LH, FSH, total testosterone (T), free testosterone (FT), androstenedione (A), dehydroepiandrostenedione sulfate (DHEAS), prolactin, and thyroid function tests:
      (i) In PCOS, one or more of the androgens (FT, A, or DHEAS) are elevated; the usual LH/FSH ratio of 1 is increased to >2.5, and prolactin may be increased (in ~25 per cent). FT as well as T need to be checked, as T may be affected by several AEDs and FT is the functionally relevant parameter (see section on AEDs and hormonal functioning).
      (ii) In hypothalamic hypogonadism, LH, FSH, and estradiol are all low.
      (iii) In hyperprolactinemia, remember psychotropic medications as well as TLE as a possible cause.
      (iv) Hypothyroidism is a common cause of menstrual irregularities.
   b. During mid-luteal phase, e.g. menstrual cycle day 22: progesterone and estradiol:
      (i) In inadequate luteal phase syndrome of all causes, progesterone level is low, less than the normal 5 ng/ml. In PCOS, estradiol is normal.
      (ii) In HH, both estradiol and progesterone are low.

3. Radiological evaluation:
   MRI of the brain (coronal views for the hypothalamus and the pituitary) for HH and hyperprolactinemia, to be done only if history and examination point to structural causes of HH and hyperprolactinemia.

How does epilepsy affect women's sexuality?

Hyposexuality is seen more commonly in epileptic women than in the general population; 25–65 per cent of women with TLE are estimated to be affected.[47] As with epileptic men, it is seen much more commonly with TLE than with primarily generalized epilepsy. Hyposexuality is characterized by lack of libido and difficulty in achieving orgasm. The disorder may result from a number of factors, including psychosocial disability, medication (intravenous, i.v.) and epilepsy-related dysfunction of limbic structures, in particular of the amygdala. In this respect hyposexuality occurs more commonly with right-sided TLE. In that setting, it is associated with hypothalamic hypogonadism and low serum LH levels.[34] By contrast, it has been our experience that women with left-sided TLE are rarely hyposexual.

How do seizures affect reproductive endocrine function in men?

Case 2: a 29-year-old man with TLE

A 29-year-old man with seizures complained of diminished libido and potency. He began to have partial seizures with rare secondary generalization at the age of 27, five years after head trauma that resulted in a left frontal lobe cyst and scarring. He was treated with DPH. At approximately the same time, his sexual appetite diminished, as did his ability to achieve erections both during intercourse and in sleep. His testosterone level was normal at 634 ng/dl (normal in our laboratory: 270–1100), but his free testosterone level was low at 0.9 ng/dl (normal 1.5–3.5). In addition, the percentage of his bioavailable testosterone was low at 11.67 per cent (normal 12.3–63 per cent). His sex hormone binding globulin was low at 44 nmol/l. Estradiol level was normal at 30 pg/ml (normal 0–40). He was started on intramuscular depotestosterone injections of 400 mg every three weeks. His libido returned to normal, but after three months began to decline again. At that time, testosterone, free testosterone and bioavailable testosterone levels were all normal (762 ng/dl, 2.1 ng/dl and 12.8 per cent, respectively), but his estradiol level was elevated at 47 ng/l. The aromatase inhibitor, testolactone, 150 mg t.i.d., was added to the depotestosterone. His libido and potency returned to normal. His estradiol level dropped to 23 ng/l, with testosterone of 588 ng/dl, free testosterone of 2.8 and bioavailable testosterone of 24 per cent. He has remained seizure-free and free of sexual symptoms during a two-year follow up.

This patient illustrates the most common hormonal problem in men with epilepsy, namely hyposexuality. Hyposexuality is often the cause of great concern, and, not infrequently, of marital difficulties. Its recognition is thus important, particularly because it is usually treatable.

Hyposexuality is present in one third to two thirds of all men with TLE.[48–51] Causes include hypogonadotropic hypogonadism (~25 per cent), hypergonadotropic hypogonadism (~10 per cent), and hyperprolactinemia (~10 per cent).[50] Reproductive dysfunction may be confined to the patient's sexuality, with repro-

ductive potential remaining normal. Unlike women with epilepsy, men with epilepsy have mostly normal fertility, although isolated cases of infertility have been observed.[35,48,50] In most epileptic men with sexual dysfunction, the dysfunction is one of hyposexuality; rarely, hypersexuality is observed.[50,51] Both impotence with normal libido and global hyposexuality with decline in both libido and potency are seen.[49,50]

The pathogenesis of sexual dysfunction in epileptic men, as in epileptic women, is likely to be multifactorial. Alteration of temporal lobe function by an underlying pathological lesion, alteration of temporal limbic structures by ictal or interictal discharges, associated neuroendocrine changes and medication effects may all play a part.

In lesional TLE, the underlying pathological process may be important. In cases of TLE secondary to neoplasm, for instance, hyposexuality has been noted to precede the onset of seizures by several months.[49]

Although several antiepileptic drugs can cause hyposexuality (a detailed discussion follows), epilepsy-related alteration of limbic structures may be directly involved. Thus, hyposexuality is commonly seen in TLE but not in other types of epilepsies,[51] may occur in patients with untreated TLE,[50] and may improve with AED treatment even if it involves higher AED dosing.[49,51]

Sexual behavior is controlled by the sexually dimorphic regions of the hypothalamus and the amygdala[46]—the same regions that regulate reproductive endocrine physiology. Alteration of function of these structures by ictal or interictal epileptiform discharges may affect both the behavioral and the endocrine aspects of sexual behavior.

Hormonally, sexual behavior is promoted by LH and androgens in men and women and by estradiol in women; it is inhibited by prolactin. Men with TLE who have reproductive and sexual dysfunction tend to have right-sided lateralization of seizures,[52] reduced LH pulse frequency compared with men with left-sided TLE (unpublished personal observation), and increased risk of hypogonadotropic hypogonadism and hyposexuality. Thus, epilepsy may alter temporolimbic modulation of the frequency of LHRH and LH pulses in relation to the lateralization of the paroxysmal discharges and thus affect gonadal androgen secretion and androgen-dependent sexual behavior. Moreover, this behavior may depend not only on the serum levels of androgens, but also on the responsiveness to androgens by brain structures such as the androgen receptor-containing amygdala.[46] It is possible that alteration of these structures by ictal or inter-ictal epileptiform discharges could alter their responsiveness to androgens, resulting in hyposexuality or hypersexuality.

In addition, elevated prolactin levels may also be a contributing factor to hyposexuality in epileptic men. Chronic hyperprolactinemia in non-epileptic men is associated with decreased libido and impotence.[53] Men with both complex partial and primary generalized seizures have increased prolactin levels interictally.[54] Prolactin antagonizes LHRH release from the hypothalamus, with a resulting reduction in LH and FSH secretion. Epilepsy-associated hyperprolactinemia could thus result in hypogonadotropic hypogonadism with associated hyposexuality.

In our patient, it was unclear whether his hyposexuality was due to his seizures, to DPH, or to both. Because his seizures had been unstable, we chose not to change his AED. Instead, we treated his hyposexuality hormonally. Evaluation and treatment of hyposexuality are discussed below in the section on effects of AEDs on hormonal function.

What effects do seizures have on hormone production acutely, and what clinical relevance does this have?

Transient post-ictal elevation of serum prolactin occurs after primary or secondarily generalized tonic–clonic seizures and after complex partial seizures, but rarely after simple partial seizures.[55,56] Prolactin rises within 10–30 min after the seizure, the prolactin level gradually returning to normal over the subsequent hour. The elevation occurs in 80 per cent of tonic–clonic, 45 per cent of complex partial, and 10 per cent of simple partial seizures.[56] Depth electrode recordings in patients with partial seizures show that a rise in serum prolactin is always associated with complex partial seizures involving the temporal lobes and often with simple partial seizures with high frequency discharges and widespread involvement of the mesial temporal limbic structures.[57] The prolactin elevation after simple partial seizures is about 45 per cent lower than that seen after complex partial seizures.[57]

Transient post-ictal serum prolactin elevation has been used clinically to distinguish primary or secondarily generalized tonic–clonic seizures and complex partial seizures of temporal lobe origin from pseudoseizures (non-epileptic seizures). Prolactin levels, unlike cortisol levels, are infrequently elevated in non-epileptic seizures. Earlier studies had shown that serum prolactin levels increased twofold or less after non-epileptic seizures, a degree of elevation that occurs also with stress and postprandially, but threefold or more after tonic–clonic seizures or complex partial seizures involving the temporal lobe.[55,56] However, in a study using 10-min blood sampling over 8 h, we have found that significant elevation of prolactin levels (three- and tenfold elevation above baseline in normal subjects and in patients with TLE, respectively) may occur interictally in the absence of epileptiform discharges or seizures.[58] Thus, the potential for false positive and false negative errors limits the usefulness of post-ictal prolactin assays in differentiating seizures from pseudoseizures.

Are any other hormonal systems clinically affected by partial seizures?

The function of the hypothalamo-pituitary-adrenal axis may be altered chronically as well as acutely in seizure patients.[59] Cortisol has been shown to be elevated interictally in some studies,[60] but not in others.[54] Corticotrophin (ACTH) is also elevated interictally in patients with temporal lobe seizures,[60] a finding that appears to be related specifically to abnormal functioning of the anterior temporal lobe,[60] where the amygdala is located, and to be limited to TLE that involves the amygdala. For instance, stimulation of the amygdala in TLE patients[61] as well as in animals[62] leads to a rise in serum corticosteroids and ACTH, but stimulation of the hippocampus inhibits their secretion.[61]

ACTH is secreted by the anterior pituitary in response to corticotropin releasing hormone (CRH) produced by neurons in the paraventricular nucleus of the hypothalamus. These neurons receive direct input from CRH-containing neurons in the amygdala.[63] Post-ictal and interictal elevation of ACTH and cortisol after seizures is thus most likely due to activation of the hypothalamic-adrenal axis by the amygdala as a result of ictal and interictal epileptiform discharges.

What are the clinical consequences of this activation? Few have been appreciated to date, but that may be because they have not been specifically sought. We have reported three cases of reversible Cushing's syndrome and myopathy in patients with refractory complex partial seizures. The Cushing's syndrome and myopathy fluctuated in parallel to seizure exacerbations and remitted with normalization of glucocorticoid levels upon treatment with ketoconazole, an inhibitor of adrenal steroidogenesis.[64] Ketoconazole also successfully treated the seizures.

How do AEDs affect hormonal functioning?

Anticonvulsant medications may affect endocrine function in a number of different, clinically significant ways. The most prominent effects are those on reproductive function, chiefly on sexuality.

What is the effect of AEDs on sexuality in men and women, and on reproduction in men?

The hepatic enzyme-inducing AEDs, namely phenobarbital, primidone, CBZ and DPH may all contribute to or cause reproductive and sexual dysfunction in men with epilepsy.[65,66]

Androgens are important in regulating potency and libido.[67] Testosterone (T) is the most important androgen; its serum concentration is affected by the barbiturates, DPH, and CBZ. Serum testosterone exists in three forms: free testosterone (FT, 2–3 per cent of total), albumin-bound (55 per cent), and sex hormone-binding globulin (SHBG)-bound (43–45 per cent).[68] The SHBG-bound fraction is not biologically active, but the albumin-bound and free fractions are. Reduction in free but not total testosterone is associated with diminished libido and potency,[65,66] as occurred in our Case 2 patient. Testosterone increases potency and libido, whereas estradiol lowers it.[68] Although estradiol constitutes only 1 per cent of male gonadal steroids, it exerts almost 50 per cent of the negative feedback on male LH secretion.[68] Hepatic enzyme-inducing AEDs lower the amount of free or biologically active testosterone available to stimulate sexual function and at the same time they increase the serum level of estradiol which actively inhibits it.

Barbiturates, DPH and CBZ affect serum testosterone and estradiol levels by at least four distinct mechanisms:[68]

1. CBZ and DPH act directly on the testis to inhibit testosterone synthesis by the Leydig cells of the testis.[69]
2. Barbiturates, CBZ, and DPH induce the hepatic p-450 enzymes that catabolize both AEDs and testosterone. Induction of those enzymes leads to increased clearance of testosterone from the body and lowering of its level.
3. These drugs induce liver production of SHBG.[65,66] Thus, serum SHBG is elevated, more of the total testosterone is bound to SHBG, and less testosterone remains available as free or biologically active testosterone. The increase in SHBG-bound T may result in normal or even elevated levels of total testosterone, even while the concentration of free or bioactive testosterone is reduced.[65,66] Clinically manifest hyposexuality corresponds to the duration of AED therapy, being more likely to occur after five or more years of treatment with CBZ or DPH.[70] The reason may be that SHBG levels increase progressively over time during chronic treatment with these medications.[70]
4. These drugs induce the liver production of the enzyme aromatase, which converts testosterone to estradiol (the last step of estradiol production). Its induction by the AEDs leads

to elevated serum level of estradiol[71] and, by shunting of FT to estradiol, to further reduction of serum-free tesosterone. Thus, the ratio of free testosterone to estradiol (FT–E2) is lower in epileptic men with hyposexuality than in sexually normal epileptic patients or in normal controls.[72] Because estradiol exerts a potent negative feedback upon male LH secretion, suppression of LH secretion leads to hypogonadotropic hypogonadism. Estradiol may also produce premature aging of the hypothalamic arcuate nucleus,[68] and, with it, hypothalamic hypogonadism. Both these effects may result in impaired testosterone secretion. Moreover, estradiol stimulates SHBG synthesis, whereas testosterone inhibits it. Thus, AED-induced elevation of estradiol could have a downward-spiraling effect of decreased testosterone and T–E2 ratio, stimulating SHBG synthesis with resultant further depression of bioactive T over time.

Laboratory findings in hyposexual patients on AED therapy may show, as in our patient, normal, or occasionally even elevated serum total testosterone levels.[65] However, levels of free testosterone or biologically active T,[73] are reduced. Serum estradiol is frequently elevated. In summary, the laboratory findings show: usually normal serum total testosterone; reduced serum free or biologically active testosterone; elevated SHBG; often elevated serum estradiol.

In practical terms, the following endocrinological tests should be checked in hyposexual men who are receiving AEDs: total testosterone, free testosterone and estradiol levels in all patients; and bioactive testosterone in those patients in whom the former two tests are normal.[73] In addition, serum LH and FSH should also be checked to evaluate the possibility of hypothalamic hypogonadism.

Treatment of AED-related hyposexuality consists of several options, and is usually successful. Obviously, changing anticonvulsant medications from the hepatic enzyme-inducing category to hepatic enzyme-inhibiting ones such as sodium valproate can be considered. However, in patients with previously hard-to-control seizures, which are well controlled with the hyposexuality-causing AEDs such as our Case 2 patient, changing AEDs may not be desirable. In those patients, treatment with testosterone to restore normal free testosterone levels (aiming for the high end of the normal range) would be the first step. Intramuscular depotestosterone, usually at 400–600 mg every 2–3 weeks, or the more expensive cutaneous androderm patch, applied daily, can be used. This may be sufficient treatment. Rarely, aggressive tendencies may develop with T. In some patients, however, there may be no response or, more commonly, initial improvement may be followed by a relapse. Relapse may be caused by rising levels of serum estradiol after testosterone treatment, because more testosterone is available for conversion to estradiol via the enzyme aromatase. If a relapse occurs, addition of the aromatase inhibitor testolactone to the testosterone will lower the serum estradiol level and restore normal libido and potency.[73] In some patients, lowering estradiol levels with testolactone may even lead to improved seizure control.[73] Treatment with the antiestrogen, clomiphene, may restore sexuality as well as improve seizure control[74,75] (see also the text that follows). Finally, symptomatic treatment with sildenafil citrate (Viagra) may also be successful.

What additional effects may AEDs have on reproductive function in women?

Sodium valproate may be associated with increased occurrence of PCOS.[76] PCOS is a condition of anovulatory cycles with hyperandrogenism, characterized by hirsutism and menstrual disorders. It is more frequent in obese women.[38,77] Isojarvi et al. have noted PCOS to be more common in epileptic women treated with sodium valproate (~45 per cent) than in those who are treated with CBZ (20 per cent).[76] They suggest that valproate causes weight gain, insulin resistance and hyperinsulinemia, which then cause hyperandrogenism,[78] and leads to PCOS. Hyperinsulinemia may indeed cause hyperandrogenism by directly stimulating ovarian steroidogenesis[38] and by inhibiting the synthesis of SHBG with a consequent increase in the availability of bioactive androgens. In valproate-treated women with epilepsy and PCOS, switching from valproate to another AED such as lamotrigine may reverse the hyperandrogenism and normalize ovarian morphology.[79]

On the other hand, we have argued that PCOS is related to the underlying epilepsy (see previous section) and that the difference in the incidence of PCOS between valproate-treated women and women treated with other AEDs may be due to a beneficiary effect upon PCOS by hepatic enzyme-inducing AEDs such as barbiturates, DPH and CBZ.[77] Thus, PCOS is less common in treated (13 per cent) than in untreated (30 per cent) women with TLE when treatment does not include sodium valproate.[34] Hepatic enzyme-inducing AEDs lower biologically active androgen levels while valproate does not. AEDs other than valproate, therefore, may treat epilepsy-related hyperandrogenism and thus PCOS, whereas valproate therapy may not. This mechanism could contribute to the higher occurrence of PCOS in valproate-treated women with epilepsy.[77]

Other effects of valproate on reproduction may include amenorrhea and pubertal arrest, seen transiently after initiation of valproate therapy.[80,81]

Hepatic enzyme-inducing AEDs such as barbiturates, DPH and CBZ lower the efficacy of hormone contraceptives, including oral contraceptives, i.m. medroxyprogesterone and subcutaneous levonorgestrel implant (Norplant). This occurs because an increase in steroid hormone metabolism by *p*-450 enzymes and an increase of hepatic synthesis of steroid hormone-binding globulin result in a decrease of exogenous estrogen and progesterone levels.[82] Failure rate of oral contraceptives doubles in women treated with such AEDs. Topiramate also lowers the efficacy of oral contraceptives, although the mechanism is uncertain. Valproic acid, gabapentin, lamotrigine and tiagabine do not affect oral contraceptive treatment efficacy. In women receiving enzyme-inducing AEDs or topiramate who desire effective contraception, therapeutic choices include oral contraceptive preparation with higher steroid content, e.g. 50 μg ethinyl estradiol; addition of a non-hormone-based form of contraception such as the double barrier method; or changing AED to valproic acid, lamotrigine, gabapentin or tiagabine.

Hormonal treatment in epilepsy

Endocrine treatment of seizures may rationally be aimed at those endocrine aspects of seizures that act either to exacerbate or to ameliorate them. On the basis of hormonal effects discussed above, treatment with progesterone, estrogen antagonists and medications that suppress the activity of the hypothalamo-pituitary-adrenal axis may prove to be useful adjunctive therapy in appropriate epilepsy patients.

Progesterone

As noted previously, low progesterone levels or rapid withdrawal of progesterone may be a factor in the increased seizure frequency seen during the premenstrual and early follicular phase of women with catamenial epilepsy and normal ovulatory cycles, and during the entire luteal phase of women with anovulatory cycles.[1,2,19] Progesterone may be expected to be beneficial in these women.

Synthetic progestin therapy may be considered. Little or no benefit has been seen in a number of studies noted with oral forms[83,84] although occasional benefits have been described in single case reports. In one study of women with refractory partial seizures and normal ovulatory cycles, medroxyprogesterone (MP) doses large enough to induce amenorrhea (i.e. 120–150 mg every 6–12 weeks intramuscularly (i.m.) or 20–40 mg orally daily) resulted in 40 per cent average seizure reduction from an average of eight to five seizures per month.[83] It is unclear whether the effect was due to direct antiepileptic activity of MP or to the hormonal consequences of the MP-induced amenorrhea. We have found weekly doses of 400 mg i.m. depomedroxyprogesterone to be more effective. Potential side effects include depression, sedation, breakthrough vaginal bleeding and delay in the return of regular menstrual cycles.[83]

Natural progesterone may be an effective treatment.[32] In an open-label trial of 25 women with catamenial exacerbation of complex partial seizures of temporal lobe origin, 11 with C1 pattern and 14 with C3 pattern of seizures, 72 per cent of the women improved, with a 55 per cent decline in average daily seizure frequency, from 0.39 to 0.18.[32] Progesterone was administered as lozenges 200 mg t.i.d. on days 23–25 of each menstrual cycle to the C1 women; and on days 15–25 of each menstrual cycle, with taper over days 26–28, for C3 women.[32]

Natural progesterone is available as soybean extract in lozenge, micronized capsule, cream and suppository form. The usual daily regimen to achieve physiological luteal range serum levels is 100–200 mg three times daily.[32] The synthetic progestins are not equivalent because the natural progesterone is metabolized to allopregnanolone, which has potent GABA-α mimetic and anticonvulsant action[15,16] whereas synthetic progestins are not metabolized in this way. Potential side effects may include sedation, depression, weight gain, breast tenderness and breakthrough vaginal bleeding—all readily reversible upon discontinuation of the hormone or lowering of the dose.

Neuroactive steroids

The experimental and animal data on the cellular effects of GABA-mimetic neuroactive steroids such as allopregnanolone, suggest that these compounds may have a potent antiepileptic effect.[85] Ganaxolone, a form of allopregnanolone synthetically modified so as to minimize allopregnanolone's sedative side effects and prolong its half-life, showed initial promise in early open-label studies in children and adolescents with refractory partial or generalized seizures.[86] Unfortunately, a double-blind placebo-controlled trial of adult patients with refractory complex partial seizures taken off all other AEDs did not show significant benefits.[87] No further clinical studies are currently in progress.

Clomiphene

Clomiphene citrate is an estrogen analogue with both estrogenic and antiestrogenic effects that are dose-dependent. In its clinical use, it acts primarily as an antiestrogen at the hypothalamic and pituitary level to stimulate gonadotropin secretion, ovulation and fertility. It exerts an anticonvulsant effect in rats in a dose-related fashion.[11] Remarkable reduction

in seizure frequency has been reported in a number of isolated cases in both men and women.[74,75,88] In one series of 12 women with complex partial seizures and menstrual disorders (polycystic ovarian syndrome or inadequate luteal phase cycles) who were given clomiphene, ten improved, often dramatically, with an 87 per cent average seizure frequency decline.[88] Improvement in seizure frequency was associated with normalization of the menstrual cycle and of luteal progesterone secretion. The only two women who did not improve continued to have menstrual abnormalities.[88]

Clomiphene may be a useful adjunct antiepileptic treatment in women with menstrual disorders. It is administered in doses of 25–100 mg daily on days 5–9 of each menstrual cycle in women and 25–50 mg daily in men. Side effects can be significant and include risk of unwanted pregnancy, ovarian hyperstimulation syndrome, transient breast tenderness and pelvic cramps. Furthermore, seizure frequency may increase during the enhanced preovulatory increase in serum estradiol levels in some women. Clomiphene should therefore be restricted to women who have irregular anovulatory cycles that cannot be normalized readily with cyclic progesterone use. It should not be administered in cases of suspected pregnancy or in the absence of adequate birth control measures unless it is used in conjunction with a consultation with a gynecologist as part of a fertility program. It may be tried in men with refractory partial seizures and hyposexuality.

Testolactone

We have reported notable improvement in seizures in a couple of patients whose AED-related hyposexuality was treated with testosterone and testolactone, an inhibitor of the enzyme aromatase, which inhibits the conversion of estrogens and androgens.[73] Treatment with testosterone alone was ineffective. The successful treatment was associated with normalization of previously elevated estradiol levels, suggesting that the anticonvulsant effect of testolactone may be due to a reduction of the proconvulsant effects of estrogen.

LHRH agonists

Lowering of estrogen levels by induction of menopause could be expected to improve seizure control. Medical menopause can be achieved by chronic usage of one of the long-acting LHRH analogs. Long-term suppression of gonadotropin and ovarian secretion develops after an initial 3–4-week long phase of reproductive endocrine stimulation. One patient with severe refractory seizures that were exacerbated perimenstrually was reported to have improved markedly after treatment with the LHRH agonist goserelin.[89] In one open-label study of goserelin, 8 out of 10 patients with refractory catamenial seizures improved, including three patients who became seizure-free.[90] Adverse effects, mainly hot flushes and headache, also occurred in 8 out of 10 patients. Our observations in a few cases suggest that seizure control may improve, but that seizure exacerbation during the first month stimulation phase may preclude the use of LHRH analogs in some cases. Moreover, the immediate and long-term effects of hypoestrogenism need to be considered.

Adrenal steroid-based treatments

Both ACTH and prednisone have been used extensively in the treatment of refractory infantile spasms and other primary generalized seizures of childhood.[91] They have been successfully used in another childhood epileptic syndrome, the Landau–Kleffner syndrome of acquired aphasia and seizures,[91] but not in other forms of partial epilepsy.

As mentioned previously, we have seen three patients with refractory seizures and hypercortisolemia whose seizures became controlled upon normalization of cortisol levels by ketoconazole.[64] Wider use of ketoconazole and other potential enzymatic inhibitors of cortisol synthesis have not been explored.

Summary

In recent years, major advances have been made in our understanding of how gonadal and adrenal hormones and related neuropeptides affect seizures and how epilepsy affects endocrine functions. Diverse evidence shows that steroidal hormones have neuroactive effects which may facilitate or blunt seizure occurrence. This provides a basis for the use of hormones for the treatment of seizures. Our growing understanding of the effects of seizures on reproductive endocrine functions enables us to better manage reproductive endocrine disorders associated with epilepsy.

References

1. Laidlaw J. Catamenial epilepsy. *Lancet* 1956;**271**:1235–7.

2. Herzog AG, Klein P, Ransil B. Three patterns of catamenial epilepsy. *Epilepsia* 1997;**38**:1082–8.

3. Newmark NE, Penry JK. Catamenial epilepsy: a review. *Epilepsia* 1980;**21**:281–300.

4. Klein P, Herzog AG. Hormonal effects on epilepsy in women. *Epilepsia* 1999;**39**(Suppl 8):S9–S16.

5. Jones GS. The luteal phase defect. *Fertil Steril* 1976;**27**:351–6.

6. Wong M, Moss RL. Long-term and short-term electrophysiological effects of estrogen on the synaptic properties of hippocampal CA1 neurons. *J Neurosci* 1992;**12**:3217–25.

7. Woolley CS, Schwartzkroin PA. Hormonal effects on the brain. *Epilepsia* 1999;**39**(Suppl 8):S2–S8.

8. Lothman EW. Seizure circuits in the hippocampus and associated structures. *Hippocampus* 1994;**4**:286–318.

9. Hom AC, Buterbaugh GG. Estrogen alters the acquisition of seizures kindled by repeated amygdala stimulation or pentylenetetrazol administration in ovariectomized female rats. *Epilepsia* 1986;**27**:103–8.

10. Logothetis J, Harner R. Electrocortical activation by estrogens. *Arch Neurol* 1960;**3**:290–7.

11. Nicoletti F, Speciale C, Sortino MA, et al. Comparative effects of estradiol benzoate, the antiestrogen clomiphene citrate and the progestin medroxyprogesterone acetate on kainic acid-induced seizures in male and female rats. *Epilepsia* 1985;**26**:252–7.

12. Woolley DE, Timiras PS. The gonad–brain relationship: effects of female sex hormones on electroshock convulsions in the rat. *Endocrinology* 1962;**70**:196–209.

13. Teresawa E, Timiras P. Electrical activity during the estrous cycle of the rat: cyclic changes in limbic structures. *Endocrinology* 1968;**83**:207.

14. Logothetis J, Harner R, Morrell F, et al. The role of estrogens in catamenial exacerbation of epilepsy. *Neurology* 1959;**9**:352–60.

15. Majewska MD, Harrison NL, Schwartz RD, et al. Steroid hormone metabolites are barbiturate-like modulators of the GABA receptor. *Science* 1986;**232**:1004–7.

16. Paul SM, Purdy RH. Neuroactive steroids. *FASEB* 1992;**6**:2311–22.

17. Landgren S, Backstrom T, Kalistratov G. The effect of progesterone on the spontaneous inter-ictal spike evoked by the application of penicillin to the cat's cerebral cortex. *J Neurol Sci* 1978;**36**:119–33.

18. Backstrom T, Zetterlund B, Blom S, et al. Effects of intravenous progesterone infusions on the epileptic discharge frequency in women with partial epilepsy. *Acta Neurol Scand* 1984;**69**:240–8.

19. Backstrom T. Epileptic seizures in women related to plasma estrogen and progesterone during the menstrual cycle. *Acta Neurol Scandinav* 1976;**54**:321–47.

20. Smith SS, Gong QH, Hsu FC, et al. GABA-A receptor α4 subunit suppression prevents withdrawal properties of an endogenous steroid. *Nature* 1998;**392**:926–9.

21. Shavit G, Lerman P, Korczyn AD, et al. Phenytoin pharmacokinetics in catamenial epilepsy. *Neurology* 1984;**34**:959–61.

22. Roscizewska D, Buntner B, Guz I, et al. Ovarian hormones, anticonvulsant drugs and seizures during the menstrual cycle in women with epilepsy. *J Neurol Neurosurg Psychiatry* 1986;**49**:47–51.

23. Morrell MJ, Hamdy S, Seale CG, Springer EA. Self-reported reproductive history in women with epilepsy: puberty onset and effects of menarche and menstrual cycle on seizures. *Neurology* 1998;**50**:A448.

24. Knight AH, Rhind EG. Epilepsy and pregnancy: a study of 153 pregnancies in 59 patients. *Epilepsia* 1975;**16**:99–110.

25. Schmidt D, Canger R, Avanzini G. Change in seizure frequency in pregnant epileptic women. *J Neurol Neurosurg Psychiatry* 1985;**46**:751–5.

26. Sallusto L, Pozzi O. Relations between ovarian activity and the occurrence of epileptic seizures. Data on a clinical case. *Acta Neurol (Napoli)* 1964;**19**:673–81.

27. Beaussart M, Faou R. Evolution of epilepsy

with Rolandic (centrotemporal) paroxysmal foci. *Epilepsia* 1978;**19**:337–42.

28. Panayiotopoulos CP. Benign childhood epilepsy with occipital paroxysms: a 15-year prospective study. *Ann Neurol* 1989;**26**:51–6.

29. Longo LPS, Saldana LEG. Hormones and their influences in epilepsy. *Acta Neurol Latinoam* 1966;**12**:29–47.

30. Rosciszewska D. The course of epilepsy at the age of puberty in girls. *Neurol Neurochir Pol* 1975;**9**:597–602.

31. Harden CL, Jacobs A, Pulver M, Trifiletti R. Effect of menopause on epilepsy. *Epilepsia* 1997;**38**(Suppl 8):133.

32. Herzog AG. Progesterone therapy in women with complex partial and secondary generalized seizures. *Neurology* 1995;**45**:1660–2.

33. Sharf M, Sharf B, Bental E, et al. The electroencephalogram in the investigation of anovulation and its treatment by clomiphene. *Lancet* 1969;**1**:750–3.

34. Herzog AG, Seibel MM, Schomer DL, et al. Reproductive endocrine disorders in women with partial seizures of temporal lobe origin. *Arch Neurol* 1986;**43**:341–6.

35. Dansky LV, Andermann E, Andermann F. Marriage and fertility in epileptic patients. *Epilepsia* 1980;**21**:261–71.

36. Cummings LN, Giudice L, Morrell MJ. Ovulatory function in epilepsy. *Epilepsia* 1995;**36**:353–7.

37. King JC, Anthony ELP, Fitzgerald DM, et al. Luteinizing hormone-releasing hormone neurons in human preoptic/hypothalamus: differential intraneuronal localization of immunoreactive forms. *J Clin Endocrinol Lab* 1985;**60**:88–97.

38. Carr BR. Disorders of the ovary and female reproductive tract. In: Wilson JD, Foster DW, eds. *Williams textbook of endocrinology*. Philadelphia: W.B. Saunders, 1992:733–99.

39. Drislane FW, Coleman AE, Schomer DL, et al. Altered pulsatile secretion of luteinizing hormone in women with epilepsy. *Neurology* 1994;**44**:306–10.

40. Maeda K, Tsukamura H, Okhura S, et al. The LHRH pulse generator: a mediobasal hypothalamic location. *Neurosci Biobehav Rev* 1995;**19**:427–37.

41. Canteras NS, Simerly RB, Swanson LW. Organization of projections from the medial nucleus of the amygdala: a PHAL study in the rat. *J Comp Neurol* 1995;**360**:213–45.

42. Reynaud LP. Influence of amygdala on the activity of identified neurons in the rat hypothalamus. *J Physiol* 1976;**260**:237–52.

43. Zolovnick AJ. Effects of lesions and electrical stimulation of the amygdala on hypothalamic-hypophyseal regulation. In: Eleftheriou BE, ed. *The neurobiology of the amygdala*. New York: Plenum Press 1972:745–62.

44. Bilo L, Meo R, Valentino R, et al. Abnormal patterns of luteinizing hormone pulsatility in women with epilepsy. *Fertil Steril* 1991;**55**: 705–11.

45. Herzog AG. A relationship between particular reproductive endocrine disorders and the laterality of epileptiform discharges in women with epilepsy. *Neurology* 1993;**43**:1907–10.

46. Simerly RB, Chang M, Muramatsu M, et al. Distribution of androgen and estrogen receptor mRNA-containing cells in the rat brain: an in situ hybridization study. *J Comp Neurol* 1990; **294**:76–95.

47. Morrell MJ, Guldner G. Self-reported sexual function in women with epilepsy. *Epilepsia* 1994;**35**(Suppl 8):108.

48. Taylor DC. Sexual behavior and temporal lobe epilepsy. *Arch Neurol* 1969;**21**:510–16.

49. Hierons R, Saunders M. Impotence in patients with temporal lobe lesions. *Lancet* 1966;**2**: 761–4.

50. Herzog AG, Seibel MM, Schomer DL, et al. Reproductive endocrine disorders in men with partial seizures of temporal lobe origin. *Arch Neurol* 1986;**43**:347–50.

51. Blumer D. Changes of sexual behavior related to temporal lobe disorders in man. *J Sex Res* 1970;**6**:173–80.

52. Bear DM, Fedio P. Quantitative analysis of interictal behavior in temporal lobe epilepsy. *Arch Neurol* 1977;**34**:454–67.

53. Carter J, Tyson J, Tolis G. Prolactin-secreting tumors and hypogonadism in 22 men. *N Engl J Med* 1978;**299**:847–52.

54. Molaie M, Culebras A, Miller M. Nocturnal plasma prolactin and cortisol levels in epileptics with complex partial seizures and primary generalized seizures. *Arch Neurol* 1987;**44**:699–702.

55. Trimble MR. Serum prolactin in epilepsy and hysteria. *Br Med J* 1978;**2**:1682.

56. Wyllie E, Luders H, Macmillan JP, et al. Serum prolactin levels after epileptic seizures. *Neurology* 1984;**34**:1601–4.

57. Sperling MR, Pritchard PB, Engel J, et al. Prolactin in partial epilepsy: an indicator of limbic seizures. *Ann Neurol* 1986;**20**:716–22.

58. Herzog AG, Klein P, Jacobs A, et al. Abnormal interictal prolactin elevations particularly among men and women with complex partial seizures of right temporal origin. *Epilepsia* 1997;**38**(Suppl 8):48.

59. Abbot RJ, Browning MCK, Davidson DLW. Serum prolactin and cortisol concentrations after grand mal seizures. *J Neurol Neurosurg Psychiatry* 1980;**43**:163–7.

60. Gallagher BB, Murvin A, Flanigin HF, et al. Pituitary and adrenal function in epileptic patients. *Epilepsia* 1984;**25**:683–9.

61. Mandell AJ, Chapman LF, Rand RW, et al. Plasma corticosteroids: changes in concentration after stimulation of hippocampus and amygdala. *Science* 1963;**139**:1212.

62. Dunn JD, Whitener J. Plasma corticosterone responses to electrical stimulation of the amygdaloid complex: cytoarchitectural specificity. *Neuroendocrinology* 1986;**42**:211–17.

63. Gray TS, Carney ME, Magnusson DJ. Direct projections from the central amygdaloid nucleus to the hypothalamic paraventricular nucleus: possible role in stress-induced adrenocorticotropin release. *Neuroendocrinology* 1989;**50**:433–46.

64. Herzog AG, Sotrel A, Ronthal M. Reversible proximal myopathy in epilepsy-related Cushing's syndrome. *Ann Neurol* 1995;**38**:306–7.

65. Toone BK, Wheeler M, Nanjee M, et al. Sex hormones, sexual activity and plasma anticonvulsant levels in male epileptics. *J Neurol Neurosurg Psychiatry* 1983;**46**:824–6.

66. Isojarvi JIT, Pakarinen AJ, Ylipalosaari PJ, et al. Serum hormones in male epileptic patients receiving anticonvulsant medication. *Arch Neurol* 1990;**47**:670–6.

67. Davidson JM, Camargo CA, Smith ER. Effects of androgens on sexual behavior in hypogonadal men. *J Clin Endocrinol Metab* 1979;**48**:955.

68. Herzog AG. Hormonal changes in epilepsy. *Epilepsia* 1995;**36**:323–6.

69. Kuhn-Velten WN, Herzog AG, Muller MR. Acute effects of anticonvulsant drugs on gonadotropin-stimulated and precursor-supported testicular androgen production. *Eur J Pharmacol* 1990;**181**:151–5.

70. Isojarvi JIT, Repo M, Pakarinen AJ, et al. Carbamazepine, phenytoin, sex hormones and sexual dysfunction in men with epilepsy. *Epilepsia* 1995;**36**:364–8.

71. Herzog AG, Levesque L, Drislane F, et al. Phenytoin-induced elevations of serum estradiol and reproductive dysfunction in men with epilepsy. *Epilepsia* 1991;**32**:550–3.

72. Murialdo G, Galimberti CA, Fonzi S, et al. Sex hormones and pituitary function in male epileptic patients with altered or normal sexuality. *Epilepsia* 1995;**36**:364–8.

73. Herzog AG, Klein P, Jacobs AR. Testosterone versus testosterone and testolactone in the treatment of reproductive/sexual dysfunction in men with epilepsy and hypogonadism. *Neurology* 1998;**50**:782–4.

74. Herzog AG. Seizure control with clomiphene therapy: a case report. *Arch Neurol* 1988;**45**:209–10.

75. Login IS, Dreifuss FE. Anticonvulsant activity of clomiphene. *Arch Neurol* 1983;**40**:525.

76. Isojarvi JIT, Laatikainen TJ, Pakarinen AJ, et al. Polycystic ovaries and hyperandrogenism in women taking valproate for epilepsy. *N Engl J Med* 1993;**329**:1383–8.

77. Herzog AG. Polycystic ovarian syndrome in women with epilepsy: epileptic or iatrogenic? *Ann Neurol* 1996;**39**:559–61.

78. Isojarvi JIT, Laatikainen TJ, Knip M, et al. Obesity and endocrine disorders in women taking valproate for epilepsy. *Ann Neurol* 1996;**39**:579–85.

79. Isojarvi JIT, Rattya J, Myllyla VV, et al. Valproate, lamotrigine and insulin-mediated risks in women with epilepsy. *Ann Neurol* 1998;**43**:446–51.

80. Margraf JW, Dreifuss FE. Amenorrhoea following initiation of therapy with valproic acid. *Neurology* 1981;**31**:159.

81. Jones TH. Sodium valproate-induced menstrual disturbances in young women. *Hormone Res* 1991;**35**:82–5.

82. El-Sayed Y. Obstetric and gynecologic care of women with epilepsy. *Epilepsia* 1999;**39**(Suppl 8):S17–S25.

83. Mattson RH, Cramer JA, Caldwell BV, et al. Treatment of seizures with medroxyprogester-

one acetate: preliminary report. *Neurology* 1984;**34**:1255–8.

84. Dana-Haeri J, Richens A. Effect of norethisterone on seizures associated with menstruation. *Epilepsia* 1983;**24**:377–81.

85. Klein P, Herzog AG. Emerging applications of hormonal therapy of paroxysmal central nervous system disorders. *Exp Opin Invest Drugs* 1997;**6**:1337–49.

86. Dodson WE, Bourgeois B, Kerrigan J, et al. An open label evaluation of safety and efficacy of ganaxolone in children with refractory seizures and history of infantile spasms. *Epilepsia* 1997; **38**(Suppl 8):179.

87. Monaghan EP, Harris S, Blum D, et al. Ganaxolone in the treatment of complex partial seizures: a double-blind, presurgical design. *Epilepsia* 1997;**38**(Suppl 8):179.

88. Herzog AG. Clomiphene therapy in epileptic women with menstrual disorders. *Neurology* 1988;**38**:432–4.

89. Haider Y, Barnett D. Catamenial epilepsy and goserelin. *Lancet* 1991;**2**:1530.

90. Bauer J, Wildt L, Flugel D, Stefan H. The effect of a synthetic GnRH analogue on catamenial epilepsy: a study in ten patients. *J Neurol* 1992;**239**:284–6.

91. Snead OC. ACTH and prednisone: use in seizure disorders other than infantile spasms. In: Levy RH, Mattson RH, Meldrum BS, eds. *Antiepileptic Drugs*. New York: Raven Press, 1995:941–48.

33

Subacute focal encephalitis

Olivier Dulac

Introduction

Subacute focal encephalitis (Rasmussen's syndrome) was first identified as a specific condition in 1958 when Rasmussen et al reported three cases with very peculiar clinical and histopathological characteristics.[1] The next major step forward was the detailed monograph edited by Andermann.[2] From then on, the problem of selecting appropriate therapy based on presumed aetiologies has been discussed, but without much scientific basis or evidence of improved outcome for patients.

The disorder combines intractable focal motor seizures, progressive neurological deterioration, focal cortical atrophy mainly involving perisylvian areas and an inflammatory process resulting in perivascular cuffs of round cells, microglial nodules and mild meningitis. Several cases have been preceded by unilateral uveitis.[3] One half of the patients exhibit epilepsia partialis continua (EPC).[2] The disorder is unilateral in most instances, but cases with either clinical or neuropathological evidence of bilateral involvement have been reported.[2,4] In most of the latter cases, the disorder appears to be clinically unilateral and contralateral involvement is a neuropathological discovery.

The electro-encephalographic (EEG) findings are focal discharges arising from multiple independent foci within a wide epileptogenic zone, discharging in a subcontinuous fashion. Over a period of a few months or years, the area of the body that is clinically affected by the discharges widens. Functional imaging shows increased rolandic, and eventually, thalamic metabolic activity and cerebral blood flow, even during the early stage of the disorder, when no atrophy can be disclosed on conventional imaging.[5,6] Electrocorticography recordings disclose multiple, independent epileptogenic foci. Stereo-EEG and magneto-encephalography recordings have shown that seizures and jerks do not originate from the same area of the motor strip—motor seizures are triggered by the convexity, and jerks by the cortex located in the depth of the rolandic fissure (see Chapter 28).

Diagnosis

One of the most difficult issues associated with this disorder is accurate diagnosis. Indeed, focal encephalitis can only be demonstrated on histology. However, examination of resected tissue shows that inflammatory cells seem to disappear from the centre of the lesion and progressively involve its periphery, thus explaining the progressive character of the neurological defect and of the epilepsy. For this reason, a targeted biopsy often produces negative findings, which delays the diagnosis. Other conditions that may also produce EPC comprise inborn errors of metabolism, particularly mitochondrial diseases diagnosed on the basis of increased lactate concentrations in the cerebrospinal fluid (CSF). In Alpers disease, hepatic failure occurs late in the course of the disorder, although the presence of diffuse spike–wave activity over the most affected hemisphere gives the clue at an earlier stage.[7] The cause of EPC that is most difficult to identify is cortical dysplasia affecting the rolandic area.[8] This diagnosis may be particularly challenging when the lesion is not obvious on neuroradiology studies. There may be several types of seizures, with seizures persisting also in sleep. However, the age of seizure onset is younger than in patients with subacute focal encephalitis and the ictal EEG pattern is characteristic, showing rhythmic and regular paroxysmal activity.

Treatment

Conventional treatment with various antiepileptic drugs (AEDs) alone or in combination is ineffective in subacute focal encephalitis. Clinical observations suggest that topiramate may reduce the frequency of seizures originating from the rolandic area, and piracetam has a mild effect, as in other kinds of cortical myoclonus.[9] Patients experience repeated episodes of worsening of seizures that often culminate in status epilepticus.

The aetiology of focal encephalitis remains unknown. An immunological process is strongly suggested by the neuropathological findings and CSF studies. Infiltration by inflammatory cells is usual; in contrast, such infiltration is seldom observed in children with severe epilepsy undergoing resective surgery, except when the seizure disorder is clearly related to remote encephalitis or bacterial meningitis. In one half of the patients with Rasmussen's syndrome, electrophoresis of the CSF proteins shows oligoclonal bands similar to those seen in multiple sclerosis.[10] Preliminary

reports claimed positive findings from polymerase chain reaction studies for various viruses including Epstein–Barr virus and cytomegalovirus, but further investigations failed to confirm these findings.

Based on histopathological studies and CSF protein electrophoresis, an autoimmune pathogenesis was suggested and steroid treatment advised.[4] Later, an animal model was developed by immunizing rabbits against the GluR3 protein, which produced a clinical pattern characteristic of Rasmussen's syndrome, both from the clinical and neuropathological points of view. Indeed, there were inflammatory cells within the cerebral cortex.[11] In addition, the authors could identify antibodies against GluR3 fusion protein in two of three patients with Rasmussen's syndrome, compared with only one of 21 control patients with other kinds of epilepsy, and there were no antibodies against GluR1 or GluR6 receptors. Two GluR-negative patients with Rasmussen's syndrome had undergone hemispherectomy 2 years earlier and they no longer suffered from seizures. If this finding is confirmed, the precise mechanism by which the disease is unilateral and progressive, and by which antibodies enter the brain will have to be determined. The increased permeability of the blood–brain barrier produced by seizures could give a clue to the unilateral pathological involvement. Unfortunately, the findings regarding GluR3 could not be reproduced by other groups.

On the basis of these reports, antiviral treatments and treatments affecting the immunological status of patients have been attempted. Zidovudine[12] and gancyclovir[13] have both been tried with moderate success in one patient, although the disorder later affected the contralateral side. Immunoglobulins were also tried, but with no or only transient effect.[14] The dose was either 400 mg/m^2 for 5 days or 1 g/m^2 for 2 days, repeated monthly. In one patient reported by Rogers et al, plasmapheresis was performed in order to remove the abnormal antibodies, without persistent beneficial effect, although the procedure was claimed to be initially effective with an 80 per cent decrease in seizure frequency over the 7 weeks of exchange.[11] Unfortunately, this result could not be reproduced in several other patients treated but not reported in the literature.

Conflicting results were reported regarding high dose steroids. One multicenter retrospective study reported lack of efficacy with a time-limited treatment schedule given to 16 patients from Canada, the UK and Argentina with quite advanced conditions.[15] On the other hand, one prospective open study included eight patients receiving high dose steroids with monthly pulses of methylprednisolone combined with oral prednisone in decreasing doses for >6 months. In five patients with unilateral involvement and in whom steroid treatment was started within the first 15 months of the disease, EPC resolved within a mean of 6 months.[4] Motor improvement followed resolution of EPC. Four patients later showed episodes of transient relapse lasting 3–4 weeks, every 3–4 months, with a follow-up of 3–5 years, but without worsening of neuroradiological abnormalities. These episodes were eventually triggered by fever.

Surgery

Surgery is only effective when disconnection of the affected hemisphere can be performed, whereas focal resection and callosotomy are either ineffective or produce very transient effects. Indeed, partial resection, even when guided by corticography, fails to produce any long-lasting effect because the disorder extends centrifugally. According to Vining et al,[16] surgical disconnection of the abnormal hemisphere should be performed as early as possible once the diagnosis is made. Although two of the three patients for whom Honavar et al performed subpial transection had early favourable outcome, follow-up periods were very short.[17] In two patients in our series submitted to subpial transection, the benefit did not exceed 1 year, and more extensive disconnection had to be performed.

The current clinical challenge is to determine the most appropriate time for surgery, given the fact that loss of the function of the contralateral hand and transient deterioration of language are possible risks that have to be accepted by the family (if they have not already occurred). Some patients benefit considerably from surgery even despite the loss of function produced by this treatment. From the technical point of view, it is preferable to avoid removing the hemisphere in order to prevent the late occurrence of haemosiderosis. For this reason, hemispherotomy that totally disconnects the hemisphere without removing more than the biopsied cortex and underlying white matter (that gives access to the basal ganglia) was developed by Delalande et al,[18] following encouraging results obtained by functional hemispherectomy.[19]

Summary

The value of immunological treatment of subacute focal encephalitis remains speculative, mainly because whether there is an autoimmune basis to this disorder remains unknown. There seems to be a role for high dose steroid treatment, provided that it is performed early, for example, within the first year of the disorder. As soon as lack of efficacy becomes evident, the issue of hemispheric disconnection should be raised so that the potential benefit of this procedure to the patient's quality of life is not delayed.

References

1. Rasmussen T, Olszewski J, Lloyd-Smith D. Focal seizures due to chronic localised encephalitis. *Neurology* 1958;8:435–45.

2. Anderman F, ed. *Chronic focal encephalitis and epilepsy. Rasmussen's syndrome.* Boston: Butterworth-Heinemann, 1991.

3. Fukuda T, Oguni H, Yanagaki S, et al. Chronic localized encephalitis (Rasmussen's syndrome) preceded by ipsilateral uveitis: a case report. *Epilepsia* 1993;35:1328–31.

4. Chinchilla D, Dulac O, Robain O, et al. Reappraisal of Rasmussen's syndrome with special emphasis on treatment with high doses of steroids. *J Neurol Neurosurg Psychiatry* 1994;57:1325–33.

5. Hajek M, Antonini A, Leenders KL, Wieser HG. Epilepsia partialis continua studied by PET. *Epilepsy Res* 1991;9:44–8.

6. Sztirha L, Pavios L, Ambrus E. Epilepsia partialis continua: follow-up with 99m Tc-HMPAO-SPECT. *Neuropediatrics* 1994;25:250–4.

7. Harding BN. Progressive neuronal degeneration of childhood with liver disease. *J Child Neurol* 1990;5:273–87.

8. Kuzniecky R, Powers R. Epilepsia partialis continua due to cortical dysplasia. *J Child Neurol* 1993;8:386–8.

9. Obeso JA, Artieda J, Luquin MR, et al. Antimyoclonic effect of piracetam. *Clin Neuropharmacol* 1986;9:58–64.

10. Dulac O, Dravet C, Plouin P, et al. Aspects nosologiques des épilepsies partielles continues chez l'enfant. *Arch Fr Pediatr* 1983;40:689–95.

11. Rogers SW, Andrews PI, Gahring LC, et al. Autoantibodies to glutamate receptor GluR3 in Rasmussen's encephalitis. *Science* 1994;265:648–51.

12. De Toledo JC, Smith DB. Partially successful treatment of Rasmussen's encephalitis with zidovudine: symptomatic improvement by involvement of the contralateral hemisphere. *Epilepsia* 1994;34:352–5.

13. McLachlan RS, Levin SD, Blume WT, et al. Rasmussen's encephalitis: treatment with the antiviral drug gancyclovir. *Epilepsia* 1995;(Suppl 4):107.

14. Walsh P. Treatment of Rasmussen's syndrome with intravenous immunoglobulin. In: Andermann F, ed. *Chronic focal encephalitis and epilepsy: Rasmussen's syndrome* Boston: Butterworth-Heinemann, 1991.

15. Hart Y, Cortez M, Andermann F, et al. Medical treatment of Rasmussen's syndrome (chronic encephalitis and epilepsy): effect of high dose steroids or immunoglobulins in 19 patients. *Neurology* 1994;44:1030–6.

16. Vining EPG, Freeman JM, Brandt J, et al. Progressive unilateral encephalopathy of childhood (Rasmussen's syndrome): a reappraisal. *Epilepsia* 1993;34:639–50.

17. Honavar M, Janota I, Polkey CE. Rasmussen's encephalitis in surgery for epilepsy. *Dev Med Child Neurol* 1992;34:3–14.

18. Delalande O, Pinard JM, Jalin C, et al. Surgical results of hemispherotomy. *Epilepsia* 1995;36 (Suppl 3):241.

19. Villemure JG, Andermann F, Rasmussen TB. Hemispherectomy for the treatment of epilepsy due to chronic encephalitis. In: Andermann F, ed. *Chronic focal encephalitis and epilepsy: Rasmussen's syndrome* Boston: Butterworth-Heinemann, 1991.

34

Vagal nerve stimulation

Steven C Schachter

Introduction

Despite the recent introduction of new antiepileptic drugs, a significant proportion of patients with partial-onset seizures either continue to have seizures or experience unacceptable side effects from pharmacotherapy. In the past, several non-pharmacological treatments were used for refractory seizures, including epilepsy surgery, cerebellar stimulation, thalamic stimulation and the ketogenic diet. Of these treatment modalities, only epilepsy surgery is widely considered efficacious and safe, particularly for adults.[1] However, some patients are opposed to having intracranial surgery and others are not candidates based on the localization of their seizures.

Vagal nerve stimulation (VNS) is a new non-pharmacological therapy for adults with treatment-resistant partial seizures who are unable to function to the best of their abilities because of seizures or medication side effects. The Neurocybernetic Prosthesis (NCP; Cyberonics, Inc.) was approved on July 16, 1997 by the Food and Drug Administration in the US for use as adjunctive VNS therapy for adults and adolescents aged over 12 years, whose partial-onset seizures are refractory to antiepileptic medications. VNS is also approved in numerous European Union countries for use in reducing the frequency of seizures, in patients whose epileptic disorder is dominated by partial seizures, and in Canada for similar patients who do not have adequate seizure control with antiepileptic drug therapy. As of November 1998, over 3400 patients had been implanted with the NCP system worldwide, with a total cumulative exposure to VNS of over 3800 patient-years.

This chapter reviews the NCP system, the surgical techniques used for its implantation, the possible mechanisms of action of VNS, the results of adjunctive efficacy studies, and the safety and tolerability profile of VNS.

The NCP system and implantation procedure

The NCP system (Figure 34.1) consists of a programmable pulse generator, a bipolar VNS lead, a programming wand with accompanying software, a tunneling tool and hand-held magnets.[2,3]

The pulse generator is implanted in the patient's upper left chest and is powered by a lithium thionyl chloride battery, which produces charge-balanced waveforms at constant current. The current version of the hermetically sealed titanium generator weighs 65 mg, and is 55 mm in diameter and 13.2 mm deep.

The bipolar stimulating electrodes directly connect the generator to the left vagus nerve, and thereby convey the electrical signal produced by the generator to the vagus nerve. The two connector pins at one end are plugged into the generator. At the other end are two

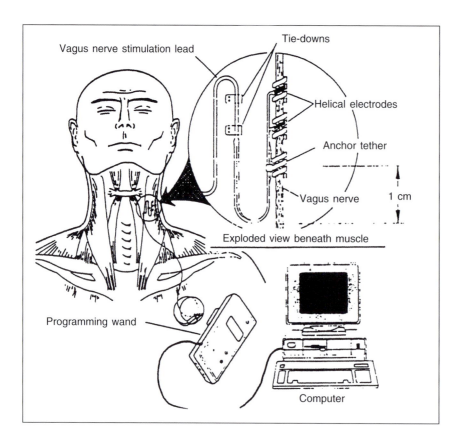

Figure 34.1
Components of the Neurocybernetic Prosthesis (NCP) system. Adapted from Michael et al (1993).[53]

separate helical silicone coils. Each helix has three turns; on the inside of the middle turn is a platinum ribbon coil that is welded to the lead wire. The helical shape of the coils enables the surgeon to place the coils around the nerve non-traumatically, so that the middle coil with the platinum ribbon maintains mechanical contact with the nerve.

The programming wand uses radiofrequency signals to communicate with the generator under the control of computer software. In this manner, the physician can program the following stimulation variables: output current (clinically tolerated range 0.25–4 mA in 0.25-mA steps), signal frequency (1–145 Hz), signal pulse width (130, 250, 500, 750, 1000 μs), signal on-time (7, 14, 21 s and 30–270 s in 30-s steps), and signal off-time (0.2, 0.3, 0.5, 0.8, 1.1, 1.8, 3 min and 5–180 min; 5–60 min in 5-min steps, 60–180 min in 30-min steps). In addition, magnet-activated stimulus parameters—pulse width, output current, and on-time—are also programmable (a supplied hand-held magnet turns on stimulation when briefly held against the chest, over the generator). Using this wand, the physician can also perform diagnostic checks of wand-generator communications, lead impedance, programmed current, or estimated remaining generator battery life.

The implantation procedure is performed as same-day surgery at some centers,[4] whereas, at other facilities, patients remain in the hospital

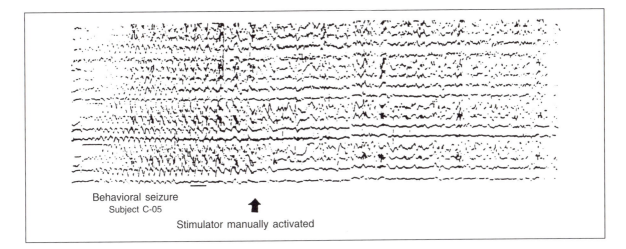

Behavioral seizure
Subject C-05

Stimulator manually activated

Figure 34.2
Effect of manual activation of vagal nerve stimulation in terminating an electrographic and behavioral seizure in a human subject. Adapted from Hammond et al (1992).[9]

the night after the implantation. The procedure lasts approximately 1–2 h and is typically performed under general anesthesia to minimize the possibility that a seizure will disrupt the operation,[5–7] though regional cervical blocks have also been used.[8]

The procedure begins by exposing the vagus nerve using an approach similar to that used for a carotid endarterectomy. The first incision is made over the anterior border of the left sternocleidomastoid muscle, centered between the mastoid process and the clavicle. The vagus nerve is then identified in the carotid sheath in a posterior groove between the carotid artery and the jugular vein. At least 3 cm of the nerve is mobilized using vessel loops to facilitate attachment of the helical coils. The second incision, for the generator, is made either in the left upper chest (8 cm inferior to the clavicle, centered under the mid-point of the clavicle),

or further laterally, near the axilla. The generator is placed into a subcutaneous pouch that is made above this incision.

A tunneling tool is used to advance the electrode pins subcutaneously from the base of the cervical incision to the thoracic incision. The helical coils are then carefully attached to the exposed vagus nerve; subsequently, the generator is brought into the surgical field and attached to the electrode connector pins.

Before the generator is placed into the subcutaneous pouch and both incisions closed, diagnostic tests are performed to check the system for proper operation. At most centers in the US, the generator's output current is then set to 0 mA for the first two postoperative weeks, after which ramping-up of the output current is initiated. Some centers, particularly those in Europe, begin stimulation in the operating room or the day after implantation.

The ramp-up procedure and settings for intermittent stimulation are individualized according to patient tolerance. A typical treatment regimen consists of adjusting the current output to tolerance over several weeks using a 30-Hz signal frequency with a 500 µs pulse width for 30 s of generator on-time and 5 min of off-time. These are the same settings that were found to be efficacious in the double-blind, controlled studies. The generator delivers intermittent stimulation until the battery wears out, which typically occurs after 4 years of operation.

Besides intermittent stimulation, on-demand stimulation may be brought on by the patient or a companion through placement of the supplied magnet on the patient's chest over the generator for several seconds. The stimulator settings employed for on-demand stimulation usually utilize a higher current and pulse width than those used for intermittent stimulation. Some patients have reported that on-demand stimulation interrupts a seizure or reduces its severity if administered at the onset of the seizure (Figure 34.2).[9]

Mechanism of action of VNS

The mechanism of action of VNS remains unknown, although it is clearly different from that of pharmacotherapy, which involves effects on neuronal membrane ionic conductance or neurotransmitters and their receptors.[10] Clarifying the mechanism of action of VNS will potentially help clinicians individualize VNS therapy more effectively and determine which medications, if any, could work synergistically with VNS. As it is likely that the mechanism of action of VNS pertains to its anatomical connections and associated physiology, these topics are reviewed.

The vagus nerve is a mixed nerve, in terms of both fiber size and direction of nerve transmission. Most fibers are small-diameter, unmyelinated C fibers; the rest are intermediate-diameter, myelinated B fibers and large-diameter, myelinated A fibers. Just as for other peripheral nerves, there are direct relationships between vagal fiber diameter and conduction velocity, and between fiber diameter and stimulation threshold. As discussed below, the anticonvulsant effect of VNS in experimental animals generally requires C-fiber stimulation. The threshold for C-fiber activation is 10–100 times higher than for A-fiber activation.

Vagal efferents

Special visceral vagal efferents innervate the larynx and pharynx. For example, the recurrent laryngeal branches of the vagus nerve innervate the larynx. The general visceral efferents provide parasympathetic innervation of the heart (resulting in slowing of the heart rate), lungs (bronchial constriction and pulmonary secretions), and gastrointestinal tract (increased peristalsis and secretions).

During development, the right and left vagal efferents acquire somewhat asymmetric visceral connections.[11,12] For example, the right vagus innervates the cardiac atria, whereas the left is more closely associated with the ventricles.[12] Innervation of the ventricles is less dense than that of the atria; this may explain why left vagal stimulation is less likely to affect cardiac conduction than right vagal stimulation.[13]

Vagal afferents

Sensory afferents, which comprise 80 per cent of vagal fibers, carry visceral sensation from the head, neck, thorax and abdomen.[14,15] The cell bodies are located in the nodose ganglion and project to the nucleus of the solitary tract

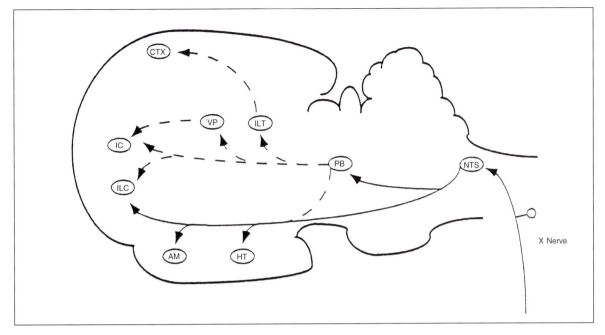

Figure 34.3
*Schematic of the ascending pathways relaying information from the vagus nerve to the forebrain. All
afferents in the vagus nerve (nerve X) synapse in the nucleus of the solitary tract (NTS). The NTS
provides an ascending pathway to the parabrachial nucleus (PB). The output from the PB is then
supplemented by the additional axons from the NTS in providing input to the hypothalamus (HT), bed
nucleus of the stria terminalis and amygdala (AM), and the infralimbic cortex (ILC). These pathways
allow vagal inputs to interact with autonomic, endocrine and emotional control. A second pathway
from the PB goes directly to the thalamus and cortex. Some axons go to a visceral sensory relay
nucleus in the ventroposterior thalamic complex (VP), which relays information about the internal
body to the visceral sensory cortex in the insular area (IC). This is probably the pathway that relays
sensation from the vagal stimulation to conscious perception. Other axons from the PB go to the
thalamic intralaminar and midline nuclei (ILT), which have extensive and diffuse projections
throughout the cerebral cortex (CTX). This latter pathway may represent the point at which vagal
stimulation interacts with pathways traditionally believed to control cortical synchronization and
desynchronization. Reproduced with permission from Schachter and Saper (1998), published by
Lippincott Williams & Wilkins.[13]*

(NTS; Figure 34.3). The NTS, in turn, relays
the sensory information to autonomic pregan-
glionic and related somatic motor neurons
located in the medulla and spinal cord,[16,17] as
well as to the medullary reticular formation
and the forebrain.

Most of the output of the NTS is relayed via
the parabrachial nucleus (PBN), which is
located in the dorsal pons lateral to the locus
ceruleus.[18] The PBN provides direct input to
several components of the thalamus, such as
the ventroposterior parvocellular nucleus,
which acts as a relay for visceral sensation to
the insular cortex.[19] In addition, the PBN also
projects to the intralaminar nuclei of the thalamus,[20] which probably exert widespread effects

on cortical activity. Finally, the PBN and the NTS project to the hypothalamus, amygdala and basal forebrain. Both the lateral hypothalamus and basal forebrain, in turn, project diffusely to the cerebral cortex and influence overall cortical activity.[21]

Attempts have been made with studies of *fos* immunoreactivity to determine which aspects of vagal anatomy and connectivity are influenced by VNS. *Fos* is a nuclear protein that signals gene transcription; its expression is used as a functional marker for neurons that become activated under controlled experimental conditions. Increased *fos* expression is seen in several areas of rat forebrain in association with left VNS, including posterior cortical amygdaloid nucleus, cingulate and retrosplenial cortex, and ventromedial and arcuate hypothalamic nuclei; *fos* induction is also observed in the habenular nucleus of the thalamus, the vagus nerve nuclei, and in the noradrenergic nuclei of the A5 and the locus ceruleus.[22]

The influence of vagal physiology on cortical and subcortical function has been studied *in vivo* with EEG[23-26] and evoked responses. Mechanical vagal stimulation, such as pressure on the carotid sinus, induces EEG slowing in experimental animals[26-28] and in humans undergoing carotid surgery (independent of cardiovascular effects).[29]

Early studies showed that repetitive vagal stimulation in anesthetized animals either synchronized or desynchronized the EEG, depending on the stimulus frequency and current strength (i.e., which fiber types in the vagus nerve were recruited).[30-32] The mechanism underlying the effect of VNS on the EEG was studied by directly stimulating the NTS in animals. High-frequency stimulation (> 30 Hz) resulted in EEG desynchronization, whereas slower stimulation (1–17 Hz) caused synchronization.[26] Others identified evoked responses in the ventroposterior complex and intralami-

nar regions of the thalamus associated with vagal nerve stimulation, which suggested that vagal effects on the EEG were probably mediated by the NTS–parabrachial–thalamic pathway.[24]

As reviewed by Rutecki[33] and Woodbury,[34] EEG rhythms became synchronized in the animal models when myelinated nerve fibers were stimulated, and desynchronized when slower conducting, unmyelinated, vagus nerve fibers were activated. As seizures are associated with excessive cortical synchronization, these observations led to the hypothesis that vagal stimulation disrupts the spread of seizures in animals by desynchronizing interconnected cortical regions. Further, these results suggested that each subpopulation of vagal afferent exerted its own influence on thalamic–forebrain regulation.

Several recent physiological studies in humans showed that VNS produces cortical evoked potentials, although its effect on the waking EEG background rhythms or power spectrum is very slight.[35,36] Other studies have failed to demonstrate an effect of left VNS on EEG rhythms in awake and freely moving rats,[37] or in patients who are awake, asleep, or under general anesthesia—even patients whose seizures have responded to VNS.[9,38]

The effect of VNS on activation of human forebrain structures has also been assessed using positron emission tomography (PET), though the findings have been inconsistent.[39,40] Henry et al found relationships between stimulation parameters, as well as chronicity of stimulation and the volume of activation and deactivation sites as measured by PET.[41,42] High-resolution techniques, such as functional magnetic resonance imaging, may further delineate the cerebral structures that are activated in patients by VNS.

Despite studies that show measurable effects of VNS on *fos* activation, EEG, evoked potentials and PET scans, the direct link between vagal functional anatomy and VNS mechanism of action has not yet been conclusively made. Recent, unconfirmed work suggests that the locus ceruleus is critically involved in the anticonvulsant effects of VNS, possibly through the release of norepinephrine.[43]

Efficacy of VNS in animal models of epilepsy

VNS has been investigated in several animal models of epilepsy. In most of these studies, stimulation was applied just before or immediately after seizures occurred, because the mechanism of action of VNS was presumed to be transient desynchronization of cortical rhythms for the reasons discussed above.[34,44-46] Other studies have evaluated the relationship between the cumulative duration of vagal stimulation and the temporal persistence of anticonvulsant effects,[37,47] i.e. the preventive effect of intermittent VNS.

In experiments in male rats, Woodbury and Woodbury showed that vagal stimulation prevented or reduced clonic seizures induced by intraperitoneal pentylenetetrazol (PTZ) and 3-mercaptopropionic acid (an inhibitor of γ-aminobutyric acid or GABA synthesis and release), as well as tonic–clonic seizures caused by maximal electroshock.[34,45] The best effect was achieved with stimulus frequencies and pulse widths of 10–20 Hz and 0.5–1 μs, respectively. The effectiveness of VNS directly correlated with the fraction of C fibers stimulated, and inversely with the delay of stimulus relative to seizure onset—the greater the delay before vagal stimulation, the greater the seizure duration; therefore, stimulation worked best when applied as soon as possible after a seizure began.

A dog model of strychnine-induced generalized seizures and PTZ-induced muscle tremors

confirmed the results in the rat model. VNS stopped the seizures and tremors within 0.5–5 s when acutely applied.[46] Further, VNS protected against seizures for a period that was four times longer than the duration of stimulation. Stimulation frequencies over 60 Hz were less effective than slower frequencies, consistent with the work of Woodbury and Woodbury that the anticonvulsant effect of VNS in animals required stimulation of small-diameter, slower-conducting, unmyelinated fibers. In further support of this hypothesis, stimulation of vagal C fibers for 20 s reduced penicillin-induced, focal, interictal spikes in male rats by 33 per cent.[44]

In another study that more closely paralleled human treatment with intermittent VNS for partial-onset seizures, right VNS was administered at the onset of each spontaneous seizure, or at least every 3 h for 40 s in an alumina-gel monkey model of spontaneous partial and secondarily generalized seizures.[47] Seizures were completely controlled in two of four monkeys and decreased in frequency in the other two, even though no diminishment of interictal spikes was observed. Further, the prophylactic anticonvulsant effect persisted into a stimulation-free period.

Takaya et al demonstrated that VNS protected against induced seizures, even when discontinued before seizure onset, suggesting to the authors that VNS caused long-term changes in neural activity.[37] In addition, the relationship between the cumulative duration of VNS and its anticonvulsant effect was studied. Although 60 min of continuous VNS protected awake and freely moving rats from PTZ-induced seizures more effectively than 60 min of intermittent VNS with the same stimulation settings, intermittent stimulation was more effective than a single 1-min stimulus. The anticonvulsant effect was nearly half-maximal 5 min after VNS was discontinued. Although it is impractical to apply continuous electrical stimulation to the vagus nerve because of safety considerations and limitations in battery life, these results suggest that the intermittent stimulation protocol of 30 s on, 5 min off, utilized for human epilepsy is a reasonable compromise with respect to efficacy, safety and feasibility.

Efficacy studies in patients

The first patient was treated with VNS in 1988 as part of a pilot, single-blind trial of patients who had refractory partial seizures but were not candidates for epilepsy surgery.[8] The first pivotal trial of VNS was the E03 study, a multi-center, double-blind, randomized, parallel, active control trial of VNS in 114 patients with predominantly partial seizures.[48–51] The second pivotal clinical study was the E05 study, a multi-center, double-blind, randomized, parallel, active control trial of VNS in 199 patients with complex partial seizures.[52] In 1991, a compassionate use trial enrolled 124 patients with all types of intractable seizures (the E04 study).

The study designs as well as the efficacy results of the E03 and the E05 trials are discussed in detail. Efficacy for other seizure types and in childhood epilepsies are then presented.

Add-on, double-blind, active-control, parallel-design trials

Study designs
The E03 and E05 studies were multi-center, blinded, randomized, active control trials that compared two different VNS stimulation protocols for the treatment of partial-onset seizures: high stimulation (30 Hz, 30 s on, 5 min off, 500 μs pulse width) and low stimulation (1 Hz, 30 s on, 90–180 min off, 130 μs

pulse width). The low stimulation treatment was felt to be less effective than high stimulation treatment.

Study candidates were followed over a 12–16-week prospective baseline period, during which seizures were counted and changes in antiepileptic drug dosages were allowed only to maintain appropriate concentrations or in response to drug toxicity. Patients who satisfied all inclusion and exclusion criteria were then implanted with the NCP system. Two weeks later, patients were randomized to receive either high or low stimulation. Over the next 2 weeks, those randomized to the high group had their generator output current increased as high as could be tolerated, whereas those randomized to the low group had the current increased only to the point that the patient could perceive stimulation. Efficacy was then assessed during the remaining 12 weeks of the treatment phase. At the conclusion of the study, patients were eligible to enter long-term open studies.

Enrollment information
Patients enrolled in the E03 and E05 studies were at least 12 years old, had at least six seizures per month, and were taking one to three antiepileptic drugs. In the E05 study, patients had to have partial seizures with alteration of consciousness to enroll.

In the E03 study, 125 patients were enrolled; 114 completed the prospective baseline and were implanted. The average duration of epilepsy was 23 years for patients in the high group ($n = 54$) and 20 years for the low group ($n = 60$). Patients in both groups were taking a mean of 2.1 antiepileptic drugs at study entry.

In the E05 study, 254 patients were entered, including 55 who were discontinued from baseline for failing protocol eligibility; 199 patients were implanted; one patient was not randomized as a result of device infection, and two randomized patients (one in each treatment group) were excluded from the analysis for administrative reasons. The baseline characteristics for patients in the high group (*n* = 94) and those in the low group (*n* = 102) were similar and consistent with the E03 study.

Results

In both studies, the primary efficacy analysis was the percentage change in total seizure frequency during treatment relative to baseline, comparing the high and low stimulation groups. In the E03 study, the high stimulation group had a mean reduction in seizure frequency of 24.5 per cent, versus 6.1 per cent for the low stimulation group (*p* = 0.01). In the E05 study, the mean percentage decreases in seizure frequency during treatment compared with baseline were 28 per cent and 15 per cent for the high and low groups, respectively. The between-group comparison was statistically significant in favor of high stimulation (*p* = 0.039).

Secondary efficacy measures in both studies showed statistically significant effects in favor of high stimulation. In the E03 study, 31 per cent of patients in the high group had at least a 50 per cent reduction in seizures compared with 13 per cent of patients in the low group (*p* = 0.02). In the E05 study, 11 per cent of patients in the high group had a reduction in seizure frequency greater than 75 per cent, versus 2 per cent for patients in the low group (*p* = 0.01). In addition, both the high and the low groups showed a statistically and clinically significant difference in within-group mean percentage change in seizure frequency during treatment compared with baseline (*p* < 0.0001).

There are suggestions that efficacy further improved after the initial 3-month treatment period for patients who completed the E03 and E05 studies, but these results should be interpreted cautiously because ongoing therapy with VNS was unblinded, and concomitant antiepileptic drugs could be adjusted.[50,53–55]

Efficacy in other seizure types

Adjunctive VNS may have potential for other seizure types and epilepsy syndromes, including symptomatic generalized epilepsies characterized by mixed generalized seizures.[56] Anecdotal reports in patients with the Lennox-Gastaut syndrome are encouraging.[57,58]

Efficacy in children

There is limited published experience with VNS in children.[59] In one series of 12 children aged 4–16 years with medically and surgically refractory seizures who were implanted with the VNS, five had a greater than 90 per cent reduction in seizure frequency and four were able to reduce the number of antiepileptic drugs used.[60] In another series of 16 children aged 4–19 years, six experienced at least a 50 per cent reduction in seizure frequency during months 10 to 12 of VNS.[61]

Safety and tolerability

Mechanical and electrical safety

Although high-frequency stimulation may be associated with tissue damage,[3] there is no evidence that the vagal stimulation protocols in present clinical use cause damage to the vagus nerve.[5,62] The NCP system has several built-in safety and tolerability features. For example, a clamping circuit within the generator prevents more than 14 V from being delivered to the vagus nerve. In addition, patients may turn off stimulation at any time by keeping the supplied magnet over the generator. This may become necessary if stimulation becomes uncomfortable, or if the patient anticipates a prolonged period of speaking and does not wish to experience hoarseness or voice change from stimulation.

Environmental considerations

The antenna within the generator is controlled by radiofrequency signals transmitted by the programming wand. None the less, neither the generator nor the electrode leads are affected by microwave transmission, cellular phones, or airport security systems. Some restrictions do apply to magnetic resonance imaging (MRI) testing, however. As the heat induced in the electrode leads by a body MRI could theoretically cause local tissue injury, body MRI scans are contraindicated. Brain MRI testing performed with a head coil appears to be safe under certain conditions, as described in the July 1997 *Physician's Manual* supplied by Cyberonics, Inc.

Safety and tolerability in the E03 and E05 studies

In the E03 study, safety and tolerability were evaluated with interviews, physical and neurological examinations, vital signs, EKG rhythm strips, Holter monitoring (in a subset of 28 patients), gastric acid monitoring (in 14 patients), and antiepileptic drug concentrations. Similarly, safety and tolerability were evaluated in the E05 study with interviews, physical and neurological examinations, vital signs, Holter monitoring, pulmonary function tests, standard laboratory tests and urinalysis.

In the E03 study, the adverse events (side effects) that occurred in at least 5 per cent of patients in the high group during treatment were hoarseness (37 per cent), throat pain (11 per cent), coughing (7 per cent), dyspnea (6 per

cent), paresthesia (6 per cent), and muscle pain (6 per cent). Hoarseness was the only adverse event that was reported significantly more often with high stimulation than with low stimulation.

In the E05 study, none of the serious adverse events that occurred during the treatment phase were judged to be probably or definitely caused by VNS. Implantation-related adverse events all resolved and included left vocal cord paralysis (two patients), lower facial muscle paresis (two patients), and pain and fluid accumulation over the generator requiring aspiration (one patient). The peri-operative adverse events that were reported by 10 per cent or more patients included pain (29 per cent), coughing (14 per cent), voice alteration (13 per cent), chest pain (12 per cent), and nausea (10 per cent). After randomization, the adverse events that were reported by patients in the high group at some time during treatment, and which were significantly increased compared with baseline, were voice alteration/hoarseness, cough, throat pain, nonspecific pain, dyspnea, paresthesia, dyspepsia, vomiting and infection. The only two adverse events that occurred significantly more often in the high group than in the low group were dyspnea and voice alteration. Adverse events in both treatment groups were rated as mild or moderate 99 per cent of the time. There were no cognitive, sedative, visual, affective, or co-ordination side effects. No significant changes in Holter monitoring or pulmonary function tests were noted.

Two E05 patients had VNS discontinued during the treatment. One patient in the high group had two episodes of Cheyne–Stokes respiration post-ictally; after the device was deactivated, two more episodes were reported and the patient's mother requested that the device be reactivated. One patient in the low group had the device deactivated as the result of a group of symptoms that the patient had experienced pre-implantation, as well as subsequent to device deactivation. No deaths occurred during either study.

Laboratory values

As would be predicted from a non-pharmacological therapy, there were no changes in hematology values or common chemistry values in either study. Similarly, there were no changes seen with antiepileptic drug concentrations.

Long-term safety and tolerability

Among a cohort of 444 patients who elected to continue receiving VNS after participating in a clinical study, 97 per cent continued for at least 1 year, and 85 per cent and 72 per cent continued for at least 2 and 3 years, respectively.[63] The most commonly reported side effects at the end of the first year of VNS were voice alteration (29 per cent) and paresthesia (12 per cent), at the end of 2 years, voice alteration (19 per cent) and cough (6 per cent), and at 3 years, dyspnea (3 per cent).

The mortality rates and standardized mortality ratios of 791 patients treated for 1335 person-years with VNS were contrasted with those of other epilepsy cohorts.[64] These rates and ratios were comparable with those of other young adults with refractory seizures who were not treated with VNS. Additionally, the incidence of definite and probable sudden unexpected death in epilepsy was 4.5 per 1000 person-years, which was consistent with other non-VNS epilepsy cohorts.

Several anecdotal reports of complications of VNS have appeared as the number of patients treated with VNS has grown rapidly. These reports include posture-dependent stimulation of the phrenic nerve[65] and transient asystole in one patient during intraoperative testing of the NCP system.[66]

Six patients from VNS clinical studies and two patients who were implanted after approval became pregnant while receiving VNS.[67] Five of the pregnancies resulted in full-term, healthy infants, including one set of twins. There was one spontaneous abortion, one unplanned pregnancy was terminated by an elective abortion, and another pregnancy ended with an elective abortion because of abnormal fetal development that was attributed to antiepileptic drugs.

The possible relationship of VNS to swallowing difficulties[61] was studied by barium swallow in a series of eight children.[68] Laryngeal penetration of barium was present in three patients without stimulation, and was caused by VNS in one other patient. Results from another small series of children treated with chronic VNS suggest that some children with severe mental disability and motor impairment who are dependent on assisted feeding, may be at increased risk for aspiration while being fed during VNS.[69]

Clinical use of VNS

Clinicians must now decide how to integrate VNS into the growing armamentarium for partial seizures. At this time, the successful application of VNS presents three practical problems: first, there is no measurable physiological response to VNS with which to monitor and adjust stimulation individually; second, patient- and epilepsy-related variables that can be used prospectively to identify good candidates for VNS are not yet known; and third, the initial cost is high. These limitations and others have prompted a discussion of the appropriate role of VNS in the treatment of epilepsy.[70] Yet, despite these limitations, VNS therapy may be considered reasonable and necessary for patients whose partial-onset seizures adversely affect quality of life and cannot be controlled after appropriate anticonvulsant medications, alone or in combination, have failed. Furthermore, the high initial cost of VNS treatment is more than offset by reductions in direct medical expenses resulting from epilepsy within the first 2 years after implantation in some patients.[71]

Some clinicians experienced with VNS alter the 'high' stimulation protocols used in the E03 and E05 studies if satisfactory seizure reduction is not obtained after 3–6 months of therapy. For example, VNS efficacy may be improved in some patients by reducing the stimulation off-time from 5 min to 1.8 min.[72]

Summary

VNS is effective, safe and well-tolerated in patients with long-standing, refractory, partial-onset seizures.[73] The most frequently encountered adverse effects typically occur during stimulation; these are usually mild to moderate in severity and resolve either with reduction in current intensity or spontaneously over time. Conspicuously absent with VNS stimulation therapy are the typical CNS side effects of antiepileptic drugs. There are no apparent effects of VNS on vagally mediated visceral function or antiepileptic drug serum concentrations. There has been no indication of tolerance to therapeutic effect in long-term, open studies. Efficacy results for other seizure types and in children are encouraging.

Although the precise mechanism of action of VNS remains unknown, the introduction of effective stimulation therapy for epilepsy ushers in a new, non-pharmacological era in the treatment of seizures. Further controlled studies should be performed to explore the use of VNS for other seizure types and epilepsy syndromes. In addition, future controlled studies should demonstrate: (1) how VNS therapy can be individualized to maximize its effectiveness, either with intermittent stimulation or acutely with the magnet; (2) whether VNS complements antiepileptic drugs or those that are not antiepileptic, with particular mechanisms of action; (3) how to identify patients prospectively who are the most likely to benefit from VNS and for whom VNS is cost-effective; and (4) the efficacy and tolerability of adjunctive VNS compared with adjunctive AED therapy.

References

1. Fisher RS, Uthman BM, Ramsay RE, et al. Alternative surgical techniques for epilepsy. In: Engel J, ed. *Surgical treatment of the epilepsies.* New York: Raven Press, 1993:549–64.
2. Terry R, Tarver WB, Zabara J. An implantable neurocybernetic prosthesis system. *Epilepsia* 1990;**31**(Suppl 2):S33–7.
3. Terry RS, Tarver WB, Zabara J. The implantable neurocybernetic prosthesis system. *Pacing Clin Electrophysiol* 1991;**14**:86–93.
4. Schaefer PA, Rosenfeld WE, Lippmann SM. Same-day surgery for implanting vagal nerve stimulators: safe and decreased cost. *Epilepsia* 1998;**39**(Suppl 6):193.
5. Tarver WB, George RE, Maschino SE, Holder LK, Wernicke JF. Clinical experience with a helical bipolar stimulating lead. *Pacing Clin Electrophysiol* 1992;**15**:1545–56.
6. Reid SA. Surgical technique for implantation of the neurocybernetic prosthesis. *Epilepsia* 1990;**31**:(Suppl 2):S38–9.
7. Landy HJ, Ramsay RE, Slater J, Casiano RR, Morgan R. Vagus nerve stimulation for complex partial seizures: surgical technique,

safety, and efficacy. *J Neurosurg* 1993;78: 26–31.

8. Penry JK, Dean JC. Prevention of intractable partial seizures by intermittent vagal stimulation in humans: preliminary results. *Epilepsia* 1990;31(Suppl 2):S40–3.

9. Hammond EJ, Uthman BM, Reid SA, Wilder BJ. Electrophysiological studies of cervical vagus nerve stimulation in humans: I. EEG effects. *Epilepsia* 1992;33:1013–20.

10. Schachter SC. Review of the mechanisms of action of antiepileptic drugs. *CNS Drugs* 1995;4:469–77.

11. Prechtl JC, Powley TL. Organization and distribution of the rat subdiaphragmatic vagus and associated paraganglia. *J Comp Neurol* 1985; 235:182–95.

12. Saper CB, Kibbe MR, Hurley KM, et al. Brain natriuretic peptide-like immunoreactive innervation of the cardiovascular and cerebrovascular systems in the rat. *Circ Res* 1990;67: 1345–54.

13. Schachter SC, Saper CB. Progress in epilepsy research: vagus nerve stimulation. *Epilepsia* 1998;39:677–86.

14. Foley JO, DuBois F. Quantitative studies of the vagus nerve in the cat. I. The ratio of sensory and motor fibers. *J Comp Neurol* 1937;67: 49–97.

15. Agostini E, Chinnock JE, Daly MD, Murray JG. Functional and histological studies of the vagus nerve and its branches to the heart, lungs, and abdominal viscera in the cat. *J Physiol (Lond)* 1957;135:182–205.

16. Loewy AD, Burton H. Nuclei of the solitary tract: efferent projections to the lower brain stem and spinal cord. *J Comp Neurol* 1978; 181:421–50.

17. Ruggiero DA, Cravo SL, Arango V, Reis DJ. Central control of the circulation by the rostral ventrolateral reticular nucleus: anatomical substrates. *Prog Brain Res* 1989;81:49–79.

18. Saper CB. The central autonomic system. In: Paxinos G, ed. *The rat nervous system,* 2nd edn. San Diego: Academic Press, 1995:107–31.

19. Cechetto DF, Saper CB. Evidence for a viscerotopic sensory representation in the cortex and thalamus in the rat. *J Comp Neurol* 1987; 262:27–45.

20. Fulwiler CE, Saper CB. Subnuclear organization of the efferent connections of the parabrachial nucleus in the rat. *Brain Res Rev* 1984; 7:229–59.

21. Saper CB. Diffuse cortical projection systems: anatomical organization and role in cortical function. In: Plum F, ed. *Handbook of physiology. The nervous system V.* Bethesda: American Physiological Society; 1987:169–210.

22. Naritoku DK, Terry WJ, Helfert RH. Regional induction of *fos* immunoreactivity in the brain by anticonvulsant stimulation of the vagus nerve. *Epilepsy Res* 1995;22:53–62.

23. Bailey P, Bremer F. A sensory cortical representation of the vagus nerve. *J Neurophysiol* 1938;1:405–12.

24. Dell P, Olson R. Projections thalamiques, corticales, et cerebelleuses des afferences viscerales vagales. *C R Soc Seances Soc Biol Fil* 1951;145:1084–8.

25. Zanchetti A, Wang SC, Moruzzi G. The effect of vagal stimulation on the EEG pattern of the cat. *EEG Clin Neurophysiol* 1952;4:357–461.

26. Magnes J, Moruzzi G, Pompeiano O. Synchronization of the EEG produced by low frequency electrical stimulation of the region of the solitary tract. *Arch Ital Biol* 1961;99: 33–67.

27. Bonvallet M, Dell P, Hiebel G. Tonus sympathetiques et activite electrique corticales. *EEG Clin Neurophysiol* 1954;6:119–44.

28. Garnier L. EEG modifications produced by gastric distention in cats. *C R Seances Soc Biol Fil* 1968;162:2164–8.

29. Bridgers SL, Spencer SS, Spencer DD, Sasaki CT. A cerebral effect of carotid sinus stimulation. Observation during intraoperative electroencephalographic monitoring. *Arch Neurol* 1985;42:574–7.

30. Chase MH, Sterman MB, Clemente CD. Cortical and subcortical patterns of response to afferent vagal stimulation. *Expl Neurol* 1966; 16:36–49.

31. Chase MH, Nakamura Y, Clements CD, Sterman MB. Afferent vagal stimulation: neurographic correlates of induced EEG synchronization and desynchronization. *Brain Res* 1967; 5:236–49.

32. Chase MH, Nakamura Y, Clemente CD, Sterman MB. Cortical and subcortical EEG patterns of response to afferent abdominal

vagal stimulation: neurographic correlates. *Physiol Behav* 1968;3:605–10.

33. Rutecki P. Anatomical, physiological, and theoretical basis for the antiepileptic effect of vagus nerve stimulation. *Epilepsia* 1990; **31**:(Suppl 2):S1–6.

34. Woodbury DM, Woodbury JW. Effects of vagal stimulation on experimentally induced seizures in rats. *Epilepsia* 1990;**31**:(Suppl 2):S7–19.

35. Hammond EJ, Uthman BM, Reid SA, Wilder BJ. Electrophysiologic studies of cervical vagus nerve stimulation in humans: II. Evoked potentials. *Epilepsia* 1992;33:1021–8.

36. Salinsky MC, Burchiel KJ. Vagus nerve stimulation has no effect on awake EEG rhythms in humans. *Epilepsia* 1993;34:299–304.

37. Takaya M, Terry WJ, Naritoku DK. Vagus nerve stimulation induces a sustained anticonvulsant effect. *Epilepsia* 1996;37:1111–16.

38. Salinsky MC, Burchiel KJ. Vagus nerve stimulation has no effect on awake EEG rhythms in humans. *Epilepsia* 1993;34:299–304.

39. Garnett ES, Nahmias C, Scheffel A, Firnau G, Upton ARM. Regional cerebral blood flow in man manipulated by direct vagal stimulation. *Pacing Clin Electrophysiol* 1992;15:1579–80.

40. Ko D, Heck C, Grafton S, et al. Vagus nerve stimulation activates central nervous system structures in epileptic patients during PET $H_2^{15}O$ blood flow imaging. *Neurosurgery* 1996; 39:426–31.

41. Henry TR, Bakay RAE, Votaw JR, et al. Brain blood flow alterations induced by therapeutic vagus nerve stimulation in partial epilepsy: I. Acute effects at high and low levels of stimulation. *Epilepsia* 1998;39:983–90.

42. Henry TR, Votaw JR, Bakay RAE, et al. Vagus nerve stimulation-induced cerebral blood flow changes differ in acute and chronic therapy of complex partial seizures. *Epilepsia* 1998;**39** (Suppl 6):92.

43. Krahl SE, Clark KB, Smith DC, Browning RA. Locus coeruleus lesions suppress the seizure-attenuating effects of vagus nerve stimulation. *Epilepsia* 1998;39:709–14.

44. McLachlan RS. Suppression of interictal spikes and seizures by stimulation of the vagus nerve. *Epilepsia* 1993;34:918–23.

45. Woodbury JW, Woodbury DM. Vagal stimulation reduces the severity of maximal electroshock seizures in intact rats: use of a cuff electrode for stimulating and recording. *Pacing Clin Electrophysiol* 1991;14:94–107.

46. Zabara J. Inhibition of experimental seizures in canines by repetitive vagal stimulation. *Epilepsia* 1992;33:1005–12.

47. Lockard JS, Congdon WC, DuCharme LL. Feasibility and safety of vagal stimulation in monkey model. *Epilepsia* 1990;31(Suppl 2): S20–6.

48. Ben-Menachem E, Manon-Espaillat R, Ristanovic R, et al. Vagus nerve stimulation for treatment of partial seizures: 1. A controlled study of effect on seizures. *Epilepsia* 1994; 35:616–26.

49. Ramsay RE, Uthman BM, Augustinsson LE, et al. Vagus nerve stimulation for treatment of partial seizures: 2. Safety, side effects, and tolerability. *Epilepsia* 1994;35:627–36.

50. George R, Salinsky M, Kuzniecky R, et al. Vagus nerve stimulation for treatment of partial seizures: 3. Long-term follow-up on first 67 patients exiting a controlled study. *Epilepsia* 1994;35:637–43.

51. The Vagus Nerve Stimulation Study Group. A randomized controlled trial of chronic vagus nerve stimulation for treatment of medically intractable seizures. *Neurology* 1995;**45**: 224–30.

52. Handforth A, DeGiorgio CM, Schachter SC, et al. Vagus nerve stimulation therapy for partial-onset seizures; a randomized, active-control trial. *Neurology* 1997; (submitted).

53. Michael JE, Wegener K, Barnes DW. Vagus nerve stimulation for intractable seizures: one-year follow-up. *J Neurosci Nurs* 1993;25: 362–6.

54. Salinsky MC, Uthman BM, Ristanovic RK, Wernicke JF, Tarver WB. Vagus nerve stimulation for the treatment of medically intractable seizures. Results of a 1-year open-extension trial. *Arch Neurol* 1996;53:1176–80.

55. DeGiorgio CM, Handforth A, Schachter S. Multicenter double-blind crossover and 6-month follow-up study of vagus nerve stimulation for intractable partial seizures. *Epilepsia* 1998;**39**(Suppl 6):69.

56. Labar D, Nikolov B, Tarver B, Fraser R. Vagus nerve stimulation for symptomatic generalized epilepsy: a pilot study. *Epilepsia* 1998;39: 201–5.

57. Helmers SL, Al-Jayyousi M, Madsen J. Adjunctive treatment in Lennox–Gastaut syndrome using vagal nerve stimulation. *Epilepsia* 1998;**39**(Suppl 6):169.

58. Murphy JV, Hornig G. Chronic intermittent stimulation of the left vagal nerve in nine children with Lennox–Gastaut syndrome. *Epilepsia* 1998;**39**(Suppl 6):169.

59. Hornig G, Murphy JV. Vagal nerve stimulation: updated experience in 60 pediatric patients. *Epilepsia* 1998;**39**(Suppl 6):169.

60. Murphy JV, Hornig G, Schallert G. Left vagal nerve stimulation in children with refractory epilepsy. Preliminary observations. *Arch Neurol* 1995;**52**:886–9.

61. Lundgren J, Amark P, Blennow G, Stromblad LG, Wallstedt L. Vagus nerve stimulation in 16 children with refractory epilepsy. *Epilepsia* 1998;**39**:809–13.

62. Agnew WF, McCreery DB. Considerations for safety with chronically implanted nerve electrodes. *Epilepsia* 1990;**31**(Suppl 2):S27–32.

63. Morris G, Pallagi J. Long-term follow-up on 454 patients with epilepsy receiving vagus nerve stimulation therapy. *Epilepsia* 1998;**39**(Suppl 6):93.

64. Annegers JF, Coan SP, Hauser WA, Leestma J, Duffell W, Tarver B. Epilepsy, vagal nerve stimulation by the NCP system, mortality, and sudden, unexpected, unexplained death. *Epilepsia* 1998;**39**:206–12.

65. Leijten FSS, Van Rijen PC. Stimulation of the phrenic nerve as a complication of vagus nerve pacing in a patient with epilepsy. *Neurology* 1998;**51**:1224–5.

66. Asconape JJ, Moore DD, Zipes DP, Hartman LM. Early experience with vagus nerve stimulation for the treatment of epilepsy: cardiac complications. *Epilepsia* 1998;**39**(Suppl 6):193.

67. Ben-Menachem E, Ristanovic R, Murphy J. Gestational outcomes in patients with epilepsy receiving vagus nerve stimulation. *Epilepsia* 1998;**39**(Suppl 6):180.

68. Schallert G, Foster J, Lindquist N, Murphy JV. Chronic stimulation of the left vagal nerve in children: effect on swallowing. *Epilepsia* 1998;**39**:1113–14.

69. Lundgren J, Ekberg O, Olsson R. Aspiration: a potential complication to vagus nerve stimulation. *Epilepsia* 1998;**39**:998–1000.

70. McLachlan RS. Vagus nerve stimulation for treatment of seizures? Maybe. *Arch Neurol* 1998;**55**:232–3.

71. Vonck K, Nieuwenhuis L, Boon P, Vandekerckhove T, D'Have M, O'Connor S. Cost–benefit analysis of vagal nerve stimulation. *Epilepsia* 1997;**38**:(Suppl 8):109.

72. Naritoku DK, Handforth A, Labar DR, Gilmartin RC. Effects of reducing stimulation intervals on antiepileptic efficacy of vagus nerve stimulation (VNS). *Epilepsia* 1998;**39**(Suppl 6):194.

73. Ben-Menachem E. Vagus nerve stimulation for treatment of seizures? Yes. *Arch Neurol* 1998;**55**:231–2.

XI

THE TEAM APPROACH TO THE TREATMENT OF EPILEPSY

35

Patient satisfaction and patient advocacy in epilepsy

Ann Jacoby and Gus A Baker

Introduction

Recent advances in understanding of the genetic, structural, metabolic and biochemical processes involved in the group of conditions referred to as epilepsy, while offering enormous potential for their future management, also serve to highlight their complexity. Significantly increased pharmacological and neurosurgical options both offer more solutions and pose more questions about their treatment. A large part of the present volume has been devoted to consideration of the challenges for everyday clinical practice that such technological advances raise. In this, the penultimate chapter, we turn attention away from problem-solving from the viewpoint of the clinician to focus on the needs of the people with epilepsy themselves. Although most people with epilepsy may well embrace innovations in the management and treatment of their condition as eagerly as their clinicians, this cannot be assumed. Given the increasingly complex range of possible options, the importance of providing care that is not only appropriate but also acceptable to its recipients should not be overlooked.

Examining the acceptability of care from the viewpoint of users rather than providers poses its own problems, both conceptual and methodological, which we discuss below. However, the current political agenda emphasizes the importance of patient perspectives on medical care, not only in relation to its positive and negative impacts on their quality of life, but also in relation to their expectations about it and the level of their satisfaction; it therefore behoves us to try to resolve these problems. Although, to date, there has been relatively little systematic research to explore the issue of patient satisfaction with epilepsy care, we summarize the key findings from those studies that have been done and the main messages, as we see it, for future clinical practice and service provision. We also focus on the issue of advocacy in medical care and identify whom we see as the main advocates in epilepsy and their role in ensuring that the needs of people with epilepsy are met and that the care provided for them is optimal.

Patient satisfaction: conceptual and methodological issues

The arguments for assessing patient satisfaction with health care parallel those for assessing health-related quality of life from the patient's perspective. Taking account of the views of users with regard to the quality of their health care is in part a response to the wider consumer movement in Western societies.[1] At the same time, cultural and philosophical developments through the 20th century have emphasized a holistic approach to patient care, within which the views of patients themselves have acquired increased significance. The change in patterns of disease is also of relevance, because patients affected by a chronic illness or disability are inevitably called upon to take a more active part in the management of their condition than those experiencing an acute one. Lastly, the emphasis on patient satisfaction may also be seen as a response to economic exigency, which demands evidence of the cost-effectiveness of health service provision. Donabedian,[2] the so-called 'guru' of quality assurance in health care, states that:

> Client satisfaction is of fundamental importance as a measure of the quality of care because it gives information on the provider's success at meeting those client values and expectations which are matters on which the client is the ultimate authority.

In the UK, successive government reports have enthusiastically embraced the idea of 'client' surveys, and as a result research activity around the topic of patient satisfaction has flourished. At the same time, a number of authors have expressed reservations about both the concept of satisfaction and the reliability with which levels of satisfaction among patients can be gauged. One problem is that, like quality of life, the term 'satisfaction' has rarely been defined either by the researchers using it or to the patients asked to think about it.[3] Although the concept of patient satisfaction, again like that of quality of life, has been operationalized as the gap between expectations and experience, Calnan[4] argues that this is problematic, given that 'expectations develop during the process of health care delivery and are revised in the light of experience'. Calnan,[5] suggests that, rather than focusing on the relationship between expectations and satisfaction, a more fruitful line of investigation would

be to explore patients' motives for seeking medical care, because these will determine the demands they make and so, in turn, their evaluations of how well or otherwise those demands are met. Williams[6] goes further, arguing that patient satisfaction surveys provide only the 'illusion of consumerism' because they rest on a series of unjustified assumptions, among which are: that satisfaction is determined by the attributes of care only and not by any external factors; that satisfaction is the product of fulfilled values and expectations about care; and that the users of health care services have clearly articulated values and expectations in the first place. Williams suggests that these assumptions need to be questioned, because in reality the expression of satisfaction may reflect the nonexistence of opinion, passivity on the part of patients, and expectations only about what *should not* happen rather than about what *should* happen.

Surveys of patient satisfaction have focused on a number of different dimensions of health care, including its accessibility and availability, the physical environment in which it is provided, its continuity and its interpersonal aspects. Interestingly, such surveys relatively rarely ask patients to make judgements about the technical aspects of care, the underlying assumption being that they lack the knowledge and expertise necessary to do so. Calnan,[5] however, argues that patients do in fact have clear criteria both for evaluating medical procedures and for judging the abilities of their doctors, and there is research that supports this. For example, Ware and colleagues[7] asked patients to view videotapes of simulated consultations during the course of which interpersonal attributes were held constant while the technical content was manipulated; they found that patients rated more highly those consultations that were also considered technically better by physicians. And West[8] studied encounters between doctors and the parents of children with epilepsy and reported that, though the parents were initially passive and uncritical, they became increasingly more critical and willing to challenge the authority and expertise of the doctor as their own knowledge and experience increased.

The concern has been voiced by a number of authors that surveys of patient satisfaction, whatever topics they focus on, almost uniformly report high levels of expressed satisfaction, and so support the status quo. One potential problem[6] is that the reductionism inherent in the quantitative methods employed in most published studies of patient satisfaction may mask important differences lying behind the responses of those surveyed. Thus, patients describing themselves as satisfied may indeed be so; alternatively, they may be dissatisfied but unable or unwilling to criticize; or they may be unable to make a sensible evaluation but happy to trust in the abilities of the staff caring for them. The limitations of quantitative approaches to the measurement of patient satisfaction are also illustrated by research showing that, when patients are given the opportunity to express themselves in their own words, rather than in response to structured questions, they are more likely to be critical, as they are when asked to evaluate individual aspects of the care rather than making global evaluations.[3] Further, it has been shown that whether statements are worded positively or negatively in structured satisfaction questionnaires may significantly influence reported levels of satisfaction.[9]

Like and Zyzanski[10] highlight a number of other features of patient satisfaction studies that may significantly influence the responses elicited from those taking part. These include: whether patients are asked to think about a specific health care professional or clinical encounter, as opposed to health care profes-

sionals and the health care system in general; whether their opinions are elicited during an episode of ill health when they are actively seeking care or when they are well; and whether the data are collected in the health care setting under scrutiny or in a neutral environment. To this list, we can add whether the researcher is seen by the respondent as operating independently or as closely aligned to the service being researched, and, as it has been shown that perceptions of the quality of care tend to change over time, the timing of data collection. There is also evidence that high ratings of satisfaction by patients may reflect a combination of factors external to the quality of the care provided, including their self-assessed health status,[11] psychological functioning,[12] low expectations, ignorance of the alternatives and underlying positive disposition towards the health professional involved in their care.[13]

Perhaps because of the various conceptual and methodological problems outlined above, studies that have tried to identify factors influencing satisfaction have been singularly unsuccessful in accounting for the variance in satisfaction scores. For example, a study by Thompson[14] of satisfaction with hospital care included a wide range of potential influencing factors—patients' demographic and personal characteristics, personal experience, attitudes and expectations, the characteristics of the disease for which they were treated, duration of hospital stay and the health care outcome, the physical resources of the hospital, institutional characteristics and the organizational aspects of care. Taking all these factors into account, Thompson was still able to explain only 20 per cent of the variance in satisfaction scores. Although he concluded that unmeasured attributes must explain the bulk of the variance, he was unable to shed light on what these unmeasured attributes might be.

Given all these caveats, the reader may be forgiven for wondering about the value of conducting studies of patient satisfaction; but it is worth remembering that support for such activity comes not only from government but from clinicians themselves. One[15] describes satisfaction surveys as 'the start of an emerging science' and concludes that 'at a time when anger and distrust seem ubiquitous in the health systems of so many countries, asking patients to report on the quality of their care may bring clinicians and those they serve closer together'. And even those who question whether patients' answers to questions about their care should always be taken at face value, none the less acknowledge the importance of growing interest in their views.[16] In the next section, we turn to consider what this emerging science has to tell us about patient satisfaction with epilepsy care.

Patient satisfaction studies in epilepsy: what do they tell us?

To date, there have been relatively few studies of the views of users of epilepsy services. It would appear that interest in patient satisfaction, as in patient-perceived quality of life, has lagged behind in this clinical area compared with others. In the UK, however, four separate studies, including our own, have recently been published, all employing a core set of questions about epilepsy care.[17–20] The four studies were carried out in four different health regions and between them include over 2000 patients, identified from primary care physicians' medical records. In our own study,[17] patients aged 16 and over were sent questionnaires by post, which included a series of questions about their views and experiences of their

primary and secondary epilepsy care. The focus of this quantitative investigation was determined by analysis of qualitative data obtained from in-depth interviews with patients at the pilot phase of the project. Specifically, respondents were asked their opinions about the interpersonal skills and technical knowledge of the clinicians treating them, the communication and informational aspects of their care, the continuity of their care and their overall satisfaction.

For both primary and secondary care physicians, there was a highly significant association between each of the items relating to the doctor's interpersonal skills and expertise and patients' overall satisfaction (Table 35.1). However, as in other studies of patient satisfaction, external factors were also important: patients whose seizures were well controlled were more likely to describe their care as excellent or good than were those with frequent seizures; women were more critical of the quality of their care than men; and older people were more likely than younger people to assess their care favourably.

If we compare the views and experiences of people with epilepsy about their care across the four UK surveys, a number of trends emerge. For example, in each of them around 80 per cent of respondents described their primary care physician as easy to talk to and as knowing enough about epilepsy, and 60 per cent as always taking their views into account (Table 35.2). However, around a third in each study felt that they were provided with insufficient information by their primary care physician, and only around a third assessed the quality of their care overall as 'excellent'. Respondents in all four surveys were more likely to have discussed clinical than social aspects of epilepsy with their primary care physician (Table 35.2), despite recognition[21] that, as a result of the natural history of the

Patients' views of clinicians	Patients describing care as excellent/good (%)	
	Primary physician care	Secondary care
Easy to talk to?		
very/fairly easy	83 (*n*=397)	82 (*n*=157)
not very/not at all easy	38 (*n*=64)	47 (*n*=51)
Takes patient's views into account?		
always/usually	85 (*n*=371)	84 (*n*=147)
sometimes/never	37 (*n*=78)	46 (*n*=59)
Amount of information given?		
right	92 (*n*=309)	93 (*n*=115)
not enough	46 (*n*=152)	48 (*n*=90)
Knows enough about epilepsy?		
yes	89 (*n*=341)	81 (*n*=172)
no	38 (*n*=89)	32 (*n*=34)

p value = < 0.00001 in all cases.

Table 35.1
Relationship between patient satisfaction with care overall and perceptions of clinicians' skills and expertise.

Percentage of patients who:	UK region			
	Mersey	Yorkshire	South-west	Inner London
described physician as easy to talk to	86	86	85	–
felt physician knew enough about epilepsy	80	80	78	–
felt physician always took views into account	61	61	–	–
felt they were given sufficient information	67	67	63	65
had discussed with physician:				
causes of epilepsy	42	50	42	–
type of seizures	49	54	46	–
AED side effects	49	–	43	51
drug interactions	50	53	51	–
driving	48	48	49	59
employment/education	31	31	23	–
social life/activities	22	29	17	–
self-help groups	9	17	14	10
assessed care overall as excellent	36	36	–	–

Information not reported.
AED, antiepileptic drug.

Table 35.2
Patients' views of primary physician care for epilepsy.

condition, the latter may become more significant for patients than the former. This finding seems to support the view[22] that physicians are more interested in 'those aspects of patient rationalisation that promise to facilitate diagnosis or management, but not in the process of rationalisation *per se*'.

In each of the four surveys, patients generally expressed a preference for receiving care for their epilepsy in a primary setting. The most oft-cited reasons for this preference were that primary-based care was more personal, more holistic and offered greater continuity. This finding supports the current emphasis in the UK on the primary physician as the key in the ongoing management of chronic conditions such as epilepsy.[23–25] Despite this preference, in three of the four UK surveys fewer than 20 per cent of respondents had any regular arrangement to see their primary care physician about their epilepsy. It is also worth noting that, in our own survey, among the 120 patients who had been seen by both their primary and secondary care physicians in the preceding 12-month period and who were therefore in a position to compare the quality of care received from each, the former were judged to do better in relation to interpersonal skills, but the latter in relation to technical ones.

Another aspect of the management of epilepsy that has been investigated from the point of view of the patient is that of surgery.[26–28] Wheelock et al[28] examined the relationship between expectation and satisfaction in 79 patients undergoing anterior temporal lobectomy, all of whom had medically intractable seizures. Those taking part were asked to rate how satisfied they would be with four different surgical outcomes: complete elimination of their seizures, a 50–75 per cent reduction in seizure frequency; a less than 50 per cent reduction; and no change in seizure activity. The authors then computed a score

representing the degree to which patients' expectations were met 2 months and a year postoperatively (where a score of 1 meant that their expectations were not met at all, through to a score of 7, where their expectations were fully met). Scores on the expectations-met variable were 6.35 and 6.41 at the two time points for those who became seizure-free, compared with 3.13 and 4.13 for those with continuing seizures: in other words, when their expectations about the clinical outcome of surgery were met, patients were more likely to report being satisfied. Although this may seem self-evident, it is important to note that patients whose expectations were not met also indicated greater distress on a number of measures of psychological and psychosocial functioning postsurgically. The authors conclude that it is vitally important that clinicians help patients to be realistic in their expectations of the outcome of surgery, in order to reduce the negative impact of less than complete success.

A second study to address the issue of epilepsy surgery outcome is that by Wilson et al.[27] Using semi-structured interviews, the authors asked patients to identify their preoperative expectations for surgery. These fell into two broad categories: those that were practical and so more easily realizable, such as the elimination of seizures, reduction or cessation of medication, and changes in driving and employment status; and those that were less tangible, such as improvements in self-image, psychological well-being and lifestyle. Postoperatively, those who regarded their operation as successful were found to have had expectations that fitted into the first category only, whereas those who regarded it as unsuccessful had held both types of expectations. These findings led Wilson and colleagues to concur with the authors above that 'patients require clear and detailed counselling about the type of gains that can be realistically expected post-operatively', in order to maximize the level of their satisfaction with treatment outcomes. An important point emerging from both these studies is that, in contrast to Williams'[6] hypothesis that patients are generally uncertain about their expectations for health care, patients have very clearly articulated expectations for epilepsy surgery, which generally rest on an assumption that seizure freedom will be achieved.

Finally, two randomized studies that have examined the issue of patient satisfaction with epilepsy care also deserve brief mention here. In the first, the authors examined the impact on patients' care of the routine use of a generic health status measure.[29] Though the group of patients who completed the measure more frequently believed that their physician took account of their emotional status and daily functioning in developing a management plan, there were no significant differences between them and the control group in reported levels of satisfaction with their care. Clearly, there were many factors other than this one that influenced their perceptions. The second examined the impact on the quality of primary care of the introduction of an epilepsy specialist nurse, working across a number of primary care practices.[30] Patients in the practices served by the specialist nurse were found to be more likely to have discussed a range of aspects of their epilepsy with their clinician and to rate their care as excellent—though there were no observable differences in either their health status or perceived quality of life.

In summary, then, patient satisfaction surveys in epilepsy provide consistent evidence that people with epilepsy attach great importance to having care that is technically proficient. They also place high value on having a clinician who is not only knowledgeable about their condition, but also approachable and

communicative, and on receiving adequate information about the various aspects of their condition. Their apparent failure to achieve these goals and consequent dissatisfaction with their epilepsy care may well reflect what had been described as a 'clash of perspectives',[31] and offers support for Scambler's[22] proposed criteria for good quality care. He suggests that, in addition to providing a technically competent service, physician–patient encounters should embody the following principles: first, that patients be seen as co-participants in their care; second, that there should be an open agenda within which patients have the opportunity to raise issues that they themselves define as important; third, that there should be a less biomedical orientation, with the emphasis on informing and advising and not just managing disease; and fourth, that doctors develop their counselling as well as their technical skills. The current gaps in service provision identified by its recipients would at least be narrowed if providers moved some way towards this counsel of perfection.

Non-adherence as patient dissatisfaction

The question of whether patient satisfaction is simply a measure of the process of health care or a health outcome in its own right is one that has been debated in the literature. Fitzpatrick[32] argues for the latter, and that it is an important one because it predicts the likelihood of patients adhering to prescribed treatment regimens,[33] their reattendance for treatment[34] and improvements in their health status.[35] In this section, we explore the first of these scenarios—the relationship between patient satisfaction and treatment adherence—more closely. Non-adherence is a critical issue in the management of seizures, because missed or altered drug dosages can significantly increase the risk of seizure recurrence.[36,37] Despite this, failure to follow prescribed regimens is known to be fairly widespread,[38,39] and factors known to influence this include: the perceived efficacy of treatment and associated short- and longer-term adverse effects; the stigma potential inherent in taking medication; and the ease with which medication regimens can be accommodated within patients' everyday lives. In addition, a number of the factors highlighted above as being of importance in determining levels of satisfaction with health care have also been linked to the likelihood of patients adhering to treatment. For example, Freeman et al[40] showed that patients were more likely to take their medication as prescribed when they perceived their physician as being easy to talk to and concerned. Stockwell Morris and Schulz[41] go further, suggesting that the meaning patients attach to their medication is based on their perception of the nature of their relationship with their physician; thus:

> Medication can become a token of the physician's caring. . . [or] may be viewed by some as a dismissal, indicating that the physician does not have the time or desire to talk with the patient. Taking or not taking the medication can be viewed as a non-verbal communication to the physician.

In another much-quoted qualitative study of the experience of epilepsy from the patient's perspective,[42] patients accused their clinicians of lacking the skill, time or inclination to show empathy about the psychosocial problems that their condition imposed, while focusing too heavily on issues around its medical management. These 'unrecognised or unaddressed divergences' between clinician and patient perspectives can, Scambler maintains,[22] render good communication between them almost impossible—and so in turn heighten dissatisfaction. However,

good interpersonal skills on the part of the physician are not of themselves sufficient to guarantee adherence. In our recent community study,[43] we showed that patients who thought that it was unimportant to take medication as prescribed were also less likely to adhere to the prescribed regimens. This finding emphasizes that patients also need to be provided with information that increases their understanding about the importance of doing so.

The epilepsy patient as active co-participant

We would like briefly to take up Scambler's call that patients become more active co-participants in epilepsy care, as it relates to their involvement in research into its quality. Despite the accompanying rhetoric, the role of patients in evaluations of their health care—such as those described above—has so far largely been limited to answering questions that researchers or service providers have formulated. As their perspectives and concerns are not necessarily the same as either of these other groups of research stakeholders, it seems obvious that patients should also be involved in helping to set the research agenda, and in determining how research is funded, designed and monitored.[44,45] Yet, more often than not, they are excluded from all these other stages of the research process, thus severely limiting their potential contribution:[13] and also, we suggest, helping to perpetuate the problems discussed above in conceptualizing and operationalizing the issue of patient satisfaction. Despite the barriers to service users becoming more involved in research, this is an issue that is currently receiving increasing attention and there is now a clear political mandate for them to do so.[46,47] That they can do so effectively is amply illustrated by reference to other areas of health care,[45,48] though the dangers of 'token consumerism' should not be disregarded.[46,49]

Patient advocacy: a political agenda

Historically, people with epilepsy have received less than ideal health care, a problem that can be attributed at least in part to the stigma associated with the condition. In the UK, for example, epilepsy has had relatively low priority within the health care system, and services remain sparse and fragmented,[50] despite a series of reports that have highlighted their shortcomings and made clear recommendations about their development.[51] Scambler[22] has identified an important limitation of the various documents that address the issue of how services can be tailored to meet the needs of people with epilepsy better, as illustrated in the studies quoted above. This is that need is defined from the medical rather than the patient perspective. One way to redress this imbalance is through advocates working together with and on behalf of people with epilepsy, both individually and as a group. An advocate is one who 'pleads for another' (*Concise Oxford Dictionary*, 1982) and Ganz[52] suggests that the key functions of the patient advocate must be to ensure that he or she has access to medical care, and that the quality of that care is optimal and enhances survival, rehabilitation and psychological adaptation. This begs the question of who can best act as advocate for the patient with epilepsy.

The concept of the nurse as patient advocate is one that has become popular in both the UK and North America over the last decade,[53] and which nurses themselves see as involving elements clearly related to the issue of patient satisfaction, namely informing, supporting and representing.[54] It could be argued that the epilepsy specialist nurse is well placed to take on this role. For example, Ridsdale[55] suggests that the epilepsy nurse 'could act as an agent, initiating demands for advice', and Appleton and Sweeney[56] identify a role for him or her in working with school and community health personnel and with the general public 'to address the frequent misconceptions and misunderstandings which are prevalent'. There is considerable debate, however, in the nursing literature about the legitimacy and appropriateness of the nurse acting in the capacity of advocate. Though they may be the person best placed within the health care team to do so, their position there also presents potential for conflict[53,57] and so makes advocacy a risky role for them to adopt.[58]

If not the nurse, who else can act as advocate for the patient with epilepsy? Bastian[49] suggests that it is the consumer groups that best fit this role and, in the UK at least, there are a number of such groups for epilepsy. The British Epilepsy Association, the leading UK patient organization, defines, as one of its key functions, political lobbying at the national and local level to encourage better services and establish acceptable standards of care.[59] The umbrella organization for the UK support groups, the Joint Epilepsy Council, pursues a parallel political agenda. At an international level, the International Bureau for Epilepsy sets, among its objectives, the promotion of a broader understanding of the nature of epilepsy and the needs of the person with epilepsy. Other non-epilepsy organizations may also be able to function as advocates for epilepsy. In the UK, for example, the community health councils were created in the 1970s to represent the public's interest in the National Health Service. They both network with the voluntary organizations and draw on their own work with individual complainants to identify important concerns and hold NHS bodies to account, as well as highlighting the health care needs of their community.[60] Although many people with epilepsy will have access to the resources required to be 'active co-participants' in their care, and so will be happy to act as their own advocates, there are also many less able to do so,[61] to whose care organizations such as these can make a significant contribution.

Summary

Although there are acknowledged conceptual and methodological difficulties in assessing patient satisfaction that need to be more rigorously addressed, the importance of the patient perspective is now firmly on the research and political agendas. Despite the proliferation of patient satisfaction studies generally, there have been relatively few to date in the field of epilepsy, and this is an area worthy of further investigation. Nevertheless, studies into patient satisfaction with epilepsy care confirm clinical anecdotal experience that patients are more likely to feel satisfied with their care if the following criteria are met: access to good quality technical care which enables them to achieve optimal seizure control with minimal adverse treatment effects; information about the various aspects of their condition adequate to their individual needs; a positive therapeutic relationship with their clinician within which they have the opportunity to be active co-participants; a clinician who is well informed, understanding of and responsive to their needs; and, in as far as it is possible within the constraints of the system, care that is continuous.

People with epilepsy have a right to be satisfied with the care that they receive. Given that there is research that supports the relationship between satisfaction and other health outcomes, it also behoves those providing that care to ensure that optimal standards are delivered. A number of organizations already exist that can and do act as advocates for people with epilepsy. They must continue to campaign for the right to play a much more integrated role in the planning and delivery of services at a local and national level.

References

1. Jones L, Leneman L, MacLean U. *Consumer feedback for the NHS*. London: King Edward's Hospital Fund; 1987.
2. Donabedian A. *Explorations in quality assessment and monitoring*: Vol. 1. *The definitions of quality and approaches to its assessment*. Ann Arbor, MI: Health Administration Press, 1980.
3. Locker D, Dunt D. Theoretical and methodological issues in sociological studies of consumer satisfaction with medical care. *Soc Sci Med* 1978;**12**:283–92.
4. Calnan M. Why take into account patient views about health care. *Br J Health Care Management* 1996;**2**:328–30.
5. Calnan M. Towards a conceptual framework of lay evaluation of health care. *Soc Sci Med* 1988;**27**:927–33.
6. Williams B. Patient satisfaction: is it a valid concept? *Soc Sci Med* 1992;**38**:509–16.
7. Davies AR, Ware JE. Involving consumers in quality of care assessment. *Health Affairs* 1988;**7**:33–48.
8. West P. The physician and the management of childhood epilepsy. In: Robinson D, Wadsworth M, eds. *Studies in Everyday Medical Life*. London: Martin Robertson, 1976.
9. Cohen G, Forbes J, Garraway M. Can different patient satisfaction survey methods yield consis-

tent results? Comparison of three surveys. *BMJ* 1996;**313**:841–4.

10. Like R, Zyzanski SJ. Patient satisfaction with the clinical encounter: social psychological determinants. *Soc Sci Med* 1987;**24**:351–7.

11. Linn LS, Greenfield S. Patient suffering and patient satisfaction among the chronically ill. *Med Care* 1982;**20**:425–31.

12. Rosenberg SJ, Peterson RA, Hayes JR, Hatcher J, Headen S. Depression in medical in-patients. *Br J Med Psychol* 1988;**61**:245–54.

13. Martin EM. Consumer evaluation of human services. *Social Policy and Administration* 1986;**20**, 3:185–99.

14. Thompson AGH. The soft approach to quality of hospital care. *Int J Quality Reliability Management* 1986;**3**:59–67.

15. Delbanco TL. Quality of care through the patient's eyes. *BMJ* 1996;**313**:832–3.

16. Sensky T, Catalan J. Asking patients about their treatment. *BMJ* 1992;**305**:1109–10.

17. Buck D, Jacoby A, Baker GA, Graham-Jones S, Chadwick D. Patients' experiences of and satisfaction with care for their epilepsy. *Epilepsia* 1996;**37**:841–9.

18. Ridsdale L, Robins D, Fitzgerald A, Jeffery S, McGee L. Epilepsy monitoring and advice recorded: general practitioners' views, current practice and patients' preferences. *Br J Gen Pract* 1996;**46**:11–14.

19. Mills N, Bachmann M, Harvey I, McGowan M, Hine I. Patients' experience of epilepsy and health care. *Family Practice* 1997;**14**:117–23.

20. Rogers, D. and Taylor, M. *Don't fit in front of your workmates*. Doncaster: Doncaster Medical Audit Advisory Group, 1996.

21. Commission for the Control of Epilepsy and its Consequences. *Plan for nationwide action on epilepsy*. DWEH Public. No. NIH 78-276. Washington, DC: US Government Printing Office, 1978.

22. Scambler G. Patient perceptions of epilepsy and of doctors who manage epilepsy. *Seizure* 1994;**3**:287–93.

23. Department of Health and Social Security. *Report of the working group on services for people with epilepsy*. London: HMSO, 1986.

24. White P. Structured management in primary care of patients with epilepsy. *Br J Gen Pract* 1996;**46**:3–4.

25. Brown S, Betts T, Chadwick D, Hall B, Shorvon S, Wallace S. Clinical review: an epilepsy needs document. *Seizure* 1993;**2**:91–103.

26. Guldvog B. Patient satisfaction and epilepsy surgery. *Epilepsia* 1994;**35**:579–84.

27. Wilson SJ, Saling MM, Kincade P, Bladin PF. Patient expectations of temporal lobe surgery. *Epilepsia* 1998;**39**:167–74.

28. Wheelock I, Peterson C, Buchtel HA. Presurgery expectations, postsurgery satisfaction, and psychosocial adjustment after epilepsy surgery. *Epilepsia* 1998;**39**:487–94.

29. Wagner AK, Ehrenberg BL, Tran TA, Bungay KM, Cynn DJ, Rogers WH. Patient-based health status measurement in clinical practice: a study of its impact on epilepsy patients' care. *Quality of Life Research* 1997;**6**:329–41.

30. Mills N, Bachman M, Harvey I, Hine I, McGowan M. Effect of a primary care based epilepsy specialist nurse service on quality of care from the patients' perspective: quasi-experimental evaluation (unpublished paper).

31. Friedson E. *Profession of medicine: a study of the sociology of applied knowledge*. New York: Russell Sage Foundation, 1970.

32. Fitzpatrick R. Surveys of patient satisfaction: I – important general considerations. *BMJ* 1991; **302**:887–9.

33. Kincey J, Bradshaw P, Ley P. Patients' satisfaction and reported acceptance of advice in general practice. *J R Coll Gen Practit* 1975;**25**: 558–66.

34. Roghmann K, Hengst A, Zastowny T. Satisfaction with medical care: its measurement and relation to utilisation. *Med Care* 1979; **17**:461–77.

35. Fitzpatrick R, Hopkin A, Harvard-Watts O. Social dimensions of healing: a longitudinal study of outcomes of medical management of headaches. *Soc Sci Med* 1983;**17**:501–10.

36. Mattson RH, Cramer JA, Collins JF. VA Epilepsy Cooperative Study Group. Aspects of compliance: taking drugs and keeping clinic appointments. In: Schmidt D, Leppik IE, eds. *Compliance in epilepsy*. Amsterdam: Elsevier, 1988.

37. Stanaway L, Lambie DG, Johnson RH. Non-compliance with anticonvulsant therapy as a cause of seizures. *N Z Med J* 1985;**98**:150–2.

38. Eisler J, Mattson RH. Compliance in anticonvulsant drug therapy. *Epilepsia* 1975;**16**:203.

39. Cramer JA, Mattson RH. Monitoring compliance with antiepileptic drug therapy. In: Cramer JA, Spilker B, eds. *Patient compliance in medical practice and clinical trials.* New York: Raven Press, 1991.

40. Freeman B, Negrete V, Davis M, Korsch B. Gaps in doctor–patient communication: doctor–patient interaction analysis. *Pediatr Res* 1971; 5:298–311.

41. Stockwell Morris L, Schulz RM. Medication compliance: the patient's perspective. *Clin Ther* 1993;**15**:593–606.

42. Scambler G. *Epilepsy.* London: Tavistock, 1989.

43. Buck D, Jacoby A, Baker GA, Chadwick DW. Factors influencing compliance with antiepileptic drug regimes. *Seizure* 1997;**6**:87–93.

44. Goodare H, Smith R. The rights of patients in research. *BMJ* 1995;**310**:1277–8.

45. Liberati A. Consumer participation in research and health care. *BMJ* 1997;**315**:499.

46. NHS Executive Research Development Directorate. Research: what's in it for consumers? 1st Report of the Standing Advisory Group on Consumer Involvement in the NHS R&D Programme to the Central Research & Development Committee 1996/97. Wetherby: Department of Health, 1998.

47. Entwistle VA, Renfrew MJ, Yearley S, Forrester J, Lamont T. Lay perspectives: advantages for health research. *BMJ* 1998;**316**:463–6.

48. Chalmers I. What do I want from health research and researchers when I am a patient? *BMJ* 1995;**310**:1315–18.

49. Bastian H. The power of sharing knowledge: consumer participation in the Cochrane collaboration. The Cochrane Collaboration. 1994:1.

50. Chadwick DW. *Quality of life and quality of care in epilepsy. RSM Round Table Series No. 23.* London: Royal Society of Medicine, 1990.

51. Thompson P. The Cohen Report onwards. In: Chadwick DW, ed. *Quality of life and quality of care in epilepsy.* 1990.

52. Ganz PA. Advocating for the woman with breast cancer. *Cancer J Clin* 1995;**45**:114–26.

53. Mardell A. Advocacy: exploring the concept. *Br J Theatre Nursing* 1996;**6**:34–6.

54. Watt E. An exploration of the way in which the concept of patient advocacy is perceived by registered nurses working in an acute care hospital. *Int J Nursing Pract* 1997;**3**:119–27.

55. Ridsdale L. Matching the needs with skills in epilepsy care. *BMJ* 1995;**310**:1219–20.

56. Appleton RE, Sweeney A. The management of epilepsy in children: the role of the clinical nurse specialist. *Seizure* 1995;**4**:287–91.

57. Norrie P. Ethical decision-making in intensive care: are nurses suitable patient advocates? *Intens Critical Care Nursing* 1997;**13**:167–9.

58. Mallik M. Advocacy in nursing: a review of the literature. *J Adv Nurs* 1997;**25**:130–8.

59. *British Epilepsy Association Annual Review 1996.* Leeds: British Epilepsy Association, 1996.

60. Harris T. Do we still need CHCs? *Health Matters* 1998;**33**:6–7.

61. Baribeault JJ. Clinical advocacy for persons with epilepsy and mental retardation living in community-based programs. *J Neurosci Nurs* 1996;**28**:359–72.

36

The team approach to treating epilepsy: when do we need it?

Warren T Blume

Introduction

As epilepsy impacts upon multiple medical and non-medical aspects of a patient's life, it is axiomatic that integrated care by more than one type of professional is needed. Accurate diagnosis of the epilepsy that the seizures represent and the provision of optimum medical care are essential. Epilepsy usually strikes patients in their formative years, and thus can distort the development of a favourable self-image. Low self-esteem will equip a patient poorly for the vocational and social challenges of life. A team approach will more effectively manage these medical, psychological and social aspects more effectively than any single care provider. Active participation in patient care by an interacting team maximizes the effectiveness of each professional and minimizes avoidable consequences of this often chronic, yet treatable, disorder.

This chapter surveys the components of a team approach. Hopefully, the reader will conclude that 'we always need it'.

The managing physicians

The neurologist

As epilepsy is the most common neurological disorder affecting young people,[1,2] at least one evaluation by a neurologist familiar with epilepsy would be optimal. Manpower short-ages may prevent this in many areas of the world.

The first task of the neurologist is to diagnose the paroxysmal events as epileptic seizures or as representing some other condition.[3,4] Several conditions may mimic epileptic seizures, such as syncope, cardiac irregularities, migraine, transient ischaemic attacks and some movement disorders.

A second task for the neurologist is to determine which epilepsy syndrome or neurological disease the epileptic seizures represent. As neurologists, Loiseau et al[5] were able to classify 97 per cent of 986 consecutive patients into one of the epilepsy syndromes. In contrast, primary care physicians were able to place only 34 per cent of newly diagnosed epileptic patients into a syndrome in one study.[6] Epilepsy syndrome determination helps to indicate which ancillary diagnostic tests are indicated and which can be avoided. Moreover, prognosis varies markedly among syndromes. For example, only about 10 per cent of patients with Lennox–Gastaut syndrome become seizure-free.[7] In contrast, only about 2 per cent of persons with benign Rolandic epilepsy of childhood proceed to chronic epilepsy.[8] Syndromic classification may also guide in the selection of antiepileptic drugs (AEDs). For example, valproate is the most effective drug for juvenile myoclonic epilepsy.[9]

The neurologist may be more alert to the long-term side effects of some AEDs. For example, phenytoin may be associated with progressive kyphosis, facial morphological changes and peripheral neuropathy.[10] Although innumerable possible drug interactions exist, stemming from the vast array of therapeutic options currently on the market, the neurologist–epileptologist will be aware of the more common ones occurring among AEDs, and between AEDs and medications prescribed for other conditions.

Finally, the neurologist should understand the impact of epilepsy on the patient's lifestyle, job search and interpersonal relationships. Untoward effects on these aspects and the existence of avoidable stressors increase the seizure tendency. I tell patients that happiness is an excellent antiepileptic 'medication'.

The general physician

Patients with epilepsy receive far better care when the general physician enters actively into the management process. He or she may become a valuable colleague for the neurologist in this respect.

As the general medical health of the patient interacts either favourably or unfavourably with the epileptic condition, the general physician's management in this area may be most helpful.

Most patients are better known to the general physician than to the neurologist because of a longer acquaintance and a closer look at lifestyle. This enables the general physician to better assess the impact of the seizure disorder upon the patient's life. He or she may more immediately assess the favourable or unfavourable effects of medication changes suggested by the neurologist and make prompt adjustments within a therapeutic framework. Compliance can be monitored and encouraged.

Many general physicians are understandably concerned about entering into the treatment process. I have found that management of one or two patients with moderately severe epilepsy by a general physician equips him or her with the principles of the treatment of epilepsy. This emboldens the general physician to participate more actively in such care and to welcome the addition of other patients with epilepsy to his or her practice.

Electroencephalography and the technologist

Electroencephalography (EEG) is the most valuable laboratory test for patients with a chronic seizure disorder. EEG helps to determine the seizure type and also the epilepsy syndrome which the seizures represent. The value of this latter determination was outlined above.

The following is a sample of relevant aspects of EEG recordings. Precipitating factors for seizures may be revealed by EEG: profuse polyspike waves with photic stimulation suggest that generalized tonic–clonic (grand mal) seizures may be so precipitated; afferent stimuli to hand or foot may elicit focal rolandic polyspikes. Polygraph recordings may unravel the mechanism of myoclonus. As epileptiform potentials (spikes) occur intermittently, more than one recording may be required to reveal their presence. This situation occurs occasionally in patients with temporal lobe epilepsy. A knowledgeable technologist will allow sleep to occur. This may elicit many types of epileptiform potentials, including those of benign Rolandic epilepsy of childhood. Anterior temporal spikes and occipital spikes or polyspikes are other examples that may be seen principally in sleep.

EEG may assist in the differential diagnosis of epilepsy. Rapid descent into non-rapid eye movement (non-REM) sleep may indicate that intermittent attacks of impaired awareness represent excessive daytime sleep arising from various causes. Suggesting that a recorded seizure would be diagnostically useful may evoke a pseudoseizure, i.e. a non-epileptic paroxysmal event mimicking a seizure but without cerebrally originating EEG changes.

EEG technologists acquire considerable knowledge about epileptic disorders, and therefore may take a knowledgable history. As the patient may be more relaxed talking to a technologist than to a physician, significant medical, psychological or social details may emerge.

Neuroradiology

The second most useful laboratory examination for epilepsy is magnetic resonance imaging (MRI). Unfortunately, this modality is often employed indiscriminately because the following thought process is pursued: seizure, therefore brain disorder, therefore scan. The most common benefit of this sequence is a legally more defensible position for the practitioner, but it does lead to avoidable pitfalls. A consequence of such thought processes is false identification of irrelevant MRI anomalies as possibly epileptogenic.

A more fruitful use of neuroimaging is the initial creation of a concise list of possible epileptogenic areas and aetiologies derived from neurological assessment and EEG. These data will probably indicate some particular areas and types of lesions for scrutiny such as mesial temporal sclerosis and subtle frontal cortical malformations.

Neuroimaging laboratories that emphasize profit over quality should be avoided,[11] as some health care systems permit only a single neuroimaging study. Often the subtle nature of epileptogenic lesions requires high quality

scanning for their demonstration. Neuroradiology of epilepsy is emerging as a subspecialty; its advantages are better detection of epileptogenic lesions and identification of their nature.

Neuropsychology

In addition to assessment of overall cognitive abilities, the array of tests administered by neuropsychologists may indicate which areas of the brain are dysfunctional. Such areas may be epileptogenic. Of particular importance is assessment of memory, which is perhaps the most common cognitive impairment recognized by patients with epilepsy. The neuropsychologist may quantify such impairment and advise the patient as to mechanisms to circumvent the difficulty. Assessment of memory is a crucial step when epilepsy surgery is considered, particularly if resection of the temporal lobe dominant for language is an option. Patients with preoperatively normal memories risk their partial loss by the procedure.[12]

Clinical psychology and psychiatry

The behavioural, emotional and psychosocial implications of epilepsy are becoming increasingly realized. Thus, the clinical psychologist performs an essential role in the management of many patients under care in an epilepsy unit.

The clinical psychologist assesses personality, ability to cope with stress and relationship problems among patients with chronic epilepsy. This enables the identification of various psychopathologies in patients with a chronic disorder such as epilepsy. Appropriate psychological intervention may be thus provided. The foregoing helps to identify emotional disorders requiring assessment and possible treatment by a psychiatrist. For example, Manchanda et al[13] found DSM-III-R disorders in 47 per cent of patients undergoing evaluation for epilepsy surgery.

Such assessment is particularly crucial when epilepsy surgery is under consideration. The consideration of life after surgery is an essential component of the presurgical evaluation. Coping with the acute disappointment that results when the epilepsy team concludes that surgery is not a reasonable option also needs to be addressed. Adjustment to life after epilepsy surgery, irrespective of its effectiveness, forms a significant role for the clinical psychologist with respect to all patients. Paradoxically, such adjustment may be more difficult when surgery eradicates seizures than when it fails to do so. Expectations placed upon a newly seizure-free patient by others will suddenly increase. Loss of the sedative effect of antiepileptic medications may lead to transient irritability and insomnia. Although health-related quality of life may improve significantly after temporal lobectomy in most patients, this does not apply in all instances.[14] In fact, at 2 years after epilepsy surgery, those with >90 per cent reduction in seizure frequency reported significant improvements in quality of life whereas those with <90 per cent seizure reduction experienced its deterioration.[15]

Identifying and treating the depression which daunts many epileptic patients forms a most significant aspect of clinical neuropsychology. Such depression may occur in many circumstances, including transiently after epilepsy surgery, particularly when it succeeds!

Assessment of patients with possible pseudoseizures is another significant role of the clinical neuropsychologist. The Minnesota Multiphasic Personality Inventory (MMPI), as restandardized (MMPI-2),[16] was able to accurately classify 92 per cent of patients with pseudoseizures, particularly the scales for hypochondriasis, depression and hysteria.

Community organizations

These organizations work closely with the above-mentioned members of the epilepsy team, particularly the clinical psychologists and neurologists, to maximize quality of life for epilepsy patients.

Epilepsy usually begins in early life and therefore impacts upon the personality during its formation. Epilepsy may be a life-long condition whose consequences vary with seizure control and medication effects, therefore, a support group that integrates these factors with components of the patient's life, will serve to enhance its quality. This involves familiarizing family, teachers, employers, vocational counsellors and social service providers with respect to the impact of the aforementioned factors upon the patient. Epilepsy community organizations bring people with epilepsy together; the sharing of problems and their solutions benefits most patients participating in activities sponsored by these organizations. Many patients learn much about epilepsy from each other, a knowledge that in some respects is beyond what any health care team can impart.

Issues of daily life may be addressed by the community organizations. The first of these involves creation of a medically beneficial lifestyle including adequate sleep, exercise and nutrition. Seizure-related injury or death may be avoided by advice concerning bathing, smoking and cooking.

As adults suffering from epilepsy are underemployed, epilepsy community organizations may aid in the approach to employment.[17]

Increasing public awareness of epilepsy forms a major role of community organizations. This features education of teachers and public school students so that the injurious prejudice against epilepsy and patients with epilepsy can be minimized.

Clinical AED trials

The many potentially new marketable AEDs require clinical trials to verify their efficacy and safety. As many patients attending an epilepsy unit outpatient or inpatient facility are candidates for such drug trials, a new component of epilepsy care has been generated.

As AED trial protocols demand frequent visits to the same team, the patient receives more frequent attention than usual. Several benefits arise from this situation. The nature, frequency and aggravating factors concerning the seizures become better known to the epilepsy team. The patient becomes more confident in the competence of the team. His or her knowledge about the epileptic condition increases. Serum levels of standard and new AEDs can be monitored. Adverse events of all types are realized. Importantly, the full impact of epilepsy upon their associates may be realized by the health care team.

Above all, such drug trials regenerate hope— an essential ingredient for enduring any chronic illness.

Acknowledgements

The following persons assisted in the preparation of this chapter: Ms Lisa Brown, Dr Paul Derry, Ms Jo Anne DePace, Dr Michael Harnadek and Dr Donald Lee. Maria Raffa carefully prepared the manuscript.

References

1. Blume WT. Temporal lobe epilepsy surgery in childhood: rationale for greater use. *Can J Neurol Sci* 1997;**24**:95–8.
2. Shields WD, Duchowny MS, Holmes GL. Surgically remediable syndromes of infancy and early childhood. In: Engel J Jr, ed. *Surgical treatment of the epilepsies.* New York: Raven Press, 1993:35–48.
3. Blume WT. Differential diagnosis of epileptic seizures. In: Wada JA, Ellingson RJ, eds. *Handbook of electroencephalography and clinical neurophysiology. Clinical neurophysiology of epilepsy (Revised series, Vol. 4).* Amsterdam: Elsevier, 1990:407–31.
4. Schmidt D, Lempert T. Differential diagnoses in adults. In: Dam M, Gram L, eds. *Comprehensive epileptology.* New York: Raven Press, 1991:449–71.
5. Loiseau P, Duche B, Loiseau J. Classification of epilepsies and epileptic syndromes in two differ-
ent samples of patients. *Epilepsia* 1991;**32**: 303–9.
6. Manford M, Hart YM, Sander JWAS, Shorvon SD. The national general practice study of epilepsy. The syndromic classification of the International League Against Epilepsy applied to epilepsy in a general population. *Arch Neurol* 1992;**49**:801–8.
7. Beaumanoir A, Dravet C. The Lennox–Gastaut syndrome. In: Roger J, Bureau M, Dravet C, et al, eds. *Epileptic syndromes in infancy, childhood and adolescence.* London: John Libbey, 1992:115–32.
8. Sander JWAS, Sillanpää M. Natural history and prognosis. In: Engel J Jr, Pedley TA, eds. *Epilepsy: a comprehensive textbook.* Vol 1. Philadelphia, PA: Lippincott-Raven Publishers, 1998:69–86.
9. Janz D, Durner M. Juvenile myoclonic epilepsy. In: Engel J Jr, Pedley TA, eds. *Epilepsy: a*

comprehensive textbook, Vol 3. Philadelphia, PA: Lippincott-Raven, 1998:2389–400.

10. Bruni J. Phenytoin. Toxicity. In: Levy RH, Mattson RH, Meldrum BS, eds. *Antiepileptic drugs, 4th edn.* New York: Raven Press, 1995:345–50.

11. McBride MC, Bronstein K, Bennet B, Berg MG. The futility of non-epilepsy centre neuroimaging in intractable temporal lobe epilepsy. *Epilepsia* 1996;**37**:188.

12. Seidenberg M, Hermann B, Wyler AR, et al. Neuropsychological outcome following anterior temporal lobectomy in patients with and without the syndrome of mesial temporal lobe epilepsy. *Neuropsychology* 1998;**12**:303–16.

13. Manchanda R, Schaefer B, McLachlan RS, et al. Psychiatric disorders in candidates for epilepsy surgery. *Epilepsia* 1996;**37**(Suppl 5):120.

14. Rose KJ, Derry PA, Wiebe S, McLachlan RS. Determinants of health-related quality of life after temporal lobe epilepsy surgery. *Qual Life Res* 1996;**5**:395–402.

15. McLachlan RS, Rose KJ, Derry PA, et al. Health-related quality of life and seizure control in temporal lobe epilepsy. *Ann Neurol* 1997;**41**:482–9.

16. Derry PA, McLachlan RS. The MMPI-2 as an adjunct to the diagnosis of pseudoseizures. *Seizure* 1996;**5**:35–40.

17. Hauser WA, Hesdorffer DC. *Epilepsy: frequency, causes and consequences.* New York: Demos Publications, 1990.

Index

Page numbers in *italic* refer to the illustrations.